ENVISIONING A BRIGHT FUTURE

Interventions that Work for Children and Adults with Autism Spectrum Disorders

Patricia S. Lemer, MEd, NCC, Editor

Optometric Extension Program Foundation

The OEP Foundation, founded in 1928, is an international non-profit organization dedicated to continuing education and research for the advancement of human progress through education in behavioral vision care.

OEP Foundation, Inc.
1921 E. Carnegie Ave., Suite 3-L
Santa Ana, CA 92705
www.oep.org

Managing editor: Sally Marshall Corngold
Cover design: Bill Greaves

Library of Congress Cataloging-in-Publication Data

Envisioning a bright future : interventions that work for children and adults with autism spectrum disorders / Patricia S. Lemer, editor.
    p. ; cm.
 Includes bibliographical references and index.
 ISBN 978-0-929780-17-5 (alk. paper)
 1. Autism. 2. Visual training I. Lemer, Patricia S. II. Optometric Extension Program Foundation.
 [DNLM: 1. Autistic Disorder--rehabilitation. 2. Child Development Disorders, Pervasive--rehabilitation. 3. Sensory Art Therapies--methods. WM 203.5 E61 2008]
 RC553.A88E58 2008
 616.85'88206--dc22

                                                   2008012246

****

Optometry is the health care profession specifically licensed by state law to prescribe lenses, optical devices and procedures to improve human vision. Optometry has advanced vision therapy as a unique treatment modality for the development and remediation of the visual process. Effective vision therapy requires extensive understanding of:

- the effects of lenses (including prisms, filters and occluders)
- the variety of responses to the changes produced by lenses
- the various physiological aspects of the visual process
- the pervasive nature of the visual process in human behavior

As a consequence, effective vision therapy requires the supervision, direction and active involvement of the optometrist.

****

Acknowledgements

This book represents the gigantic joint efforts, knowledge and support of so many people. I simply could have not done it without them.

The authors and contributors, listed in the beginning of the book. Thank you for sharing your expertise, time and skills.

My Optometric mentors: Amiel Francke and Irwin Suchoff. You pushed me to speak and write in the world of optometry, where I found a new family.

DDR Board members, past and present: Teresa Badillo, Kelly Dorfman, Margaret Britt, Sanford Cohen, Mary Coyle, Eileen Culhane, Meredith Ficca, Farrel Gerber, Kim Kubistek, Audrey Kuhlenschmidt, Robin Mumford, Melissa McNeese, Jayme Lewin Rich, Scott Theirl, Bobbi Wade, Lynn Williamson. I have learned so much from you. Thank you all for being there for me.

My Editors and dear Friends: Len Press for reading the entire book word by word to assure optometric accuracy and clarity. Mary Rentschler, the ultimate editor's editor. Jeannie Tower for opening my eyes to the energetic world.

The Staff and Board at OEP: Bob Williams who offered me this opportunity, and always believed in me. Your generosity is unmatched. How can I ever repay Sally Corngold, whose indefatigable efforts set up the pages of this book to meet my endless demands? Kathleen Patterson, who shared her ideas about cover designs. Paul Harris for making sure everything read "just right."

My designers: Bill Greaves for the beautiful cover, and Robin Mumford for recommending him. Llouise Altes for teaching me about kerning and layout.

My officemates in Pittsburgh: Franne Berez, Jane Critchfield, Donna Klonko, Mary Magan, Rachel Walton. Thank you for your support.

My brother Bill and his family for listening. I just couldn't allow my "baby brother" to be the only published author in the family!

My assistants along the way: Kristen Johanson who worked as my right hand for five years, Katie Grunst, my first intern from the Ellis School, who got this book off the ground.

Colleagues who offered suggestions, located references and solved problems: Lynn Balzer-Martin, Donna Embree, Priscilla Freisen, Diana Henry, the late Lorna Jean King, Diana Sava.

To one and all I extend my humble gratitude and thanks.

Patricia S. Lemer

Dedication

This book is dedicated to four strong women in my family.

Two who came before and have supported me throughout my life:
My grandmother Connie Strassburger and my mother Martha Heyman

And two who are the bright future:
My daughter Elizabeth Day and my granddaughter, Penelope

Table of Contents

Foreword

After almost five years I am very proud to offer you what I believe is the most comprehensive book on autism treatments presently available. You may be wondering why a book on autism for optometrists was edited by someone who is not an optometrist. The answer is that for much of my 35-year career as a counselor I have served as a bridge between the autism and optometric communities. In many ways my entire career has been pointing towards this book. I have been extremely fortunate to have learned from some of the best in many fields: neurology, psychology, occupational therapy, speech-language therapy, medicine, and, of course optometry.

As a newly degreed graduate student in counseling psychology, I was hired by a Boston hospital as a junior psychologist whose job was to evaluate and treat children with such diverse problems as chicken pox encephalitis and head injuries sustained falling 25 feet from a tree. No autism, no ADD, no learning disabilities. My work as a play therapist was very frustrating; I continuously wondered why certain children demonstrated aberrant behaviors. Luckily, I was a member of a multi-disciplinary team. While no optometrist was on the team, the doctors, occupational therapists (OTs) and speech language pathologists (SLPs) all seemed to be getting results where I was failing. Special diets stopped seizures, brushing programs calmed kids down, movement got them talking. I started thinking. Maybe I was just treating symptoms. They were treating the underlying causes.

I soon moved to the Washington, DC area, where the reading, writing and spelling problems about which I consulted with parents and teachers seemed benign compared to the severe disabilities I had seen at the Boston hospital. Yet, similarities existed. Now, as a member of a team of educators rather than medical professionals, I was again treating symptoms: letter reversals, handwriting issues and slow, dysfluent reading. I often suggested to parents that they have their children's eyes checked. One day I got lucky. A mother called me so excited that she could hardly contain herself, "You were right. My child can see, but she has vision problems!" She went into a long explanation of why 20/20 was not enough. I quickly asked for the name of the eye doctor who had evaluated her child. "Dr. Robert Kraskin," she replied, giving me his telephone number.

That was in 1979. I had no idea how profoundly that phone call would change my professional life. I visited the Kraskin office and learned about optometry. Why hadn't I heard about any of this before? Growing up in Pittsburgh my family had taken my brother and me to ophthalmologists exclusively. I got my first pair of glasses in second grade when I could hardly see the E at the top of the chart, and my hyperopic three-year-old brother giggled as he read all the way to the bottom. "She needs glasses, and he won't need them until he is 40," pronounced the doctor.

My next encounter with optometry was as a career counselor at George Washington University. A student came to me seeking guidance on choosing a major. He explained that he had vision issues that had caused him some learning difficulties, and that he was resolving them with a wonderful doctor whose office was nearby. I asked the name, and the next day met the remarkable Amiel Francke. I'll never forget sharing a brown bag lunch with him at his impeccable office. I recall only that he downed more vitamins than lunch. I was fascinated by his approach to adults with long-standing vision issues. Not only did he recommend vision activities, but dietary and lifestyle changes as well. He invited me to attend both his monthly informational seminar and one of his therapy sessions. I was amazed at the lawyers, politicians and high functioning individuals I saw there.

Amiel and I got to know each other well over the next couple of years. He taught me how vision affects all aspects of behavior. Caught up in my little world of cognitive, achievement and personality testing, I was amazed at the power of vision in each realm. Professionally and ethically, I could no longer determine IQ levels without considering vision. Likewise for reading, writing, arithmetic. How can one separate out personality from visual perception? I could no longer interpret a Rorschach without knowing a person's visual status.

One day in the mid 1980s, Amiel invited me to his office and told me about the Optometric Extension Program's (OEP's) Regional Clinical Seminar (RCS) program, which he had developed. He explained that experienced optometrists traveled to different parts of the country and presented weekend workshops on subjects of interest to optometrists. The seminars were practical, with one of the primary goals to put material learned to use on Monday morning. He invited me to be the first non-optometrist to offer an RCS on psychological and educational testing. I was to show optometrists how each test relied upon vision, and teach them how to interpret test scores. They could then communicate intelligently with school psychologists, occupational therapists and others with whom they shared patients.

My first reaction was, "Do I have enough material to speak for two entire days?" I shared my concerns with Amiel and Dr. Bob Greenberg, another strong influence, both of whom agreed that this seminar could easily cover two days. I eventually presented the material about a dozen times, both as an RCS, and at Eastern States and Great Lakes Congresses.

Becoming a Regional Clinical Seminar presenter was my introduction to the Optometric Extension Program (OEP), its Executive Director Bob Williams, and the organization's Board of Directors. Bob helped strengthen my role as a bridge between optometry and the public. Throughout the 1980s and 90s, he sent me to conferences on learning disabilities and occupational therapy as a spokesperson for optometry, and to optometric meetings to distribute OEP educational materials.

During this time, I attended my first Skeffington Symposium, now called the Kraskin Invitational Skeffington Symposium on Vision (KISS). I loved being a part of the optometric family. The Kraskins, Lewises and others from the East and West Coasts who have attended for more than 50 years embraced me. My new optometric family was one where I was understood, accepted, and not considered a "heretic," like I was in the world of psychology and education.

My role as a bridge continued in Washington, DC, where a group of professionals had just founded Washington Independent Services and Educational Resources (WISER). I was elected as the Program Chair. For eight years my committee and I arranged about 10 programs a year on various subjects. Of course, optometry was prominent. In those years, DC area educators discovered the importance and power of optometry through the lectures of Jeff Kraskin, Harry Wachs, Nancy Lewis, Stan Appelbaum, Walter Kaplan, Amiel and others. I had also arranged for GN Getman to speak. Unfortunately, two nights before his scheduled speaking engagement, he passed away.

In the late 1980s, at Eastern States, I noticed a man in the audience taking copious notes, and shaking his head affirmatively when I was speaking. I quickly learned his identity, as he followed me as the next speaker. Dr. Irwin Suchoff took the microphone from me, and picked up right where I had left off. A colleague had told me that he was speaking at the conference and I should look him up. Little did I know that, once again, I would find a mentor, who would push me further, by insisting that I write about, and not just speak about, what I knew.

As the newly appointed Editor of the *Journal of Behavioral Optometry (JBO)*, Irwin invited me to join his Peer Review Board and submit articles for publication. I have now written five articles for the JBO, three of which have won awards from the Optometric Editors Association. Two articles, "From ADD to Autism, What Optometrists Need to Know" and "Treatments for Those on the Autism Spectrum" developed into the outline for a chapter I wrote for a book on autism for occupational therapists, published in 2001 by the American Occupational Therapy Association (AOTA). After the publication of that book, Bob Williams asked me to expand the chapter into a book on the same subject for optometrists. I had the idea to ask experts to write the chapters, and agreed to serve as the book's editor. That was almost five years ago.

Soon after I met Irwin, I was so excited about the synergistic relationship between optometry and occupational therapy that I decided to put together a symposium on OT/OD collaboration. The OT/OD symposiums were held in Washington, DC and Anaheim, CA in the late 1980s. In these two day workshops, Irwin presented a one-day lecture on vision for OTs, and an occupational therapist taught ODs about sensory integration. During the second day OT/OD pairs demonstrated how they worked collaboratively to evaluate and treat patients with cerebral palsy, learning disabilities, head injury and autism. It was during this time that I met and learned from other amazing optometrists, including Beth Ballinger, Lynne Hellerstein, Bob Sanet and Don Getz. I understand that the OT/OD Symposiums spawned several multi-disciplinary practices that are still going strong.

In the early 1990s, while sitting through a not-very-interesting conference on attention deficits, I decided to look at the symptoms of ADD as defined by the Diagnostic and Statistical Manual (DSM). Symptoms such as "Often fails to give close attention to details" or "makes careless mistakes" and "Often has difficulty organizing tasks and activities" clearly could be caused by undiagnosed visual dysfunction. I decided to determine whether a child with visual problems could satisfy the criteria for an ADD diagnosis. The result is my OEP published pamphlet entitled "Attention Deficits: A Developmental Approach," in which I show that kids with allergies/nutritional deficits, sensory integration issues AND kids with vision issues all could be misdiagnosed as having ADD.

The culmination of my work as a counselor is the co-founding of Developmental Delay Resources, the non-profit organization I have run since 1994. After meeting nutritionist Kelly Dorfman, I realized that understanding the relationship between the body and the mind is not complete without knowing about diet, vitamins, minerals, proteins and all those tiny particles that we eat, drink and breathe. Knowing Kelly took me back to my early work in Boston, where I watched dietary changes stop seizures. Kelly was applying the same knowledge to the autism epidemic in the nineties.

Through DDR, now a nationally recognized group composed of thousands of professionals, families and organizations world-wide, I have met many more optometrists. Many recalled hearing me speak at various meetings or had read my articles in the *JBO*. I am grateful that they are DDR members, and impressed with how they integrate so much from other professions into their practices.

Becoming a part of the optometric family has helped me understand both myself and my clients. Vision therapy opened my eyes to possibilities and ideas. I can only imagine how different my brother's and my lives would have been if our childhood doctor had prescribed some early vision therapy for me and some plus lenses for my brother. I guess he would not be the "visionary" he is today, and this book would never have been written. I use this opportunity to extend my profound gratitude to my mentors in optometry and all the optometrists who have made this book possible. Little did I know how long it would take!

INTRODUCTION
Autism Spectrum Disorders:
How Medical, Societal, Educational & Environmental Changes
Have Contributed to an Epidemic

In the late 1980s an epidemic of autism spectrum disorders began, and it continues today. Skeptics suggest that identification of an increasing number of affected children is a result of diagnostic substitution and more comprehensive categories.[1] Many in the field now agree that triggers, such as Thimerosal in vaccines are clearly devastating to genetically vulnerable children with compromised immune systems and faulty detoxification pathways.[2] This book details convincingly how a clash of genetic susceptibility with an infinite number of environmental triggers, in complex combinations with other load factors, must accumulate to put many children at risk, and push others over their personal limits.

In the past 40 years as a counselor, I have watched the world change. While we cannot go "back to the future," we can be conscious about how "progress" may not be so "progressive" in terms of children's health and development. I strongly believe that environmental changes, so prominent in the news today, are not sufficient, however to cause such alarming changes. Slow, subtle modifications in medical, societal and educational practices are also contributing to the autism epidemic.

Identifying how these factors may impede a child's growth and putting mitigation into place could assist families on the road to recovery. What if, along with starting expensive, intensive, early intervention with skilled therapists and health care specialists, doctors, schools and families instituted practices aimed at counteracting the negative effects of these changes which so profoundly affect today's children?

Changes in Medicine
Medicine has "progressed" markedly since the 1950s. While doctors have extended the life span by utilizing remarkable technology diagnostically, and applying high level biochemistry therapeutically, many agree that personal care often gets lost. Here are some differences that are certainly not in the best interest of today's children.

- *From house calls to managed care* In the past, the family doctor knew a family personally, and came to the home to minister to a sick child's needs. He took the time to chat with the parents and learn what preceded the onset of symptoms. Today's child is a part of a huge managed care conglomerate, "with cost-cutting strategies that have shortened office visits and threatened to reduce the traditional doctor-patient covenant to a business contract."[3] Most families see a different physician at each visit, with the latest doctor relying on the previous one's scribbled notes. Physician assistants take only limited time for history-taking, let alone establishing a personal relationship. The goal is "alleviate the symptom," not find the cause.

- *Over-use of antibiotics* Antibiotics are miracle drugs that have saved the lives of millions of people. However, recently the bugs are outsmarting them by mutating.[4] Physicians claim parents demand prescriptions for today's medications, which are atom bombs compared to early versions, such as penicillin.

  No one yet knows what antibiotic overuse is doing to children's immune systems short- or long-term. When an antibiotic does the job, the body's immune response becomes lazy and under-reactive.[5] Women are familiar with yeast infections which result from antibiotic overuse. Many children with developmental problems also suffer from yeast overgrowth in their guts.[6] If their bodies are fighting colonies of yeast, little energy is available for learning and development. Many months of returning good bacteria to their damaged digestive tracts are necessary to produce normal stools. Once the body is healthier, language, learning and behavior all improve spontaneously.

Could long-term use of antibiotics starting in childhood be contributing to the rise in autism spectrum disorders in childhood as well as to more auto-immune diseases later in life?

- ***Increase in the numbers of vaccines*** Today's children are mandated to receive over 50 vaccines before entering school,[7] compared to a single shot for smallpox 50 years ago. As the number of vaccines has increased, so has the incidence of autism spectrum disorders. One doctor, who wishes to remain anonymous, called the American Academy of Pediatrics vaccine schedule one of the largest medical experiments ever. The mercury-containing preservative thimerosal and other toxic ingredients include metals such as aluminum, and poisons, such as formaldehyde.[8] Just like with antibiotics, we are only beginning to understand possible long-term devastating effects of vaccines.

Changes in the Environment and Society

- ***Increase in environmental toxins*** Few would argue that we now live in a toxic world. The now classic Body Burden study by the Environmental Working Group (EWG)[9] proved that harmful chemicals are showing up in umbilical cord blood. Is health only the lack of symptoms? Are there degrees of health? Truly "healthy" people are taking daily measures such as buying organic food and filtering air and water to protect their bodies from neurotoxic chemicals that did not exist 50 years ago. To eliminate environmental toxins that they inadvertently eat, drink and breathe, they are detoxing with saunas and supplements.

- ***Increase in food additives*** Label reading is now an inherent part of grocery shopping. In the past 50 years, artificial colors, flavors and preservatives have crept into most foods to enhance their taste, smell and shelf-life. Many like monosodium glutamate and aspartame are "excitotoxins" which activate the nerves so much that they literally excite themselves to death.[10] Today's kids are drinking gallons of sodas and eating colored cereals and baked goods that have virtually no nutritional value. Consumption of fresh fruits and vegetables is waning as the amount of processed foods consumed rises.

- ***Increase in electronic and wireless technology*** Enter the electronic baby sitter. Television, DVDs, cell phone screens and iPods have replaced the local teenager. Today's kids entertain themselves and their friends by playing video games, watching movies, listening to music plugged into their ears and bouncing off their brains, and by instant messaging. Do they have shorter attention spans because their eyes are constantly trying to focus on moving objects?

Gone are the days of playing ball against the steps in the neighborhood and coming home when the street lights came on. Richard Louv believes that many kids suffer from what he has termed "Nature-deficit Disorder."[11] Few are permitted to venture out into the woods (if they can find any woods) for safety reasons. Even if they were, they would probably be connected to home by a cell phone, "just in case."

- ***Changes in sleeping practices*** Doctors now encourage back sleeping to prevent sudden infant death syndrome (SIDS).[12] Only with adequate 'tummy time" can head, neck, shoulder and upper body muscles develop and primitive reflexes emerge and become integrated. Are the plethora of learning and behavioral problems in this generation of kids due in part to retained reflexes and weakened hands which have difficulty holding pencils and cutting with scissors? Occupational therapists must provide hand strengthening and reflex integration so that kindergartners can accomplish these simple tasks.

- *Increased safety measures restrict movement* In attempts to keep kids safe, society now severely restricts their movements from the day they are born. We place them in car seats, back packs, play pens and walkers. In addition to further impeding the emergence and integration of reflexes, these modern day pieces of equipment limit children's natural sensory needs to touch and move. Restricting and limiting touch and movement secondarily limit kids' innate abilities to know where they are in space and to use their bodies purposefully.

Changes in Schools

Any seasoned elementary school teacher will tell you that curriculum and expectations in today's schools are different than they were 50 years ago. These changes may not be in the best interest of today's kids.

- *An accelerated academic curriculum* The first grade curriculum of last generation is now taught in kindergarten. Our youngest students are expected to "sit still and pay attention." Many of them still have poor control over their own bodies, let alone pencils and scissors. Despite the fact that they have not had the experience of sitting through a 15-minute meal, they are expected to sit through 30 minutes of circle time in kindergarten and a 60-minute lesson in first grade. Many stare out the window for visual relief, or wiggle and squirm to keep alert.
- *Early reading initiatives* The "No Child Left Behind" (NCLB) initiative has hastened the teaching of reading and writing to a generation of children who cannot sleep through the night, tie their shoes or speak in complete sentences. Our Federal government's lack of understanding of normal childhood development has mandated unrealistic expectations for many young children. Pushing them ahead academically without a strong foundation of motor, sensory-motor and language skills, forces them to learn by rote, at best. At worst, they are labeled "learning disabled" or as having an "attention deficit disorder."
- *Recess and P.E. are becoming extinct* "Learning is not all in your head,"[13] says educator Carla Hannaford. Kids must move and use their senses to learn! Developmental specialists recognize that movement is food for the nervous system, and that young students' bodies need movement as much as a nutritious breakfast. Unfortunately, today's schools have seriously decreased opportunities for movement, and some are eliminating recess and physical education altogether.
- *Decrease in time for art and music* The arts are being replaced by computer time and foreign language study to enlarge the worlds of students, many of whom know little geography, and cannot find their home towns on the map. Kids need "free" time to use their imaginations with paints, paper, scissors and musical instruments. Lessons in music and drawing are not the same as providing materials and allowing freedom of expression.
- *Increase in class size* Today's teachers must contend with up to 30 children of varying abilities and achievement levels in their classrooms, often without the assistance of an aide. As schools are cutting back on their budgets, classes can also span two or more grades. If a system has 40 first graders and 20 second graders, they might make a one-two combination. Placing higher level first graders with lower functioning second graders is a questionable practice.
- *Increase in inclusion* Research shows that both students with disabilities and those without benefit from inclusion.[14] However, many safeguards must be in place for inclusion to be successful. These include extensive teacher training and support, or "mainstreaming" can put a further burden on already stressed-out teachers. The common solution of instituting an aide or "shadow" for the student can help. However, sometimes aides act as policemen, keeping students with developmental delays "on task," further squelching their needs to move and touch.

Changes in Families

- *Decrease in the number of stay-at-home moms* For many reasons, primarily financial, stay-at-home moms have become the exception rather than the rule. Consequently, grandparents, nannies, day care centers and babysitters have assumed parenting roles. Arguments can be made for the benefits of both parents having a life outside of the home. Research shows that children in day care are just as well adjusted as those who are raised at home with both parents.[15] The problems stem from the stress that arises from parents who think about their children while at work, and who attend to work responsibilities while at home. The most successful families I know keep strict boundaries between these two parts of their lives.

- *Distance separates close relations* The support of having relatives in the same town, let alone a bike ride away, as I did, is ancient history. Many children of this generation hardly know their parents' siblings and parents because few aunts, uncles, and grandparents live nearby. Spending a few precious days with them during holidays and school vacations in a whirlwind of ice cream, movies and other Disneyland treats is not the same as a day-to-day relationship.

- *Increase in fast food and eating out* Today, food is available almost everywhere, not just at home, in the grocery store and at school. Vending machines are ubiquitous, and dining at bookstores, coffee houses and sports events constitutes a "meal." The number of meals eaten out has doubled from 16% in 1978, to over 30% in 2005.[16] The rare family eats more than three meals a week together at home, according to my informal surveying. Compare that to three meals a day I ate with my family when growing up.

Children are missing out on home-cooked foods and all the nutrients they contain, as well as on the experiences that accompany them, such as waiting for dessert, passing the peas, and seeing who gets the last bite of mashed potatoes. One kindergarten teacher suggested that sitting through a 15-minute dinner with the family should be a pre-requisite to circle time at school. Eating micro-waved Chinese beef and broccoli from a take-out container in front of the television or in the car on the way to soccer is not the same as a sharing meat loaf and broccoli at the table. Mom's version is made with virgin olive oil, fresh onions and love.

- *Less time for unstructured play* Group sports and lessons have replaced "free" play, even for our youngest children. Over-zealous parents, hoping to raise the next Tiger Woods, Venus Williams or Sasha Cohen start three year olds on golf, tennis or ice skating lessons. By requiring children's bodies to conform to motor poses and their minds to rules of the game, few are learning how to control their bodies spontaneously and by trial and error. Instead, they are acquiring "splinter" athletic skills and playing games by rote.

- *More reliance on technology reduces inter-personal interactions* Busy parents use television, DVDs and movies to keep kids entertained while they check their e-mail and participate in teleconferences. What happened to board games such as Clue, Checkers and Monopoly? Playing games teaches so much: how to wait your turn, anticipate, strategize, lose, count, sequence, think. Zoning out in front of a screen implants many of the wrong kinds of images in the mind's eye. Some youngsters cannot fall asleep after watching frightening scenes. Which brings us to the last item.

- *Sleep deprivation* According to experts, school-aged children need 10-12 hours of sleep a night, teenagers 8½ - 9 hours, and adults 7- 8½ hours.[17] Sleep deprivation impairs metabolism, immune function and motor skills. It increases stress hormones, and cripples sugar metabolism.[18] One study found that a majority of children diagnosed with

Attention Deficit Disorder (ADD) no longer qualified for that label once they caught up on their sleep.[19]

We can neither turn back the clock nor undo these changes, a few of which have benefit as well as being detrimental. Even though medical, environmental, societal, educational, and familial factors alone cannot account for the rise in the numbers of kids with issues, collectively their synergistic interactions are working against this generation of children.

In Chapter 3, DDR co-founder and nutritionist Kelly Dorfman and I discuss the cumulative effect or "total load" of individual assaults on the body as a whole. Recognizing load factors and limiting them can often result in a huge benefit for children with autism spectrum disorders.

Total Load Theory

Dorfman labels the cumulative effect of individual assaults on the body as a whole as "total load."[20] Each individual has a personal load limit, as does a bridge. When that limit is exceeded, immunological, digestive, respiratory, skin, language, motor and attention symptoms occur. These issues co-exist with developmental, cognitive, sensory and social/emotional problems, and their relationship is very complex.

While early signs of stress on the immune system, such as allergies and infections are the most prominent, many prenatal conditions add to the total load. Babies who endured complications of pregnancy, or had subtle birth trauma, such as oxygen deprivation or breech presentation, and are born to mothers with a large number of "silver" dental amalgams, or have conditions such as thyroid problems, severe allergies, chronic fatigue syndrome or fibromyalgia, are much more at risk for later developmental problems.

The following chapters cover other relevant areas of pathology and treatment:

Chapter 4 looks at the significant role of **Vaccines** and their additives, including thimerosal

Chapter 5 – A Biomedical Approach to Autism Spectrum Disorders

Chapter 6 – The Defeat Autism Now! Movement both cover treatments that boost the immune system, including dietary modification, nutritional supplementation, and detoxification

Chapters 7 - 10 are on sensory therapies

Chapter 7 covers problems and treatments that focus on **Sensory Integration and Processing**

Chapter 8 addresses problems with and therapy for retained **Primitive Reflexes**

Chapter 9 focuses on **Vision Therapy**

Chapter 10 reports on **Sound-based Therapies**

Chapter 11 details **Therapies that address Communication and Social-emotional issues through Play**, including Greenspan's FloorTime, Gutstein's RDI and Son-Rise

Chapter 12 covers classical and sequential **Homeopathy**, as well as homotoxicology

Chapter 13 is on **Educational Kinesiology** (Brain Gym)

Chapter 14 describes **Applied Behavioral Analysis (ABA)** and **Neurofeedback**, therapies that are based on Operant Conditioning

Chapter 15, Healing with Animals, including horses, dogs and dolphins

Chapter 16 is **Dr. Dietrich Klinghardt's autism protocol**

Chapter 17 presents a systematic approach to **Prioritizing Therapies**

When reading through the chapters, make mental notes about healthy changes you and your family can make in your daily life, without resorting to expensive therapies and consultations. You will be surprised at what a difference just a few "tweaks" can make!

References

1. *Newschaffer CJ, Curran LK. Autism: an emerging public health problem. Public Health Rep. 2003 Sept-Oct;118:393–99.*

2. *Bock K. Healing the New Childhood Epidemics: Autism, ADHD, Asthma, and Allergies: The Groundbreaking Program for the 4-A Disorders. New York, Ballantine Books, 2007.*

3. *Seaman B. Charting the doctor-patient relationship. www.spiralnotebook.org (Accessed December 5, 2007)*

4. *Shnayerson M, Plotkin MJ. The Killers Within: The Deadly Rise of Drug Resistant Bacteria. Boston: Little Brown, 2002.*

5. *Levy SB. The Antibiotic Paradox: How Miracle Drugs are Destroying the Miracle. New York: Plenum, 1992.*

6. *Shaw W. Biological Treatments for Autism and PDD. Lenexa, KS, Great Plains Laboratory, 2002.*

7. *Recommended Childhood and Adolescent Immunization Schedule. American Academy of Pediatrics. www.aap.org (Accessed June 19, 2006)*

8. *Kirby D. Mercury in Vaccines and the Autism Epidemic: A Medical Controversy. New York: St. Martin's Press, 2005.*

9. *http://www.ewg.org/reports/bodyburden1/methodology.php (Accessed May 20, 2006)*

10. *Blaylock RL. Excitotoxins: The Taste That Kills. Santa Fe, NM: Health Press, 1997.*

11. *Louv R. Last Child in the Woods: Saving Our Children from Nature-Deficit Disorder. New York, NY: Workman Publishing, 2005.*

12. *Safe Sleep for Your Baby: Ten Ways to Reduce the Risk of Sudden Infant Death Syndrome. National Institute of Child Health and Human Development. Bethesda, MD: NIH Pub No. 05-7040: 2003.*

13. *Hannaford C. Smart Moves: Why Learning Is Not All In Your Head. Arlington, VA: Great Ocean Publishers, 1995.*

14. *http://http://www.kidstogether.org/inclusion/benefitsofinclusion.htm. (Accessed Februbary 14, 2008)*

15. *Ceglowski D, Bacigalupa C. Keeping current in child care research, annotated bibliography: an update. Early Childhood Res Pract 2002;4:1.*

16. *Farner B. Eating Out Healthy. University of Illinois Extension. June, 2005, www.urbanext.uiuc.edu (Accessed December 9, 2007)*

17. *Your Child's Sleep Needs. www.parenting.ivillage.com. (Accessed December 9, 2007)*

18. *The Effects of Sleep Deprivation. www.familymatters.tv (Accessed December 9, 2007)*

19. *Van der Heijden KB, Smits MG, Gunning, WB. Sleep-related disorders in ADHD: a review. Clin Pediatr 2005;44:1-10.*

20. *Dorfman K. Why so many children have developmental problems: the total load theory. New Developments newsletter 1996 Winter;1:3-4.*

Editor

Patricia S. Lemer, MEd, NCC, MS Bus is a co-founder and the Executive Director of Developmental Delay Resources (DDR), a non-profit organization integrating conventional and holistic therapies for children with autism spectrum disorders. She received a Bachelor of Science degree in Psychology and Mathematics (Psychological Testing) from Simmons College, Boston, MA. She holds a Master of Education in counseling and learning disabilities from Boston College and a Master of Science in Business from Johns Hopkins University. She is a National Certified Counselor (NCC), is licensed in the state of Pennsylvania (LPC) and practiced as an educational diagnostician and counselor for over 30 years, helping parents choose and prioritize appropriate interventions for their children.

Ms. Lemer is the author of "Alternative and Complementary Approaches in the Treatment of Autism" in *Autism, A Comprehensive Occupational Therapy Approach*, the OEP pamphlet "Attention Deficits: A Developmental Approach," and "Diagnosis: Autism, What Families Can Do" (Mothering Magazine, May-June 2000). Her published articles in the *Journal of Behavioral Optometry (JBO)* include "Education for All Handicapped Children Act: Public Law 94-142: What Optometrists Need to Know" (1:6, 1990), "Disabilities and the Law: What Optometrists Need to Know" (4:5, 1994), "From Attention Deficit Disorder to Autism: A Continuum" (7:6, 1996), "Treatments for Those on the Autistic Spectrum" (9:2, 1998), and "How Recent Changes have Contributed to an Epidemic of Autism Spectrum Disorders" (17:3, 2006). Ms. Lemer's great interest in vision and the role of visual dysfunction in autism led to the writing of this book.

Ms. Lemer lectures internationally about using a trans-disciplinary approach to the diagnosis and treatment of autism spectrum disorders, including AD(H)D and learning disabilities. She is on the Peer Review Board of the Journal of Behavioral Optometry (JBO), and has been honored by the Optometric Editors Association on three occasions. She is also a member of the Advisory Board of the US Autism & Asperger Association.

Ms. Lemer lives in Pittsburgh, PA and is the mother of an adult daughter and the grandmother of Penelope, born in August, 2006.

Authors and Contributors

Sidney MacDonald Baker, MD – Co-founder of the Autism Research Institute's Defeat Autism Now! project. Author of *Detoxification and Healing, The Circadian Prescription*, and co-author with Jon Pangborn of *Autism: Effective Biomedical Treatments*. Founder of Medigenesis <www.medigenesis.com>. Maintains private practice in Long Island, New York.

Samuel Berne, OD, FCOVD, FCSO – Optometric educator on vision, reflexes, and nutrition. Maintains private practice in Santa Fe, New Mexico. Author of *Without Ritalin* and *From ADD to Autism*, a DVD. Trained in CranioSacral therapy. <sberneod@cybermesa.com>

Barbara Brewitt, PhD – Medical scientist. Founder, CEO and Chief Scientific Officer of Biomed Comm® Inc., in Seattle, WA. Expert on homeopathic growth hormone and growth factors. Holds nine patents. Also holds Master of Divinity degree. <www.biomedcomm.com>

Judy Chiswell, EdD, OTR – Occupational therapist and EEG neurofeedback specialist interested in mind/body interactions, the developing brain and sensory integration. Private practice in Buffalo, NY. <hemispheres@adelphia.net>

Dorinne Davis, MA, CCC-A, F-AAA – Educational and rehabilitative audiologist with 30+ years experience. President and Founder of The Davis Center for Hearing, Speech, & Learning, Inc., in Mt. Arlington, NJ. Author of *Sound Bodies Through Sound Therapy* and *Every Day a Miracle: Success Stories with Sound Therapy*. <www.thedaviscenter.com>

Kelly Dorfman, MS, LND – Nutritionist and health program planner with over 25 years of clinical experience with autism and developmental delays. Maintains private practice in suburban Washington, DC. Co-founder with Patricia Lemer of Developmental Delay Resources (DDR). <www.kellydorfman.com>

Stephen M. Edelson, PhD – Psychologist and Director of the Autism Research Institute (ARI). Past President Society for Auditory Integration Therapy (SAIT). Editor of Recovering Autistic Children. <www.autism.com>

Barbara Loe Fisher – President and co-founder National Vaccine Information Center (NVIC). Co-author *DPT: A Shot in the Dark* and author of *The Consumer's Guide to Childhood Vaccines*. <www.nvic.org>

Melvin Kaplan, OD, FCOVD – Director of The Center for Visual Management in Tarrytown, NY. Specializes in the management of patients with visual spatial learning differences, including perceptual, psychological, autistic, and traumatic brain injury dysfunction. Author of *Seeing Through New Eyes*. <www.autisticvision.com>

Dietrich Klinghardt, MD, PhD – Physician and healer, originally from West Germany. Has synthesized traditional and alternative medicine for more than 30 years. Made many innovative contributions, including the development of Autonomic Response Testing (ART). Offers workshops throughout the United States and Europe. Treats patients in Bellevue, WA, where he collaborates with **Elizabeth Hesse Sheehan, DC, CCN**, a chiropractic physician, specializing in both traditional and low force chiropractic techniques, as well as clinical nutrition, natural medicine and ART. <www.neuraltherapy.com> and <www.drsheehan.com>

Carol Marusich, OD, MS, FCOVD – Optometric physician with private practice in Eugene, Oregon for over 25 years. Specializes in developmental vision and eye health care for infants, children and adults. Author of DVD: *Integration of Primitive Motor Reflexes: Why Should I Care ?* <www.lifetimeeyecare.net>

Brendan O'Hara – Accomplished musician and international lecturer on kinesiology, primitive and postural reflexes, and righting them through movement aided by bean bags. Author of *The Children's Music CD & Songbook, Wombat and his Mates CD & Songbook,* and *Beanbag Ditties CD.* <www.movementandlearning.com/au>

Siegfried Othmer, PhD – Physicist and Chief Scientist at the EEG Institute in Los Angeles, CA. Founder of EEG Spectrum, the largest neurofeedback service delivery organization in the world. Co-author of *ADD: The 20-Hour Solution.* <www.eeginstitute.com>

Jon Pangborn, PhD – Holds doctorate in chemical engineering. Founder of Bionostics, Inc. Co-founder of the Autism Research Institute's Defeat Autism Now! project, and co-author with Sid Baker of *Autism: Effective Biomedical Treatments.* Holds 9 U. S. patents. Author of over 200 publications and presentations.

Judyth Reichenberg-Ullman, ND, DHANP, LCSW and Robert Ullman, ND, DHANP – Licensed naturopathic physicians and board-certified diplomates of the Homeopathic Academy of Naturopathic Physicians. Co-authors of *A Drug-Free Approach to Asperger Syndrome and Autism, Prozac-Free, Ritalin-Free Kids, Rage-Free Kids, Homeopathic Self-Care,* and *The Patient's Guide to Homeopathic Medicine.* Maintain private practices in Edmonds, WA. <www.healthyhomeopathy.com> and <www.drugfreeasperger.com>

Mary Rentschler, M. Ed. – Special educator, licensed Brain Gym consultant, Masgutova Method Integration Specialist, and co-founder of The Systemic Constellations Group. Training with Dietrich Klinghardt, M.D. Presents nationally on Educational Kinesiology, reflexes and related topics. Maintains private practice working with adults and children in Washington, DC. <wren@pipeline.com>

Bernard Rimland, PhD (1928-2006) – Research psychologist and pioneer in understanding the relationship between nutrition and retardation, hyperactivity, learning disabilities, delinquency and autism. Founder of the Autism Society of America and Autism Research Institute. Editor of the *Autism Research Review International,* Author of *Infantile Autism: The Syndrome and Its Implications for a Neural Theory of Behavior.* <www.autism.com>

Randy Schulman, OD, MS, FCOVD – Behavioral optometrist and expert in autism and related disorders. Director of Total Learning & Therapy Center and in private practice in Connecticut. <www.tltc.org>

Anju Usman, MD – Board certified Family Practice physician specializing in treating biochemical imbalances in children and adults with ADD and autism. Director of True Health Medical Center in Naperville, IL. A Defeat Autism Now! doctor who has researched copper/zinc imbalances, metallothionein dysfunction and promotion therapy, and uses nutrition, homeopathy, herbals, flower essences & far infra-red sauna with her patients.

Susan Varsammes, MA Ed – Special educator and expert in Applied Behavior Analysis. Owner and Director Holistic Learning Center in Eastchester, NY. Author of several articles and publications in the field of educating, advocating for, and providing services the population with learning and Autism Spectrum Disorders. <www.hlcinfo.com>

Chapter 1
Autism Spectrum Disorders: Overview
Patricia S. Lemer, MEd, NCC

Introduction

Optometrists are seeing an increasing number of patients with diagnoses of autism, pervasive developmental disorders, attention deficits and learning disabilities. Most readers would agree that all of these patients manifest visual dysfunction to some degree, if they apply a developmental definition of "vision."

Lorna Wing, a British psychiatrist, was among the first to consider the above diagnoses not as discrete entities, but rather as part of a continuum of disorders. She entitled this continuum "The Autistic Spectrum."[1] Diagnoses range from Attention Deficit Disorder (ADD) at the mild extreme to autism as the most severe impairment. Attention deficit disorder with hyperactivity (ADHD), learning disabilities (LD), non-verbal learning disabilities (NLD), pervasive developmental disorders (PDD) and Asperger syndrome (AS) lie between the extremes, as moderate degrees of disability. Figure 1-1 illustrates the concept.

ADD AD(H)D LD NLD Asperger Syndrome PDD PDD-NOS Autism		
Least severe	More severe	Most severe

Figure 1-1. The Autism Spectrum of Disorders (ASD)

While each of these disorders has very specific diagnostic criteria, two clinicians may or may not agree upon a diagnosis, because determining the presence or absence of symptoms requires subjective judgment. Asperger syndrome is a case in point. It is presently described as an autism spectrum disorder. Uta Frith describes AS individuals as "having a dash of autism."[2] Some professionals use AS, NLD and "high functioning autism" (HFA) synonymously, while others believe that AS and NLD are discrete syndromes. AS also shares many of the characteristics of PDD-NOS. Because Asperger syndrome was virtually unknown until a few years ago, many individuals with AS either received an incorrect diagnosis or remained undiagnosed. It is not at all uncommon for a child to be initially diagnosed with ADD or ADHD, and later to be re-diagnosed with AS. In addition, some individuals who were originally diagnosed with HFA or PDD-NOS are now being given the AS diagnosis. Some even have a dual diagnosis of Asperger syndrome and High Functioning Autism.

People with the same diagnosis can have a broad range of cognitive, social, language and attentional deficits. An infinite number of combinations of strengths and weaknesses inherent in all of these diagnoses make their precise placement on a linear chart difficult and easy to debate. Imagine the frustration of a parent searching for the "right" diagnosis.

An Historical Perspective

Autism The term "autism" derives from two Greek roots: auto (self) and ismos (condition), and was first used by psychiatrist Eugene Bleuler in 1913.[3] A few years earlier, however, Theodore Heller, a special educator in Vienna, Austria, wrote about some seemingly normal children whose behavior and learning deteriorated or was arrested in the second year of life. Heller proposed the term "dementia infantilis" to describe these children.[4]

The discovery of autism is traditionally attributed to Leo Kanner who, in the 1940s, considered it to be a psychiatric disorder.[5] Also called "childhood schizophrenia," it was thought to be the result of a "refrigerator mother" by followers of Bruno Bettelheim in the 1960s and 70s. Most professionals no longer subscribe to this belief. Until near the end of the 20th century, Kanner's, or "classic" autism, was the only type described in the literature. Autism was rare, one in only 500,000. Patients so diagnosed were considered unfortunate and untreatable, so the medical establishment simply ignored them and their families.[6]

In the early 1990s, physicians and nurses began to see a number of these patients, as well as their own children and grandchildren, showing signs of regressive autism. This regression followed a series of immunizations containing thimerosal, a mercury-containing preservative. Some like retired pediatrician Edward Yazbak and Congressman Dan Burton (R-IN) have become outspoken advocates for changes in medical practice and policy because of their personal stories. Burton has held numerous Congressional hearings with government agencies and physicians and scientists to get to the bottom of why the world's second most toxic substance, mercury, is knowingly added to a vaccination that is supposed to prevent illness, not cause it.

Today's doctors could not suggest that families were simply unaware of their children's early signs of autism, because they could show videos of normal babies waving at the camera on their first birthdays and ignoring their surroundings a year later. Heller's syndrome, dormant for almost a century, had reappeared. This new group of vocal professionals and parents of children with regressive autism could not be ignored.

Tenacious families found each other on the new communication tool: the Internet. They exchanged information in chat rooms, discovered similarities in their stories, and began researching together. Regressive autism was the epidemic of the 90s. Something was harming children; what? Was it the vaccines themselves, the thimerosal, or something more complex? The story of the "Autism-Vaccine Connection" is in Chapter 4.

They looked for answers from anyone who would entertain their hypotheses. Two professionals who listened were Kelly Dorfman, a nutritionist, and this author, an educational counselor, both in private practice in suburban Washington, DC. In 1994 they met with the mother of a three-year-old twin just diagnosed with autism. She was astonished to discover that her child's health history and subsequent autism diagnosis was not unique. She declared, "If there are other children like mine, let's start a registry." This meeting was the catalyst for the formation of the non-profit organization Developmental Delay Registry (DDR), later re-named Developmental Delay Resources.

DDR founders compiled a survey of questions for parents, asking what they thought had gone wrong. Dorfman and Lemer had their own hypotheses. The children they saw in their practices had many commonalities in their early health histories: reflux, frequent ear infections, allergies, many rounds of antibiotics, yeast infections, thrush, eczema, diarrhea, constipation, immunization reactions, among others. They asked questions about these and other factors in the survey.

Surprisingly, parents not only completed the lengthy survey, but attached health and immunization records as well as passionate letters thanking them for their interest. In 1994 DDR ran a statistical analysis of the responses, completed by a self-selected group of parents of 449 children with autism spectrum diagnoses and 247 normally developing children. Comparisons between affected and non-affected children showed that:
- Children with developmental delays were 27% more likely than the unaffected kids to have had more than three ear infections
- Children with delays were almost four times as likely to have had a negative reaction to an immunization

- Children who took 20 or more rounds of antibiotics were 50% more likely to be developmentally delayed than those who had not

About the same time as this survey was being done, some of these parents had found willing ears in a prominent group of researchers and physicians who had long been involved in debunking Bettleheim's myth. This group, the Autism Research Institute (ARI), founded in the 1950s by Dr. Bernard Rimland, a psychologist and father of a son with autism, held a think tank called "Defeat Autism Now!" in Dallas in January, 1995. The attendees were approximately 30 physicians and scientists from the United States and Europe who have special expertise in autism research and treatment. Psychiatry, neurology, immunology, allergy, biochemistry, genetics and gastroententerology were among the fields represented. A number of the attendees, like Dr. Rimland, were parents of children with autism.

In February, 1996, Defeat Autism Now! published its first protocol co-authored by Dr. Sidney Baker, a Yale educated physician, and former Director of the Gesell Institute and Dr. Jon Pangborn, a chemist, parent of an autistic son, and President of Doctor's Data, a major medical laboratory. Updated five times and grown from 40 to over 300 pages, this publication has become the "bible" of parents and professionals determined to unearth the causes of this autism epidemic.[7] An unstoppable movement that was to have a profound effect on the medical, educational and political establishments had begun. The remarkable story of Defeat Autism Now! appears in Chapter 6.

Attention deficit disorder (ADD and ADHD) The concept of a disorder of attention debuted at the turn of the twentieth century as "a morbid defect of moral control." Fifty years later, children who were inattentive were thought to have an organic brain syndrome. In the 60s, the disorder acquired a name: minimal brain dysfunction. Gradually, focus shifted from a very narrow, medically-based model to a much broader, more inclusive and subjective category, incorporating an increasing number of symptoms and subsets. Soon, today's definitions of attention deficit disorder, with and without hyperactivity emerged, pathologizing more and more children.[8]

Learning disabilities (LD) Learning problems are hardly new. As early as 1867, Heinrich Stotzner, a German teacher of the deaf, recognized children who did not have mental retardation, but had memories too weak to retain letters and fingers too poorly coordinated to write.

A Scottish eye surgeon named James Hinshelwood was one of the first to suggest that there was such a thing as dyslexia, a specific learning disability.[9] In 1907, Hinshelwood was called in to diagnose four brothers who, unlike their seven siblings, had "experienced the greatest difficulties in learning to read." Hinshelwood offered that, in his opinion, the boys had "congenital word-blindness." Because the reading problems were clustered in a normal family, and all four boys had normal intelligence, lacked visual problems, and had good visual memory except for letters and words, it was "evident that their defect was cerebral, probably hereditary, and caused by a defective language-related area of the brain.[10] It is fascinating that an eye surgeon should initiate the misunderstanding about the relationship between vision and learning.

During the first half of the 20th century, psychiatrists and psychologists perpetuated Hinshelwood's concept of "word blindness." Most educators attribute the term "learning disabilities" to Samuel Kirk. In the early 60s he described children with "disorders in development of language, speech, reading, and associated communication skills" as "learning disabled."[11]

Kirk and his contemporaries, Newell Kephart and William Cruickshank supported programs of perceptual motor activities to remediate the visual issues inherent in their students' educational problems. Many of their prescriptions were similar to some of today's home and office based vision therapy protocols. The role of the optometrist in a multi-disciplinary to learning disabilities is attributed to G.N. Getman.[12]

How Are Autism Spectrum Disorders Diagnosed?

The holistic model in this book focuses on treatments for underlying causes, not for symptoms or by diagnosis. However, it is certainly helpful for the reader to have an understanding of the different characteristics of the various diagnoses and how their determination is made.

Before one can fully understand the similarities among the disorders, it is necessary to learn the symptoms that define them. The tool used most frequently by clinicians for this purpose is the *Diagnostic and Statistical Manual, Fourth Edition* (DSM-IV)[13] the "bible" of the American Psychiatric Association. Professionals and parents alike, especially those involved in the new movement, are often shocked to learn that the diagnostic determination for all of these disabilities is psychiatric.

The DSM-IV lists the most common diagnoses in the autism spectrum along with their diagnostic standards. Each diagnosis has strict criteria with guidelines for frequency, duration and severity of symptoms. Symptoms must manifest themselves consistently and sometimes in more than one environment. Diagnosis requires clear evidence of clinically significant impairment in social, academic and occupational functioning. The most common use of the DSM diagnosis at the present time is, not surprisingly, by health insurance companies to allow or deny coverage for a given treatment.

Some of the more frequently used diagnoses are discussed below. This overview is hardly exhaustive. The autism spectrum could also include some "psychiatric" diagnoses, such as panic and anxiety disorders, Tourette syndrome and obsessive compulsive disorder.

ADD and ADHD The DSM-IV lists nine symptoms of inattention and nine of hyperactivity. To qualify as having ADD, an individual must satisfy six symptoms of inattention. To add the "H," an additional six of hyperactivity must be present for at least six months and to a degree that is maladaptive and inconsistent with the person's developmental age. Attention deficits cannot be caused by other disorders, such as anxiety or psychosis. The symptoms of ADD and ADHD appear in Tables 1-1 and 1-2 respectively.

Table 1-1 Symptoms of Attention Deficit Disorder (ADD) (At least six are necessary)	Table 1-2 Symptoms of Hyperactivity and Impulsivity (AD(H)D) (At least six necessary)
• Often fails to give close attention to details or makes careless mistakes • Often has difficulty sustaining attention in tasks or play activities • Often does not listen when spoken to directly • Often does not follow through on instructions or fails to finish work • Often has difficulty organizing tasks and activities • Often avoids, dislikes or is reluctant to engage in tasks requiring sustained mental effort • Often loses things • Often distracted by extraneous stimuli • Often forgetful in daily activities	• Often fidgets with hands or feet or squirms in seat • Often has difficulty remaining seated when required to do so • Often runs or climbs excessively • Often has difficulty playing quietly • Often "on the go" • Often talks excessively • Often has difficulty awaiting turn • Often interrupts or intrudes on others • Often blurts out answers to questions before they have been completed

Learning disabilities (LD) The DSM-IV puts learning disabilities into three broad categories:
- Developmental speech and language disorders
- Academic skills disorders
- "Other," a catch-all that includes certain coordination disorders and learning handicaps not covered by the other terms

Each of these categories includes a number of more specific disorders. Since so much has been written about LD, it will not be elaborated upon here.

Non-verbal learning disabilities (NLD) First appearing in the literature in the late 60s, NLD has become a frequently used diagnosis. Although not in the DSM-IV, NLD is diagnosed symptomatically by the same professionals who diagnose other learning disabilities. An NLD may be called a developmental coordination disorder, a disorder of written expression or dysgraphia. To complicate matters further, NLD can be easily confused with Asperger syndrome (see below) and is sometimes used synonymously with the dual diagnosis of gifted/learning disabled.

NLD describes a cluster of deficits in motor, visual-spatial, social and sensory arenas combined with strengths in vocabulary, rote memory and attention to detail. This syndrome results in sensory overload and varying difficulty with cognition, academics and relationships.

Most people diagnosed with NLD demonstrate motor and sensory deficits in the first year of life. They may have never crawled, walked early or late, or adopted idiosyncratic movement patterns. They also have early histories of tactile defensiveness, vestibular disturbance and low tone, which preclude having well-integrated touch and movement experiences. To cope, they rely more heavily on what they hear than on what they sense, do or see. Audition and language skills predominate over vision and the more primitive senses early on. As language becomes ever more proficient, the NLD individual becomes less able to use vision to focus on and give meaning to what he sees. Avoidance and fear perpetuate the problems, and then can take on a life of their own as more serious psychological disorders, such as panic attacks.

Readers of this definition would be correct in thinking, "This sounds to me like a learning-related vision problem." NLD is essentially a developmental visual processing disorder that starts early in life. While many professionals from other disciplines who take a developmental point of view recognize it as such, and refer to behavioral optometrists, there are still some psychologists and educators who do not understand that NLD requires an optometrist on their teams.

Autism Autistic disorder is one of five developmental disorders falling under the umbrella of Pervasive Developmental Disorders (PDD). The others are Asperger syndrome (AS), Childhood Disintegrative Disorder (CDD), Rett syndrome, and Pervasive Developmental Disorder, not otherwise specified (PDD-NOS).

PDDs are characterized by "severe and pervasive impairment in social interaction and communication in the presence of repetitive and stereotyped behavior, interests and activities."[13] In order to satisfy the diagnosis of autism, a person must have a total of at least six items from the three areas.

1. Impairment in social interaction
- Inappropriate eye contact or facial expression
- Failure to develop peer relationships
- Lack of spontaneous sharing of enjoyment or interests
- Lack of social or emotional reciprocity

2. Impairment in communication
- Delayed or non-existent language development
- Poor conversational abilities if language is present
- Stereotypic, repetitive language or idiosyncratic language
- Lack of make-believe or social imitative play

3. Repetitive and stereotyped behavior, interests and activities
- Abnormally intense preoccupation with one or more interests
- Seemingly inflexible adherence to routines or rituals
- Mannerisms such as hand or finger flapping or twisting or whole body movements
- Preoccupations with object parts

Asperger Syndrome or Asperger's Disorder is named for a Viennese physician, Hans Asperger. In 1944 Asperger published a paper describing a pattern of behaviors in several young boys who had normal intelligence and language development, but who also exhibited autistic-like behaviors with marked deficiencies in social and communication skills.[14] Despite publication of his paper in the 1940s, it wasn't until 1994 that Asperger syndrome (AS) was added to the DSM-IV. Only in the past few years has AS been recognized by professionals and parents as a subset of autism.

Individuals with AS can exhibit a variety of characteristics and the disorder can range from mild to severe. Asperger individuals show marked deficiencies in social skills, have difficulties with transitions or changes and prefer sameness. They often also have obsessive routines and may become preoccupied with a particular subject of interest.

By definition, those with AS have a normal IQ and many individuals (although not all) exhibit exceptional skill in a specific area. These talents include, but are not limited to, perfect pitch, amazing drawing skills, the ability to perform complex arithmetic calculations without pencil and paper, and the "party skill" of telling the day of the week for any given day of any year. Recently, some highly accomplished individuals, viewed as "odd" by others, including Thomas Jefferson and Albert Einstein have been "diagnosed" with AS.[15]

While language development in Asperger syndrome is, by definition, not delayed, individuals with AS often have deficits in pragmatics and prosody. Vocabularies may be extraordinarily rich and some children sound like "little professors." However, persons with AS can be extremely literal and have difficulty using language in a social context.

AS individuals are often highly sensitive to sounds, tastes, smells and sights. In the words of one very articulate 18 year old who is now lecturing about growing up with high-functioning autism, "The pain of lights, sounds and the bees and motorcycles in my head were really bad... The hardest thing to process was snow. Having it land on you was absolutely overwhelming. Processing it changing from cold snow to liquid on my skin drove me out of my mind. I could not tell how deep it was... I felt like I was going to keep falling and the crunching sound made it feel like I would disappear under it."[16]

They may prefer soft clothing, eat only certain foods, and be bothered by sounds or lights no one else seems to hear or see. Parents, teachers and others may perceive their heightened responses to sensory experiences as rudeness or inappropriate behavior.

Many children diagnosed with AS after age 10 manage to develop age-appropriate self-help skills, adaptive behaviors (other than social interaction), and curiosity about the environment. As they get older, it becomes apparent that they often have a great deal of difficulty reading nonverbal cues (body language) and determining proper body space. It is important to remember that the person with AS perceives the world very differently. Many behaviors that seem odd or unusual are due to their unique combination of a high degree of functionality and social naiveté. They are therefore often viewed as eccentric and can easily become victims of teasing and bullying.

The sensory deficits and social difficulties inherent in AS are described in graphic detail by Temple Grandin[17] and Donna Williams,[18] two very successful adult women with high functioning autism, who have written about their experiences growing up.

Childhood Disintegrative Disorder (CDD) The DSM-IV describes CDD as a pattern of progressive deterioration in language, social interest, toileting and self-care after at least two years of apparently normal development. The child gradually begins to develop autistic-like behaviors. Often some specific trigger or neuro-pathological process is apparent. Given the new thinking about possible causes of autism spectrum disorders, this sub-type is today being likened to "regressive" autism or Heller's syndrome.

Rett Syndrome Rett syndrome was first recognized by Andreas Rett in 1966 and affects only females. Girls with Rett syndrome often exhibit autistic-like behaviors, such as repetitive hand movements, prolonged toe walking, body rocking and sleep problems.

In addition to the typical characteristics of autism, those with Rett syndrome demonstrate shakiness of the torso (and possibly the limbs), an unsteady, stiff-legged gait, breathing difficulties (including hyperventilation, apnea and air swallowing), seizures, teeth grinding and difficulty chewing, retarded growth, hypo-activity, and a cognitive functioning level in the severely to profoundly mentally retarded range. In most cases, there is continuous regression in cognition, behavior, social and motor skills throughout their lifetime.[19]

Pervasive Developmental Disorder, Not otherwise Specified (PDD-NOS) If none of a the other diagnoses fits a particular child, the diagnosis PDD-NOS (atypical autism) has become the catch-all. In other words, it looks like autism but does not satisfy sufficient criteria. Children with "atypical autism" may have deficits in only two of the three areas, and not to the degree required for the full blown "autism" diagnosis.

Medical or Educational?

While the medical community was using the *Diagnostic and Statistical Manual*[13] as their diagnostic tool, school systems discovered that they too needed guidelines for determining who was eligible for what services. Traditionally, students with physical disabilities, such as cerebral palsy, blindness and deafness, and mental retardation were "closeted" at home. Schools systems never had to worry about educating them.

By the 1960s an increasing number of children were entering schools classified as "learning disabled." In 1969, with the passage of the Children with Specific Learning Disabilities Act, federal law finally mandated support services for students with learning disabilities. A specific learning disability is defined as "...a disorder in one or more of the basic psychological processes involved in understanding or in using language, spoken or written, that may manifest itself in an imperfect ability to listen, think, speak, read, write, spell, or do mathematical calculations, including conditions such as perceptual disabilities, brain injury, minimal brain dysfunction, dyslexia, and developmental aphasia."[20]

In 1975, Congress passed Public Law 94-142 or the Education for All Handicapped Children Act (EHA).[21] This landmark decision by the U.S. Congress, re-enacted in 1990 as the Individuals with Disabilities Education Act (IDEA), assures a free and appropriate education to school-aged children with a dozen handicapping conditions. The doors of public schools were now legally open to those previously kept at home: the blind, deaf, retarded, and physically disabled.

Under this act, up for re-authorization every five years, public schools are required to design and implement an Individualized Educational Program (IEP) tailored to each child's specific needs. In 1991 IDEA was amended to extend services to developmentally delayed children down to age five. This law makes it possible for young children to receive help even before they begin school.

Another law, the Americans with Disabilities Act of 1990 (ADA),[22] extends services beyond secondary school into college and the workplace. The ADA requires publicly funded colleges and universities to remove barriers that keep out learning disabled students. Students with learning disabilities can arrange to take college entrance exams orally or in rooms free from distraction. Once accepted, colleges must provide recorded books and lectures, an isolated area to take tests, permission to tape record rather than write reports, depending upon a student's individual needs. Many colleges have created special programs to specifically accommodate these students.

ADA also guarantees equal employment opportunity for people with learning disabilities and protects disabled workers against job discrimination. Employers may not consider the learning disability when selecting among job applicants. Employers must also make "reasonable accommodations" to help workers who have handicaps do their job. Such accommodations may include shifting job responsibilities, modifying equipment or adjusting work schedules.

"Specific learning disability" (SLD) is one of 14 categories qualifying children for special education services. Today, students with learning disabilities make up a majority of those receiving special education services in our schools.

What about AD(H)D and autism? Neither made the list of handicapping conditions included under IDEA or ADA. In 1991, a movement of zealous professionals tried desperately to make attention deficit disorder qualify. After much debate lawmakers determined that students with AD(H)D usually qualified for services as either "learning disabled" or "seriously emotionally disturbed." If neither of those categories worked, then the student could be eligible under "other health impaired." This category was originally established for students with accepted medical conditions, such as AIDS, cystic fibrosis and muscular dystrophy, which affect their stamina and thus their ability to function in school. However, a loophole in the definition states that "if the medical condition is a chronic or acute health problem resulting in limited alertness, which adversely affects educational performance," then the student qualifies as "other health impaired."[23] Many advocates are applying this definition to those with AD(H)D.

Autism, on the other hand did not enter the list until 1990. Because the number of students prior to that date had been so few, no one had even considered the need for autism as a separate handicapping condition.

Prevalence

Once considered rare, autism is now epidemic. Prevalence studies prior to 1985 estimate four to five individuals per 10,000 were diagnosed with autism.[24] All studies agree that males are about three to four times more likely to be affected with autism spectrum disorders than females.

Today, according to a *U. S. News and World Report* article in June 2000,[25] one of every six children in America is either autistic, learning disabled or has an attention deficit. An estimated one in 166 children is autistic. That works out to one in 68 families having a child with autism, and an estimated 26,846 new diagnoses in the past year.

The Autism Society of America estimates that more than one-half million people in the U.S. today have autism or some form of pervasive developmental disorder, making autism one of the most common developmental disabilities.[26] According to a report released in April, 2000 by the Centers for Disease Control (CDC), it is more common than childhood cancer, diabetes and Down syndrome. The autism epidemic is not limited to the United States. In 1992, there was no Arabic word for "autism." In Kuwait, there are now over 3000 children diagnosed with autism, most of who were born during or after the Gulf War.[27]

Attention deficit disorders and the various types of learning disabilities have also increased, but not as dramatically as autism. According to estimates, as many as four million individuals with ADD and 10 million with learning disabilities attend our schools. ADD prevalence is approximately 3-7% of school-age children and 3% of adults.[28] According to the 2006 Annual Report of the National Center for Learning Disabilities:

- About 6% of K-12 students are formally identified as learning disabled
- Almost 3 million students with LD attend public schools
- About 15 million individuals with LD live in the United States[29]

It is possible that autism, ADD, LD and other ASD are over-diagnosed. Many suggest that the rise in numbers is due to a combination of increased awareness, better diagnostic skills and record keeping, as well as broader diagnostic categories. That is extremely unlikely. It is not possible that so many children with seriously handicapping conditions would go unnoticed for so long, that well-educated parents would remain silent for so long, and that professional awareness would suddenly increase dramatically, and all at the same time!

California Leads the Way

In 1998, Rick Rollens, father of Russell, was suspicious that his son was not the victim of a rare disorder, but rather one that had become quite common in children. Russell, a previously healthy boy, had became autistic following a series of DPT, Hib and MMR vaccinations. A former Secretary of the California Senate, co-founder of Families for Early Autism Treatment (FEAT) and the University of California (UC)-Davis Mental Illness and Neuroscience Discovery Institute (M.I.N.D.), Rollens persuaded the California legislature to fund an investigation and analyze the history of autism in the state.

In an April 1999 report,[30] the Department of Developmental Services (DDS) found a 273 percent increase between 1987 and 1998 in the numbers of new children entering the California developmental services system with a professional diagnosis of autism. The report concluded that "the number of persons with autism grew markedly faster than the number of persons with other developmental disabilities (cerebral palsy, epilepsy and mental retardation)" and "compared to characteristics of 11 years ago, the present population of persons with autism are younger (and) have a greater chance of exhibiting no or milder forms of mental retardation." The California legislature, recognizing that the increase in numbers was real, voted to appropriate one million dollars to the UC-Davis M.I.N.D. Institute to investigate possible environmental and biological factors including vaccine use.[31]

After the California report documented the dramatic increases in autism in the past decade, the California legislature voted to appropriate one million dollars to the UC-Davis M.I.N.D. Institute to look for possible environmental and biological factors, including vaccine use, that could have contributed to this autism increase. In January 2008 researchers from the California State Department of Public Health found that the autism rate in children continued to rise during the 12-year period from 1995 to 2007.[32]

Skeptics claim better diagnostic criteria. Some say that broader categories, including the concept of autism as a spectrum, account for the increase. Others cite increased awareness and better record-keeping. However, the 2001 M.I.N.D. Institute study proved that the increase in numbers was real.

Other States Follow

With the confirmed surge in autism in California, many other states, spurred on by concerned parents, began to check their statistics.

- The 1998 Maryland Special Education Census Data revealed that the state experienced a 513% increase in autism between 1993 and 1998, while the general Maryland population from 1990 to 1998 increased just seven percent.[33]
- According to a study conducted by the National Center on Birth Defects and Developmental Disabilities (NCBDDD), published in the January 1, 2003 edition of the *Journal of the American Medical Association (JAMA)*,[34] the prevalence of autism in metropolitan Atlanta is 3.4 per 1,000, approximately 10 times higher than the rates from studies conducted in the United States 10 years ago.

According to FightingAutism, an autism advocacy and research foundation, school year 2001-2002 figures show 98,589 students with autism, while school year 2002-2003 shows an 870% increase to 118,669 nationwide (50 states, DC and PR). This rate of increase is almost 50 times higher than the rate of increase of 28.4% for all disabilities. Numbers continue to increase. At the time of publication, an estimated 250,000 children ages three to 22 in the United States are diagnosed with autism.[35]

What Is the Etiology of Autism Spectrum Disorders?

The list of proposed causes of autism, PDD, LD and AD(H)D is extensive. Initially, the emphasis was on psychological factors such as the "refrigerator mother" theory (see Chapter 4),[36] which held tight for 25 years and was then discredited.[6] Next, attention and the bulk of research has focused on the neurology of these disorders. Those interested in this interpretation are referred to *The Neurobiology of Autism*,[37] *The Neurobiology of Reading and Dyslexia*,[38] *The Biology of the Autistic Syndromes*,[39] and *Driven to Distraction*.[40]

Viewing autism as simply a neurological "disease" is now losing favor and being replaced by an "environmental" hypothesis. Today's families are simply not content with being told that their children's brains have "faulty wiring" when they suspect something iatrogenic. Concurrent with the wave of new autism cases in the 1990s, scientists began looking at changing medical and environmental factors which could be contributors. Readers interested in learning more about these are referred to *Children with Starving Brains*,[41] *Healing the New Childhood Epidemics*,[42] and *Changing the Course of Autism*.[43]

The problem with the "neurological abnormalities" hypothesis is that neurological dysfunction is inferred from observing a child's behavior. Both the DSM-IV and schools base their diagnostic criteria on observed behaviors, which are biased by both the observer and the circumstances. No other factors are taken into account. This is akin to saying that all headaches are the same and require aspirin, whether they are caused by a nagging mother-in-law, a deadline at work, food poisoning or a brain tumor.

Where does this alleged neurological dysfunction come from? Just as it is wrong to assume that those with the same diagnosis have similar characteristics, it is improbable that the symptoms of all those with autism spectrum disorders emanate from a common source.

Nature? Scientists have historically focused on genetics as the primary source of autism spectrum disorders, describing "these affected children" as victims of some clearly defined medical syndrome. Yet, research has yielded only minimal evidence to support this premise. The gene for Rett syndrome was located in 1999 by Dr. Huda Zoghbi and her colleagues on one of the two X chromosomes that determine sex. Zoghbi noted that Rett syndrome results from the mutation of the gene that makes methyl cytosine binding protein, resulting in excessive amounts of this protein.[44] Then is not the cause excessive methyl cytosine, not the gene mutation?

Despite the lack of substantiation, the alleged genetic basis for other forms of autism, for learning disabilities and for attention problems has taken on the authority of proven fact.[45] For the past decade, this "fact" has inspired many government agencies and grass-roots non-profit organizations to invest millions of dollars in research searching for those elusive genes.

Several organizations have been committed to genetic research. Cure Autism Now (CAN) and the National Alliance for Autism Research (NAAR) awarded millions in grants in the past 10 years. In 2006, they merged with Autism Speaks, now the world's richest autism association. Autism Speaks spent $30 million, mostly on genetically related research, in 2007.[46] Unfortunately, many professionals and parents do not feel that Autism Speaks speaks for them.

The National Institutes of Health (NIH) support two major programs under the umbrella "Autism Research Network:" The Collaborative Programs of Excellence in Autism (CPEA) and Studies to Advance Autism Research and Treatment (STAART).[47] This network funded $93 million for autism research in 2003, and will spend an estimated $108 million (the same as in 2006 and 2007) in 2008.[48] Most of the research is genetic in nature.

Despite the prodigious efforts of these organizations, little headway has been made in understanding the causes of autism through the avenue of genetics. Sophisticated brain imaging techniques do show structural,[49] size[50] and activity level differences[51] between the brains of typical and autistic and learning disabled individuals, but not the etiology of their neurological differences. Furthermore, it is still impossible to identify any of these supposed neurological abnormalities through any form of medical examination or test.

Nurture? Families have changed from the traditional model with mom at home and Dad at the office. Rumors have spread that 80% of families having one or more children with autism divorce.[52] When a child has two parents, most likely both work. These parents may or may not be the same sex, race, culture or religion.

Parents are easy scapegoats, as few schools educate teens on how to raise children in this crazy new world. Many parents believe that they are doing their job by providing for their children's physical needs and following the advice of trusted medical professionals and professional educators. What are they to do if their pediatricians insist upon strict adherence to one size-fits-all vaccination schedules and teachers demand medications and "time out" for their children who cannot conform to an accelerated and sedentary curriculum?

Some parents blame teachers rather than their children. One expert recommended that the term "learning disabilities" be replaced by the term "teaching disabilities."[53] Another coined the word "dysteachia" to describe children exposed to inappropriate teaching. Thomas Armstrong, an outspoken critic of both the LD and the ADD diagnoses, wrote, "our schools are selling millions of kids short by putting them into remedial groups or writing them off as underachievers, when in reality they are disabled only by poor teaching methods."[54]

Almost a century ago, when Hinshelwood diagnosed the four brothers with learning disabilities, he rejected or ignored the roles that school, family and other environmental conditions may have played. As Coles points out in *The Learning Mystique*,[45] even then there were other very plausible explanations for the boys' reading difficulties.

Both? The classic "nature/nurture" question is at the heart of the matter in autism. Neither alone appears to be the cause. Most in the field believe that autism is extremely complex and a result of far more than genes, bad parenting or poor teaching.

In November, 2003 U.S. government officials unveiled a three-stage, seven-to-10 year plan to fight the epidemic of autism. The three-pronged proposal sets goals for more coordinated biomedical research, earlier screening and diagnosis and effective therapy. For the first time, collaboration among scientists, clinicians, educators and policymakers from an array of federal agencies will be a reality.[55] But what about today's kids, born since the early 1990s? This effort is too late to help them.

We are just beginning to understand the concept of genes being turned on or off. Autism, and probably learning disabilities and attention deficits, too, are the result of the complex interaction between heredity and environment. Genetics might "load the gun," while it is probably an environmental insult that "pulls the trigger."

In other words, individuals with autism spectrum disorders are increasingly thought to have a genetic propensity or pre-disposition that manifests itself only when triggered by the "right" combination of environmental factors. Moreover, the more "right" the genetic material combined with the more "right" environmental insults, the more severe the disability. Those on the lesser end of the spectrum with attention problems have fewer genetic variables combined with fewer environmental insults. Those on the autism end are unfortunate enough to have a larger number of the each factor.

Environmental? If autism runs in families who live in the same house, eat the same food, and breathe the same chemicals coming out of new cabinets and carpeting, shouldn't we be looking at what everyone is eating, drinking and breathing, as well? Surely these and other environmental factors play some role. Why do some get sick and have autism, learning disabilities and attention problems, and others do not?

At no point in history have there been such dramatic changes in the physical environment. The 20th century has brought with it genetically altered and preserved foods, polluted air, electro-magnetic fields, treated and tainted water and depleted soil. Rachel Carson shocked the world in her 1962 classic, *Silent Spring*.[56] This frightening expose about how pesticides, chemicals and other poisons have disrupted the bodies of all creatures on earth was a "wake-up call" to everyone. In 1997, in *Our Stolen Future*,[57] Theo Colburn confirmed that another generation later, things were getting worse, not better.

Chemical exposure can profoundly affect the development of both the unborn child by disrupting the thyroid gland and the entire endocrine system and the hormones it produces. Research shows that higher than normal levels of polychlorinated biphenyls (PCBs) in the mother's blood and breast milk directly correlate with children's deficits in intelligence, memory and attention.[58] PCBs have been banned for the past 20 years; however, they remain in the soil, water and air forever.

Polybrominated Diphenyl Ethers (PBDEs), the "sons" of PCBs, are flame retardants which have been used in polyurethane foam, plastics for computers and electronics, and car parts, as well as for stain-proofing textiles, since the 1970s. They look like PCBs chemically, behave like PCBs environmentally and have the same toxic effects as PCBs biologically. They are in dumps everywhere, persistently contaminating the food chain, making their way into human bodies where they act as endocrine disrupters.[59]

Research shows PBDEs in the bodies and breast milk of nursing mothers, where they are passed on to babies during critical stages of development. The results: impaired intelligence, motor skills, nervous systems and thyroid hormone balance: critical for proper brain development. North American women have the highest levels of these chemicals in their breast milk, with levels doubling in the US population every two to five years.[60] The United States lags behind Europe in reducing human exposure to these chemicals. The European Union banned two of the worst kind of PBDEs in 2002. Maine, California, New York, Massachusetts, Minnesota and Wisconsin are the only states that have passed bills banning different types PBDEs.[61]

If you have any question about the role of toxins in damaging the bodies, brains, and behavior of our children, read Doris Rapp's, *Our Toxic World*.[62] Exhaustively documented, this volume will shake up anyone questioning why we are in the midst of an autism epidemic.

Along with environmental problems came a new field of medicine: clinical ecology. This term was coined by Theron Randolph an allergist, who saw allergic-type reactions in his patients who were exposed to chemicals and certain foods. He is attributed to recommending food labeling.[63]

Clinical ecology has evolved into the integrative medicine of today. Most physician/parents of children with autism recognize environmental factors as key to their children's difficulties. Treatments to remove the toxins and the damage they have caused are discussed in Chapter 5.

None of the Above? For many years, some in the field, have presented the heretical idea that ADD and LD do not even exist. Over-diagnosis of ADD is so prevalent that one article proposed that the acronym stood for "**A**ny **D**ysfunction or **D**isorder."[64] Dr. Jan Strydom and Susan du Plessis in a "must-read," exhaustive *History of Learning Disabilities*[65] suggest that the idea of a learning disability is an invention of physicians and educators.

Thomas Armstrong, previously mentioned as questioning the ADD diagnosis, wrote that he quit his job as a learning disabilities specialist because he no longer believed in learning disabilities. "After teaching for several years in public and parochial special education classes in the United States and Canada, I realized I was going nowhere with a concept that labeled children from the outset as handicapped learners. I also began to see how this notion of learning disabilities was handicapping all of our children by placing the blame for a child's learning failure on mysterious neurological deficiencies in the brain..."[54]

Others agree that the behavioral symptoms of autism, learning disabilities and attention deficits are real, but question their cause. Szasz in *The Myth of Mental Illness*,[66] Coles in *The Learning Mystique*,[45] and Schrag and Divoky in *The Myth of the Hyperactive Child*,[67] all challenge the wisdom of blaming a child's brain.

More Disabilities, More Programs

No one anticipated the giant "market" that was to grow from the needs of those with autism. Suddenly, school systems required new curricula for students with ADD, LD, PDD, Asperger's and autism, training programs for teachers and funding for both. Lawyers discovered a new specialty, mental health professionals, speech language pathologists, occupational therapists, and optometrists, had a new and ready niche market in dire need of their expertise. The handicapped enterprise "soon became an enormous machine — indeed a factory — with attending cottage industries, fueled by legal, socio-political, educational and entrepreneurial energy."[45 (page 4)]

Neither the medical nor educational establishment was prepared for the enormous costs associated with diagnosing and servicing those with autism spectrum disorders. The government's new 10-year plan has no price tags.[55] The motor, sensory-motor, language, social-emotional and academic deficits inherent in these children's diagnoses were destined to bankrupt even the flushest insurance companies and suburban school systems. The tab for mandated services has become a "hot potato" that continues to be tossed back and forth. The real losers are neither the companies nor the school districts, but the millions of children whose educational and medical needs are not being met.

How are Autism Spectrum Disorders Treated?

Because autism spectrum disorders are defined both medically and educationally, their primary care occurs in both the health-care and educational arenas. These two environments provide optometrists with considerable opportunities to work as members of multidisciplinary teams to evaluate and treat each child. Optometrists working with children on the autism spectrum need to be aware of the enormous variety of treatment options, as parents searching for appropriate alternatives may question them.

In the 21st century, tried and true interventions of the past continue to take precedence over some exciting, innovative new techniques and methods which are showing some efficacy. The government's research plan includes objectives such as developing teaching methods that can allow 90% of autistic children to speak and finding effective drugs for the symptoms of autism.[68] "Treatment" in the eyes of researchers almost always focuses on pathology in the child, not the environment. The possibility that problems relating to the home, school or other social conditions are affecting the child is generally ignored. We just test and treat the child, not his/her environment.

The multi-disciplinary approach usually recommended by physicians, mental health professionals and educators consists of pharmaceutical intervention, special education, counseling, and applied behavior management. These approaches focus on the assumed neurological and observed behavioral, language, psychological, and academic deficits, not their possible causes.

The ultimate goal of treatment is to eliminate undesirable behaviors such as hyperactivity, attentional difficulties, anxiety, depression, mood swings, agitation, aggression, self-injurious behavior, insomnia, perseveration and impulsivity, while increasing desirable outcomes such as relatedness, eye contact, self-control, attention span and confidence. Although the traditional treatments certainly have palliative affects, they fail to address underlying physiological issues. In addition they are frequently accompanied by undesirable side effects.

Medications According to C.T. Gordon, one of the leading psychiatrists in treating autism pharmacologically, and the father of a son with autism, "The ultimate goal of medication in an individual who has autism is to prepare the brain's physiology to take optimal advantage of other aspects of treatment. In other words, pharmacologic intervention should typically be viewed as only one part of a multi-modal treatment plan for an individual with autism. The goal of medication, as well as all other treatments in autism, is to maximize the individual's functioning."[68]

Gordon suggests that medications be prescribed one at a time so that effectiveness and side effects can be accurately determined. "There are certainly times when a patient benefits from a combination of medications, but excessive poly-pharmacy should be avoided to minimize side effects and prevent drug interactions."[68] Unfortunately, clinicians often use several drugs together to balance out one another's side effects. For instance, Anafranil can cause insomnia, so Clonodine may be added to induce sleep.

Since they were introduced 60 years ago, medications for behavioral and learning problems have become more specialized and powerful. At the present time, five classes of drugs are being prescribed for children on the autistic spectrum of disorders (See Table 1-3).

Table 1-3			
Common Medications Used with Children on the Autistic Spectrum			
CLASS	**DRUGS**	**BENEFIT**	**SIDE EFFECTS**
Anti-psychotics or Neuroleptics	Haldol Mellarill Stelazine Thorazine	Reduce agitation, anxiety, aggression, hyperactivity, stereotypic and self-stimulatory behaviors, and temper outbursts	Addiction **Blurred vision** Dyskinesia Psychosis Sedation, Tremors
Typical Neuroleptics	Abilify Clozaril Geodon Risperdal Seroquel Zyprexa	Reduce aggression, agitation, self-injurious behavior	Agitation Increased appetite Lowers white blood cell count Tardive dyskinesia
Anti-depressants	Anafranil Celexa Elavil Lexapro Luvox Paxll, Prozac Tofranil Wellbutrin Zoloft	Raise serotonin levels Reduce anxiety Reduce obsessive-compulsive & ritualistic behaviors	Arhythmias **Blurred vision** Constipation Dry mouth Dizziness Hyperactivity & Impulsivity Lowered threshold for seizures Sleep disturbances
Anti-anxiety agents	Ativan Buspar Klonapin Valium Xanax	Reduce anxiety	**Abnormal eye movements** Crying Disinhibition Irritability
Stimulants	Adderol Cylert Daytrona patch Dexedrine Focalin Ritalin	Affect dopamine Improve focus and regulation Monitor arousal system Decrease impulsivity	Depression Increase in perseveration & repetitive behaviors Irritabililty Palpitations Sleep disturbance
Anti-hypertensives	Clonodine Tenex	Calm and improve sleep Decrease hyperactivity & impulsivity	Irritability Lower blood pressure Sedation
Anti-convulsants/ Mood stabilizers	Depakote, Dilantin Keppra Phenobarbitol Tegretol Trileptal	Calm behavior Lessen mood swings, outbursts	Affects kidney function **Vision impairments such as rapid eye movements**
Norepinephrine re-uptake inhibitor	Strattera	Reduces inattention, hyperactivity & impulsivity	Possibly bipolar disorder

Adapted from Medication Fact Sheets, 2003-2004 edition
Dean Konopasek, Sopris West. Frederick, CO. www.cambiumlearning.com

The research on medications for patients with autism is sketchy at best. Because until the mid-seventies some considered autism to be a childhood form of schizophrenia, it was natural to try anti-psychotic drugs. Also called neuroleptics, because of their sedating effect, these medications have the largest body of studies. Although effective in their reduction of negative behaviors, their side effects are potentially irreversible. Tardive dyskinesis, a Parkinsonian-like tremor disorder, was the trade-off for symptom reduction in many patients in our mental hospitals of old.

The newer neuroleptics replaced the anti-psychotics in the nineties, although some of the original drugs are still prescribed. Like the anti-psychotics they reduce undesirable behaviors, but with drastically reduced neurological side effects. The potential for tardive dyskinesia is as yet unclear, since risperidone has not been on the market long enough for it to be fully assessed. The most studied neuroleptic is Risperdal. A large-scale study, funded by the NIMH, found the drug to be useful in symptom reduction.[69] Gordon reports that there are, to date, no published studies on individuals with autism for any of the other atypical neuroleptics.

The anti-depressants with the most research in autism are Anafranil, Luvox and Prozac. With these medications, symptom reduction is significant, but is accompanied by a long list of side effects. Are sleep disturbances, constipation, seizures and potentially fatal heart problems acceptable trade-offs for increased attention and decreased aggression? The most disturbing research is about Paxil. First banned in the United Kingdom because of increased suicides in children, it has also been recently disallowed for children in the United States.[70]

Anti-anxiety agents have been studied little with patients diagnosed with autism. Stimulants have long been used for those with the attention deficits on the less severe end of the spectrum, but have not been studied much in individuals with autism. Yet their use is widespread across the spectrum. Strattera, the new miracle drug, has few studies behind it, as well.

Minor to severe health-related side effects are inevitable with almost all drugs. In this arena, Ritalin helps attention, but could possibly set off a tic disorder, such as Tourette's syndrome, in vulnerable children.[71] It is important to be aware that, in addition to the undesirable problems with these drugs listed above, their patients may also have subtle to serious visual side effects. By taking an extensive health history, including a patient's use of medications, and by becoming familiar with the side effects of individual drugs used in autism by reading the Physicians Desk Reference (PDR), professionals will recognize that it is possible that problems such as lack of focus or abnormal eye movements could be drug-related.

Since 1967, the Autism Research Institute has been collecting parent ratings of the behavioral effects of over 40 drugs on individuals with autism. These statistics representing responses from over 25,000 children, are presented in Table 1-4.

With the majority of drugs, parents reported improved behavior less than 50% of the time. And at what cost?

Special Education, Counseling and Behavior Management Traditional treatment plans generally include special education services and psychological counseling or behavioral management in addition to medication. Unquestionably, children with autism spectrum disorders require specialized teaching and their parents need psychological support to address the social and emotional issues of raising a child with special needs.

While medications, special education and counseling can clearly help, these treatments mask behavioral symptoms of autism rather than address possible underlying causes. In addition, all of these supports have other drawbacks. Their benefits are short term at best. At worst, benefits may not outweigh side effects. While applied behavior management and special education provide external methods of monitoring and handling behavior, children may not learn from experience how to develop internal controls. Also of great concern is the aforementioned huge financial burden placed on both the health-care and the educational systems, which were not designed to manage so many children.

PARENT RATINGS OF BEHAVIORAL EFFECTS OF BIOMEDICAL INTERVENTIONS
Autism Research Institute ● 4182 Adams Avenue ● San Diego, CA 92116

The parents of autistic children represent a vast and important reservoir of information on the benefits—and adverse effects—of the large variety of drugs and other interventions that have been tried with their children. Since 1967 the Autism Research Institute has been collecting parent ratings of the usefulness of the many interventions tried on their autistic children.

The following data have been collected from the more than 26,000 parents who have completed our questionnaires designed to collect such information. For the purposes of the present table, the parents responses on a six-point scale have been combined into three categories: "made worse" (ratings 1 and 2), "no effect" (ratings 3 and 4), and "made better" (ratings 5 and 6). The "Better:Worse" column gives the number of children who "Got Better" for each one who "Got Worse."

DRUGS	Got Worse[A]	No Effect	Got Better	Better: Worse	No. of Cases[B]
Aderall	43%	25%	32%	0.8:1	775
Amphetamine	47%	28%	25%	0.5:1	1312
Anafranil	32%	38%	30%	0.9:1	422
Antibiotics	33%	53%	15%	0.5:1	2163
Antifungals[C]					
Diflucan	5%	38%	57%	11:1	653
Nystatin	5%	44%	50%	9.7:1	1388
Atarax	26%	53%	22%	0.9:1	517
Benadryl	24%	50%	26%	1.1:1	3032
Beta Blocker	17%	51%	31%	1.8:1	286
Buspar	27%	45%	28%	1.0:1	400
Chloral Hydrate	41%	39%	20%	0.5:1	459
Clonidine	22%	31%	47%	2.1:1	1525
Clozapine	37%	44%	19%	0.5:1	155
Cogentin	19%	54%	27%	1.4:1	186
Cylert	45%	36%	20%	0.4:1	623
Deanol	15%	57%	28%	1.9:1	210
Depakene[D]					
Behavior	25%	43%	32%	1.3:1	1071
Seizures	11%	33%	56%	4.8:1	705
Desipramine	34%	35%	31%	0.9:1	86

DRUGS	Got Worse[A]	No Effect	Got Better	Better: Worse	No. of Cases[B]
Dilantin[D]					
Behavior	28%	49%	23%	0.8:1	1110
Seizures	15%	37%	48%	3.3:1	433
Felbatol	20%	55%	25%	1.3:1	56
Fenfluramine	21%	52%	27%	1.3:1	477
Haldol	38%	28%	34%	0.9:1	1199
IVIG	10%	44%	46%	4.5:1	79
Klonapin[D]					
Behavior	28%	42%	30%	1.0:1	246
Seizures	25%	60%	15%	0.6:1	67
Lithium	24%	45%	31%	1.3:1	463
Luvox	30%	37%	34%	1.1:1	220
Mellaril	29%	38%	33%	1.2:1	2097
Mysoline[D]					
Behavior	41%	46%	13%	0.3:1	149
Seizures	19%	56%	25%	1.3:1	78
Naltrexone	20%	46%	34%	1.8:1	302
Paxil	33%	31%	36%	1.1:1	416
Phenergan	29%	46%	25%	0.9:1	301
Phenobarb.[D]					
Behavior	47%	37%	16%	0.3:1	1109
Seizures	18%	43%	39%	2.2:1	520

DRUGS	Got Worse[A]	No Effect	Got Better	Better: Worse	No. of Cases[B]
Prolixin	30%	41%	29%	1.1:1	105
Prozac	32%	32%	36%	1.1:1	1312
Risperdal	20%	26%	54%	2.8:1	1038
Ritalin	45%	26%	29%	0.7:1	4127
Secretin					
Intravenous	7%	49%	44%	6.3:1	468
Transderm.	10%	53%	37%	3.6:1	196
Stelazine	28%	45%	26%	0.9:1	434
Steroids	35%	33%	32%	0.9:1	132
Tegretol[D]					
Behavior	25%	45%	30%	1.2:1	1520
Seizures	13%	33%	54%	4.0:1	842
Thorazine	36%	40%	24%	0.7:1	940
Tofranil	30%	38%	32%	1.1:1	776
Valium	35%	41%	24%	0.7:1	865
Valtrex	6%	42%	52%	8.5:1	65
Zarontin[D]					
Behavior	35%	46%	19%	0.6:1	153
Seizures	19%	55%	25%	1.3:1	110
Zoloft	35%	33%	32%	0.9:1	500

BIOMEDICAL/ NON-DRUG/ SUPPLEMENTS	Got Worse[A]	No Effect	Got Better	Better: Worse	No. of Cases[B]
Calcium[E]	3%	62%	35%	14:1	2097
Cod Liver Oil	4%	45%	51%	13:1	1681
Cod Liver Oil with Bethanecol	10%	54%	37%	3.8:1	126
Colostrum	6%	56%	38%	6.1:1	597
Detox. (Chelation)[C]	3%	23%	74%	24:1	803
Digestive Enzymes	3%	39%	58%	17:1	1502
DMG	8%	51%	42%	5.4:1	5807
Fatty Acids	2%	41%	56%	24:1	1169
5 HTP	13%	47%	40%	3.1:1	343
Folic Acid	4%	53%	43%	11:1	1955
Food Allergy Trtmnt	3%	33%	64%	24:1	952
Hyperbaric Oxygen Therapy	5%	34%	60%	12:1	134
Magnesium	6%	65%	29%	4.6:1	301
Melatonin	8%	27%	65%	7.8:1	1105
Methyl B12 (nasal)	15%	29%	56%	3.9:1	48
Methyl B12 (subcut.)	7%	26%	67%	9.5:1	170
MT Promoter	13%	49%	38%	2.9:1	61
P5P (Vit. B6)	12%	37%	51%	4.2:1	529
Pepcid	12%	59%	30%	2.6:1	164
SAMe	16%	63%	21%	1.3:1	142
St. Johns Wort	18%	66%	16%	0.9:1	150
TMG	15%	43%	42%	2.8:1	803

BIOMEDICAL/ NON-DRUG/ SUPPLEMENTS	Got Worse[A]	No Effect	Got Better	Better: Worse	No. of Cases[B]
Transfer Factor	10%	48%	42%	4.3:1	174
Vitamin A	2%	57%	41%	18:1	1127
Vitamin B3	4%	52%	43%	10:1	927
Vit. B6/Mag.	4%	48%	48%	11:1	6634
Vitamin B12 (oral)	7%	32%	61%	8.6:1	98
Vitamin C	2%	55%	43%	19:1	2397
Zinc	2%	47%	51%	22:1	1989
SPECIAL DIETS					
Candida Diet	3%	41%	56%	19:1	941
Feingold Diet	2%	42%	56%	25:1	899
Gluten- /Casein-Free Diet	3%	31%	66%	19:1	2561
Removed Chocolate	2%	47%	51%	28:1	2021
Removed Eggs	2%	56%	41%	17:1	1386
Removed Milk Products/Dairy	2%	46%	52%	32:1	6360
Removed Sugar	2%	48%	50%	25:1	4187
Removed Wheat	2%	47%	51%	28:1	3774
Rotation Diet	2%	46%	51%	21:1	938
Specific Carbo-hydrate Diet	7%	24%	69%	10:1	278

A. "Worse" refers only to worse behavior. Drugs, but not nutrients, typically also cause physical problems if used long-term.
B. No. of cases is cumulative over several decades, so does not reflect current usage levels (e.g., Haldol is now seldom used).
C. Antifungal drugs and chelation are used selectively, where evidence indicates they are needed.
D. Seizure drugs: top line behavior effects, bottom line effects on seizures.
E. Calcium effects are not due to dairy-free diet; statistics are similar for milk drinkers and non-milk drinkers.

Table 1-4 "Parent Ratings of Behavioral Effects of Drugs and Nutrients"
Autism Research Institute Survey (Reprinted with permission)

Biomedical Interventions Contributing environmental factors are now receiving a great deal of attention. Many researchers are investigating the causes of "emerging symptoms" of autism:

- Gastro-intestinal abnormalities, such as reflux, diarrhea, constipation and abdominal pain[72,73]
- Altered metabolic processes, such as the impaired ability to metabolize toxic chemicals[74,75]
- Immune system abnormalities, such as multiple ear, strep and yeast infections and allergies to common foods,[76,77] and the most emotionally-charged possibility
- Vaccines and thimerosal, the mercury-containing preservative in some of them[73]

Studies are continuing to focus on what environmental factors are major contributors. Possible sources of toxic metal exposure include seafood, the individual vaccines themselves (the flu shot and Hepatitus B vaccine),[78] dental amalgams,[79] rhogam (mercury),[80] flame retardants (antimony), cookware and cans (aluminum)[81] and pesticides.[82]

Conclusion

Autism, attention deficits, learning disabilities and a number of other psychiatric disabilities are now being considered as components of a spectrum of disorders called the autism spectrum (ASD). While basically ignored since its discovery in the beginning of the twentieth century, autism is considered the epidemic of the 1990s with prevalence in as many as one in 68 families. The alarming rise in numbers has resulted in increased interest in research funding, educational programs and new treatment options.

A movement of health care professionals and parents are looking beyond traditional medical and educational management to reverse regression in children who were seemingly normal and then became autistic. Within the context of an historical prospective, the optometrist working with children on the autistic spectrum has a professional obligation to learn about autism basics and become conversant about new diagnostic and treatment options. He/she must learn how to recognize when biomedical issues can interfere with vision and develop a network of appropriate referral sources for their patients. Conversely, those working with biomedical issues must learn to recognize visual issues in their patients diagnosed with any of the spectrum disorders.

Subsequent chapters in this book expand upon each new area of concern, its relationship to vision and efficacious treatment options that complement vision therapy by ameliorating underlying problems. The reader is encouraged to explore each patient's unique case history to determine an appropriate treatment plan.

References

1. Wing L. *The Autistic Spectrum – A Guide for Parents and Professionals. Philadelphia PA: Trans-Atlantic Publications, 1996.*

2. Frith U. *Autism and Asperger Syndrome. Cambridge Univ. Press, 1991:111.*

3. Bleuler E. *Autistic Thinking. Am J Insanity 1913; 69:873-886.*

4. *http://info.med.yale.edu/chldstdy/autism/cdd.html (Accessed 1/2/08)*

5. Marohn S. *The Natural Medicine Guide to Autism. Charlottesville, VA:Hampton Roads Publishing, 2002, 15.*

6. Rimland B. *Infantile Autism, Upper Saddle River, NJ: Prentice-Hall, 1964:43.*

7. Pangborn J, Baker S. *Autism: Effective Biomedical Treatments. (Have we done everything we can for this child?) Individuality in an Epidemic. San Diego, CA: Autism Research Institute (ARI), September, 2005.*

8. *http://add.about.com (Accessed June 23, 2004)*

9. Opp G. *Historical roots of the field of learning disabilities. J Learn Disabil January 1994:10.*

10. Hinshelwood J. *Four cases of congenital word-blindness occurring in the same family. British Med J 1907;2:1229-32.*

11. Kirk SA. *Behavioral diagnosis and remediation of learning disabilities. In Proceedings of the Conference on the Exploration into the Problems of the Perceptually Handicapped Child. Evanston, IL: Fund for the Perceptually Handicapped Child, 1963.*

12. Getman GN. *The visuomotor cortex in acquisition of learning skills. In: Hellmuth J, ed. Learning Disorders, vol 1. Seattle, WA: Special Child Publications, 1965.*

13. American Psychiatric Association. *Diagnostic and Statistical Manual of Mental Disorders, Fourth Edition (DSM-IV) Washington, DC: American Psychiatric Association, 2000.*

14. Asperger H. *Die "autistischen Psychopathen" im Kindesalter. Berlin:Archiv für Psychiatrie und Nervenkrankheiten, 1944;117:76-136.*

15. Morgan J. *John Schneider promotes Asperger's Syndrome awareness. USA Today 2003 Apr. 15.*

16. Curtin M. *Personal communication, June 22, 2004.*

17. Grandin T. *Emergence: Labeled Autistic. New York: Warner Books, 1996.*

18. Williams D. *Nobody Nowhere: The Extraordinary Autobiography of an Autistic. New York: Harper Collins, 1992*

19. Edelson S. *Rett Syndrome. http://www.autism.org/rett.html (Accessed 1/2/08)*

20. *34 Code of Federal Regulations §300.7(c) (10), 1969.*

21. *Individuals with Disabilities Education Act (IDEA). 20 U.S.C. § 1401 (3) (26) §300, 1997.*

22. *Americans with Disabilities Act. (ADA) 42 U.S.C. §§12101-12213,, 1990.*

23. *http://www.wrightslaw.com/law/code_regs/OSEP_Memorandum_ADD_1991.html Accessed 1/02/08)*

24. Wing L. *The definition and prevalence of autism: a review. Eur Child Adolescent Psychiatry 1993;2:61-74.*

25. Kaplan S, Morris J. *Kids at Risk. U. S. News and World Report 2000 June 19;128:47-53.*

26. *www.autism-society.org . (Accessed January 2, 2008)*

27. *www.q8autism.com (Accessed January 2, 2008)*

28. *http://newideas.net/adhd/about_attention_deficit/prevalence_of_adhd. Accessed January 3, 2008.*

29. *www.ncld.org 2006 Annual Report. (Accessed January 3, 2008)*

30. *Changes in the population of persons with autism and pervasive developmental disorders in California's developmental services system: 1987-1998. A report to the legislature. California Health and Human Services. Dept. of Developmental Services, April, 1999.*

31. Schafer L. *Autism and vaccines: A new look at an old story. January 15, 2001. FEAT Daily newsletter. www.vaccinationnews.com (Accessed January 3, 2008)*

32. Schechter R, Grether JK. *Continuing increases in autism reported to California developmental services system. Arch Gen Psychiatry 2008 Jan;65:19-24.*

33. Blaxill M, Baskin D, Spitzer W. *The changing prevalence of autism in California. J Autism Dev Dis 2003; 33:223-26.*

34. Yeargin-Allsopp M, Rice C, Karapurkar T, Doernberg V. et al. *Prevalence of autism in a US metropolitan area. JAMA 2003;289:49-55.*

35. *www.fightingautism.org (Accessed January 3, 2008)*

36. Bettelheim B. *The Empty Fortress – Infantile Autism and the Birth of the Self. New York, NY: The Free Press, 1967.*

37. Bauman ML, Kemper TL. *The Neurobiology of Autism. Baltimore: Johns Hopkins University Press, 1994.*

38. Shaywitz SE, Shaywitz BE. *The Neurobiology of Reading and Dyslexia. Focus on Basics 2001:5A.*

39. Gillberg C. Coleman M. *The Biology of the Autistic Syndromes, 3rd ed. London: MacKeith Press, 2000.*

40. Hallowell E. *Driven to Distraction: Recognizing and Coping with Attention Deficit Disorder from Childhood through Adulthood. New York, NY: Touchstone Press, 1995.*

41. McCandless J. *Children with Starving Brains: A Medical treatment Guide for Autism Spectrum Disorder. Revised edition. Putney, VT: Bramble Books, 2007.*

42. Bock, K. *Healing the New Childhood Epidemics: Autism, ADHD, Asthma, Allergies. New York, NY: Ballantine Books, 2007.*

43. Jepson B. *Changing the Course of Autism: A scientific approach for parents and physicians. Boulder, CO: Sentient Publications, 2007.*

44. *http://www.autism.com/autism/behavior/rett.htm (Accessed January 3, 2008)*

45. Coles G. *The Learning Mystique. New York, NY: Random House, 1989, xii.*

46. *www.autismspeaks.org (Accessed January 3, 2008)*

47. *http://www.autismresearchnetwork.org/AN/default.aspx (Accessed January 3, 2008)*

48. *http://www.nih.gov/news/fundingresearchareas.htm (Accessed January 3, 2008)*

49. Casanova MF,. Buxhoeveden DP,. Switala AE, Roy E. Mincolumnar pathology in autism. Neurology 2002; 58:428-32.

50. Piven J. Bailey J. Ranson BJ, Arndt S. An MRI study of the corpus callosum in autism. Am J Psychiatry 1997;154:1051-56.

51. Eden GF, Van Meter JW, Ramsey J, et al. Abnormal processing of artistic talent in dyslexia revealed by functional brain imaging. Nature 1996: 82:66-69.

52. www.nationalautismassociation.org. Press release. (Accessed January 16, 2008)

53. Bateman B. Educational implications of minimal brain dysfunction. Reading Teacher. 1974;27:662-68.

54. Armstrong T. In their Own Way: Discovering and Encouraging Your Child's Personal Learning Style. New York, NY: Jeremy P. Tarcher/Putnam (Penguin-Putnam), 2000:40.

55. Fox M. US Government Teams with Advocates Against Autism. New York Times, 11/19/03.

56. Carson R. Silent Spring. Boston, MA: Houghton Mifflin Co., 1962.

57. Colburn T, Dumanoski, D, Myers JP. Our Stolen Future. New York: Penguin Books, 1997.

58. Jacobson J, Jacobson SW. Intellectual impairment in children exposed to polychlorinated biphenyls in utero. N E J Med 1996 Sept;335:11.

59. Vos JG, Becher G. Van den Berg M, de Boer J., et. al Brominated flame retardants and endocrine disruption. Pure Appl Chem 2003;75:2039-46.

60. WHO. Levels of PCBs, PCDDs and PCDEs in breast milk: Results of WHO-coordinated interlaboratory quality control studies and analytical field studies. Yrjanheikki EJ, ed. Environmental Health Series Report 34. Copenhagen:WHO Regional Office for Europe, 1989.

61. www.computertakeback.com (Accessed January 16, 2008)

62. Rapp D. Our Toxic World. Buffalo, NY: Environmental Medical Research Foundation, 2003.

63. Randolph TG, Moss RW. An Alternative Approach to Allergies: The New Field of Clinical Ecology Unravels the Environmental Causes of Mental and Physical Ills. New York, NY, Harper and Row, 1979.

64. Goodman G, Poillion MJ. ADD: Acronym for any dysfunction or difficulty. J Special Ed 1992 Spring;26(1):37-56

65. http://audiblox2000.com/book2.htm (Accessed June 24, 2004)

66. Szasz T. The Myth of Mental Illness: Foundations of a Theory of Personal Conduct. New York: Harper and Row, 1974.

67. Schrag P, Divoky D. The Myth of the Hyperactive Child and Other Means of Child Control. New York,NY: Penguin Books, 1975.

68. Gordon CT. Pharmacological treatment options for autism: Part 1. J Natl Alliance Autism Res 2003 Spring;8.

69. McCracken JT, McGough J, Shah,B, Cronin P.et al. Risperidone in children with autism and serious behavioral problems. N E J Med 2002 Aug;347:314-21.

70. FDA: Teens, children shouldn't use Paxil. Reuters News Service 2003 June 19, 1:38PM

71. Gadow KD, Sverd J, Sprafkin J, Nolan EE, Grossman S. Long-term methylphenidate therapy in children with comorbid attention-deficit hyperactivity disorder and chronic multiple tic disorder. Arch Gen Psychiatry 1999 Apr;56:330-36.

72. Horvath K. Papadimitriou J. Rabsztyn A, et al. Gastro-intestinal abnormalities in children with autism disorder. J Pediatrics 1999;135:559-63,.

73. Wakefield A. Murch S. Anthony A, et al. Ileal-lymphoid-nodular hyperplasia, non-specific colitis, and pervasive developmental disorder in children. Lancet 1998;351:637-41.

74. Alberti A. Pirrone, P. Elia M. et al. Sulphation deficit in low functioning autistic children: a pilot study. Biological Psychiatry 1999;46:420-24.

75. Deth R, Waly M. Effects of mercury on methionine synthase: Implications for disordered methylation in autism. Fall Defeat Autism Now! 2003 Conference, Portland, Oregon, October 3-5, 2003.

76. Singh V. Fudenberg H, Emerson D, Coleman M. Immunodiagnosis and immunotherapy in autistic children. Annals New York Academy of Science 1988;540:602-04.

77. Gupta S. Immunological treatments for autism. J Autism Dev Dis 2000;30:475-79.

78. Geier MR, Geier DA. Neurodevelopmental disorders after thimerosal-containing vaccines: A brief communication. Silver Spring, MD: The Genetic Centers of America, 2002.

79. Adams JB, Holloway CE, Margolis M, George F. Heavy metal exposures, developmental milestones and physical symptoms in children with autism. Spring Defeat Autism Now! 2004 Conference, April 16, 2004.

80. Holmes AS, Blaxill MF, Haley BE. Reduced levels of mercury in first baby haircuts of autistic children. International Journal Toxicology 2003;22:4.

81. Tennakone K. Wickramanayake S. Aluminum leaching form cooking utensils. Nature 1987;325:270-72.

82. Weiss B. Pesticides as a source of developmental disabilities. Mental Retard Dev Dis Res Rev 1997; 3:246-56.

Chapter 2
Optometry's Role in
Autism Spectrum Disorders
Randy Schulman, MS, OD, FCOVD

As recently as 10 years ago optometrists saw only a few patients a year with autism spectrum diagnoses; today these individuals are far more common. New books on autism, the press, television news and other media coverage advise readers about vision therapy, listing both the College of Optometrists in Vision Development (COVD) and the Optometric Extension Program (OEP) as resources. Parents network extensively via support groups, conferences and the Internet, informing each other of optometrists who have helped their children.

Many of the behavioral characteristics of those falling within the autism spectrum involve the visual system. Poor eye contact, staring at lights or spinning objects, side viewing, and general difficulties attending are often symptoms of visual dysfunction. Thus, any individual with a diagnosis of autism, PDD, learning disability, speech-language delay, sensory integration dysfunction, Asperger's syndrome, non-verbal learning disability or psychological problems should undergo a thorough examination by a developmental optometrist.

Individuals on the autism spectrum are extremely diverse, given the range of severity of their symptoms. They present a multitude combination of delays and idiosyncratic behaviors involving their motor systems, sensory processing, audition, language and socialization. Because each individual is unique, it is impossible to offer a description that applies to everyone. However, when the optometrist notes, respects and understand the similarities and differences among individuals on this spectrum, she can successfully design an evaluation and treatment program for her patients.

The earlier children with autism undergo a visual examination and begin visual intervention, the faster the improvement and the longer lasting the gains and overall chances for success. The American Optometric Association (AOA) recommends that all children undergo visual exams by six months of age. If parents complied with this guideline, optometrists would certainly note many visual aberrations in these young, yet undiagnosed children.

For those with autism spectrum diagnoses, an immediate developmental exam is essential. A vision examination can be the first step in preventing compensatory behaviors such as turning or tilting the head, gaze avoidance and side looking, as well as in improving visual function and overall development. For example a child who has difficulty making eye contact may end up with long lasting difficulties in interpersonal relationships not only because of speech and language difficulties but also because of poor eye contact.

A Review of the Literature on Vision and Autism
Not surprisingly, scant research on the presence of visual dysfunction in children with autism exists. More is available on those with less severe diagnoses, such as learning disabilities and attention deficits.

John Streff was one of the first to write about optometric care for a child with autism in the *Journal of the AOA* in 1975.[1] He described a case history of an almost five-year-old boy who he had evaluated at the Gesell Institute. First, Streff used 15 diopters base-up and base-down prism lenses as a home program with excellent success. He then added base-left and base-right along with bi-nasal occluders. Finally, he added +1.50 sphere without occlusion to be used alternately with his previous prescription. He noted significant gains in language understanding and output, as well as socialization.

Due to lack of interest in autism over the next 20 years, the next research paper published on vision and autism was in the early 1990s. In 1992, Janice Scharre, OD, MA, and Margaret Creedon, PhD, FAClinP, assessed 34 individuals with autism, aged 2 to 11 years for ocular alignment, refractive error, visual acuity, oculomotor skills and stereopsis.[2] They found a 21% rate of strabismus using the cover test at far and 18% at near. Although all of the subjects exhibited appropriate saccadic eye movements while moving their eyes from one place in space to another, 31 of the 34 had atypical optokinetic nystagmus and only five demonstrated voluntary pursuit movements. Most of the subjects revealed an intermittent exotropia. Independent research in private practice by this author found similar results.

A study of 266 patients at the Ratner Eye Center, University of California, San Diego, by David B. Granet, MD, Director, and Maria Lymberis, MD, clinical professor of psychiatry, University of California at Los Angeles, showed that children with convergence insufficiency are three times as likely to be diagnosed with AD(H)D as children without the disorder.[4] An article in the New York Times, "Not Autistic or Hyperactive: Just Seeing Double at Times," reported that convergence insufficiency can easily be missed or mis-diagnosed.[5]

Researchers at Harvard University and Beth Israel Hospital in Boston reported that, for those with dyslexia, information in the transient and sustained pathways arrive at the visual centers of the brain out of sequence.[6] As a result, printed words seem to move chaotically and may appear reversed. Transient vision deficits appear to impact most upon reading skills. For those interested in an in-depth discussion of and research documenting the role of vision in learning disabilities and dyslexia, read "Clinical Practice Guidelines: Care of the Patient with Learning Related Vision Problems."[7]

Merrill Bowan, OD, wrote a review of the literature on learning disabilities and vision, which was published in the September, 2002 issue of *Optometry*, the Journal of the AOA.[8] This document includes over 300 references affirming a positive relationship between learning problems and the following: poor saccadic skills, convergence insufficiency, faulty binocular vision, hyperopia, amblyopia, poor visual processing, weak visual motor skills, and suppression. Bowan contends that much of the literature suggests that a significant portion of individuals with learning disabilities and dyslexia have low-threshold problems that ophthalmologists would ordinarily consider as sub-clinical. In addition, his literature review supports benefit for patients diagnosed with dyslexia and other learning problems with prisms and spectacle lenses, filters and other vision therapy techniques for the following co-existing problems: accommodative disorders, amblyopia, convergence insufficiency and intermittent exotropia.

Motor, Sensory, Language and Cognitive Development

Children with autism spectrum disorders (ASD) have motor, sensory, language and social-emotional delays that affect visual processing. Likewise visual problems affect cognitive, speech-language, social-emotional and perceptual development. Whichever delay is primary, it is essential that optometrists understand development in each of these areas and the relationships between each of these systems and vision.

Motor Developmental histories of those on the autism spectrum often reveal delayed or skipped motor milestones, as well as red flags such as an unusual or absent crawl, very early or late walking, or difficulty navigating stairs and/or playground equipment. All can negatively affect binocular development and function. Children with autism often have delays in both gross and fine motor abilities. They may exhibit poor upper body, torso or hand strength, as well as generalized low tone. The optometrist can informally observe these problems by looking at gait, posture and hand use, as well as whether the mouth is open or shut while at rest. These children may lack a well-developed pincer grasp or the ability to hold and drink from a cup. They may not be able to use utensils at even four years of age. Toilet training is often a very significant issue with bladder and bowel control not developed by even elementary school age.

Billye Ann Cheatum, PhD, an adaptive physical education teacher who spent her career working with children on the autism spectrum, describes the movement patterns in autistic children as either excessive or repetitive, but rarely, just right.[9] She believes they use movement as a calming technique, stimulating their tactile and proprioceptive systems at the same time.

Sensory In addition to significant motor delays, children on the spectrum are functioning at a very low sensory level, often preferring less typically used senses of taste and smell to gain information. They smell or taste inedible objects, and use touch instead of vision to give meaning to what they see. Vision develops according to a hierarchy, and vision development will be delayed by immature oral and motor development.

These young children may be hypo- or hyper-sensitive to what they taste, smell or feel. Most are very picky eaters, rejecting many foods because of their flavors, odors or textures. A child may sniff everything or be nauseated by the odors from a garbage truck a block away. Many children are extremely sensitive to touch, insisting upon the same soft, loose sweat pants every day. Others crave deep touch and pressure (proprioception), requesting massage, and climb into their parents' laps, pressing their faces to the mothers' face, neck and hair. Some whose systems receive poor information from their muscles and joints move and wiggle constantly. They are giving the brain feedback about where their bodies are in space. They touch other people and objects around them in an attempt to get a sense of how they relate to their environment.

Most children with ASD have vestibular problems. These could be a result of lack of appropriate prenatal stimulation, or an unfortunate consequence of the continuous ear infections and rounds of antibiotics many endure in the first two years of life. In any case, because the vestibular system is key to good digestion, emotional function, expressive language and eye movements, when it is dysfunctional, so are those other areas. These children present with both under- and over-responsive movement systems, either craving spinning, swinging and other movement activities, or throwing up in the car practically before it is out of the driveway.

Many children with ASD are extremely sound sensitive. Just as the scraping of nails on the blackboard can be very disturbing to many of us, the sound of a dripping faucet, the hum of the refrigerator, forced air heat or air conditioning, a ringing telephone or even rain on the roof can be profoundly disturbing to these children. Non-verbal children may cover their ears, or generate their own louder noises by banging or humming, for protection. Those with language can communicate their sensitivities, stating, "Not too loudly; you'll make my ears creak," if someone speaks much over a whisper.

Sometimes when multiple sensory stimuli compete for the body's attention, one sense may be hyper-sensitive, while another under-respond, as a method of preservation. There are an infinite number of sensory combinations. For instance, a child who demonstrates tactile defensiveness on a "bad" day and screams bloody murder at the hairdresser, may tolerate a haircut if she is feeling better on another.

Reflexes A reflex is an involuntary movement that a person makes in response to a stimulus. Babies are born with many reflexes. Primitive reflexes account for most of the movement patterns during the first few months of life. In the first year, the more primitive reflexes should integrate and disappear, so that the baby can develop increasingly more complex motor skills, such as sitting, creeping, crawling, walking and running. Other reflexes remain, preparing the body for even more advanced movement patterns. Eventually, voluntary movement and motor skills replace most of the reflexes.

Many children on the autism spectrum still retain some primitive reflexes. These can interfere with the development of the complex motor skills listed above and their retention can account for odd movement and behavior patterns. Four reflexes that commonly affect vision development are the asymmetrical tonic neck reflex (ATNR), the tonic labyrinthine reflex (TLR), the Moro reflex and the symmetrical tonic neck reflex (STNR). (For more information on reflexes and how they affect vision development see Chapter 8.)

Language Sound sensitivities and misperceptions can certainly affect language development. Thus, children on the autism spectrum not only have difficulties processing sound, but also show delays with most aspects of receptive and expressive language. They may appear oblivious to the call of their name or appear not to understand what was said. Yet, many often understand language at a much higher level than they can produce it. Some do not call people by name and have great difficulty with personal pronouns. They often call themselves by proper name, rather than use the pronouns "I" or "me." For example, one might hear, "Danny want juice" instead of "I want juice."

Those on the severe end show significant language delays with little or no expressive speech at age three or four. What little they say may be unintelligible, showing severe articulation difficulties. Their vocabularies are limited, consisting of necessary words such as *juice, milk or cookie*. Echolalia is also common, with repetition of the last word(s) heard. Even non-verbal children with autism communicate, but at a very basic level. They often have such poor visual skills that at times, they may not even be aware of others. They may even treat family members as inanimate objects, except when it is necessary to facilitate their everyday needs. Then, they may grab someone's hand, leading them to what they want: food, drink or a favorite toy. But for the most part, they seem to be in their own little worlds.

Lower functioning children sometimes make high-pitched and/or nasal vocalizations or blurt out inappropriate and nonsensical utterances, often quite loudly. Theresha Szypulski, a speech-language pathologist who is an expert on the oral-motor issues of children with autism, believes that these guttural sounds and the jaw/teeth clenching that accompany them, serve a real purpose by giving the child sensory feedback in the jaw, lips and throat, as well as auditorially.[10]

Those with mid-range disabilities may have had some language, but lost it. They may use words inappropriately because they heard only part of what was said. For example, the word *bag* may be used in place of *go* if a child associates it with leaving, after hearing his mother say, "Let me get my bag and then we'll go."

At the less severe end, language may appear typical, but is often "scripted." Although a child may have an abundance of words, little is said. What one often hears are the words from favorite videos, books or songs-verbatim. Those with Asperger's syndrome have an especially difficult time making conversation, even though they have large vocabularies. Small talk is a foreign concept; but they may be able to speak with great knowledge about a favorite subject such as computers, science fiction or the Civil War.

Cognitive The cognitive profiles of children with autism spectrum disorders range from profoundly retarded to gifted. Their sensory, motor, language and vision issues often interfere with the psychological and educational testing necessary to determine overall cognitive levels of functioning.

In general, most have stronger language than non-verbal skills on cognitive measures. Those who can complete a *Wechsler Intelligence Scale* show huge discrepancies between high Verbal scores and low scores on the Performance sections. The latter subtests all involve visual function to some degree, so optometrists can point to the discrepancy as evidence of visual problems, including tracking, focusing, understanding of visual spatial relationships and visual-motor skills.

Social-Emotional Development Inflexible sensory processing leads to inflexible behavior. Patients with ASD tend to be very resistant to change. Going to a new place can be very traumatic and temper tantrums can occur if a well-meaning eye doctor disrupts routine. The more familiar one is with how children with ASD interact, the better the chances are for success in the examination and treatment.

Socialization is a major issue, and the one that is often of most concern to parents. It can be embarrassing to family members if a child does not look at someone when speaking, does not respond to a question, or has his hand in his pants. It reflects on the parent as a teacher of manners and appropriate behavior. Assuring families that the optometrist is not judgmental about a child's inappropriate behaviors often puts them at ease.

Eye contact with new people in new surroundings is fleeting, at best. Some children appear "shy," clinging to a parent for dear life; others may explore and destroy the office quickly if left on their own for a period of time. They may crawl under a table or into a corner, and tear up every magazine on the reading rack, or line up trucks, soldiers or dolls linearly (end-to-end) across the room, viewing their parade with only one eye, while lying on the side.

These unusual behaviors are usually attributed to the lack of skills related to imaginary play. Another interpretation is that the child lacks vergence eye movements, which are more complicated and develop later than version eye movements, which are easier to use. Another favorite way to play with toys and other objects is to drop them down a grate, out a window, or placing them along the side of sofas, tables or chairs. They seem to have a fascination with the edges of objects, scaring everyone by walking precariously along the edges of rooftops or on balcony railings.

Children with less significant delays exhibit some of the same visual behaviors but to a lesser degree. They are aware, but disinterested in playing with toys, exhibiting a very short attention span for any activity. Those with sensory issues may never actually play with toys, but rather, just walk around clutching onto them, refusing to look at or give them up.

Therapists with a wide range of training and skills can address motor, sensory, language and social-emotional concerns Optometrists need to know when and where to make referrals for physical, occupational, and speech-language therapy, as well as Brain Gym, chiropractic, nutritional, cranio-sacral work and biofeedback. As an inherent part of an interdisciplinary team, optometrists are professionally responsible to have some knowledge of these interventions. (Look in the Table of Contents for later chapters covering treatment modalities designed to remediate deficits in all of these areas.)

Vision Development
Obviously, if children have developmental delays, they are going to have delays in vision. Specifically, delays in oculomotor function, focusing and binocular abilities can affect gross

and fine motor abilities and language acquisition. Sensory problems result when vision does not coordinate with the vestibular and proprioceptive systems properly, or if there is poor synchronization between the central and peripheral visual systems. Poor visual awareness negatively affects socialization and poor visualization can hinder the development of skills for imaginative play.

Parents are often thrilled to discover that the optometrist has the training to recognize problematic visual issues even in the most involved patients with ASD. Furthermore, they may not understand the relationship between visual dysfunction and behavior. When they discover that visual remediation has the potential to positively affect every aspect of learning and behavior, their amazement is palpable.

The reader should be familiar with how vision develops, so this chapter will not review general vision development. (For a good overview, read *Vision: Its Development in Infant and Child.*)[11] What is important is that the time period from age 18 months to four years of age, when autism is usually diagnosed, is an extremely important window of development for vision, as well as language, socialization and other crucial areas.

During this very critical time frame, vision should begin to dominate the movement system, and to coordinate the proprioceptive, vestibular and tactile systems. As vision combines with the other senses, central or focal vision should emerge. If there is faulty information processing in any of the other sensory and motor systems, including further complicated by retained primitive reflexes, visual dysfunction is inevitable. These patients then still need to touch and move to experience their environment because their visual systems are so inefficient. Some of their "aberrant" behaviors such as flapping and other self-stimulatory hand and arm gestures, may actually serve the purpose of allowing them to interact with their world, and tell the brain where the body is in space.

One of the most significant issues for people with autism spectrum disorders is difficulty coordinating central and peripheral vision. They tend to use one or the other, but not both simultaneously. The efficient integration of central and peripheral vision is the essence of Skeffington's four circles.[12] (Figure 2-1.)

Those whose vision is primarily focal can fixate on a central point of focus for excessive periods of time. These are the patients who play with specks of dust in the carpet or who become obsessed with details or staring at a wand or stick in their central visual field. Perhaps individuals who demonstrate savant abilities in a particular field are solely central to the exclusion of any peripheral distracters in their area of expertise.

Many utilize only their peripheral processing centers, spending hours staring at spinning objects or staring at high contrast, moving, colorless targets, such as lights, shadows, machinery parts or shiny objects. When asked to follow an object visually, they are unable fixate on it centrally; but rather scan it or look out of the side of their eyes at it instead.

Poor integration of central and peripheral vision can lead to difficulties in focusing, attention, spatial organization and visual perception. These visual problems lead the individual to develop compensatory techniques to deal with their faulty view of the world. Examples of compensatory behaviors include toe walking and walking while touching or holding onto the walls.

Most individuals on the less severe end of the spectrum, generally show more subtle, but very significant visual processing problems. Patients with attention deficits and learning disabilities are often very attracted to external, highly charged visual stimulation. They love to play video games and are generally highly skilled with computers. These traits lead

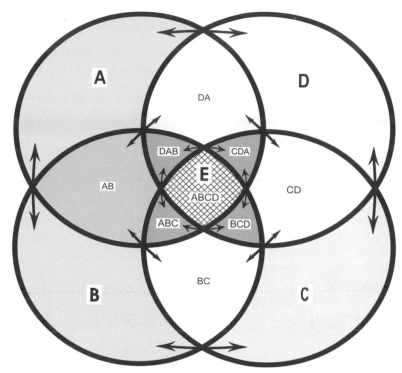

Figure 2-1. Skeffington's Four Circles
A. Centering, B. Anti-gravity, C. Speech-Auditory, D. Identification, E. VISION

to the misunderstanding by well-meaning adults that vision is an area of strength. Often it is these kids who are then labeled "visual learners" because they learn best when they can touch and see the materials. The real crime is that this misunderstanding about vision often prevents them from seeing any eye doctor, let alone one who can make a profound difference in their functioning. Optometrists must enlighten educators and parents about vision as a developmental process that must work with other systems in a coordinated manner. Just because the visual system is "strong" does not necessarily mean that it is operating in an efficient manner.

The literature supports that a very high percentage of children with autism spectrum disorders demonstrate eye movement disorders and a high incidence of strabismus.[2 (p.438),13] Some on the lesser end have had one or more surgeries with poor success.

Many children with autism also have a variety of competing stressors on their bodies during the critical second year of life. Inadequate or inappropriate sensory stimulation and health problems, ranging from food allergies to ear infections and asthma can all disrupt vision development. Whether the health or the vision issues are primary, visual concerns are real, and parents and professionals must pay attention to them. Even when health issues subside, and behavior, attention, and even eye contact improve, underlying visual delays often remain, and optometric intervention is necessary. Those with ASD simply have gaps in sensory, motor and visual areas so enormous that they cannot be closed without therapy.

Presentation of Vision Problems

In order to work productively with autism spectrum patients, optometrists should become familiar with how these patients present at the time of the examination, so that they can play a key role in the diagnosis of visual dysfunction and be an effective part of subsequent treatment. Obviously those on the less severe end of the continuum, such as those with attention deficits and learning disabilities, will generally be easier to examine, while those with the more severe forms of autism will offer the optometrist the biggest challenges.

Children on the autism spectrum typically bring a number of unusual visual behaviors or concerns to the optometrist. The most common are listed in Table 2-1.

Table 2-1 Signs of Visual Problems in Individuals with ASD
• Squints or closes an eye
• Stares at certain objects or patterns
• Looks through hands
• Flaps hands, flicks objects in front of eyes
• Looks at objects sideways or with quick glances
• Shows sensitivity to light (photophobia)
• Becomes confused at changes in flooring or on stairways
• Pushes or rubs eyes
• Has difficulty making eye contact
• Widens eyes or squints when asked to look
• Bumps into objects
• Is fascinated by lights and shadows
• Touches walls or tables while moving through space

Most patients seek vision care for abnormal behaviors such as squinting, blinking, closing one eye, side looking, frequent rubbing of the eyes, an apparent lack of interest in looking at things, or difficulties with depth perception. Parents complain also about poor attention, lack of focus, distractibility and difficulties with reading, writing or arithmetic. Interestingly enough, most families do not seek vision care for the most common behavior of those on this spectrum: poor eye contact.

Some present with visual sensitivities and close or cover their eyes or insist on wearing baseball caps outdoors or in fluorescent lighting, others appear to crave visual stimulation. Repetitious, visual stimulatory behaviors are also common. Many children rapidly flick their hands, a stick or piece of string in front of or at the sides of their eyes, especially when upset. Side looking is often one of the more distressing signs that alerts a parent to the possible need for vision care.

A change in gait or apparent confusion upon encountering junctions in the floor or a stairway could indicate problems with spatial orientation and depth perception. Parents may report fear of heights, stairs, or tunnels, and alternatively, an apparent fearlessness that strands them in trees and at the top of monkey bars on the playground.

Fearless behavior is both disturbing and reassuring to parents because, obviously, the child can see. While such performance could demonstrate adequate visual-motor coordination, it may not necessarily indicate good visual-spatial skills. A fearless child may be simply unaware of any danger because of poor integration of central and peripheral processing. It may be that balance and movement are highly tuned while central attention is absent.

Parents, teachers and other professionals assume that most behaviors seen in ASD are simply a result of the disorder, not a by-product of vision problems. They are astonished to learn that poor eye contact, repetitive stimulatory behaviors, and practically every other behavioral symptom, could be caused by poor fixation, accommodation, or eye teaming abilities. Fortunately, that scenario is gradually changing as most parents are very motivated to learn all that they can about their child's problems and are educating themselves by reading and talking with professionals.

Vision Examination

The examination begins when the parent calls for an appointment. (See "New Patient Form" at end of chapter.) The initial phone consultation is an opportunity both to learn about the patient and the referral source, and to share some information about behavioral optometry. With this knowledge, the optometrist will gain a sense of what length appointment is needed. When scheduling, make certain that it is a good time of day for the child, not near nap or mealtime. Set aside 45 minutes to one hour, and be on time, so the family does not have to wait.

Mail intake forms prior to the examination appointment, and ask that they be completed and returned with adequate time to be read. Learn whether there is a family history of vision problems and what, if any, other vision intervention that the child has received. A sample intake form, appropriate for patients on the autism spectrum is at the end of this chapter. This form includes a checklist of some of the more unique visual behaviors seen in this population as well as the standard list of visual complaints of most school-age children. The optometrist must rely on his interpretation of reported behaviors such as in Table 2-1 to make conjectures about possible vision problems.

In addition to questions about vision, the form inventories milestones and all aspects of general development. Understanding the possible impact of the mother's health upon her child, including allergies, asthma, medications, diet, drug, cigarette or alcohol use, may be helpful to the optometrist. Included on the history form is a place to list complications of pregnancy including gestational diabetes, immunizations, infections and bed-rest. Next, the form lists questions about birth weight, length of gestation, delivery complications, such as Caesarian section, forceps or vacuum aspiration and Apgar scores.

The answers to some of these questions may not be available for adopted children. Many children adopted from foreign countries suffered from significant sensory deprivation and malnutrition in orphanages and foster homes. Sometimes these early experiences have irreversible visual consequences because they turn off essential centers of the brain.

The child's health history is often very revealing. Risk factors for visual problems include frequent illness, particularly ear and strep infections, and their treatment with antibiotics. Many children with ASD have been on, had reactions to, or are presently taking medications for behavior and allergies. Refer to Chapter 1, Table 3 for an understanding of these and their possible visual side effects. Many have food allergies and may be on special diets or take supplements. These generally do not interfere with visual function and may, in fact, improve it.

Next, look at developmental milestones, being aware of delays in motor, speech, language, social and cognitive development. Learn about all other interventions that a child has or is receiving, and from whom. Most have had occupational, physical, speech, behavioral and nutritional therapy, as well as bodyworks, including cranio-sacral, chiropractic and osteopathy. Some have even had music therapy, hippotherapy (therapeutic horseback riding), biofeedback, Brain Gym or auditory integration training. Find out the names of local resources and invite them to visit your office, and to collaborate with you on patients you have in common. The intake form concludes with the parent's general description of the child. This part is very valuable as it gives the optometrist an idea of what to expect from both the patient and his parents, and what the parents' expectations of the optometrist and their child are.

Remember each case is unique and must be treated as such. Learn about where others believe the patient's problems lie; then make observations and figure out the role vision is playing. Vision problems may be the number one priority or secondary to motor and sensory issues. Most important, however, are the parents' most pressing concerns, because they mirror their motivation and desire for change.

Formal Testing

Start testing in the exam room; this part of the evaluation should take approximately 15 to 20 minutes.

Acuity An accurate acuity examination is often difficult, but sometimes a parent can make it easier by explaining the procedure to the child. It is sometimes beneficial to start at near to familiarize the child with the shapes, even pointing out the birthday cake, bird, etc. and naming each one. Then ask the child to point to smaller and smaller birds or cakes. It might be necessary to block off a single row or a few rows or even isolate individual letters or pictures so as to eliminate competing items that might be distracting. Unfortunately, sometimes pointing does not work because a child has significant fine motor issues and simply cannot coordinate the finger to point.

Next, attempt standard acuity tests such as the American Optical (AO) picture charts, Lighthouse cards or even the Snellen chart. Sometimes the Snellen is surprisingly useful, as often kids with ASD who do not communicate know all of their letters and numbers.

If standard procedure fails with a non-verbal patient, ask him to point to the object seen at distance on the near chart. Many children in a behavioral or ABA program (See Chapter 14.) are able to match pictures or letters. If that, too, is unsuccessful, attempt using Lea gratings (similar to the Teller cards but handheld and inexpensive).

The first visit may not yield much in the way of acuity measures. More often than not acuity and refraction will appear fairly normal. This finding is consistent with parents' reports that their child can spot a bird miles away (if it is a plane, be careful, it may be the sound that the child orients to), or can spot and pick up a piece of lint on the carpet.

Ocular motilities Most children with ASD have considerable oculomotor difficulties, so the optometrist has to be very creative to complete a full pursuit and saccadic fixation evaluation. Patients may either show no interest in the Wolff wand (reflective steel ball on a shaft), or grab it and become distracted or absorbed by it. Use treats such as raisins, gluten-free pretzels, a pacifier or goldfish crackers as alternatives for tracking. Be sure that your stimulus is fully natural and conforms to special gluten-, dairy-, sugar- and additive-free diets.

Attempt both monocular and binocular motilities. Both may not be possible, as often the children are extremely disrupted by attempts to cover one eye. Differences in resistance to attempts to cover either the right or left eye may reveal an underlying asymmetry that should be probed further. Often, eye movements tend to be saccadic in nature and are not necessarily accurate. Saccades tend to be hypometric, and often are accompanied by compensatory head and/or body movement.

The large majority of patients demonstrate frequent loss of fixation or no fixation at all upon initial evaluation. Rarely do these children demonstrate good grasp, release, and re grasp of fixation. Mostly they have fair to poor fixation ability with very poor ability to maintain fixation. Pursuit eye movements are also poor with frequent saccadic intrusions. Pursuits may be better than ability to hold fixation, but usually not by much.

At this point in the exam, take a look at visual motor integration with fixation testing. Ask the child to touch the target. Note first of all if he or she even attempts to touch it. Then, look at accuracy in all positions of gaze, and note differences on the right, left and center and ability to cross midline. Also note the dominant hand, and whether or not the child uses the whole hand or can isolate a single finger. If a child uses his entire hand in a groping manner, ask him to touch with one finger and demonstrate how. Keep the instruction simple such as "Do this" and point with your own finger. Depending on the age of the child, the inability to touch a target with one finger may be a significant delay. This test is also a useful performance test to demonstrate to the parent both faulty eye hand coordination and possible difficulties with depth perception and spatial judgments.

Refraction Next, take a look at refraction and accommodation. This part of the exam might also be challenging because of patients' aversion to or obsession with lights. Consider doing a Mohindra technique; even though fixation may be unreliable, with this procedure, a fixation on lights can be an advantage.

Do retinoscopy quickly, if necessary. Try flashing the lenses over the eye quickly and make a guesstimate. Children with ASD really do not like being in a strange, darkened room with an unfamiliar doctor peering into their eyes, even at a distance, with a light wand that they may associate with something threatening or that they didn't like, such as an otoscope. As soon as a loose or flipper lens is placed over an eye, children with ASD tend to grab it. They will probably not sit there smiling cooperatively, because they want to remove whatever is over their eyes and clutch it in their hands, put it in their mouths, or throw it on the floor. If there is reliable fixation during retinoscopy, try displaying the 20/400 cake and ask the child to blow the candles out or count them. To keep a patient's interest, place the red and green slide over the cake and ask what colors he sees. As an alternative, use an appropriate video or moving toy.

Interestingly enough, even though poor fixation and inattention complicate exams, results consistently show that most patients with ASD have little refractive error. Using both dynamic and static retinoscopy techniques, the majority of these patients are emmetropic or mildly farsighted, demonstrating hyperopia between +0.50 and +1.00 D. A handful are more hyperopic; very few are myopic or astigmatic.

Accommodation One way to assess near accommodation is with Bell retinoscopy. Most patients demonstrate considerable lags of up to +1.00 D or more. Again, sometimes the Bell does not work, because of poor fixation, no interest and no against motion at all. Frequently there are asymmetries as large as a 2″ to 4″ difference between the right and left eye, even upon test repetition.

Another near retinoscopy measurement that can be helpful in this population is stresspoint retinoscopy. Consider using the child's favorite book or toy. Be persistent, making observations, whenever possible, when the child is engaged.

Cover test Cover testing is a real challenge; it can be quite revealing if successful. The optometrist must overcome not only poor fixation, but also poor acceptance of cover. To assess alternate and unilateral cover, a high interest target is essential. Use the Hirschberg images. Frequently, an eye turn can be noted.

My experience is that assessing eye alignment precisely can be quite difficult. The first reason is that many of these children will not look at a single object in primary gaze and allow the interposition of the cover for long enough to permit the optometrist to make an accurate assessment. The second reason is that they often have such significant developmental delays in fixation control and in refixation following the shift of the cover that they may appear to have misalignments that turn out to be pseudo turns once their visual development reaches appropriate levels.

Additional binocular testing Most optometrists working with children on the autism spectrum report a high incidence of strabismus, primarily because they are seeing patients who exhibit a high number of visual symptoms. The turn is usually intermittent in nature, so testing for near point of convergence and stereopsis is often successful.

On the near point of convergence (NPC) try using a puppet or penlight. It is often difficult to get a recovery finding, however. These children break at 8″ to 10″, or more, if they are exophores, or they look off to the side or the eye remains stuck in, if they are esophores.

Stereopsis responses are evident in more than half of these patients, with typically a positive response to the stereofly on initial testing. Random dot stereograms including the Butterfly are often harder to elicit a response. If a child is able to respond to the Stereo Fly, more than half are also able to identify two or three of the animals correctly on stereopsis testing. Unfortunately, many are not able to respond to "touch the animal that is closer, jumping, different or real." Even if they can understand the question, they may not be able to actually point to the target. They may also demonstrate tactile defensiveness to the Polaroids, so it is helpful to use stereoscopic targets that do not require Polaroids.

After all this testing, attempting phorometric tests, Keystone skills, cheiroscope and the Van Orden Star may be nearly impossible. Try to assess binocular skills using a prism bar at distance and near, base-out and base-in, looking at eye movements for loss of vergence and recovery.

Prism bar testing is a very gross assessment, but it does give some additional information as to binocular status and sustaining ability. Often, only objective measurements can be made with the prism bar. Subjective responses are difficult and the child may merely echo two after hearing "Tell me when you see two." At the very least, it is another piece of information for the record and an area that might improve with intervention.

Ocular health An examination of ocular health is best reserved until the end of the formal examination. Many kids with ASD are extremely light sensitive and can be quite volatile when a stranger comes close with the ophthalmoscope. While slit lamp exams are usually extremely difficult to do with this population, a hand held slit lamp and monocular indirect are particularly useful if available. Tonometry may be at best finger tension; again the hand-held units are appropriate. Try getting a dilated fundus examination, expecting cooperation to be very limited. The rule of thumb is "to get in, get out."

Informal Testing

By now the child is ready for some action, so go into the therapy room to make further observations. This next part of the exam normally takes me about 20 minutes. Making time and a place for informal observation is of vital importance, as it allows an opportunity to assess a child's overall functioning and to determine the role of the visual system in the profile. While optometric tools are time-tested and fairly accurate measures of visual status in this population, they may not give the optometrist all the information she needs.

The therapy room, equipped with a white board, the Marsden ball, walking rail, balance board and cabinets full of toys of all types, looks like a playroom to most children. Take out a few toys such as pegs, puzzles or balls and see if the child interacts with them on his own or with prompting.

The fact that a child is unable to comply fully with the demands of the examination probably indicates a visual problem. Yet, in cases of children with autism spectrum disorders, who have multiple challenges, it is often difficult to sort out the pieces. Is poor sensory processing disrupting visual function or vice versa? For example, are the sounds of every footstep, car, bird or voice so distracting that the patient cannot focus on the task at hand? Similarly is the sound of the bell during retinoscopy so distracting that it prevents the patient from accommodating? Or is the patient so overwhelmed visually he cannot focus on any of the instructions?

The main purpose of being in the therapy room is to somehow determine which came first, the chicken or the egg! The key is observation and a good knowledge of what is expected for the child's chronological age, not only in vision, but also in motor, speech-language and social-emotional areas, as well. The optometrist can help parents use guidelines from OEP's "Parents' Guide and Checklist"[14] or Kavner's, *Your Child's Vision*[15] as references for how far behind their child is in all areas.

Observe everything! Start out by just watching the child interact in the therapy room for as long as you are able, gaining insights into the child's behavior. Sometimes it may be for just a few minutes, sometimes longer; it depends on how impatient the child or parents are. Families often expect the optometrist to be interacting with their child all the time, or may attempt to intervene and direct the child's activity because they are concerned that if left unattended, their child could be disruptive. Explain that an uninterrupted, independent observation is precisely what you are interested in, if necessary.

What happens when you leave a child alone? Does he seek out touch, movement, pressure, taste, smell, visual or auditory stimulation? Be very aware of the involvement of all the sensory systems and especially eye movements and alignment. Take note also of a child's articulation, understanding and use of language, play skills and indications of the potential for higher cognitive ability. Finally, assess whether the child has appropriate or inappropriate social responses. Does he interact with or ignore the examiner? Is he overly friendly with everyone or trying to avoid other people?

Gross Motor Look at the body as a whole, including foot posture, general posture, shoulder and hip alignment, any rotation anteriorly or posteriorly, any indication of one side being higher/lower, or any spinal curvature. Do one or both feet turn in or out? Does the child twist the feet up when standing still or toe walk? Postural warps can mirror visual dysfunctions and asymmetries-either caused by or causing them. It is helpful to know what the posture is because it gives an indication of how embedded a visual problem is and whether or not any other intervention like orthopedic, podiatric or chiropractic is warranted.

Assess not only posture but also balance, gross and fine motor coordination, and orientation in the room. Look at general physical ability, comparing your observations with parents' comments on the intake form. Can the younger child alternately crawl or walk without support? Can a child walk smoothly without stumbling or bumping into the wall? Does he have difficulty navigating around or stepping over the toys pulled off the shelves? Is there even an awareness of the toys or the Marsden ball hanging from the ceiling? What is the reaction to bumping into it? Can an older child hop or skip?

Fine and Visual Motor Try to present as many performance tests as are necessary to assess visual motor and fine motor ability. Look informally for a good pincer grasp, comparing pointing skills to those observed in the exam room. Attempt a copy form test. Usually, all that can be elicited during the initial visit are lines and scribbles, but even scribbles give information about a dominant hand, pencil grasp, and support from the non-dominant hand.

Observe head and body posture while writing, and note if the trunk is straight or turned right or left from midline. Note working distance and preference for drawing vertical or horizontal lines. Observe if there is any organization to the scribbles and, if appropriate, ask the child to write his or her name. Again, look at organization, size of lettering and note any reversals. Have the child repeat pencil and paper tests using a slant board, noting any positive differences. A baseline here is extremely important because fine motor skills can change markedly in this population after only a few weeks of a vision therapy program using lenses and prisms.

Bubbles are a great tool for assessing visual awareness, tracking, vergence eye movements, depth awareness and visual motor coordination in the therapy room. Depending upon the age, hand the wand to the child, allowing him to blow the bubbles himself, observing oral motor and visual motor control with the task.

Another performance test to try is a puzzle, such as a form board. Look again at hand usage, speed of processing, as well as the number of attempts and types of errors involving size or shape. Next present a number of pegboard tests. The standard pegboard test is nearly impossible for most patients under five, so consider using much larger, graded wooden pegs.

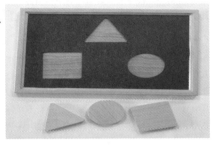

Hand the pegs to the child from different positions and assess how well he is able to reach for them. Is the child immediately aware of the peg and where it is, making a fixation towards it? Or is it necessary to tap a finger on it or move it to a different position for the child to notice it? Is there a good visual motor response? That is, does the child look as he reaches or is there no fixation but just a reaching motion? If the child reaches, how accurate is he? Does he miss or make a groping movement for the peg?

Try moving the peg in space to observe whether the child will track. Note differences in the use of the right or left hand as well as in fixations and pursuits in various positions: right, left, center, inferiorly, superiorly. Also observe the accuracy and speed with which the peg is placed in a hole and what the grasp pattern is. While placing pegs can the child sustain attention for a handful in a row or does he look away, walk away or even get frustrated and throw it away? Does the child look as she does it, or does she place the peg by feeling around for the hole? Is there any organization to the placement? For example, does the child go from left to right or is placement random? Does the child recognize color? Does he put the pegs back in the box in the color-coded and graded manner in which they came out? The chance for a child's success is dependent upon age and ability; the goal is just to get a baseline of what the child can and cannot do. Obviously if a four year old cannot fixate and feels to place the peg into the hole, he has a visual motor problem.

Sometimes children play only with toys that make sounds, or if a toy is silent, children may flick at it with their fingers, listening to the sounds they make. While this behavior may appear to be a craving for auditory stimulation, it could also be a function of extremely poor visual processing. Watch the eyes while a child plays. Is the child looking at the toy too closely or from the side? Is there a head tilt? How about a large angle alternating exotropia? Many patients rely heavily on their auditory systems because the visual systems are so inefficient and unreliable. An example of the "auditory" child is the two year old with an obvious large angle alternating exotropia 80% of the time with little to no control of eye movements. She could not trust her environment visually because if not suppressing she was seeing double much of the time and could not determine where she was in space. Her constant tapping was a way to determine where things were and how far away they were from her.

Another example is the child who puts everything in her mouth, touches, but does not play with every toy in the room, splashes in the water cooler and flicks the Venetian blinds. This child is functioning at an even lower sensory level, preferring oral and tactile stimulation. Oral fixations, mouthing, drooling and spitting are abnormal in all but the very youngest patients. These signs often indicate oral motor problems that must be addressed by an occupational or speech and language therapist trained in oral motor or sensory integration. Children who have poor oral motor skills such as sucking, blowing or swallowing ability often have convergence problems that can improve once the oral concerns have been addressed. What about visual function? In the exam room such a "sensory" child measured +3.50-1.50 x 180 and exhibited an alternating esotropia. In the therapy room she exhibited both the esotropia and an exotropia, confirmed by Hirschberg. She stumbled and tripped over the toys she had taken out but did not play with them, demonstrating poor balance and navigation around the room. She clearly did not have a stable visual world and required the more basic stimulation to give her information about her environment.

I have found it quite helpful to work with physical, occupational and speech and language therapists. Optometrists, OTs and PTs have a great deal to learn from each other. (See Chapter 7 on collaboration.) While anyone could make a case here for sensory integration based occupational therapy in the above child, because of her oral motor needs, poor balance and lack of spatial awareness, certainly an extremely disrupted visual system is contributing to all three areas.

Awareness and attention Patients' responses to all these tests impart information about two very important visual skills: awareness and attention. It is essential to note the locus of visual attention. Is the child's awareness of things around the room adequate or does he ignore some or all the toys, preferring to stare out the window? Is the child able to maintain central attention to task, while still maintaining some peripheral awareness? What is under scrutiny is the level of integration between central processing (focusing, identification and attention) and peripheral processing (binocularity, centering and spatial awareness). A child may have too much central and not enough peripheral organization or vice versa.

Typically, there is a lack of integration between the two areas. Donna Williams, an adult with autism, eloquently describes the problem of seeing parts but never the whole, in her book *Somebody Somewhere*.[16] She writes of noting the chair, bed or clothes in the room but never getting a sense that they were all in the same place. Similarly, some patients may not initially notice the animal pictures on a wallpaper border in the therapy room, but comment about them after therapy and lens work, and even understand that they were always there, and not new additions.

Lens probing At this point a fairly clear picture of the overall functioning of the child, strengths and weaknesses, and most importantly, a sound assessment of visual status should be emerging, Now is the opportunity to begin a few probes of lenses and/or prisms that testing indicates might be of benefit to the child. Keep a large number of ready-made prescriptions in children's eye sizes as probes. Optometrists should acquire a set of lenses to use as probes of visual behavior. (See Table 2-2) Consideration of various sphere and prism powers should be done carefully. Many protocols recommend prism powers in the 3 and 5 diopter range. Some will test at lower powers as well. Most prism sets should have pairs in each of the base directions: up, down, right and left. You will use some more often than others, but one can never tell ahead of time which lenses will be the ones that help a particular child, without actually trying them and observing behavior with them on.

Table 2-2
Recommended Lenses for Probing
Rotating Plano 3 Prisms or
Plano 3 Base Right
Plano 3 Base Left
Plano 3 Base Down
Plano 3 Base Up
Rotating Plano 5 Prisms or
Plano 5 Base Right
Plano 5 Base Left
Plano 5 Base Down
Plano 5 Base Up
+0.50 3 Base Right
+0.50 3 Base Left
+0.50 3 Base Down
+0.50 3 Base Up
+0.25 1 Base Up
+0.25 1 Base Down
+0.25 1 Base In
+0.50 1 Base In
+0.37 ½ Base In
+0.50 Sphere

See Table 9-1 for the effects of each of these types of lenses.

How do you know what to probe? Retinoscopy findings at distance and near as well as binocular results help you know where to start. If there is a large lag in accommodation or if convergence is off, try plus lenses with prism base-up, down or in, depending on whether there is an under- or over-convergence. If the eyes turn in, probe with base-down and if the child is very exophoric, try base-in. Reserve the base-up for the more involved cases with a large exotropia and/or hypertropia.

If a child is all over the place with no awareness of where he is in space, try base-up or in. It is usually wise to try a few prescriptions, while making some observations. Start with lower powers of plus and base in if the child is quite delayed or is very exotropic and/or peripheral and disorganized, or base-down if he is an esotrope or a toe walker.

It may be necessary to use flippers if a child does not accept glasses readily. If possible present the child with one of the visual motor tasks again, such as pegs or drawing tasks, and note differences. Or, use the Marsden ball with and without prisms and/or lenses to get a sense of performance differences. Make observations. For example, with glasses on, does the child seem to have a change in awareness, catch the ball more easily, reach out with two hands instead of letting the ball hit her body? Does the child appear less fearful or more playful with lenses on? Does tracking of the ball improve?

It is often possible to realize differences with the lenses in place, without repeating tests. Just lens application may elicit positive responses, such as improved attention, eye contact, tracking, balance and awareness. One five-year-old boy who never made eye contact with me in the examination, made it for the first time with lenses on. Another child who appeared completely unaware of the toys in the room, peeked at them through +0.50 D and smiled. He then looked around the room and went over to the table to color. This was a kid who during the exam was all over the place and could not even sit or stand still, while talking incessantly. He actually sat down quietly and scribbled on the paper and said "Mommy, I'll take these glasses home now." The glasses were prescribed and his mother reports that they are amazed with the results at school.

Unfortunately, not every case is so dramatic. Only about one third of my patients with autism respond definitively and positively to a pair of glasses on the first visit. In some cases the child is simply not capable of responding or is too involved for us to see immediate changes. If the child appears particularly disorganized and exhibits no positive response to lenses and prisms at first, try some glasses that are stronger than you would normally prescribe to see if you can at least get a response. Sometimes after an application of the stronger powers yields a positive response, weaker powers will have a similar effect.

Some children simply refuse lenses, prisms or occlusion in any form, whether they are in glasses or flippers. In cases like this, recommending a prescription on the first visit is impossible. If the parent agrees, ask to see the child again, or start the child in vision therapy first, and feel out the child's responses to lenses and prisms later. In cases where you are uncertain about an initial prescription, but are certain that there is a vision problem that requires attention, explain to the parent that a child's visual system does not always respond immediately. Just as the motor system takes time to develop, so does the visual system. Suggest a few sessions of vision therapy visits before prescribing glasses that will be accepted by and benefit the child, provide maximum improvements, and guide the system optimally.

Sometimes an optometrist will not get a second opportunity to try lenses or prisms on a child. In these cases, attempt using flippers. Some children will lean way into them or may even take them and put them up to their eyes. Even a very brief experience with lenses can elicit a positive response. If you are unsuccessful with lenses and prisms, assess responses to occlusion, even, very peripheral occlusion and note differences in right and left eye or visual fields. If time allows, also note responses to red, green, yellow and blue filters.

Consultation
Once all of the data is in, it's time for the consultation. The main purpose of this final step of the evaluation is to inform parents about the nature of the visual problems, how they relate to the family's stated concerns, and what can be done to help the child. Keep the importance of the visual system and the priority for vision intervention in perspective.

Go over each aspect of the exam, assuring the parent of the child's ocular health and ability to see clearly. Next, discuss refractive error and focusing ability, giving brief definitions of all visual skills, including tracking, fixation, convergence and divergence, and how the child did in each area. Discuss the child's skills in eye teaming, binocularity, depth perception, visual motor and visual perceptual abilities.

Be sure to relate each area to observed signs and symptoms in an effort to help the parent better understand visual functioning and how it relates to performance and behavior. For example, if the child often side looks or sights toys while lying on his side, explain that this behavior could be due to faulty binocularity. An explanation might be, "Your child has difficulty pointing his eyes in and out, and seeing clearly and singly. Looking to the side is an easier eye movement than looking straight ahead. When he lies down, he may be shutting down one eye, allowing the brain to ignore competing information from the two eyes. He thus avoids seeing double." Sometimes it is helpful to demonstrate diplopia using vertically dissociating prisms, ex., 5 BD OD, 5BU OS.

Next is the inevitable discussion of lenses and prisms, how they create changes in the light energy coming into the eye, and how they allow the brain to organize visual information in a different, hopefully easier, fashion. This conversation is obviously individualized, focusing on a child's specific observed difficulties, needs and responses to the lens and prism probes.

Discuss plus lenses and how they make it easier to focus and attend better to near tasks. Talk about expansion and magnification, which help make it easier to organize central tasks, particularly in a child who is very peripheral in his attention. Explain that prisms, too, bend the light and allow for changes in internal visual processing by expanding or compressing certain fields, emphasizing or decreasing input from competing areas. Relate how the prisms create changes that will accelerate the child's development.

In most cases vision therapy is appropriate in addition to lenses and prisms. Explain how glasses should make a difference, and more work is necessary for changes to become fully integrated and long lasting. Discuss how vision therapy, like occupational or speech therapy, is a tool to teach the visual system how to work. Offer a prognosis and estimated duration of therapy.

Most children with autism spectrum disorders require one-on-one, in-office therapy plus a home program to reinforce the work done in the office. Now is the time to suggest that, in your experience, improvements are faster if parents adhere to a home program. The frequency and duration of therapy must be determined on a case-by-case basis. Start with every other week for children under three. If the visual problems are not primary, try recommending some home activities, with once-a-month therapy. Some cases may require weekly visits initially, but within the first few months can be seen successfully every other week thereafter. The majority of cases are long term, as it may take years for a child to reach normal or maximal development.

Always offer parents a choice of care. Tell them that they can choose to do nothing, and the child may continue to develop. Explain that you view that option as risky, given the extent of the difficulties, and that visual dysfunction may be contributing to the child's overall delayed development and aberrant behavior. Help them understand that vision therapy, in addition to glasses, is optimal. If they choose the conservative approach of trying only glasses first, then insist upon a follow-up appointment within four to six weeks to determine the extent to which the glasses are helping, and whether or not vision therapy is indicated.

If, during the exam, the child did not immediately respond to lenses or prisms, consider a loaner pair for the patient to try on at home for a few weeks until the next visit. Regarding prisms, a pair with rotatable base directions allows the parent to try different orientations. For kids who have tactile defensiveness, ask the parent to spend some time trying to get the child to accept sunglass frames with the lenses popped out, or loan a pair of very inexpensive children's frames. When loaning out glasses, describe what parents should look for, with and without glasses. Observed changes include differences in posture, balance, coordination, eye alignment, eye contact, speech and language ability and general attention and awareness. Be certain to charge a fee for the loaner, and have the patient sign a contract agreeing that they are responsible for the full cost of the frames and lenses if they are lost or destroyed. A sample contract is at the end of the chapter.

Lastly, recommendations should include referrals to adjunct professionals whose interventions are indicated for a child, based on the intake form and observations from the vision exam. In most cases, if the child is not under their care already, it is very appropriate to make a referral to practitioners involved in total body health such as nutritionists, osteopaths and physicians, particularly Defeat Autism Now! practitioners. (See Chapter 6.) Behavioral optometrists should also know when it is appropriate to pass the baton to the occupational therapist or other practitioners. When doing so, it is important to contact the professional directly, of course after the parent signs the record release. In that way, the optometrist can explain the visual difficulties the child is experiencing and collaborate and direct some of the patient care. Regardless, in most incidences, after a thorough exam, some kind of optometric intervention can make a huge difference and, the earlier, the better.

Summary and Conclusions

Optometrists are seeing increasing numbers of patients with ASD and this trend is expected to continue. Research supports the presence of subtle to severe visual dysfunction in patients with attention deficits, learning disabilities, pervasive developmental disorders and autism. These individuals have a high incidence of strabismus, hyper- and hypo-reactivity to information coming in from their touch, movement and vestibular systems, gross and fine motor delays, and evidence of retained primitive reflexes. These underlying dysfunctions all impact upon visual development.

Visually, those with ASD present with aberrant behaviors, which parents sometimes do not associate with visual dysfunction. Although most have poor eye contact, this symptom is usually considered an inherent part of their disability, not a visual problem. A thorough developmental examination can be challenging and revealing. Few have significant refractive errors. Most have considerable difficulty with ocular motilities, accommodation and binocular function. A key issue is poor coordination of the central and visual processing systems, resulting in poor visual perception, spatial organization, focusing and attention.

The optometrist must be creative, observant, tenacious and skillful in both formal and informal testing. Combining the use of a thorough intake form, instrumentation and behavioral observations of free play and performance tests such as copy forms yields the most complete picture of the patient. Consulting with parents following an evaluation is an opportunity to educate the family about the role visual dysfunction plays in ASD, as well as to offer several rehabilitation options. Lenses and prisms combined with a home or in-office vision therapy program usually produces the best results.

The subsequent chapters in this book focus on what combination of factors result in the diagnosis of autism, and what therapies are part of a multi-disciplinary approach to the remediation of children with ASD. Some of the most common options are dietary modification, nutritional supplementation, sensory integration based occupational and physical therapy, body work, including chiropractic and cranio-sacral therapy, and auditory integration therapy.

Even optometrists who do not specialize in patients with disabilities need to be knowledgeable about these areas, because they too will be seeing children with ASD in their practices. All optometrists must be prepared not only to evaluate and treat those on the lesser end of the spectrum with learning disabilities and attention deficits, but also those with PDD, NLD, Asperger syndrome and autism. In addition to treating them, they need to know when and where to refer them out.

Behavioral optometrists must evaluate children at younger ages to achieve the goals of:

- preventing a visual contribution to developmental problems, including autism
- stimulating proper whole child development
- improving the chances of those with autism spectrum disorders to overcome their disabilities

In these stressful, hectic and demanding times, optometrists must position themselves as part of a growing field of practitioners involved in educating parents, teachers and other practitioners about the importance of vision development in everyday life. As optometrists dispel the myth that vision is eyesight, and that behavioral optometrists are unique in their understanding, qualifications, knowledge and tools to create changes, all those with autism spectrum disorders will experience success.

References

1. *Streff JW. Optometric care for a child manifesting qualities of autism. J Am Optom Assoc 1979;46:592-7.*

2. *Scharre JE, Creedon MP. Assessment of visual function in autistic children. Optom Vis Sci 1992;69:433-9.*

3. *Kaplan M, Edelson SM, Gaydos AM. Postural Orientation Modifications In Autism In Response To Ambient Lenses. Child Psychiatr Hum Dev 1996;27:81-91.*

4. *Granet D, Gomi C, Ventura R, Miller-Scholte A. The relationship between convergence insufficiency and ADHD. Strabismus 2005 Dec;13:163-68.*

5. *Novak L. Not autistic or hyperactive: Just seeing double at times. www.nytimes.com/2007/09/11/health/11visi.html. (Accessed January 1, 2008)*

6. *Lehmkuhle S, Garzia RP, Turner L, et al. A defective visual pathway in children with reading disability." N Eng J Med 1993; 328:989-96.*

7. *www.aoa.org/documents/CPG-20.pdf (Accessed January 5, 2008)*

8. *Bowan MB. Learning Disabilities, dyslexia and vision: a subject review. J Am Optom Assoc 2002 Sept;73(9):553-70.*

9. *Cheatum BA, Hammond AA. Physical Activities for Improving Children's Learning and Behavior: A Guide to Sensory Motor Development. Champaign, IL:Human Kinetics, 2000:14.*

10. *Szypulski TA. Oral Sensory-Motor Therapy as a Portal to Interaction in Autism. New Developments Newsletter, Developmental Delay Resources 2003 Fall;9:4.*

11. *Gesell A, Ilg FL, Bullis GE. Vision: its development in infant and child. Santa Ana, CA: Optometric Extension Program, 1998.*

12. *Shankman A. Behavioral Optometry's Birthright-Skeffingon's Four Circles. J Optom Vision Dev 1993;24:29-30.*

13. *Schulman R. Optometry's Role in the Treatment of Autism. J Optom Vis Dev 1994; 25:259-68.*

14. *Parents' guide and checklist: a reference guide for preschool children's vision development. Santa Ana, CA: Optometric Extension Program. Pamphlet #B124, 2000.*

15. *Kavner R. Your Child's Vision: A Parents Guide to Seeing, Growing, and Developing. New York: Simon and Schuster, Inc., 1985:189-92.*

16. *Williams D. Somebody Somewhere. New York: Times Books, 1994.*

NEW PATIENT FORM

Today's Date:_____

Patient Name: _____

Address: _____

City & State:_____

DOB: _____

Phone Number:_____

Insurance: _____

Referred By: Professional / Patient / Other

    Name: _____

    Street: _____

    City: _____ State: _____ Zip: _____

Additional Infor. on Patient: _____

_____

_____

Appointment Date:

Day:_____ Date:_____Time: _____

Cancellation List: _____ Sent Packet: _____

Date_____

Dear Parents:

   The development of your child's skills (such as seeing, moving and talking) is affected by family history as well as by certain illnesses. Therefore, your thorough answers to this form will help in determining how your child's vision, motor skills or speech and language skills have developed as well as allow us to use the office time for a complete examination of vision, motor skills, or speech and language skills.

Child's full name_____ Nickname_____

Address _____ City _____ State_____ Zip_____

Telephone _____ Birthday _____ Age _____

Grade _____ School_____Teacher_____

Parent's Names_____Occupations_____Email_____

Other family members at home (include ages and relationship)_____

_____

Insurance Carrier _____ Policy No._____Referred by_____

Present Situation:

Does your child seem to have any visual difficulty? _____ If yes, in what way? _____

How long has difficulty been noted?_____

Does your child seem to have any motor difficulty? _____ If yes, in what way? _____

How long has difficulty been noted?_____

Does your child seem to have any speech or language delays? _____ If yes, in what way? _____

How long has difficulty been noted?_____

Does your child ever report or appear to experience any of the following? If so, when?

   headaches _____ blurred vision _____

   double vision _____ eyes hurt or tired _____

Have you or anyone else ever noted the following? If so, when? _____

closes or covers one eye_____	poor handwriting_____	experiences car sickness or nausea_____
rubs or pushes on eyes excessively_____	confuses right and left_____	frequent frustration with near work_____
turns or tilts head often_____	avoids certain textures_____	distractible or inattentive_____
bumps into objects_____	difficulty making eye contact_____	has no interest in books_____
gets lost in books _____	difficulty trying new motor tasks_____	obsessed with books_____
bothered by light_____	looks through hands_____	is unable to write_____
eye(s) turn in or out_____	flicks or spins objects in front of face_____	articulation problems_____
moves head when reading_____	obsession with spinning_____	word retrieval problems_____
holds reading close_____	fascinated by light, shadows_____	difficulty with thought formulation_____
uses finger when reading _____	afraid of heights_____	difficulty with social skills_____
reverses words or numbers_____	shows no fear of heights_____	difficulty hearing_____
skips words or loses place_____	sights along linear objects_____	eating problems_____
poor reading comprehension_____	flicks fingers by sides of face_____	overall clumsiness_____
makes errors in copying_____	toe walks_____	sensitivities_____
avoids certain textures_____	disturbances in gait_____	difficulty coordinating hands_____
appears to be in constant motion_____	inconsistencies in balance_____	difficulty with writing_____
reads slowly_____	tends to feel his way along walls_____	difficulty manipulating utensils_____
difficulty staying attentive to tasks_____	difficulty with uneven flooring_____	difficulty interacting with others_____
difficulty organizing tasks_____		difficulty expressing self_____

Date_____

Dear Parents:

The development of your child's skills (such as seeing, moving and talking) is affected by family history as well as by certain illnesses. Therefore, your thorough answers to this form will help in determining how your child's vision, motor skills or speech and language skills have developed as well as allow us to use the office time for a complete examination of vision, motor skills, or speech and language skills.

Child's full name_____ Nickname_____

Address _____ City _____ State_____ Zip_____

Telephone _____ Birthday _____ Age _____

Grade _____ School_____Teacher_____

Parent's Names_____Occupations_____Email_____

Other family members at home (include ages and relationship)_____

_____

Insurance Carrier _____ Policy No._____Referred by_____

Present Situation:

Does your child seem to have any visual difficulty? _____ If yes, in what way? _____

How long has difficulty been noted?_____

Does your child seem to have any motor difficulty? _____ If yes, in what way? _____

How long has difficulty been noted?_____

Does your child seem to have any speech or language delays? _____ If yes, in what way? _____

How long has difficulty been noted?_____

Does your child ever report or appear to experience any of the following? If so, when?

    headaches _____   blurred vision _____
    double vision _____   eyes hurt or tired _____

Have you or anyone else ever noted the following? If so, when? _____

closes or covers one eye_____
rubs or pushes on eyes excessively_____
turns or tilts head often_____
bumps into objects _____
gets lost in books _____
bothered by light_____
eye(s) turn in or out_____
moves head when reading_____
holds reading close_____
uses finger when reading _____
reverses words or numbers_____
skips words or loses place_____
poor reading comprehension_____
makes errors in copying_____
avoids certain textures_____
appears to be in constant motion_____
reads slowly_____
difficulty staying attentive to tasks_____
difficulty organizing tasks_____

poor handwriting_____
confuses right and left_____
avoids certain textures _____
difficulty making eye contact_____
difficulty trying new motor tasks_____
looks through hands_____
flicks or spins objects in front of face_____
obsession with spinning_____
fascinated by light, shadows_____
afraid of heights_____
shows no fear of heights_____
sights along linear objects_____
flicks fingers by sides of face_____
toe walks_____
disturbances in gait_____
inconsistencies in balance_____
tends to feel his way along walls_____
difficulty with uneven flooring_____

experiences car sickness or nausea_____
frequent frustration with near work_____
distractible or inattentive_____
has no interest in books_____
obsessed with books_____
is unable to write_____
articulation problems_____
word retrieval problems_____
difficulty with thought formulation_____
difficulty with social skills_____
difficulty hearing_____
eating problems_____
overall clumsiness_____
sensitivities_____
difficulty coordinating hands_____
difficulty with writing_____
difficulty manipulating utensils_____
difficulty interacting with others_____
difficulty expressing self_____

Dear Patient,

Congratulations on receiving your loaner therapy glasses. These lens and/or prism glasses will create needed visual changes to occur. These changes will allow the visual system to process more information by aiding in development and/or relieving visual stress.

These glasses should be worn up to 1 hour per day in the first week, gradually increasing to no more than 4 to 6 hours per day. If you or your child have difficulty adjusting to them, that is okay. Because lenses and prisms are powerful tools in treating visual problems it is advisable to go at a comfortable pace with your wearing time. Even quick peeks several times throughout the day are helpful.

As the glasses work best as part of a vision therapy program we can monitor your progress at our next therapy visit. If you have not scheduled therapy, you must schedule a progress evaluation within 4-6 weeks. As these are loaner glasses we are charging a nonrefundable nominal fee of $90 for the use of the glasses. If the glasses are either not returned or are returned in poor or unusable condition, you will be charged an additional $65 for the glasses. Upon return of glasses in good condition you may apply the full fee to a new pair of glasses or receive a credit of $45.

There are a number of observations to make before and after you begin using these glasses. Please note visual symptoms and behaviors such as headaches, blurred vision, head tilting or turning, closing or covering an eye, visual fatigue and avoidance. Note general appearance of the eyes and head and pay attention to posture. As you use the glasses note changes in your posture, eye alignment and changes in intensity of visual complaints and behaviors. Be aware of changes in general attention and awareness of things around you. You may also note changes not only in visual processing but also in motor and auditory processing. Finally, note the speed of processing and the ability to sustain visual concentration.

Space for Notes and Observations:

_____
_____
_____
_____
_____
_____

I understand and agree that I am responsible for these glasses and will be asked to report on any changes occurring as a result of using the therapy glasses.

Signature_____

Date_____

Chapter 3
Total Load Theory: Why So Many Children Have Autism Spectrum Disorders

Patricia S. Lemer, MEd
with Anju Usman, MD

Introduction

Did you ever have a nasty cold, a bad day at work, get caught in traffic on the way home, and then yell at your kids for something insignificant? You experienced "total load": the cumulative effect of individual assaults on the body as a whole.[1]

Children on the autism spectrum have a huge total load of risk factors that set them up for developmental problems. Young people are far more susceptible to a load of stressors than adults, because their small, less mature systems cannot handle the assault.

Experts are increasingly able to identify the cluster of symptoms, appearing in the first two years of life, that make children high risks for one of the diagnoses on the autistic spectrum. Figure 3-1 details some of the load factors that accumulate to produce autism spectrum disorders. Each of these falls into a category covered in this and subsequent chapters. The code is as follows: c=structural, i=immune, r=reflexes, s=sensory, t=toxicity, v=vaccines.

Figure 3-1 Risk Factors for Autism Spectrum Disorders

- Premature or traumatic birth (r, c)
- Rh incompatibility (t)
- Mother with toxic exposures, such as many mercury amalgams, excessive fish consumption, or occupational hazards (t)
- Mother with chronic fatigue, fibromyalgia, or low thyroid (i)
- Mother received vaccine(s) prior to pregnancy or while nursing (i, t, v)
- Family history of auto-immune disorders (i)
- Allergies in the family, especially to cow's milk (i)
- Sensitivity to dyes, chemicals, perfume or medications (i,t)
- Yeast infections, such as severe diaper rash or thrush (i)
- Digestive problems, including colic, reflux, projectile vomiting, constipation and diarrhea (i)
- Skin problems, including eczema and pallor (i)
- Dark circles under the eyes (allergic "shiners") (i)
- Red ears or "apple" cheeks (i)
- Recurrent ear, sinus or strep infections (i, s)
- Chronic unexplained fevers (i)
- Respiratory problems, including asthma and bronchitis (i)
- Repeated use of antibiotics (i, s)
- History of immunization reaction(s) or immunizations given simultaneously with antibiotics and/or acetaminophen (i, v)
- Regression in function between 15 and 30 months (i, v, t)
- Sensory deprivation (s)
- Hyperactivity (i, t)
- Sleep disturbances (i, s)
- Mood swings (i, s, t)
- Self-injurious or violent behaviors (i, t)[2]

The developmental histories of most children with autism and related disorders show one or more of these risk factors. According to a 1994 study of almost 700 children by Developmental Delay Resources (DDR), those children who had more than 20 rounds of antibiotics were over 50% more likely to have delays. Affected children were nearly four times as likely to have had negative reactions to an immunization.[3]

The end of the second year of life is a particularly vulnerable period, when vision, language, and social skills are maturing at a rapid rate. Visually, for example, age 12-30 months is a crucial developmental stage when the child moves out of near space, increasing visual-motor manipulation and interaction with the environment. As self-awareness expands to other-awareness, in typical children, language develops and social skills emerge.[4]

Components of the Total Load
This chapter focuses on several load factors related to:
- Structural problems such as a traumatic birth or other injury, and structural therapies, including osteopathy, cranial-sacral therapy and chiropractic
- Immune system dysfunction such as allergies, eczema, rhinitis, sinusitus, sensitivities to foods, dyes and medications; bacterial, bacterial, viral and yeast infections, digestive and respiratory problems
- Toxicity from chemicals, pesticides, food additives and heavy metals, (including aluminum, antimony, arsenic, cadmium, lead and the one receiving the most attention: mercury

The Structural Connection
According to Dr. Viola Frymann, a world-renowned osteopathic physician in California, birth trauma is the most common cause of developmental problems, including autism, with at least 80% of children with an ASD diagnosis having a history of a traumatic birth. Problems in delivery, due to the temporary compression of passing through the birth canal, from which the skull and sacrum do not recover fully, use of forceps, and vacuum aspiration, can affect the brain, spinal column, and the fluids inside these organs. An imbalance in any of the organs, fluids, bones and connective tissues for any reason, can disrupt their function. Many of the underlying health issues experienced by children on the autistic spectrum cluster into specific organ and muscular systems. The nervous and digestive systems are particularly vulnerable. In addition, some children have seizure disorders and obvious motor problems.[5]

Structural Therapies
Structural therapies aid in realigning the body's internal parts. A number of treatment modalities take into account the structural and skeletal systems of the body, and their relationship to each other. These include osteopathy, chiropractic, massage, cranio-sacral therapy, and others which cluster under the umbrella of "body-works." When an osteopath, chiropractor or other structural therapist corrects structural dysfunction resulting from birth trauma early on, neurological development can progress satisfactorily. Then motor, sensory-motor, language, social-emotional, cognitive, and behavioral problems are averted by establishing or restoring optimal anatomic-physiologic integrity.

Each therapist provides his/her version of precise, gentle, restorative manipulative treatment by applying pressure, sometimes deep, sometimes light. Each type of pressure and manipulation addresses each dysfunctional system with procedures designed to reactivate that system and bring its function back into balance.[6]

Mary Ann Block, DO, an osteopathic physician who went to medical school at the age of 39 to help her daughter heal, finds that structural therapies are particularly beneficial for treating those who have chronic ear infections. She uses osteopathic manipulation to drain the fluid in the ears along with dietary modification and nutritional supplementation to enhance the immune system. Furthermore, she teaches parents who want to do something themselves to stop the ear problems, how to treat their children at home. Manipulation is an immediately effective valuable tool that could even prevent a visit to the doctor.[7] Dr. Block's multi-disciplinary approach, which supports vision and other sensory therapies, is applicable to children at both ends of the spectrum. To learn more about her and her practice, go to <www.blockcenter.com>.

Since practitioners from many disciplines are trained in manipulative techniques, families can sometimes find it difficult to determine which type of structural therapy might be beneficial for a particular child. Some occupational and speech-language therapists use cranio-sacral therapy and massage techniques to facilitate sensory-motor and language skills. The Upledger Institute provides training courses for all types of clinicians to learn cranio-sacral techniques. For locations and the broad range of courses go to <www.upledger.com>.

When cranio-sacral therapy is combined with other therapies, such as dietary modification and nutritional supplementation, synergistic benefits emerge.[8] Sally Goddard, Director of The Institute for Neuro-Physiological Psychology (INPP), in Chester, England, reports on a French study in which cranio-sacral osteopathic manipulation benefited children with abnormal reflexes. Noticeable differences were apparent after only three sessions at two week intervals over a period of six weeks. Her conjecture is that this intervention started a neurological reorganization in the body that allowed for reflex integration. She recommends that any osteopathic correction be supported by a reflex integration program, such as is described in Chapter 8.[9]

Another "hybrid" field is chiropractic neurology, which marries the biomechanical aspect of chiropractic care with the latest techniques of assessment and rehabilitation of the central nervous system. The result is a model of diagnosis and care that focuses on the two-way interaction between the sensory systems, including vision, and the central nervous system. Some treatments look similar to vision therapy, including ocular-motor activities and computer-based techniques. To find a chiropractic neurologist, go to <www.acnb.org>.

Because the underlying cause of the problem, rather than the diagnosis, is what is important, an in-depth developmental history is essential before making a referral. Many optometrists already collaborate with chiropractors, osteopathic physicians and occupational/physical therapists using cranio-sacral techniques for patients with binocular dysfunction. The benefits of these therapies in conjunction with vision therapy are well-known. These same practitioners could be appropriate referral sources for patients with autism.

The Immune System Connection
Of all the possible causes associated with autism, dysfunction of the immune system is the one that has received the most attention. Symptoms of immune system problems, designated with an (i) in Figure 3-1, comprise 20 of the 24 risk factors listed. Early studies headed by Reed Warren Ph.D. at Utah State University,[10] Sudhir Gupta, M.D., Ph.D., a professor of neurology, pathology, microbiology and molecular genetics at the University of California, Irvine,[11] and others[12,13] indicate that most children with autism have significant immune system abnormalities.

Recent evidence comes from a 2004 Johns Hopkins study in which researchers examined tissue from three different regions of the brain in 11 people with autism, ages five to 44 years, who had died of accidents or injuries. They also measured levels of two immune system proteins, called cytokines and chemokines, found in the cerebrospinal fluid - the clear substance that surrounds, bathes and nourishes the brain and spinal cord - in six living patients with autism, ages five to 12 years. Compared with normal control brains, the brains of people with autism showed evidence of an ongoing inflammatory process in different regions of the brain and produced by cells known as microglia and astroglia. Cytokine and chemokine levels in the cerebrospinal fluid also were abnormally elevated in patients with autism.[14]

Jane El-Dahr, M.D., the Head of Immunology at Tulane Medical Center, likens the immune system to the United States Government Department of Defense (DOD). Just as the Defense Department acts to keep the country safe from invaders, the body's immune system acts to defend it against harmful substances. The "ideal" immune system
- recognizes all foreign organisms
- efficiently and rapidly destroys invaders
- prevents further infection
- never causes damage to itself

Children on the autism spectrum clearly have less than ideal immune systems. Immunologists from the M.I.N.D. Institute and the National Alliance for Autism Reseaarch (NAAR) showed in 2005 that their immune systems respond differently.[15] An immune response is appropriate against bacteria, yeast, viruses, parasites and toxins. The immune systems of children with autism over-react to almost anything, including, but not limited to, molds, pollen, chemicals, metals, common foods, food additives and incompletely digested particles of food.

While the DOD has its branches of the military and an "emergency alert system," the immune system also has different ways of staying alert to protect the body and brain against all invaders.[16] The immune system's army has many types of specialized "soldiers." Researchers have identified that different types of cells help the body with different types of immune responses. Thymus 1, or Th1 cells, participate in cell-mediated immunity; Thymus 2, or Th2 cells help with antibody-mediated defenses. According to long-time autism researcher, Sudhir Gupta, MD, PhD, mentioned above, individuals with autism have more Th2 cells than Th1 cells, when compared to neuro-typical children. Gupta believes that the fewer number of Th1 cells explains why these children are more susceptible to viral and fungal infections.[11]

Most people are familiar with immediate, and sometimes life-threatening, IgE immune responses. Skin and respiratory reactions to peanuts, shrimp, animal dander, tree pollen and dust mites are of this type. Doctors can predict which children will have serious IgE allergic reactions by their elevated scores on blood and scratch tests. Traditionally, treatment is by avoidance and with antihistamines.

Less well-understood are IgG responses, which are sometimes called "intolerances" or "sensitivities" rather than allergies, because they can be delayed and are not usually life-threatening. IgG immune responses appear as chronic skin, gastro-intestinal problems, and behavioral reactions. Those with IgG reactions have eczema, thrush, diarrhea, constipation, mood swings and hyperactivity. Many children on the autism spectrum have both IgE and IgG allergic reactions.

A third type of immune response is an IgA reaction, which is indicative of inflammation, especially of the gastro-intestinal lining. Health care professionals are seeing more of this type of immune reaction in children on the autism spectrum. IgA antibodies are often a reaction to stress. Prolonged stress changes the immune system's ability to respond quickly. As less blood flows to the intestines, digestion slows and the body heals more slowly.

Bottom line: a number of immunological measures are necessary to determine the immune status of an individual with autism. Traditional IgE testing alone is not adequate to draw conclusions about the level and presence of immune responses. Which laboratory tests are appropriate for measuring immune responses are detailed at the end of this chapter.

Ear infections In the 1994 study by DDR cited above,[3] 75% of children later diagnosed with autism spectrum disorders had five or more ear infections. Frequent ear infections are a sign of a weak immune system. Some researchers even target early ear infections as major contributors to autism.[17] A classic study by Talal Nsouli, MD, an allergist at Georgetown University Hospital, showed that 78% of early childhood ear infections are related to food allergies. By eliminating the offending food from the diet over a 16-week period, he ameliorated the infections in 86% of these children. Reintroduction of the food caused a recurrence. By limiting the diet of his patients, Dr. Nsouli avoided the unnecessary use of antibiotics or insertion of ear tubes, often seen as panaceas for such chronic problems.[18] Obviously, less invasive techniques are preferable, especially since current research now shows that ear tube insertion is not beneficial.[19]

Maryland nutritionist Kelly Dorfman has coined the term "post traumatic ear infection syndrome" (PTEIS) to describe a condition in children who have had continuous ear infections, often as result of undiagnosed food allergies.[20] Many treatments with strong antibiotics may increase the child's vulnerability to damage from toxic metals, especially mercury. Dr. Boyd Haley, the world authority on mercury, found that it takes less mercury to do harm in the presence of the antibiotics ampicillin and tetracycline.[21] Allergies, ear infections, mercury and antibiotics are a potent cocktail for triggering autism, auditory processing difficulties, learning disabilities, and attention deficits. Permanent damage to the inner ear may result because of complications from immune, toxic and sensory load factors interacting.[12]

Strep infections Some children with autism spectrum disorders, especially those with Tourette syndrome and obsessive compulsive disorder, have a history of repeated strep infections. If a strep infection induces tics or obsessive-compulsive disorder (OCD), a doctor should suspect **P**ediatric **A**utoimmune **N**europsychiatric **D**isorder **A**ssociated with **S**treptococcus or PANDAS. Individuals with PANDAS experience a very sudden onset or worsening of their OCD symptoms triggered by a strep infection, followed by a slow, gradual improvement. A subsequent strep infection, might cause their symptoms to worsen again.[22]

What is thought to occur in PANDAS is that antibodies to strep cross-react with proteins in the basal ganglia of the brain which are responsible for movement and repetitive behavior, thus causing the tics and/or obsessive-compulsive symptoms. While traditional doctors might use aggressive, and/or prophylactic antibiotics for prolonged periods of time to control strep and its OCD symptoms, some with a more holistic approach find that boosting the immune system often results in the elimination of both the strep infections and behavioral symptoms.[11]

Lyme disease Dietrich Klinghardt, MD, PhD, believes that Lyme disease is very prevalent and under-diagnosed, especially in young children diagnosed with autism spectrum disorders.[23] Because symptoms like dyspraxia, speech-language issues, sensory and auditory processing problems are so similar to those of attention deficits and pervasive developmental disorders, the possibility of Lyme is often overlooked. Even without evidence of the telltale tick bite, Klinghardt tests every child with autistic-like symptoms, because he and others believe that this insidious disease can be passed between sexual partners and from mother to unborn child. (See Chapter 16 for Klinghardt's Protocol.)

Unfortunately, most lab tests for Lyme disease are not very reliable, with doctors seeing many false negatives. Klinghardt has thus designed a very complex diagnostic procedure involving muscle testing which compares the body's energy pathways to those of the pathogen. Only those trained in applied kinesiology or muscle testing can use this technique, which is also described in Chapter 16.

The role of antibiotics "Anti-biotic" translated literally, means "against life." If a baby develops any infection, allowing its immune system to fight the invader appears to strengthen immunity in the long term.[24] When the same invader reappears, the body recognizes it and fights it off. If, however, an antibiotic fights the infection, some believe that the antibiotic suppresses the immune system, causing it to fight less vigorously the next time around.[25] By the fourth or fifth infection, the immune system might not even recognize an invader as a threat, because it now depends on the antibiotic to do its job.

In the past decade, physicians and others have become concerned about the role of antibiotic over-use in the dysregulation of the immune system.[26] As bacteria become resistant to first generation antibiotics, such as penicillin, doctors are moving to stronger ones, such as ciprofloxin. Today's antibiotics are "atom bombs" compared to the "water pistols" of the previous generation. No one knows the long-term effects to the digestive, immune and other systems.

Antibiotic creams can work well topically to combat external infections. However, taken orally, antibiotics kill not only bad bugs that cause infections, but also knock out virtually all of the bacteria in the gut, including beneficial varieties. Many people experience digestive problems after taking an oral antibiotic for this reason. The gut is a host to thousands of types of flora which live together cooperatively in the healthy person. Antibiotics disrupt this symbiotic environment. The good bacteria, which antibiotics kill in addition to combating bad bacteria, exist to control the growth of yeasts and other fungi in the digestive tract. In their absence, yeasts colonize and their usually small colonies can then proliferate.[27] Intestinal overgrowth of yeast and "bad" bacteria are a well documented outcome of taking broad spectrum antibiotics.[28]

The yeast connection The late William Crook, MD, a country pediatrician for over 50 years, wrote extensively on the relationship between ear infections, antibiotics and autism.[27,29,30] As early as 1982 he noted a child named Rusty with a history of colic and ear infections in the first year of life. By the age of two Rusty, showed both hyperactivity and autistic symptoms.

Dr. Crook believed that many children on the autism spectrum, like Rusty, have yeast-connected problems, also known as candida albicans. Dr. Bernard Rimland of the Autism Research Institute also suspected a relationship between candida and autism in 1985.[31] Children who crave sugar from candy, soft drinks, fruit juices and baked goods, are highly suspect of having yeast-based problems, because yeasts feed off of sugar to grow. Thrush, vaginal or anal itching or rubbing genitals, recurrent and persistent diaper rash, colic, recurrent ear infections with repeated or prolonged antibiotic use, chronic allergies including rashes, wheezing and coughing, headaches, muscle aches, abdominal pain or digestive problems, irritability, depression, mood swings, brain fog, hyperactivity and attention problems are all red flags for yeast.

William Shaw, PhD, the former Director of Clinical Chemistry and Toxicology at Children's Mercy Hospital and the founder of Great Plains Laboratory, both in Kansas, proved Dr. Crook right in 1995. Shaw, a biochemist, with no previous experience with autism, identified very high levels of tartaric acid and arabinose, by-products of yeast overgrowth, in the gut flora of brothers who, he later learned, were autistic.[32] Aware that yeast metabolism is the source of tartaric acid and arabinose, Shaw concluded that the brothers with autism had yeast in their intestinal tracts. In the past 10 years Dr. Shaw has become one of the world authorities on yeast-based problems and their relationship to autism spectrum disorders. Thanks to his research, we now understand far more about yeasts and gut problems. To learn more about this subject, read Shaw's book, *Biological Treatments for Autism and PDD*,[33] or go to <www.greatplainslaboratory.com>.

Viruses Unlike bacteria, viruses do not respond to antibiotics. Most "colds" and the "flu" are caused by viruses. Viruses have the ability to mutate and shift within the body, wreaking havoc with function. While Lyme disease is a bacteria, and is most often treated with strong antibiotics, it acts like a virus. That's one reason it is so difficult to diagnose and control. John Martin, M.D., PhD, believes that many autistic children have acquired a "stealth virus" that the immune system does not recognize. The immune system thus puts out no antibodies against it, leading to chronic low-grade infection.[34]

Measles virus is also considered a possible contributor to autism. In 1998, British physician, Dr. Andrew Wakefield reported finding measles virus from the measles- mumps-rubella (MMR) vaccine in the small intestines of 60 children with autism, who also had inflammatory bowel disease.[35] While this study has raised a great deal of controversy, his findings have been replicated at least twice.[36,37] Wakefield has become a hero in the autism community for confirming what many parents suspected: that there is a relationship between autism, the measles virus and gut issues. Read further in this chapter and extensively in Chapter 4 on Vaccines for more about his remarkable man and his work.

Leaky gut A "leaky gut" occurs when undigested food particles and toxins produced in the digestive process pass through the weakened thin mucosal membrane that lines the intestinal wall.[38] "Leaky gut syndrome" is a nickname for increased intestinal permeability. According to Elizabeth Lipski, a nutritionist, and author of *Leaky Gut Syndrome*, a leaky gut underlies an enormous variety of illnesses and symptoms, including autism.[39] Antibiotic overuse, heavy metal toxicity, and destructive enzymes secreted by yeasts all contribute to the breakdown of the gut lining. This phenomenon is similar to ivy attaching itself to a brick house and slowly destroying the mortar. The tiny holes made by the yeast allow toxins to enter the bloodstream. The body's immediate reaction is to clear the incompletely digested particles by producing IgG antibodies against these partially digested proteins.

Dr. Michael Gershon, in his groundbreaking book, *The Second Brain*,[40] details how the gut and the brain are two branches of the nervous system that communicate, not only with each other, but with the immune system, as well. A modern pioneer in the field of neuro-gastroenterology, he has led the way to our understanding of how damage to the gut and the immune system affect brain function. Nowhere is this connection clearer than in the bodies and minds of those with autism.

Allergies, constipation and diarrhea Inflammation in the form of "allergies" is the result of IgG antibodies attempting to combat the bacteria, yeasts, and yeast by-products. As the immune system weakens, digestive and respiratory problems worsen. Children experience severe constipation, often accompanied by serious abdominal pain and bloating, frequent diarrhea, or alternating constipation and diarrhea. Some children go weeks at a time without a bowel movement; others have a five or more a day. Stools are abnormal in color, consistency and smell, as well as frequency.

Many children with autism have impacted bowels which lead to alternating diarrhea and constipation. What appears to be diarrhea, is, in fact, leakage around a hardened stool. Once measures are taken to remove the impaction, both bowel and brain function improve.

An examination by a gastro-intestinal (GI) specialist familiar with autism, is essential at this point. The doctor performs a physical exam, which includes listening to the abdomen with a stethoscope and lightly palpating it. A hard, bloated abdomen and discomfort upon palpation help determine a diagnosis.[41]

Unfortunately, few GI experts are interested in autism. One who has put his reputation and career on the line is the aforementioned Dr. Andrew Wakefield. Wakefield recently moved to the United States to direct Thoughtful House, a clinic and research center in Austin, Texas <www.thoughtfulhouse.org>. Wakefield and his colleagues perform colonoscopies and endoscopies on children with autism. They have "scoped" hundreds of children with autism, the majority of whom have inflammation of the gut lining with swelling of the lymphoid tissues.[42] Dr. Arthur Krigsman of New York University Medical Center, and now also at Thoughtful House, and Dr. Timothy Buie at Harvard University Medical Center have both confirmed Wakefield's findings in their patients with autism.[43,44] These physicians have partnered with several other University-based medical centers to found the Autism Treatment Network, a group interested in researching, diagnosing and treating the gut issues related to autism.

Dysbiosis The gut is now out-of-balance, with "bad" bacteria, yeast and/or fungi outnumbering "good" bacteria, a condition known as "dysbiosis." Unwanted bugs wreaking havoc in the gut is trouble; however, the scenario worsens. The body must now deal with additional toxins produced as waste by-products from the metabolism of the bad bacteria, yeast and fungi. Two of these, arabinose and tartaric acid, produced by the yeast, candida albacans, alerted Dr. William Shaw that something was awry in the guts of those autistic brothers. Another bug, Clostridia, produces a neurotoxin that is thought to be responsible for very erratic behavior in patients with autism.

As yeasts increase in numbers, they produce more arabinose and tartaric acid. Arabinose and tartaric acid have drastic negative effects on human metabolism. Tartaric acid inhibits and limits energy production, causing muscle weakness throughout the body. Arabinose impedes the production of vitamins essential for the production of digestive enzymes. As the gut wall breaks down further, more undigested proteins and toxins to enter the bloodstream, yeasts proliferate, further impairing the immune system, and increasing the chances of infection and antibiotic usage. The vicious cycle continues. Doctors are just beginning to understand the degree to which dysbiosis can drastically impair health.

Enzymes, sulfation and phenols Enzymes, vitally important for proper digestion, are proteins responsible for many essential biochemical reactions. Enzymes act as catalysts, breaking down carbohydrates, proteins and fats into simple forms that the body can absorb, burn for energy, or use to build or repair itself. When enzyme production is disrupted, many functions go awry.

One enzyme, phenol sulfur-transferase (PST), is necessary for "sulfation," an essential part of the detoxification process (see section on Detoxification which follows). An efficient PST sulfation pathway is necessary for the body to break down and remove certain chemicals and toxins, called phenols, from the body. If sulfation pathways are inefficient, phenols build up.[45] Dr. Rosemary Waring, a British scientist who discovered the role of the enzyme PST, found that as many as 90% or those with autism have limited PST activity.

She believes that unprocessed phenols and toxic bacteria in the gut act as internal irritants, causing "autistic" and hyperactive behavior.[46]

While all foods contain phenolic compounds, some have higher content than others. High phenolic foods that children on the autism spectrum eat frequently are apples, grapes, strawberries, bananas, almonds and vanilla. Phenols occur in foods containing salicylates, artificial colors, flavors and some preservatives. Salicylates are a naturally occurring ingredient in many fruits, including apples, berries, and oranges, in some vegetables, including tomatoes, peppers and cucumbers, and in aspirin. Most artificial dyes, colors, flavors and the preservatives Butylated Hydroxyanisole (BHA), Butylated Hydroxytoluene (BHT) and Tertiary Butlyhydroquinone (TBHQ) contain phenols,[47] which inhibit the production of PST[48] and suppress their activity in the gut.[49]

Many of the body's own chemicals are also phenolic, and need the sulfation process to metabolize properly. Hormones, including testosterone, estrogen, DHEA and others, all require efficient sulfation to maintain proper function.

Parents who are taking comfort in the fact that their children are getting some healthy products may have to think again. Often, the very foods kids crave are the most problematic. Controlled double-blind studies linking diet and hyperactivity[50-53] show significant improvements ranging from 76 – 85% in children diagnosed with AD(H)D. Only one study[54] showed a lower rate of improvement, reporting a 50% benefit.

Gluten, casein and the opioid excess theory Problems digesting wheat and/or cow's milk products are known to be related to many chronic health problems, including eczema, asthma and childhood diabetes, constipation, diarrhea, and reflux, as well as behavioral and learning problems.[55] The American Academy of Pediatrics recommends against introducing cow's milk into a baby's diet until after the first birthday for that reason.[56]

Children on the autism spectrum have some or all of the above ailments, and frequently eat a very limited diet, consisting almost entirely of wheat- and dairy-based food. They also have trouble digesting gluten, the protein found in most cereal grains, including wheat, rye, oats and barley, and casein, the protein found in milk. Cow's milk has seven times as much casein as human milk. (Cows also have four stomachs to our one.) Waring notes that children with low levels of PST also have trouble digesting gluten and casein.[46]

Twenty-five years ago, researcher Jaak Panksepp speculated that people with autism may have elevated levels of opioids because their behavior resembled that of those with drug addictions.[57] In 1990 biochemists Karl Reichelt and Paul Shattock found that 90% of a sample of children with autism had abnormally high levels of certain opioid peptides in their urine.[58] Where did these opioids come from? An incomplete breakdown of gluten and casein.[59] They proposed the opioid excess theory, which explains this phenomenon.

The main premise of the opioid-excess theory is that the body incompletely digests gluten from grains and casein from dairy products, thus creating small peptides, instead of fully broken down amino acids. These peptides pass through the intestinal membrane, made permeable by yeasts and their metabolites, and enter the central nervous system, exerting an opioid-like effect.[60] The brain has receptors for opioids, as well as many other different types of peptides, the role of which is to switch on a neuron's sensitivity to other neurotransmitters. Some opioid peptides are useful, but an overload is harmful. Excessive peptides can mimic some of the good hormones and neuro-transmitters, thus disturbing perception, behavior, mood, emotions, brain development and immune function.[61] Sound like autism?

The Toxicity Connection

Today's generation of children is exposed to far more toxins than previous ones. Toxins are in the earth where our food grows, in the water we drink and in the air we breathe. Eating, drinking and breathing toxins are now an inevitable part of life. Over two billion pounds of neurotoxic chemicals are released into the air, land or water each year. A review of the top twenty chemicals reported released under the 2000 Toxics Release Inventory (TRI) reveals that nearly half are known or suspected neurotoxins.[62]

In May 2000 the Greater Boston Physicians for Social Responsibility (GBPSR) released the 140-page booklet *In Harm's Way: Toxic Threats to Child Development*, reporting that millions of American children exhibit learning, behavioral and developmental disabilities, including AD(H)D and autism, because of over-exposure to toxic substances.[63] This booklet is available as a free download from <http://psr.igc.org/>.

Sidney Baker, MD, co-founder of Defeat Autism Now! and author of *Detoxification and Healing: The Key to Optimal Health,* categorizes toxins as
- Biologic, from plants and germs
- Synthetic, mostly from petrochemicals
- Elemental, such as lead, mercury and cadmium[64]

The previous section focuses on biological toxins as load factors in autism. The following section completes coverage of the toxic cocktail of chemicals and metals we take in. Chapter 5 proposes a general biomedical detoxification treatment plan for ridding the body of these poisons. Chapter 6 includes a summary of the Defeat Autism Now! approach to detoxification and rebuilding.

Chemicals More than 85,000 chemicals are registered for use in the United States today.[65] Synthetic chemicals add further to the body's toxic total load. We all have several hundred chemicals in our bodies that were unknown before the 20th century.[66] No baby is born today without toxic exposure in the womb. A study by the Environmental Working Group (EWG) of umbilical cord blood from 10 babies born in 2004 in U.S. hospitals, showed 287 industrial chemicals and pollutants overall, an average of over 200 per baby. Of those detected, 217 are toxic to the brain and nervous system, and 208 cause birth defects or abnormal development in animal tests.[67]

Toxic chemical exposure continues after birth. A Swedish study showed high levels of flame retardants called polybromo diphenyl ethers, (PBDEs) in breast milk.[68] Fire retardants are in hundreds of everyday products, including sleepwear, furniture, computers, TV sets and automobiles. Minute doses of PBDEs can cause deficits in sensory and motor skills, learning, memory and hearing, as well as impair attention, learning, and behavior in laboratory animals.

In a repeat of this study by the Environmental Working Group (EWG) on American babies, the average levels of flame retardants in the breast milk of 20 first-time mothers was 75 times the average found in European studies. Milk from two study participants contained the highest levels of fire retardants ever reported in the United States, and milk from several of the mothers had among the highest levels of these chemicals yet detected worldwide. Other chemicals that can invade breast milk are chlordane, DDT, lindane, dioxins, furans and PCBs. American babies appear to be exposed to far higher amounts of fire retardants than babies in Europe, where some of these chemicals have already been banned. In the United States, only California and Maine restrict the use of PBDEs.[69]

Excitotoxins Substances added to foods and beverages, such as aspartame (Equal™ and NutraSweet™), hydrolyzed vegetable protein, and monosodium glutamate (MSG), are "excitotoxins." These ubiquitous additives are in almost all processed foods; their sole purpose is to alter taste. Both solid and liquid forms are toxic, but the liquids are worse, because the body absorbs them more rapidly. In solid form excitotoxins are sometimes disguised as "natural flavoring," "spices," "yeast extract," "textured" and "soy protein," and a host of other non-food products.[70] As liquids they are added to soups, gravies, diet sodas, ice cream, candy, cigarettes, cheese products, chewing gum, gelatin, infant formulas, and other "unexpected" places, like vaccines.[63]

MSG in Vaccines? Yes, in the form of processed free glutamic acid, described as a "stabilizer:" an ingredient to keep the virus alive. According to Dr. Joseph Mercola, at one time the chicken pox and Measles/Mumps/Rubella (MMR) vaccines made by Merck contained "free glutamic acid." To see if they still do, Mercola recommends calling Merck's National Service Center at (800) NSC-MERCK.[71]

The negative effects of excitotoxins are subtle and develop over a long period of time. They gradually stimulate neurons to death, causing varying degrees of damage to all parts of the nervous system, including the brain.[70] MSG's effects on vision go far beyond autism. Japanese researchers found that MSG binds to receptors on retinal cells, destroying them, and causing secondary reactions that reduce the ability of the remaining cells to relay electrical signals. As an aside, it is also implicated as a factor in glaucoma.[72]

Optometrists should consider adding questions about consumption of foods and drinks containing excitotoxins to their patient questionnaire. This measure could be helpful in pinpointing a possible cause of a variety of visual and other neurological disturbances, as well as raise awareness of potential health hazards in patients who drink diet sodas and use many processed foods.

Chemicals as endocrine disruptors According to Theo Colburn, main author of *Our Stolen Future*,[73] chemicals such as PBDEs disrupt the endocrine system of the body, setting off a cascade of unnatural reactions, leading to sickness and even death. Other chemical offenders are: perchlorates, substances in drinking water, which disrupt the action of the thyroid in directing brain development, and Bisphenol A, a by-product of making plastic, which activates genes involved in regulating brain growth. Excitotoxins are also endocrine disruptors. MSG, aspartame and other additives can cause damage to the hypothalamus, thus impeding its hormone-producing abilities, and thus indirectly affecting fertility.[67 (p. 80)]

Toxic metals Pre-natal exposures to toxins are not just to chemicals. The metals most implicated in autism spectrum disorders are:
- *Lead from the soil, food products and chipping paint.* According to the CDC and the U.S. Public Health Service, the devastating effects of lead on mental and physical development is one of society's most devastating environmental disease of young children.[74]
- *Aluminum from cans, cookware, antacids, anti-perspirants and vaccines.* Aluminum has no recognized biologic function. Studies relate elevated aluminum to memory and learning impairments.[75]
- *Antimony from flame-retardants in sleepwear, bedding, carpets and textiles.* All "mattresses" are required by law to be fire proof, which necessitates the use of antimony. A way to avoid this problem is buy a futon, which can be made of 100% organic cotton, because it is not officially a "mattress."
- *Arsenic from flame retardants & pressure-treated wood used in playgrounds, fungicides, herbicides, corrosion inhibitors, and in lead and copper alloys.* Arsenic is also high in some seafood, and may also come from animals, such as chickens, that are fed arsenic in their feed.
- *Cadmium from cigarette smoke and alloys used in plumbing.*[76]

Figure 3-2. Sources of Mercury[77]

Adhesives	Gas meter pressure device	Pesticides
Agricultural chemicals	Glue	Photoprocessing solutions
Air bag sensors	Gun powder	Pigments: Reds and Oranges
Air conditioner filters	Gyroscopes	Pipes
Ajax Powder	Haemophilus vaccine	Plastics
Amalgams	Hair tonics	Plants
Anti-mildew paints	Headlights	Plumbing-piping
Antiseptic	Hepatitis vaccine	Pharmaceuticals
Auto exhaust	Hepatitis B (test)	Polishes
Barometers	Hepatitis C (test)	Pollution
Batteries	HIV (test)	Porcelain
Bilirubin blue lamp	Iodine stain	Potions
Bleached flour	Influenza vaccine	Power plants
Blood Bank Saline	Insecticides	Pregnancy kit
Blood gas analyzer	Ivory Liquid	Preservatives
Bronzing	Jewelry from Mexico	Printing
Bug zapper	Joy Dishwashing Liquid	Processed foods
B5 Fixative	Lamps	Progesterone
Cajal's	Latex Paint	Quicksilver
Calomel	Laxatives	Quicksilver Maze
Cinnabar	Lysol Direct	Rabies vaccine
Cleaning bleach	Mascara	Radar
Cleaning detergent	Medical waste incinerators	Radio
Commercial cleaning soap	Mercurochrome	Scouring powder
Comet Cleaner	Mercury ammonium chloride	Shooting galleries
Cosmetics	Mercury arc	Silvering mirrors
Dental amalgams	Mercury barometer	Skin bleaching reams
Dove Soap	Mercury bromide	Sodium hydroxide
Etch-a-sketch	Mercury chloride	Sodium/Potassium
Exhaust fumes	Mercury fluoride	Soft Dish soap
Explosives	Mercury fulminate	Soft Scrub
Eye area cosmetics	Mercury iodide	Solvents
Fabric softeners	Mercury hydride	Switches
Feeding Tubes	Mercury nitrate	Auto seat belt
Felt	Mercury oxide	Takata's reagent
Fertilizers	Mercury sulfide	Talcam Powder
Finger print powder	Mercury selenide	Tanning Leather
Fish	Mercury telluride	Tattoo pigments
Fixatives	Methiolate	Telescope mirror
Electronic Ignition pilot - ranges	Miller Abbott Tubes	Tetanus vaccine
Flooring	Milton's reagent	Thermometers
Floor waxes	Mucolex	Thermostats
Flu shots	Murphy's Oil Soap	Tincture of merthiolate
Fluorescent lights	Nasal Spray	Tissue stains
FTA buffer	Neon lamps	Vaccines
Fuel cells	Nitrogen-ammonia	Vapor lamps
Exhaust hoods	Nuclear coolants	Water pollution
Eye drops	Ohlamacher fixative	Water treatment chemicals
Fungicides	Pastes	Welding
Furs	Pertussis vaccine	Wood Preservatives

And one the most toxic substances on the planet, especially to the developing brain:

• *Mercury.* Figure 3-2 details the many, many sources of mercury.

Sometime in late 1999, three families, all with children who regressed into autism, started delving into the possible sources of their children's illness. Sallie Bernard, Lyn Redwood and Albert Enayati had never met, but corresponded, comparing notes about their children. After attending a conference on biomedical approaches to autism, they came away convinced that their children were suffering from mercury poisoning. Furthermore, they believed then, as thousands of others believe now, that the main source of mercury was from vaccines their children had received. After much research, they wrote a joint paper with a physician and scientist.[78] A synopsis (see Appendix) is reprinted at the end of this chapter with permission from the authors.

Shortly after the publication of "Autism: A Unique Type of Mercury Poisoning," the authors formalized their relationship with the founding of The Coalition of SafeMinds (Sensible Action For Ending Mercury-Induced Neurological DisorderS). SafeMinds is a private, non-profit organization whose mission is to investigate and raise awareness of the risks to infants and children of exposure to mercury from medical products. The compelling story of the mercury/vaccine/autism connection was the impetus for David Kirby's best-seller, *Evidence of Harm: Mercury in Vaccines and the Autism Epidemic, a Medical Controversy*.[79] Kirby, an investigative reporter who followed the thread of this intriguing story, and the compelling congressional hearings and alleged cover-up that followed, has become yet another hero in the autism world. Read more about mercury and vaccines in Chapter 4.

Timing of toxic exposure The most sensitive time for toxic assaults to young brains of children later diagnosed as autistic is during critical periods of rapid brain development. The blood brain barrier is not fully developed in the young to protect against toxins that enter the blood. Mothers who have had years of toxic exposure themselves, pass two thirds of their toxic load through the placenta into their babies during pregnancy. The first-born child is often more severely affected than subsequent ones.[80]

An Rh-positive baby born to an Rh-negative mother who received Rhogam containing Thimerosal, and who has a mouth full of mercury-containing amalgams is exposed to many micrograms of mercury pre-natally. Even before leaving the womb, its "total load" is nearing its body's threshold. Add to this infant's load a few more micrograms of mercury within hours of birth, from the hepatitis B vaccine, and that baby has a 70% chance of having autism.[81]

Courchesne and his colleagues at the University of California, San Diego, link autism to an unusual pattern of brain growth shortly after birth. Infants who later develop autism have a slightly reduced head circumference at birth, compared to normal infants, but undergo a rapid spurt in growth during the first two years of life. By age three, autistic children's brains are larger than normal.[82] Colburn relates these findings to the possible disruption of the pace and pattern of brain development by the above-named contaminants that have become increasingly widespread over the past two decades, the same period that autism has become more common.[73]

Dosage of exposure determines toxicity Pound for pound, children eat, drink and breathe more than adults, making many infants' exposure to toxins disproportionately high. What constitutes toxicity depends upon the weight of the person. When those "trace" amounts of mercury from the thimerosal in the vaccines given to tiny babies in the first six months of life were added up, the sum equaled the effect of exposing a 200 pound man to 72 pounds of mercury![78]

As our knowledge about neurotoxic chemicals has increased, experts continuously revise "safe" thresholds of exposure downward. The legal standard for lead poisoning is well over

10 micrograms per deciliter (mg/dl) in most states. Research now shows that levels as low as 5 or 6 mg/dl can decrease a child's ability to read, write and calculate.[83]

Oxidative stress Too many load factors stress out the body through a chemical process called oxidation. Stress occurring at a cellular level is called "oxidative stress." Toxins from the environment and by-products of the body's normal metabolism can act as oxidants, and overwhelm the body's natural defenses. The body fights off oxidants with compounds called "anti-oxidants," which include vitamins and minerals from food and special enzymes which the body makes. When health is good, anti-oxidants outnumber oxidants. When oxidants prevail, cells suffer oxidative stress.[84]

Those with autism spectrum disorders are likely to have oxidative stress because they have both high levels of toxins and low levels of anti-oxidants. Most readers are probably familiar with the anti-oxidants, vitamins A, C, E and selenium. Another less well-known, but essential anti-oxidant is glutathione. More about glutathione, which is very important for removing heavy metals, follows in the section on "Detoxification."

Metallothionein (MT) disorder William Walsh, PhD, of the Pfeiffer Treatment Center, near Chicago, believes that Metallothionein (MT) disorder plays a role in autism. MT proteins are versatile chains of amino acids present in cells of the brain, skin and gastrointestinal tract. They assist in:
- Developing and pruning brain neurons
- Balancing copper and zinc levels
- Detoxifying heavy metals
- Supporting immune function
- Preventing yeast overgrowth
- Producing enzymes to break down peptides
- Improving memory and socialization
- Maintaining proper glutathione function.

Heavy metals are "enveloped" or "bound" by metallothionein (MT) proteins, which supervise and regulate metal levels in the body. The various metals in the body compete with each other for participation in chemical reactions and can displace each other depending on local concentration and their relative position in the chemical activity series. Thus, an overload or deficiency of one metal can alter the concentration and functioning of other metals. Persons with a metal-metabolism disorder accumulate, rather than eliminate, these toxins. MTs can bring zinc to a tissue or cell where the local glutathione molecules can grab it; or the reverse can occur: extra zinc is offloaded via glutathione to MT.

Consequences of MT dysfunction include:
- **Heavy metal toxicity.** MT is the body's primary protection against heavy metals: a magnet for mercury, lead and cadmium. Intestinal MT provides a barrier to absorption of ingested toxic metals. Once bound to MT, toxic metals become inactive. Without the MT barrier, heavy metals "leak" into the body.
- **Copper//Zinc imbalances.** Dr. Walsh reports that 85% of his sample of 603 patients with autism showed a significant copper overload and zinc depletion, when compared to healthy controls matched for age and gender. He found a statistical difference at a p=.0001 level. Imbalanced Cu/Zn impairs the hippocampus and amygdala, which monitor social-emotional function. Patients thus have a bio-chemical tendency for emotional meltdowns and attentional deficits.
- **Gluten/Casein sensitivities.** Digestion of casein and gluten peptides depends on zinc-dependent enzymes. Severe zinc depletion impedes the production of these enzymes. Thus a gluten-free casein-free diet is necessary.

- **Intestinal problems.** MT combats inflammation in the gut. Those with MT dysfunction experience candida overgrowth and reduced production of stomach acid. The stomach also has impaired secretin signaling and incomplete food processing.

If over-exposure to toxins at critical periods of development raises the risk of autism, why doesn't everyone who has been highly exposed become autistic, have attention deficits or learning/behavioral disorders? Because exposure is only half the story. The strength of each individual body's ability to detoxify potentially dangerous chemicals and toxins is the other half. Most people on the autism spectrum have problems related to detoxification because the immune, gastro-intestinal, nervous and detoxification systems overlap and load onto each other.

Detoxification Human bodies have built-in detoxification systems. Detoxification is the body's way of neutralizing, processing and eliminating harmful substances. The liver, an extremely complex organ involved in over 300 different functions, does most of the work.

Scientists divide the liver detoxification process into two phases. In Phase I, nutrients in the body convert toxins into less harmful substances and prepare them for elimination. Phase II is the actual elimination phase. In their book, *7-Day Detox Miracle*,[85] Bennett and Barrie compare detoxification to a two-phase wash cycle.

- *Phase One* – First, cells must be cajoled into breaking down stored toxins into intermediate forms; anti-oxidants facilitate this process. Supplementing glutathione, zinc, magnesium, taurine and other essential nutrients assist in breaking down and releasing stored-up toxins. Doctors have discovered many ways to deliver these nutrients to the cells and urge the toxins to leave. Chapter 5 covers this process in depth.

A few toxins are ready for removal at this stage, but others need a second wash cycle. If the process stops after Phase One, sickness, and even death can occur, because bad toxins are floating around wreaking havoc with all systems of the body.

- *Phase Two*, during which the goal is to excrete these toxins safely, usually in partnership with an "escort" nutrient, is more complicated. Six steps: methylation, sulfation, acetylation, glutathione conjugation, amino acid conjugation, and glucuronidation comprise Phase 2 detoxification. Five of the six pathways are dependent upon sulfur chemistry. Since this process is so very complicated, not all of it will be covered here. Those with a background in biochemistry might be interested in reading Dr. Sidney Baker's *Detoxification and Healing*.[86] For others, here are the highlights:

Methylation – The process of methylation is key to detoxification. The sulfur amino acid methionine, (considered "the queen of amino acids" by Dr. Baker), gives away a methyl group and becomes "horrible homosysteine," a potentially toxic molecule. Homosysteine is then converted to back to methionine, a process dependent upon an ample supply of methyl B-12, which many of those with autism lack. Homocysteine can also be converted to cysteine, which requires ample vitamin B_6. See Chapter 6 for references on B_6 in autism.

Sulfation – Dr. Rosemary Waring's findings of low levels of PST enzyme in patients with autism[46] are key in understanding sulfation, because an overload of phenolics from foods, hormones and neurotransmitters contribute to defective sulfation. The research of Susan Owens further documents the role of aberrant sulfur chemistry in autism spectrum disorders.[87] Owens describes sulfur as "sticky molecules" that help cells adhere to one another. When sulfur metabolism or sulfation is lacking, cells "leak." Leakiness, or excessive permeability creates different problems in different parts of the body.

Leakiness in the gut lining, or "leaky gut" has already been covered. Leaky skin creates eczema; leakiness in the joints leads to arthritis; leakiness in mucus membranes creates otitis, sinusitis and rhinitis.

Proper sulfation requires the pathway to the production of sulfates to be functioning optimally. This pathway takes the amino acid cysteine through numerous steps to make sulfite, which is then processed into sulfate through an enzyme called sulfite oxidase. Many nutrient interactions must take place for this pathway to function properly. How sulfur-containing foods and supplements benefit patients with autism is covered in Chapter 5. Experienced clinicians know that they must use these co-factors carefully, as they can exacerbate yeast overgrowth.

Glutathione conjugation – Glutathione is a tri-peptide created by every cell of the body from the amino acids glycine, glutamic acid and cysteine. Glutathione binds with hundreds of environmental toxins, including the metals cadmium, lead and mercury, dragging them out of the blood to the liver, gall bladder and gut, through which the body excretes them. Each molecule of a toxin uses up a molecule of glutathione.[88] When levels of toxins are high, the body's store of glutathione becomes depleted.

Research shows that many of those with autism have deficiencies in both cysteine and methyl B-12, thus impeding Phase Two detoxification. Dr. Jill James and her colleagues at the University of Arkansas studied blood samples from 95 autistic children and 75 healthy children, and found that the children with autism had significantly lower blood levels of glutathione. They believe that the children's stores of glutathione were depleted by their over-exposure to mercury, specifically from thimerosal-containing vaccines. Furthermore, because high levels of oxidative stress are due to low glutathione levels, low glutathione is a contributor to the neurological, gastrointestinal and immune system problems seen in these children.[89] Go to Chapter 5, "A Biomedical Approach to Autism Spectrum Disorders" to learn how health care practitioners are raising glutathione levels by supplementing with TMG, folinic acid and methyl B-12, with remarkable results.

Back to the Immune System

The genetically vulnerable defense/immune systems of children on the autism spectrum eventually becomes exhausted from continuous efforts to ward off repeated assaults. A compromised immune system trying to function in a body also affected by other load factors may not be able to purge the system completely. Residual toxins in the body start affecting other systems, which also become inflamed, distressed, and dysfunctional.[90] Reactions to foods, pollens, chemicals, and pharmaceuticals accelerate; wheezing, croup and breathing problems worsen into asthma.

Immune system load factors are intimately related to toxicity and sensory factors. Toxins, such as mercury, disrupt every system of the body.[78] The immune system, vision, touch, movement and balance are all immature at birth and compete for the body's energy during those crucial first two years of life. In the presence of high levels of toxicity, little energy is left for the demanding tasks of processing sight, sound, touch and movement, let alone for language, feelings, social emotional cues and academics. Some sensory systems become hyper-vigilant and irritable; others turn off, appearing unresponsive to stimuli.

The bodies of children with autism are in a survival mode, putting all of their energy into just staying alive. Gradually, almost imperceptibly, as the physical body becomes over-whelmed, the brain is affected; cognitive and/or behavioral problems appear.[2] This internal survival state appears outwardly as distractibility, hyperactivity or lack of responsiveness.[91]

In order to determine how dysfunctional the immune system is for an individual child, an extensive medical and developmental history is essential. This must be an exhaustive look at such pre-natal, natal, environmental and social factors as exposure to medications; vaccine reactions; use of pesticides, chemicals, or tobacco; toxic building materials; pet products; travel; changes in environment and water. Some factors may be obvious, such as moving into an older house with lead paint, but others may be subtler, such as toxic lawn treatments that are daily tracked into the home. One family became sick when the fertilizer they had been using on their farm was unknowingly "cut" with recycled radioactive material. It took an extraordinary effort to trace the cause of illness and developmental problems in children to this source.

Although history taking alone is sometimes adequate to determine an appropriate treatment plan, laboratory testing is frequently necessary to confirm suspicions about gut flora, nutritional deficiencies, or the presence of toxic agents.

Laboratory Testing

Many children on the autism spectrum have had traditional laboratory testing, such as a complete blood count (CBC) and IgE scratch tests. Obviously, these are essential. Looking for answers only with these tests, however, is like looking in the kitchen for your underwear: you are in the wrong room.

Fortunately, many specialized laboratories have developed hundreds of very sophisticated blood, urine, hair and stool tests that pinpoint exactly what has gone awry with the immune, digestive and respiratory systems and detoxification pathways. Simplified methods, such as tape-on bags for urine samples from those who are not potty-trained, and home blood tests complete with a lance to prick a finger, make sample collection fairly easy.

Hair analysis, once considered unreliable, is now better understood. This testing method is useful for the detection of recent exposure to toxic metals such as aluminum, antimony, arsenic, cadmium, lead, and mercury. In a landmark hair analysis study completed on children with autism and their typical siblings, researchers were astounded to find that the unaffected children showed higher levels of toxic metals in their hair than the affected ones. Why? Because the bodies of the normal kids had a strong ability to detoxify and excrete the poisons, while those with autism still harbored the mercury and other metals in their bodies. Only with "challenge" tests, using a chelator, which bound itself to the toxic metals, were the scientists able to show that those with autism also had high levels of toxic metals hiding in their bodies.[92]

Each health care professional has his/her favorite lab for each test. Some labs specialize in one of the tests, and do not offer others. Other labs offer all the tests. Doctors interested in which labs offer which tests should consult the *Defeat Autism Now!* manual.[93]

Most physicians order tests that measure the following:
- strength of both immediate and delayed systemic responses to various common foods,
- gluten and casein peptides
- the presence of abnormal organic acids associated with yeast, fungal and clostridia metabolism
- undesirable invaders such as intestinal parasites, bad bacteria, yeast and viruses
- amino acids and fatty acids
- unusually high antibody titers resulting from markedly abnormal responses to childhood immunizations, including MMR, DPT, and oral polio
- A$_6$ titers to various pathogens such as Lyme, Bartonella, Babesia, Mycoplasma, Strep, Cytomegalo virus, and Human Herpes virus 6.

- Xenobiotic (environmental toxin) levels
- Amonia/blood
- excessive levels of toxic metals, and deficiencies of essential minerals
- total immuno globulins and lymphocyte levels

Deciding which tests to do and which labs to use is a balancing act weighing the expense of tests with their usefulness in diagnosing the cause of symptoms. Convenience, time and expense all play a role. A doctor's prescription is necessary to run most tests. Because one approach never fits all cases, it is impossible to list a "standard" test protocol. Dr. Jacqueline McCandless, author of *Children with Starving Brains*[74] recommends the following tests for a complete look.

Comprehensive or basic IgG food allergy and inhalants (blood) – The impact of food allergies on behavior can be profound. Foods that show up as offenders on this test are often the very same ones a child craves. An IgG panel of about 100 food products, including gluten and casein proteins, can be extremely helpful. A basic test of the 10 most common allergies is also available. Most labs rate food sensitivities 0-4, where the highest number requires strict avoidance, and the lowest is no reaction. In between, foods can be consumed once in awhile, rotated, or avoided, except on occasion. Pinpointing allergies to specific inhalants, such as dust, molds, and pollens are especially beneficial for prescribing avoidance and treatment.

Organic acids test (urine) – The Organic Acids Test (OAT) is the most accurate measure of candida, which can sometimes attach to the intestinal lining, not be eliminated in the stool, and thus not show up on a stool culture test. In some cases, the sections of stool where the yeast is present are not the sections that are collected and sent in to be analyzed.

Virtually all children with autism have one or more abnormal Organic Acid compounds, due to abnormal levels of yeast and other gastrointestinal bacteria. These compounds can affect, among other things, neurological functioning, vitamin utilization, energy level, intestinal wall integrity, hormone utilization, and muscle function. In addition to identification of excessive levels of GI yeast or bacteria, the test also reveals nutritional or antioxidant deficiencies, inborn errors of metabolism, amino or fatty acid problems, exposure to solvent toxins, indications of possible diabetic conditions, deficiencies of B or C vitamins, and unusual levels of neurotransmitters. Re-test about four to six months after the start of treatment, mainly to refine the treatment.

Comprehensive stool analysis with parasitology (stool) – Tests for parasites, yeast, bad bacteria, good bacteria, inflammation, allergy markers, bile acids and proper digestion of food.

Immune deficiency panel (blood) – Immunoglobulin levels of total IgE, IgG, IgA and IgM are necessary to determine whether all aspects of the immune system are functioning properly. Tests can also include subclasses of IgG and IgA. Th1 and Th2 panels give clinicians information about both arms of the immune system. Some order antibody levels of certain bacteria, viruses and fungi to determine if the body is actively fighting infection. Many look also at antibody levels against vaccines, such as MMR, DPT, Hepatitis B and polio. A large number of those on the autism spectrum show exceptionally high numbers, indicating that their bodies are still fighting against the pathogens in the vaccines, even if it was given years prior. Other kids show no antibodies, even though they have had several booster shots.

Heavy metals (blood, hair, urine or stool) – Porphyrins, baseline and periodic metal testing is essential in determining the benefit of the various treatments in Chapter 5. Since many children with autism are showing a favorable response to various forms of removal of toxic metals,   monitoring with this test is very helpful. It also shows what the metals are doing to the minerals in the body, such as magnesium and zinc, as toxins tend to deplete the body of essential minerals.

Amino acid analysis (blood) –This test looks at essential amino acids, which are the building blocks of all proteins in the body, such as hormones, enzymes, muscles and cartilage. It also looks at amino acids and peptides, that the body produces, which are important in neurotransmitter metabolism.

Homocysteine (blood) – an important marker measuring the efficiency of methylation.

Vitamin and mineral panel (blood) – This test checks the status of vitamins A, E and beta carotene. Red blood cell testing also measures minerals such as zinc, magnesium, selenium, calcium and molybdenum actually inside the cells.

Fatty acid analysis (blood) – Most kids are deficient in omega 3 fats, and some with malabsorption may also have deficiencies in other essential fatty acids.

Thyroid function (blood or saliva) – A look at the thyroid can suggest what disruption has occurred in the endocrine system. Auto-antibodies to thyroid and low grade hypothyroidism are both common in the ASD population.

McCandless suggests that the last four can wait if finances prohibit doing all at once.

Summary and Conclusions
The concept of "Total Load" helps to bring together a coherent theory of etiology: one where each of the different aspects of autism contributes a piece to the puzzle, and none is the single cause of the disorders. Immunological, biological, neurological, toxicological, sensory, motor, language, psychological, energetic and other factors interact, affecting each other in extremely complex synergies that researchers are only beginning to understand. These pre-, peri- and post-natal factors influence all aspects of structure and function.

What we call "autism" or "PDD," "LD" or "AD(H)D" may very well be the end product of many systems of the body being stressed to their limits. The larger the load of problematic factors on the child's overall system, the more severe the attention, behavior and cognitive difficulties. With "Total Load" theory, many etiologies to the epidemic of autism are possible.

APPENDIX
Autism: A Unique Type of Mercury Poisoning
(Synopsis)
By Sallie Bernard, Albert Enayati, BS, ChE, MSME,
Teresa Binstock, Heidi Roger, Lyn Redwood, RN, MSN, CRNP, and
Woody McGinnis, MD
August 25, 2000
Reprinted with permission

Instances of mercury poisoning or "mercurialism" have been described since Roman times. The Mad Hatter in *Alice in Wonderland* was a victim of occupational exposure to mercury vapor, referred to as "Mad Hatter's Disease." Further human data has been derived from instances of widespread poisonings during the 20th Century. These misfortunes include an outbreak in Minamata, Japan, caused by consumption of contaminated fish and resulting in "Minamata Disease;" outbreaks in Iraq, Guatemala and Russia due to ingestion of contaminated seed grains; and, in the first half of the century, poisoning of infants and toddlers by mercury in teething powders, leading to acrodynia or "Pink Disease." Besides these

Summary of Mercury Exposure Variables Leading to Diverse & Non-Specific Symptomatology	
Variable	**Level of Variable**
Exposure Amount	Ranges from high doses, leading to death or near death with severe impairments, to low "safe" doses, leading to subtle neurological and other physical impairments Duration of exposure One time vs. multiple times over the course of weeks, months, or years
Dose rate	Bolus dose, daily dose
Individual sensitivity	A function of (a) the age at which exposure occurs, that is, prenatal, infant, child, adolescent, or adult, (b) genetically determined reactivity to mercury, and (c) gender
Common types of mercury	The organic alkyl forms – methyl-mercury and ethyl-mercury; and inorganic forms - metallic mercury, elemental (liquid) mercury, and ionic mercury/mercuric salt
Primary routes of exposure	Inhalation of mercury vapors, orally through the intestinal tract, subcutaneous and intramuscular injections, topically through ear drops, teething powders, skin creams and ointments, and intravenously during medical treatments

epidemics, numerous instances of individual or small group cases of Hg intoxication are described in the literature.

The constellation of mercury-induced symptoms varies enormously from individual to individual. The diversity of disease manifestations derives from a number of interacting variables which are summarized in the table below. Variables which affect individuals include age, the total dosage, dose rate, duration of exposure, type of mercury, routes of exposure such as inhaled, subcutaneous, oral, or intramuscular, and, most importantly, by individual sensitivity arising from immune and genetic factors.

Mercury (Hg) is a toxic metal that can exist as a pure element or in a variety of inorganic and organic forms and can cause immune, sensory, neurological, motor, and behavioral dysfunctions similar to traits defining or associated with autism. A review of medical literature indicates that the characteristics of autism and of mercury poisoning (HgP) are strikingly similar. Traits defining or associated with both disorders are summarized in the table immediately following. The parallels between the two diseases are so thorough as to suggest, based on total Hg injected into U.S. children, that many cases of autism are a form of mercury poisoning.

For these children, the exposure route is childhood vaccines, most of which contain thimerosal, a preservative which is 49.6% ethyl-mercury by weight. Over the last decade, the amount of mercury a typical child under two years received from vaccinations equated to 237.5 micrograms injected in several bolus (or large) doses.

The total amount injected into infants and toddlers is known to exceed Federal safety standards, is officially considered to be a "low" level; whereby only a small percentage of exposed individuals exhibit symptoms of toxicity. In fact, children who develop Hg-related autism are likely to have had a predisposition derived from genetic and non-genetic factors.

Importantly, the timings of vaccinal Hg-exposure and its latency period coincide with the emergence of autistic-symptoms in specific children. Moreover, excessive mercury has been detected in urine, hair, and blood samples from autistic children; and parental reports, though limited at this date, indicate significant improvement in symptoms subsequent to heavy-metal chelation therapy.

The pathology arising from the mercury-related variables involved in autism – intermittent bolus doses of ethyl-mercury injected into susceptible infants and toddlers – is heretofore undescribed in medical literature. Therefore, in accord with existing HgP data and HgP's ability to induce virtually all the traits defining or associated with autism spectrum disorders, we hypothesize that many and perhaps most cases of autism represent a unique form of mercury poisoning.

Summary Comparison of Characteristics of Autism & Mercury Poisoning

	Mercury Poisoning	Autism
Impairments in sociability	Social deficits, shyness, social withdrawal	Social deficits, shyness, social withdrawal
	Depression, mood swings; mask face	Depression, mood swings; mask face
	Anxiety	Anxiety
	Lacks eye contact, hesitant to engage others	Lack of eye contact, avoids conversation
	Irrational fears	Irrational fears
	Irritability, aggression, temper tantrums	Irritability, aggression, temper tantrums
	Impaired face recognition	Impaired face recognition
	Schizoid tendencies, OCD traits	Schizoid tendencies, OCD traits
	Repetitive, penseverative, stereotypic behaviors	Repetitive, penseverative, stereotypic behaviors
Speech & Language Deficits	Loss of speech, failure to develop speech	Loss of speech, failure to develop speech
	Dysarthria; articulation problems	Dysarthria; articulation problems
	Speech comprehension deficits	Speech comprehension deficits
	Verbalizing & word retrieval problems	Echolalia; word use & pragmatic errors
	Hearing loss; deafness in very high doses	Mild to profound hearing loss
	Poor performance on language IQ tests	Poor performance on verbal IQ tests
Sensory Abnormalities	Abnormal sensation in mouth & extremities	Abnormal sensation in mouth & extremities
	Sound sensitivity	Sound sensitivity
	Abnormal touch sensations; touch aversion	Abnormal touch sensations; touch aversion
	Vestibular abnormalities	Vestibular abnormalities
	Impaired visual fixation	Problems with joint attention
Motor Disorders	Involuntary jerking movements – arm flapping, ankle jerks, myoclonal jerks, choreiform movements, circling, rocking	Stereotyped movements - arm flapping, jumping, circling, spinning, rocking; myoclonal jerks; choreiform movements
	Deficits in eye-hand coordination; limb apraxia; intention tremors	Poor eye-hand coordination; limb apraxia; problems with intentional movements
	Gait impairment; ataxia – from incoordination & clumsiness to inability to walk, stand, or sit; loss of motor control	Abnormal gait and posture, clumsiness and incoordination; difficulties sitting, lying, crawling, and walking
	Difficulty in chewing or swallowing	Difficulty in chewing or swallowing
	Unusual postures; toe walking	Unusual postures; toe walking

Cognitive Impairments	Borderline intelligence, mental retardation - some cases reversible	Borderline intelligence, mental retardation - sometimes "recovered"
	Poor concentration, attention, response inhibition	Poor concentration, attention, shifting attention
	Uneven performance on IQ subtests	Uneven performance on IQ subtests
	Verbal IQ higher than performance IQ	Verbal IQ higher than performance IQ
	Poor short term, verbal, & auditory memory	Poor short term, verbal, & auditory memory
	Poor visual and perceptual motor skills, impairment in simple reaction time	Poor visual and perceptual motor skills, lower performance on timed tests
	Difficulty carrying out complex commands	Difficulty carrying out multiple commands
	Word-comprehension difficulties	Word-comprehension difficulties
	Deficits in understanding abstract ideas & symbolism; degeneration of higher mental powers	Deficits in abstract thinking & symbolism, understanding other's mental states, sequencing, planning & organizing
Unusual Behaviors	Stereotyped sniffing (rats)	Stereotyped, repetitive behaviors
	AD(H)D traits	AD(H)D traits
	Agitation, unprovoked crying, grimacing, staring spells	Agitation, unprovoked crying, grimacing, staring spells
	Sleep difficulties	Sleep difficulties
	Eating disorders, feeding problems	Eating disorders, feeding problems
	Self injurious behavior, e.g. head banging	Self injurious behavior, e.g. head banging
Visual Disturbances	Increase in cerebral palsy; hyper- or hypotonia; abnormal reflexes; decreased muscle strength, especially upper body; incontinence; problems chewing, swallowing, salivating	Increase in cerebral palsy; hyper- or hypotonia; decreased muscle strength, especially upper body; incontinence; problems chewing and swallowing
	Rashes, dermatitis/dry skin, itching; burning	Rashes, dermatitis, eczema, itching
	Autonomic disturbance: excessive sweating, poor circulation, elevated heart rate	Autonomic disturbance: unusual sweating, poor circulation, elevated heart rate
Gastro-intestinal Disturbances	Gastroenteritis, diarrhea; abdominal pain, constipation, "colitis"	Diarrhea, constipation, gaseousness, abdominal discomfort, colitis
	Anorexia, weight loss, nausea, poor appetite	Anorexia; feeding problems/vomiting
	Lesions of ileum & colon; increased gut permeability	Leaky gut syndrome
	Inhibits dipeptidyl peptidase IV, which cleaves casomorphin	Inadequate endopeptidase enzymes needed for breakdown of casein & gluten
Abnormal Biochemistry	Binds -SH groups; blocks sulfate transporter in intestines, kidneys	Low sulfate levels
	Has special affinity for purines & pyrimidines	Purine & pyrimidine metabolism errors lead to autistic features
	Reduces availability of glutathione, needed in neurons, cells & liver to detoxify heavy metals	Low levels of glutathione; decreased ability of liver to detoxify heavy metals
	Causes significant reduction in glutathione peroxidase and glutathione reductase	Abnormal glutathione peroxidase activities in erythrocytes
	Disrupts mitochondrial activities, especially in brain	Mitochondrial dysfunction, especially in brain

Immune Dysfunction	Sensitivity due to allergic or autoimmune reactions; sensitive individuals more likely to have allergies, asthma, autoimmune-like symptoms, especially rheumatoid-like ones	More likely to have allergies and asthma; familial presence of autoimmune diseases, especially rheumatoid arthritis; IgA deficiencies
	Can produce an immune response in CNS	On-going immune response in CNS
	Causes brain/MBP autoantibodies	Brain/MBP autoantibodies present
	Causes overproduction of Th2 subset; kills/inhibits lymphocytes, T-cells, and monocytes; decreases NK T-cell activity; induces or suppresses IFNg & IL-2	Skewed immune-cell subset in the Th2 direction; decreased responses to T-cell mitogens; reduced NK T-cell function; increased IFNg & IL-12
CNS Structural Pathology	Selectively targets brain areas unable to detoxify or reduce Hg-induced oxidative stress	Specific areas of brain pathology; many functions spared
	Damage to Purkinje and granular cells, brainstem, corpus callosum, basal glangia, cerebral cortex	Damage to Purkinje and granular cells, brainstem, corpus callosum, basal glangia, cerebral cortex
	Accummulates in amygdala and hippocampus	Pathology in amygdala and hippocampus
	Causes abnormal neuronal cytoarchitecture; disrupts neuronal migration & cell division; reduces NCAMs	Neuronal disorganization; increased neuronal cell replication, increased glial cells; depressed expression of NCAMs
	Progressive microcephaly	Progressive microcephaly and macrocephaly
Abnormalities in Neurochemistry	Prevents presynaptic serotonin release & inhibits serotonin transport; causes calcium disruptions	Decreased serotonin synthesis in children; abnormal calcium metabolism
	Alters dopamine systems; peroxidine deficiency in rats resembles mercurialism in humans	Possibly high or low dopamine levels; positive response to peroxidine (lowers dopamine levels)
	Elevates epinephrine & norepinephrine levels by blocking enzyme that degrades epinephrine	Elevated norepinephrine and epinephrine
	Elevates glutamate	Elevated glutamate and aspartate
	Leads to cortical acetylcholine deficiency; increases muscarinic receptor density in hippocampus & cerebellum	Cortical acetylcholine deficiency; reduced muscarinic receptor binding in hippocampus
	Causes demyelinating neuropathy	Demyelination in brain
Neuro-physiology	Causes seizures, convulsions	Abnormal EEGs, epileptiform activity
	Causes abnormal EEGs, epileptiform activity	Seizures; epilepsy
	Causes variable patterns, eg, subtle, low amplitude seizure activity	Variable patterns, eg, subtle, low amplitude seizure activities
Population-Characteristics	Effects more males than females	Male:female ratio estimated at 4:1
	At low doses, only affects those geneticially susceptible	High heritability - concordance for MZ twins is 90%
	First added to childhood vaccines in 1930s	First "discovered" among children born in 1930s
	Exposure levels steadily increased since 1930s with rate of vaccination, number of vaccines	Prevalence of autism has steadily increased from 1 in 2000 (pre1970) to 1 in 500 (early 1990s), higher in 2000
	Exposure occurs at 0 - 15 months; clinical silent stage means symptom emergence delayed; symptoms emerge gradually, starting with movement & sensation	Symptoms emerge from 4 months to 2 years old; symptoms emerge gradually, starting with movement & sensation

This conclusion that autism is a unique type of mercury poisoning has important implications for individuals with autism and their families, for other unexplained disorders with symptoms similar to those of heavy metal intoxication, for vaccine content, and for childhood vaccination programs. Due to its high potential for neurotoxicity, the authors believe that thimerosal should be removed immediately from all vaccine products designated for infants and toddlers.

References

1. Dorfman K. Why so many children have developmental problems: the total load theory. New Dev 1996 Winter;1:4.

2. Rapp DJ. Is this your child? New York, NY: Morrow, 1991.

3. Dorfman K, Lemer PS, Nadler J. What puts a child at risk for developmental delays? Unpublished survey of Developmental Delay Resources (DDR), Pittsburgh, PA, 1995.

4. Kavner RS. Your Child's Vision, New York: Simon and Schuster, 1985.

5. Frymann VM. Birth trauma: the most common cause of developmental delays. New Dev 1996 Summer; 1(4):6.

6. Caskey R. Treating candida with chiropractic kinesiology. Lecture delivered at the DDR conference, Stamford, CT, March, 1996.

7. Block MA. No More Ritalin: Treating AD(H)D without Drugs. New York, Kensington Books, 1996.

8. Upledger J. Your Inner Physician and You. Berkeley, CA: North Atlantic Books, 1991.

9. Goddard S. Reflexes, Learning and Behavior. Eugene, OR. Fern Ridge Press, 2005:129.

10. Warren RP, Margaretten N, Pace N, Foster A. Immune abnormalities in patients with autism. J Autism Dev Dis 1986;16:189-97.

11. Gupta S, Aggarwal S. Heads C. Dysregulated immune system in children with autism: beneficial effects of intravenous immune globulin on autistic characteristics. J Autism Dev Dis 1996;26(4):439-52.

12. Warren RP, Singh VK, Avere H, et al. Immunogenetic studies in autism and related disorders. Molec Clin Neuropathol 1996;28:77-81.

13. Jyonouchi H, Sun S, Itokazu N. Inate immunity associated with inflammatory responses and cytokine production against common dietary proteins in patients with autism spectrum disorders. Neuropsychobiol 2002;46:76-84.

14. Vargas DL, Nascimbene C, Krishnan C, Zimmerman AW, Pardo CA.Neuroglial Activation and Neuroinflammation in the Brain of Patients with Autism. Annals of Neurology 2005 January;57:1,67-81.

15. Children with autism have distinctly different immune system reactions compared to typical children. www.EurekAlert.org (Accessed January 7, 2008)

16. El-Dahr JM. Immunologic Issues in Autism. Lecture delivered at the Defeat Autism Now! (DAN!) Conference, April, 2004, Washington, DC.

17. Konstantareas TM, Homatidis S.. Ear infections in autistic and normal children. J Autism Dev Dis, 1987;17:585.

18. Nsouli et al. The role of food allergy in serious otitis media. Ann Allergy 1991;66:91.

19. Paradise JL, Feldman HM, Campbell TF, Dollaghan CA, et al. Tympanostomy tubes and developmental outcomes at 9 to 11 years of age. N E J Med 2007 Jan 18;356:248-61.

20. Dorfman K. Post-traumatic ear infection syndrome. New Dev 2004 Spring;93:7.

21. Haley BE. Toxic overload: assessing the role of mercury in autism. Mothering 2002 Nov/Dec;115:44-46.

22. http://intramural.nimh.nih.gov/pdn/web.htm. The official PANDAS webpage. (Accessed January 9, 2008)

23. www.neuraltherapy.com. Lyme disease: A Look Beyond Antibiotics. 1/7/05. (Accessed January 9, 2008)

24. Schmidt. Healing Childhood Ear Infections: Prevention, Home Care and Alternative Treatment. Berkeley, CA: North Atlantic Books, 1996.

25. Schmidt MA, Smith LH, Sehnert KW. Beyond Antibiotics. Berkeley, CA: North Atlantic Books, 1994.

26. Levy SB. The Antibiotic Paradox: How the Misuse of Antibiotics Destroys their Curative Power. Cambridge, MA: Perseus Books, 2002.

27. Crook WG. The Yeast Connection Handbook. Jackson, TN, Professional Books, 1996.

28. Samonis G, Gikas A, Anaissie E. Prospective evaluation of the impact of broad-spectrum antibiotics on gastrointestinal yeast colonization of humans. Antimicrobial Agents and Chemotherapy 1993;37:51-3.

29. Crook WG. The Yeast Connection. New York, Vintage Books, 1986.

30. Crook WG. *The Yeast Connection and the Woman.* Jackson, TN, Professional Books, 1994.

31. Rimland B. Candida-caused autism. *Autism Res Rev* 1985;2:2-3.

32. Shaw W, Kassen E, Chaves E. Increased excretion of analogs of Krebs cycle metabolites and arabinose in two brothers with autistic features. *Clin Chem* 1995;41:1094-104.

33. Shaw W. *Biological Treatments for Autism and PDD.* Overland Park, KS, Great Plains Laboratory, 1998.

34. http://ww.autismcoach.com/stealth_virus.htm. Stealth Virus Theory. (Accessed January 9, 2008).

35. Wakefield A. Ileal-lymphoid-nodular hyperplasia, non-specific colitis, and pervasive developmental disorder in children. *The Lancet* 1998 351:637-41.

36. Singh VK, Lin SX, Yang VC. Serological association of measles virus and human herpes virus-6 with brain auto-antibodies in autism. *Clin Immunol Immunopathol* 1998 Oct;89:105-8.

37. Bradstreet JJ, El Dahr J, Anthony A, et al. Detection of measles virus genomic RNA in cerebrospinal fluid of children with regressive autism, a report of three cases. *J Am Physicians Surgeons.* 2004 Summer;9:38-45.

38. D'Eufemia.P. Celli M, Finocchiaro R, Pacifo L, et al. Abnormal intestinal permeability in children with autism. *Acta Paediatr* 1996 Sep;85(9):1076-9.

39. Lipski E. Leaky gut syndrome.In: A Keats Good Health Guide. Los Angeles, CA: Keats Publishing, 1998:7.

40. Gershon MD. *The Second Brain.* New York: Harper Perennial, 1998.

41. Tarasuk D. The poop on poop. *New Dev* 2005 Summer;10:6.

42. www.thoughtfulhouse.com Press release, July 12, 2005. (Accessed, October 23, 2005)

43. Rimland B. Autism researchers present explosive findings. *Autism Res Rev* 2002;16:1.

44. Buie T. *Oasis 2001 Conference for Autism.* Portland, OR, November, 2001.

45. Defelice K. *Enzymes for Autism and other Neurological Conditions: A Practical Guide for Digestive Enzymes and Better Behavior.* Johnston, IA: ThunderSnow Interactive, 2002:241-3.

46. Waring R. Enzyme and sulfur oxidation deficiencies in autistic children with known food/chemical intolerances. *Xenobiotica* 1990;20:117-22.

47. Feingold B. *Why Your Child is Hyperactive.* New York: Random House, 1975.

48. Brostoff J, Gamlin L. *Food Allergy and Intolerance.* London:Bloomsbury Press, 1989.

49. Harris RM, Picton R, Singh S, Waring RH. Activity of phenylsulfotransferases in the human gastrointestinal tract. *Life Sci* 2000 September;15:67:2051-7.

50. Swanson J, Kinsbourne M. Food dyes impair performance of hyperactive children on a laboratory learning test. *Sci* March 28, 1980;207:1485-7.

51. Egger J, Stolla A, McEwen LM. Controlled trial of hyposensitization in children with food-induced hyperkinetic syndrome. *The Lancet* 1992 May;339:1150-3.

52. Boris M, Mandel F. Foods and additives are common causes of the attention deficit hyperactivity disorder in children. *Ann allergy* 1994;72:462-8.

53. Rowe KS, Rowe KJ. Synthetic food coloring and behavior: a dose response effect in a double-blind, placebo-controlled, repeated-measures study. *J Pediatr* 1994 Nov;125:691-8.

54. Kaplan BJ, McNicol J, Conte RA, Moghadam HK. Dietary replacement in preschool-aged hyperactive boys. *Pediatrics* 1989 Jan;83(1):7-17.

55. Oski F. *Don't Drink Your Milk.* Syracuse, NY, Mollica Press, 1983.

56. American Academy of Pediatrics. *Guide to Your Child's Nutrition.* New York: Villard Books, 1999.

57. Panksepp J. A neurochemical theory of autism. *Trends Neurosci* 1979;2:174-7.

58. Reichelt KL, Ekrem J, Scott H. Gluten, milk proteins and autism: dietary intervention effects on behavior and peptide secretion. *J Applied Nutrition* 1990;42:1-11.

59. Reichelt KL, et al. Biologically active peptide containing fractions in schizophrenia and childhood autism. *Advances Biochem Psychopharmacol* 1981;28:627-43.

60. Shattock P, Lowdon G,. Proteins, peptides and autism. Part 2: Implications for the education and care of people with autism. *Brain Dys* 1991;4(6):323-34.

61. McCrone J. Gut reaction. Is food to blame for autism? *New Sci* 1998 Jun 20:42-5.

62. www.epa.gov/tri/tridata. (Accessed January 10, 2008)

63. Greater Boston Physicians for Social Responsibility. *In Harm's Way: Toxic threats to child development.* Boston, MA, 2000.

64. Baker SM. *Detoxification And Healing: The Key To Optimal Health.* New York: Contemporary Books, 2003:27.

65. www.nrdc.org. (Accessed January 10, 2008)

66. www.ourstolenfuture. (Accessed January 10, 2008)

67. www.ewg.org/reports/bodyburden2. Body Burden: Pollution in newborns. (Accessed January 10, 2008)

68. Darnerud PA,. et.al. Polybrominated diphenyl ethers: occurrence, dietary exposure, and toxicology. Environmental Health Perspectives, 109, Supplement 1, 2001 Mar:49-68.

69. http://www.ewg.org/reports/mothersmilk. (Accessed January 8, 2008)

70. Blaylock RL. Excitoxins: the Taste that Kills. Santa Fe, NM, Health Press, 1997.

71. www.mercola.com. Samuels. J. The Danger of MSG and how it is hidden in vaccines. (Accessed January 8, 2008)

72. www.mercola.com. Eye Damage from MSG. Accessed October 29, 2005.

73. Colburn T, Dumanoski, D Meyers JP. Our Stolen Future. New York, Plume/Penguin, 1997.

74. McCandless J. Children with Starving Brains, 2nd ed. Putney, VT, Bramble books, 2005.

75. www.mercola. Aluminum and the Prevention of Alzheimer's Disease. Accessed October 28, 2005.

76. Buttram HE, Piccola R. Who is Looking After our Children? Quakertown, PA, Foresight America Foundation, 1990.

77. www.merccuryexposure.org (Accessed January 8, 2008).

78. Bernard S. Autism: a novel form of mercury poisoning. Med Hypotheses 2001;56(4):462-71.

79. Kirby D. Evidence of Harm. Mercury in Vaccines and the Autism Epidemic, A Medical Controversy. New York, St. Martin's Press, 2005.

80. Klinghardt D. Conference: A Biomedical Approach to Autism. Phoenix, AZ, January 21, 2006.

81. Geier DA, Geier MR. A prospective study of thimerosal-containing Rho(D)-immune globulin administration as a risk factor for autistic disorders. J Matern Fetal Neonatal Med 200720:385-90.

82. Courchesne E, Carper R, Akshoomoff N. Evidence of Brain Overgrowth in the First Year of Life in Autism. JAMA 2003;290:337-44.

83. Lanphear BP, Dietrich K, Auinger P, Cox C. Cognitive deficits associated with blood lead concentrations <10 µg/dL in US children and adolescents. Public Health Reports 2000 Nov;115:521-29.

84. McGinnis W. Oxidative stress in autism. Altern Ther Health Med. 2004 Nov-Dec;10:22-36.

85. Bennet S, Barrie S. 7-Day Detox Miracle. New York, Three Rivers Press, 2001.

86. Baker SM. Detoxification and Healing, New York, Contemporary Books, 2003:138.

87. Owens SC. Understanding the Sulfur System. Spring Defeat Autism Now! 2003 Conference Proceedings, Philadelphia PA, May 16, 2003:65-76.

88. Rogers SA. Detoxify or Die. Sarasota, FL. Sand Key Company, 2002:48-49.

89. James SJ, Cutler P, Melnyk S, Hernigan S, et al.. . Metabolic biomarkers of increased oxidative stress and methylation capacity in children with autism. Am J Clin Nutrition 2004;80(6):1611-7.

90. Bock K. Healing the New Childhood Epidemics: Autism, ADHD, Asthma, Allergies. New York: Ballantine books, 2007.

91. Dorfman K. High functioning autism. The Townsend Newsletter for Doctors and Patients 1995;140:98-101.

92. Holmes AS, Blaxill MF, Haley BE. reduced levels of mercury in first baby haircuts of autistic children. Int J Toxicol 2003;22:277-85.

93. Pangborn J, Baker SM. Autism:Effective Biomedical Treatments. San Diego, CA, Autism Research Institute, Section 4, 2005.

Chapter 4
Autism: The Vaccine Connection

Barbara Loe Fisher

Introduction

I remember the day I took my two and a half year old son to the pediatrician for his fourth diphtheria-tetanus-pertussis (DPT) shot in the fall of 1980. Except for a milk allergy that had given him colic as an infant, Chris had been a lively, precocious, contented baby who always seemed to be doing things ahead of schedule. He began saying words at seven months and was speaking in full sentences by the age of two. At two and a half he knew his upper and lowercase alphabet, numbers up to 20 and had memorized all 52 cards in the deck. It never entered my mind that the DPT shot the nurse gave him would take all that away, changing his life and mine forever.

My pediatrician didn't mention vaccine reactions and I didn't think to ask. I knew vaccines were supposed to keep healthy people healthy, and I thought they were 100 percent safe and effective. So I didn't know that the red, hard, hot lump that came up at the site of the injection and stayed for weeks after Chris's third DPT shot was a warning sign he might be sensitive to DPT vaccine. I didn't know that, because he still had slight diarrhea after finishing a round of antibiotics prescribed for a 48-hour flu three weeks earlier, Chris might be at higher risk for having a vaccine reaction the day of his fourth DPT shot.

Several hours after we got home, I walked into Chris's bedroom and found him sitting in a rocking chair staring straight ahead like he couldn't see me standing in the doorway. His face was white and his lips were slightly blue. When I called out his name, his eyes fluttered and rolled back in his head. Then his head fell to his shoulder, as if he had suddenly fallen into a deep sleep sitting up.

When I lifted Chris to carry him to his bed, he was like a dead weight in my arms. Chris stayed in bed, without moving, for hours. Later that night, when I was finally able to wake him, he couldn't sit up or walk. I had to carry him to the bathroom, where he had severe diarrhea and then fell back into a deep sleep for 12 more hours.

That was in 1980, and the American public had not been told that vaccines had been causing brain inflammation and immune system damage for more than 200 years. For generations, mothers and fathers had watched their children get sick after smallpox or DPT vaccination and either die or later exhibit mild to severe brain and immune system damage. But they never knew that the cause of their children's deaths or permanent health problems could be traced back to a vaccine reaction.

When Chris regressed in the days and weeks after his fourth DPT shot and was no longer able to identify the alphabet or count to 20; when he could not concentrate for more than a few seconds at a time and cried or got angry at the slightest frustration; when he was constantly sick with respiratory and ear infections he did not have before the shot; when he had chronic diarrhea and stopped eating and growing; when he became a totally different child physically, mentally and emotionally, I eventually came to know why.

I finally realized why my once precocious son was diagnosed with minimal brain damage that took the form of multiple learning disabilities and attention deficit disorder because I was lucky enough to see the award winning television documentary, "DPT: Vaccine Roulette," in the spring of 1981. It was the first news report in the U.S. that alerted American parents to the long hidden dangers of the DPT vaccine.

Soon after, I began searching for the truth about vaccine risks I instinctively knew that the reason Chris regressed after his DPT shot was somehow connected to my family history of autoimmunity and the fact he had just come off a round of antibiotics the day he got his fourth DPT shot. My son was both genetically and biologically vulnerable to vaccine-induced brain and immune system dysfunction. Nobody, including me, knew.

In 1980, and today, a huge vacuum of scientific knowledge exists about why and how vaccines cause injury and death for some individuals. This chapter clarifies what is and is not known about vaccine-induced brain and immune system dysfunction leading to autism and other developmental delays. The truth about vaccine-associated autism will not be fully revealed until doctors inside and outside of government want to make it a priority, and commit the resources to search for it and take action once they understand it.

In the early 1980s, the Centers for Disease Control (CDC) and American Academy of Pediatrics (AAP) alternately either (a) denied publicly that the DPT vaccine could cause serious harm or (b) said that if DPT vaccine does cause harm it occurs so rarely it cannot be measured. I soon realized that what pediatricians and public health officials were really doing was writing off children like my son as "acceptable losses" in a mass, mandatory vaccination program that fails to make allowances for genetic differences and biological factors that increase the risk of vaccine induced brain and immune system damage for some children.

My son regressed after his fourth DPT shot and stopped just short of autism. He was left with dyslexia, attention deficit disorder, auditory processing deficits, short term memory, fine, gross motor, and other developmental delays. He and I both know he could have been hurt more seriously. Perhaps he was spared more severe damage because, on that day in 1980, he only received four vaccines: oral polio (OPV) and DPT. If he had been born in 1998 and not 1978, he could have received nine vaccines on one day: OPV, DPT, hepatitis B, measles, mumps, rubella (MMR), and chicken pox. He might well have become autistic, epileptic, severely mentally retarded or never awakened from his encephalopathic state of unconsciousness and died in his bed. I might never have known why.

Today, parents, doctors and their patients, are all well aware that vaccines can cause brain and immune system dysfunction. Today in the United States, Great Britain and around the world, parents and doctors are passionately debating a possible connection between autism and vaccines.

Many parents, who witness their healthy children regressing into autism following vaccination, adamantly insist their children are vaccine injured. The CDC, AAP, Food and Drug Administration (FDA), and the Institute of Medicine (IOM) of the National Academies of Sciences, just as adamantly deny any causal association between vaccines and autism. Health officials support their stance with epidemiological research that parent advocacy groups assert is inadequate and methodologically flawed.

One positive outcome of the debate about vaccine-induced autism is that it has finally put to rest the old "refrigerator Mom" theory promoted by early autism researchers: that cold and neglectful mothers cause their children to retreat into the isolated world of autism. Enlightened physicians, who have investigated cases of vaccine-induced neuroimmune dysfunction and found ways to eliminate autistic behaviors in some children, have confirmed that autism has biological, rather than psychological, causes. They are exploring the interaction between genetic factors and external triggers, such as vaccination, prescription drugs, chemical toxins, viral or bacterial exposures in utero or during the neonatal period, nutritional deficiencies, and other environmental factors which may predispose vulnerable children to developing autism.

Child Health Report Card: Failing

The contentious debate about vaccines and autism is taking place at a time when many parents and teachers are questioning why so many highly vaccinated children are chronically ill and disabled. Mass vaccination campaigns for polio and measles may have helped to eliminate those and other acute infectious diseases in early childhood. Yet too many fully vaccinated children are "stuck on sick," requiring asthma inhalers, Ritalin, epi-pens, insulin and anti-depressants. The autism epidemic is part of a broader chronic disease and disability epidemic that began in the last quarter of the 20th century and continues to mysteriously plague a significant number of children in the U.S. and other economically and educationally advanced societies.

The connection between vaccination and the development of autistic behaviors in previously healthy children was first reported in 1985 in the book *DPT: A Shot in the Dark*, which I co-authored with medical historian Harris Coulter.[1] In the late 1990s, British gastroenterologist Andrew Wakefield, MD, and colleagues published an article on the possible biological mechanisms for vaccine induced autism after the MMR vaccination.[2]

By 2001, several parents of children born in the 1990s alleged that mercury preservatives in multiple vaccines injected into their children had poisoned them and left them with autism and other kinds of immune and brain system dysfunction.[3] A synopsis of their published hypothesis that regressive autism is a novel form of mercury poisoning is included in the previous chapter, and their stories are told in the award-winning book *Evidence of Harm: Mercury in Vaccines and the Autism Epidemic: A Medical Controversy*, by David Kirby, published in 2005.[4] That same year, Robert F. Kennedy, Jr. wrote an expose in *Rolling Stone* magazine entitled "Deadly Immunity," [5] which presents evidence of a cover-up by government health officials and vaccine manufacturers of data linking autism and thimerosal, a mercury-containing preservative.

This chapter presents evidence for a causal relationship between vaccination and autism spectrum disorders, including:

- How changes in vaccine policy and the increase in both the numbers of new vaccines and vaccine doses have paralleled the increase in numbers of children with autism and other neuroimmune disorders
- How the incidence of chronic diseases has dramatically increased as mass use of multiple vaccines has dramatically reduced or eliminated experience with infectious disease in childhood
- How vaccine-induced autism and developmental disorders are immune mediated, and may stem from an inflammatory response, via a variety of known and unknown biological mechanisms, which are unresolved in genetically vulnerable children
- How toxic vaccine additives, such as mercury and aluminum, may have contributed to the autism epidemic
- How the politics of vaccination affects vaccine safety and national vaccine policies
- How an individual's right to informed consent to vaccination, which is a medical intervention carrying an inherent risk of injury or death, is taking a back seat to mandatory, one-size-fits-all mass vaccination policies
- How parents and professionals can respond to and prevent vaccine reactions.

Vaccines and Autism

During the last two decades of the 20th century, parents of now grown vaccine injured children reported DPT reactions such as high pitched screaming, seizures and regression to the CDC and AAP. Publicly witnessing how their children regressed and were left with various kinds of brain and immune system damage after the diphtheria/pertussis/tetanus "(DPT) vaccination, a small group of parents founded a non-profit organization known today as the National Vaccine Information Center and worked with Congress on the historic National Childhood Vaccine Injury Act of 1986 (PL99-660). This public awakening to the reality of vaccine injuries and deaths, and subsequent congressional acknowledgement of the human and economic consequences of vaccine side effects, effectively launched the vaccine safety and informed consent movement in America.

After Harris Coulter and I documented in 1985 that DPT vaccine can cause a spectrum of brain and immune system dysfunction ranging from learning disabilities and attention deficit disorder to medication resistant seizure disorders, autism and severe and profound mental retardation, Dr. Coulter expanded on that evidence in his 1990 book *Vaccination, Social Violence and Criminaliity.*[6] He drew parallels between the residual learning disabilities and hyperactive/abnormal behavior caused by complications of disease or vaccine-induced encephalitis and hyperactive or other abnormal behaviors and learning disabilities.

The 1986 National Childhood Vaccine Injury Act required federal health agencies to ask the IOM to examine the literature for evidence that vaccines can kill and injure. In 1991, the IOM published the first of four reports declaring that, although there was evidence in the medical literature for a causal relation between the DPT vaccine and acute encephalopathy (brain inflammation) and shock an "unusual shock-like state," there is "no evidence to indicate a causal relation between the DPT vaccine or the pertussis component of DPT vaccine and autism."[7]

Nevertheless, for the next 15 years parents continued to report that their healthy children were regressing into autism after DPT and other vaccinations. Empirical evidence for a vaccine-autism connection continued to grow at the same time doctors and scientists inside industry, government and medical organizations continued to deny the significance of these reports.

The First "Autism Mom"

About the same time that the IOM was examining the medical literature for evidence that DPT vaccine could cause autism, a happy, healthy 13-month-old boy, Garrett Goldenberg, got his MMR vaccination in California in 1990. His mother, Cindy, witnessed her bright first-born regress, and gradually exhibit autistic behavior within two weeks of his MMR shot.

At age 18 months, Garrett got a haemophilus influenzae B (Hib) vaccination and his autistic, compulsive and hyperactive behaviors symptoms worsened. He started flapping his arms, twirling and spinning. Noise terrified him. He stopped talking. He gagged on his food, didn't see or respond to his parents, and lined up his toys.

Cindy took Garrett to doctors specializing in learning disabilities, psychology, hearing and speech disorders, desperately trying to find an answer to why her little boy had changed so dramatically. Cindy was convinced Garrett's symptoms were connected to a biological cause. She finally found a pediatrician who performed diagnostic testing, including blood tests.

All tests came back negative except for one – a blood test showing Garrett had a borderline high rubella titer. Cindy wondered why Garrett's rubella titer would be above normal a year after getting vaccinated. That one clue prompted her to delve into the medical literature on autism, rubella, vaccines and the immune system. What she found convinced her that, just as rubella infection can cause autistic behaviors in children with congenital rubella, so could the live virus rubella vaccine in the MMR shot cause autistic behaviors.[8] She also suspected that, because vaccines are injected directly into the bloodstream, they are capable of interfering with the body's primary immune system and affecting the immuno-globulin (IgG) levels which facilitate absorption of nutrients by the mucosal lining of the gastrointestinal system.

Holding fast to her conviction that the MMR vaccine had caused her son's autistic behaviors and that intravenous immune globulin intravenous infusions (IGIV) could help resolve inflammation, heal his primary immune system and lead to reduced autistic symptoms, she contacted Sudhir Gupta, MD, PhD, University of California professor of medicine and immunology. Gupta confirmed that Garrett had elevated rubella titers as well as very low IgA and IgG. After discussing options with Cindy, Dr. Gupta agreed to give Garrett IGIV infusions which, because of the known interaction between the immune and neurological system, might have a restorative effect on his immune and brain dysfunction.[9]

During IGIV therapy, Cindy eliminated milk and wheat from Garrett's diet, and gave him vitamin and nutritional supplements, such as acidophilus and globulin protein from whey, to enhance the optimal functioning of his immune and gastrointestinal system. Within weeks of the IGIV injections, dietary changes and nutritional supplement therapy, Garrett's behavior improved dramatically. As his rubella titer levels came down and his IgG and IgA levels stabilized, Garrett became less and less autistic.

By age four, gone were the repetitive behaviors, poor eye contact and limited language. Garrett was eventually weaned off the IGIV; Cindy continued dietary and nutritional therapies, and also worked round-the-clock using behavioral, sensory integrative, speech and sound therapies to help Garrett "catch-up" developmentally. Years later, Garrett graduated from high school with "A's" on his report card and attended the prom just like all the other students in his class.

Cindy was the first "Autism Mom" to recover her son from vaccine induced regressive autism through dietary and immune modulating therapies. Her voice in the early 1990s pointed doctors toward developing protocols to help heal autism, and gave new hope to a generation of parents who had been told that autism had no cure.

An "Autism Dad" Identifies An Epidemic

In the 1960s Bernard Rimland, PhD, the father of a son with autism, stepped forward and proved that autism has biological, not psychological, origins. In the late 1990s, another father of a son with autism, Rick Rollens, spoke publicly, this time, proving that there is an autism epidemic. His healthy son became autistic following a series of DPT, Hib and MMR vaccinations as a baby.

After attending the First International Public Conference on Vaccination sponsored by the National Vaccine Information Center in 1997, Rollens, the former Secretary of the California Senate, increased his efforts to persuade the California legislature to analyze the history of autism in the state. In a March 1999 report, the California Department of Developmental Services found a 273 percent increase between 1987 and 1998 in the numbers of new children entering the California developmental services system with a professional diagnosis of autism.[10]

Rollens eventually joined with three other fathers of autistic children and raised millions of dollars to build the **M**edical **I**nvestigation of **N**eurodevelopmental **D**isorders (M.I.N.D.) Institute at University of California- Davis. The M.I.N.D. Institute has become the leading medical research institution in the U.S. primarily devoted to finding the causes and cures for autism and other neuro-developmental disorders in children.

Parents of Autistic Children Organize

Much of the enhanced public awareness about autism at the beginning of the 21st century has come about because mothers and fathers have publicly witnessed how their healthy children regressed physically, mentally and emotionally after vaccination, and were eventually diagnosed with developmental delays, including autism. Independently, parents in the United States, Canada, Australia, New Zealand and Europe continue to describe in identical terms how their normally developing children are injected with one or more live virus or killed bacterial vaccines and then descend into the isolated, painful world of autism, which is marked by chronic immune and neurological dysfunction.

Those of us, who watched our children regress and become learning disabled, hyperactive, allergic, autistic, epileptic, retarded and immune impaired after DPT vaccine reactions in the 1970s and 1980s, are having a déjà vu experience today. With heavy hearts we watch a new generation of healthy, bright children regress after receiving not just one, but multiple vaccines, including hepatitis B, hepatitis A, pneumococcal, HIB, rotavirus, polio, MMR, chicken pox and the flu. The refusal a quarter century ago by vaccine manufacturers, government health agencies and pediatric organizations to seriously investigate parent reports of vaccine-associated brain and immune system damage, including development of autistic behaviors after vaccination, is reaping tragic consequences today.

The vaccine safety controversy is becoming more public and more intense because of the discrepancy between what parents are personally experiencing with their children after vaccination and the steadfast denials by medical authorities that vaccination plays any role at all in the development of autism and other developmental delays. Parents of autistic children have become more vocal as they realize they are facing lifetime support for children who will require fulltime care as adults.

Parents of young vaccine-injured autistic children have joined with older parents of autistic children and become active in established organizations such as the Autism Society of America (ASA) and Autism Research Institute (ARI). They have also founded new organizations, including Developmental Delay Resources (DDR), Families for Early Autism Treatment (FEAT), Moms Opposing Mercury, National Autism Association (NAA), No Mercury, SAFEMINDS, Southwest Autism Research and Resource Center (SARRC), The Autism Autoimmunity Project (TAAP) and Unlocking Autism. The most recently formed group, Autism Speaks has joined with 10-year-old Cure Autism Now (CAN) to form the best funded autism research organization in the world. These parent groups and the National Vaccine Information Center (NVIC), which has represented parents of vaccine injured children since 1982, are working with enlightened physicians to find the truth about the causes, cures, and ways to prevent autism.

Early History of Pediatric Vaccination in the U.S.

From the late 18th century to the mid-20th century, the only vaccine American children received was the smallpox vaccine. In the early 1940s, state-of-the-art pediatric medical care in America included only a smallpox vaccination plus a separate dose of diphtheria vaccine. In 1944, the crude, whole cell pertussis (whooping cough) vaccine developed in 1912, was recommended for babies.

By 1949, the AAP recommended routine use of the new combination DPT vaccine, followed by recommended use of killed polio vaccine in 1955. By 1958, Kanner's case files contained more than 100 cases of autism.

In 1962 the live virus polio vaccine was licensed, followed by licensing of the live virus measles vaccine in 1963, for routine use by all children. Two psychiatrists reported a dramatic upsurge of autism cases in their pediatric practice after 1964.[11] Between 1964 and 1969, the well-cared-for American child was getting DPT and live polio vaccine simultaneously at two, four, six and 18 months of age, as well as a dose of live measles vaccine at 12 months of age.

Increase in Autism Parallels Increase in Vaccines

Chapter 1 documents the dramatic increase in the numbers of American children with autism, learning disabilities and other brain and immune system disorders between 1970 and 2005. Increases in chronic disease and disability in children during this 35-year span coincided closely with (1) an increase in the total number of doses of vaccines children receive in the first few years of life; and (2) an increase in the total number of doses they receive on a single day.

By the late 1970s, public health officials, vaccine manufacturers and medical organizations escalated their efforts to add more vaccines to the mandatory child vaccination list and to raise vaccination rates in every state. Vaccine policy makers took the following actions:
- recommended all 15-month-old children get a combination live virus measles-mumps-rubella (MMR) vaccine, in addition to five doses of DPT and oral polio vaccinations each given at two, four, six, 18 months and four years of age
- provided federal grants to states to distribute free DPT, polio and MMR vaccines to children in public health clinics
- launched the National Childhood Immunization Initiative by the CDC to encourage states to enact and strictly enforce mandatory vaccination laws, and raise national vaccination rates in children to above 90 percent for all government recommended vaccines
- routinely administered live virus rubella vaccine, licensed for use in children in 1969, to hospitalized new mothers immediately after giving birth[12,13]

The 1980s brought new vaccines to the childhood schedule:
- in 1988, the CDC and AAP recommended that 18-month-old children get a dose of the newly licensed conjugated haemophilus influenza b (Hib) vaccine
- in 1989, the CDC and AAP mandated a booster measles vaccine (usually administered as MMR) for all four to six year olds because of unexpectedly high failure rates in children using only one dose of measles vaccine given between 12 and 15 months

In the 1990s, children got even more vaccines:
- in 1991, the CDC and AAP directed doctors to inject three doses of the recombinant hepatitis B vaccine, licensed in 1989, into all newborn infants, with the first dose to be given at 12 hours of age in the hospital nursery, the second dose at one month and the third dose at six months of age
- in 1991, three more doses of HIB vaccine were added to the infant schedule at two, four, and six months of age
- in 1995, the live varicella zoster (chicken pox) vaccine was put on the market and the CDC recommended it for "universal use" in all 12- to 15-month olds
- in 1996 the purified acellular DTaP vaccine was licensed to replace whole cell DPT for infants

The expansion of the childhood vaccination program continued into the new millennium:
- in 2000, the CDC and AAP added four doses of the recently licensed pneumococcal vaccine to the infant vaccine schedule at two, four, six, and 12 to 15 months of age
- in 2003, the CDC and AAP directed pediatricians to inject all children six to 23 months with flu vaccine
- in 2005, pediatricians were directed to give all 12-month olds a dose of hepatitis A vaccine
- in 2006, the CDC and AAP informed parents that their babies must get three doses of the newly licensed live oral rotavirus (diarrhea) vaccine at two, four, and six months old, as well as get annual flu vaccinations through age five
- also in 2006, the government targeted adolescents for more vaccines, including DTap, meningococcal and human papillomavirus (HPV) vaccines to prevent genital warts and cervical cancer

The bottom line is that between 1980 and 2006, doctors more than doubled the numbers of vaccines and almost tripled the number of vaccine doses given to children by age six. In 1980, the CDC and AAP recommended that children receive 23 doses of seven vaccines (DPT, polio, MMR) by age six years, with the first vaccinations given at two months. By January 2006, the CDC and AAP recommended that children receive 48 doses of 14 vaccines by age six with the first dose given at 12 hours old. By age 12, children would receive nearly five dozen doses of 16 vaccines.[14]

Today's childhood immunization schedule starts with the hepatitis B vaccine at 12 hours old in the newborn nursery, followed by seven vaccines at two months, and seven more at four months. On the six month well-baby visit, today's baby can receive as many as eight bacterial and live virus vaccines on a single day and, at age 15 months, a toddler can receive as many as 12 vaccines on a single day. By age two, most American children have received 37 doses of vaccines, including four doses each of vaccines for HIB, diphtheria, tetanus, pertussis and pneumococcal, all of which can be given during the first 12 months of life. Seven vaccines injected into a 13 lb. two-month-old infant are equivalent to 70 doses in a 130 lb. adult.[15]

While the CDC recommended childhood vaccine schedule allows the injection of seven to 13 vaccines into babies on a single day, public health officials have no science based data, either epidemiological or pathological, to demonstrate that simultaneous injection of this many live virus and inactivated bacterial vaccines will not lead to health deterioration in those who are genetically vulnerable to vaccine-induced neuoimmune dysfunction. In addition, no science based data, either epidemiological or pathological, confirms that repeated vaccination over time is not responsible for causing chronic illness and disability in those biological incapable of withstanding ongoing atypical manipulation of the immune system by vaccination.

The U.S. government and the pharmaceutical industry are creating several hundred experimental vaccines, including vaccines for AIDS, tuberculosis, malaria, cytomegalovirus, typhoid, Group B strep, syphilis, gonorrhea, hepatitis C, anthrax, parainfluenza, respiratory syncytial virus and others.[16] Many of these vaccines will undoubtedly be added to the routine childhood vaccination schedule in the future.

National Vaccination Rates Rise Along with Autism
In 1967, national vaccination rates for children under age three for DPT, polio and measles vaccine were between 60 and 80 percent, rising to 90 percent in 1999 for DPT, polio, MMR, and Hib vaccines. National vaccine coverage estimates by the CDC for the 2005-2006 school year for children entering kindergarten were above 90 percent for DTaP, polio, MMR, and hepatitis B vaccines.[17] Chicken pox vaccine coverage rates more than tripled from 1997 to 2004 and did not vary by race or ethnicity.[18]

In 2006, the CDC announced that 81 percent of all children under age three received four doses of DTaP; three or more doses of polio vaccine; one or more doses of measles containing vaccine, three or more doses of HIB vaccine and three doses of hepatitis B vaccine.[19] As a larger proportion of children received more doses of more vaccines, autism rates soared (see Chapter 1). This trend reflects a much higher uptake of multiple vaccines in very young children under three years old than in generations past.

Identifying Vaccine Reactions
Vaccination is a medical intervention usually performed on a healthy individual, for the purpose of keeping that person healthy. However, every vaccine carries a risk of injury or death, and some individuals can be at higher risk than others for suffering a vaccine reaction.

Doctors *must* discuss the signs and symptoms of a vaccine reaction with parents, so they can monitor their children closely for several weeks after vaccination, and recognize the sometimes subtle signs that a reaction has occurred.

Adverse reactions to a vaccine can begin within hours, days and weeks after vaccination, and vary from acute physical symptoms such as redness at the site of the injection, high pitched screaming, inconsolable crying, high fever, paralysis, seizures and loss of consciousness to less obvious signs, such as behavioral changes, sleep disturbances, confusion, flapping, loss of relatedness, eye contact and developmental milestones such as rolling over, sitting up or speaking, and other signs of physical, mental and emotional regression. Often regression is accompanied by symptoms of immune dysfunction such as new food and environmental allergies, asthma, digestive problems, skin disorders and chronic respiratory and ear infections. Together, these symptoms of vaccine induced brain and immune system dysfunction may persist. Later, a team of specialists makes a diagnosis of a learning disability, attention deficit or autism.

Whenever a child exhibits marked deterioration in physical, mental or emotional well being following vaccination, the possibility that the vaccine or vaccines played a role should be taken seriously. A parent who suspects that a child is having a vaccine reaction should call a doctor promptly. If the doctor is unconcerned, and the parent is worried, the child should be taken to an emergency room and the suspected reaction documented in the medical record.

Since passage of the federal National Childhood Vaccine Injury Act in 1986 (PL 99-660; 42 USC300aa 1 et seq.) doctors are required by law to:
- provide parents with information *before* a child is vaccinated explaining the benefits and risks of each childhood vaccine. The CDC publishes brief one-page vaccine information statements and drug companies are required to publish product manufacturer inserts that accompany vials of vaccine
- keep permanent records of all vaccinations given, including the vaccine manufacturer's name and lot number
- report all serious adverse events, including injuries and deaths which occur within 30 days after vaccination, to the Vaccine Adverse Event Reporting System (VAERS). ["Only a fraction of the total number of potentially reportable events occurring after vaccination are reported," with between 12,000 and 17,000 reports of adverse events, including hospitalizations, injuries and deaths following vaccination, being made annually by doctors and parents.[20]]
- inform parents, whose children suffer injury or death following vaccination, about the existence of the federal Vaccine Injury Compensation Program (VICP) created under the 1986 Vaccine Injury Act. [Between 1990 and 2006, this program awarded more than one billion dollars to more than 2500 families whose children have died or been injured after vaccine reactions,[21] even though Department of Health and Justice officials fight almost every vaccine injury claim in an attempt to minimize vaccine risks.]

Increased Vaccination Correlates with Increase in Autism
The possibility that genetically vulnerable children may suffer from repeated atypical manipulation of the immune system with multiple vaccines in early childhood is an hypothesis I first suggested to the Institute of Medicine Immunization Safety Review Committee in January 2001. I stated,
> *There is a compelling argument to be made that the dramatic increase in chronic brain and immune dysfunction in children, especially the rising number of reports of regression in previously healthy children, is due to an early exposure that is being*

experienced by all children but which is harming an expanding minority of them....
Many biological responses are at least partially under genetic control. If, for example,
adverse responses to vaccination are tied to the genes responsible for predisposition
to autoimmunity and immune-mediated neurological dysfunction, then it is possible
that the addition of more doses of vaccines to the routine schedule in the past two
decades has affected more and more children with that genetic predisposition....
Therefore, when all children only were exposed to DPT and polio vaccine in the
early 1960s, a tiny fraction of the genetically susceptible responded adversely. But
with the addition of measles, mumps and rubella to the routine schedule in 1979, and
then HIB, hepatitis B and chicken pox in the late 1980s and 1990s, far more of the
genetically susceptible have been brought into the adverse responder group.

This hypothesis could not be examined by the IOM in their 2002 report on "Multiple
Immunizations and Immune Dysfunction." After reviewing evidence in the medical literature, the IOM Immunization Safety Review Committee stated that:

The committee was unable to address the concern that repeated exposure of a
[genetically] susceptible child to multiple immunizations over the developmental
period may also produce atypical or non-specific immune or nervous system injury
that could lead to severe disability or death. (Fisher, 2001) There are no epidemio-
logical studies to address this. Thus, the committee recognizes with some discomfort
that this report addresses only part of the overall set of concerns of some of those
most wary about the safety of childhood immunization.

Class, Vaccines and Autism

Rimland, Kanner and other autism researchers noticed early on that children with autism
were often offspring of intelligent, well-educated successful professionals. Upper middle
class families in America have always sought out and received quality medical care, and
their children are the most likely to be the first to try the latest developments in medicine.
In Kanner's day, two miracle drugs of the twentieth century, antibiotics and new vaccines,
elevated trust in and reliance upon pharmaceuticals - and the medical doctors who were
prescribing them   to a new plateau.

In the 1940s and 1950s, cases of autism were concentrated in the upper and upper middle
classes. Today, the growing numbers of children affected with autism come from all social
classes because nearly everyone has access to medical care and the latest vaccines are
provided free of charge in public health clinics. Vaccination is not just a medical intervention afforded by the rich and taken advantage of by the well educated, but is an equal
opportunity extended to the rich and poor, the educated and uneducated alike in America.
Rigorous enforcement of state vaccine mandates for daycare and school entry has also
extended vaccination into all socio-economic groups in the U.S.

The CDC maintains high vaccination rates by insuring that every time it recommends a
vaccine for "universal use" in children, state health officials automatically add the vaccine
to the state's mandatory vaccination list, or join with the AAP and drug companies to lobby
state legislatures to pass laws mandating the new vaccine. The CDC awards federal grants
to states to institute mechanisms to maintain high vaccination rates with all CDC recommended vaccines. The higher the vaccination rate, the more grant money the state receives.
A "Vaccines for Children Act" (VFC), created by the CDC in 1993, guaranteed that every
American child, regardless of the family's ability to pay, would receive all CDC recommended vaccines in public health clinics.[22]

The Hygiene Hypothesis

The hygiene hypothesis, first proposed in 1989 by researcher D.E. Strachen, suggests that the reduction of early childhood infections in technologically advanced countries due to improved living conditions and sanitation, widespread vaccination and antibiotic use in the 20th century has caused an increase in chronic allergic and autoimmune diseases in children.[23] Strachen theorized that preventing children from being naturally challenged by exposure to certain viral and bacterial infections during childhood, when the immune system is maturing and learning how to successfully respond to viruses and bacteria in the environment, could weaken the immune system and make it more susceptible to immune dysfunction.

According to the Environmental Protection Agency (EPA),

> *Over the past century, the nation has basically conquered many infectious diseases that once sickened or killed thousands of people: childhood diseases such as measles and mumps, and waterborne ailments such as typhoid and cholera. Significant progress in improving sanitation and drinking water means that Americans are now relatively safe from the diarrheal diseases that imperil much of the world. Accidents are now the leading threat to children in the U.S. and most adults die from chronic illness rather than from infectious diseases. At the turn of the century, many people died from infectious diseases such as tuberculosis and influenza. Today, more than 60 percent of all U.S. deaths are attributed to cardiovascular diseases and cancer.[24]*

Lending credence to the evidence that mass use of multiple vaccines to prevent acute infectious disease in childhood may be contributing to the development of chronic disease later in life, is accumulating evidence that the hygiene hypothesis is correct.[25] In 2000, researchers at the University of Arizona examined the incidence of asthma, an autoimmune disease, in 1,035 children and found that the presence of older siblings at home protected against the development of asthma.[26] In 2005, Australian researchers investigated whether exposure or re-exposure to infections can influence the developing immune system and be protective against development of multiple sclerosis (MS), an autoimmune disease, in later life. They found that "higher infant sibling exposure in the first 6 years of life was associated with a reduced risk of MS, possibly by altering childhood infection patterns and related immune responses."[27]

In 2005, researchers at the University of Illinois at Chicago conducted a study relating asthma, hay fever, eczema and vaccination status. Working with the National Vaccine Information Center membership, researchers anonymously identified 515 never vaccinated, 423 partially vaccinated and 239 completely vaccinated children. They concluded that parents of unvaccinated children were 11 times less likely to report asthma for children with no family history of the disease and no exposure to antibiotics in infancy. Parents of unvaccinated children were 10 times less likely to report hay fever among children with no family history of hay fever. Eczema was also reported significantly less in unvaccinated children.[28]

Unvaccinated children also appear to have a lower incidence of autism, according to a 2005 investigation by UPI reporter Dan Olmsted, who looked at an unvaccinated Amish population in Lancaster, Pennsylvania. If the CDC's calculation that one in 166 children is autistic is correct, Olmsted calculated that at least 100 children in Lancaster should have autism. He found only three: a girl adopted from China, an Amish child who had been vaccinated and developed autism shortly afterwards, and another child whose vaccination status was unclear.[29]

Good Health: A Balancing Act

In Chapter 3 the authors make a strong argument for an autism-immunological relationship, as many autistic children exhibit immune dysfunction. A welcome outcome of the possibility of a vaccine-autism connection is a long overdue examination of the interaction between the developing brain and the immune system.

Humans and infectious microbes have coexisted for as long as humans have walked the earth, and the human immune system has developed an efficient way of dealing with viral and bacterial infections. When infected with a micro-organism, the body's first line of defense is for the cellular or "innate" part of the immune system to mount an inflammatory response. This response then signals the humoral or "learned" part of the immune system to produce anti-inflammatory chemicals and antibodies that resolve inflammation, so that healing can take place, and establish future resistance to re-infection. A healthy, mature immune system requires an equal balance of cellular and humoral immune system responses. A disruption in this balance can lead to development of allergy and autoimmune disorders, including neuroimmune disorders.[30-32]

Vaccination attempts to fool the body into believing it has come in contact with the real microorganism that causes infection. But vaccination does not exactly mimic the natural infection progress, and often by-passes cellular immunity in favor of humoral immunity.[33] Most live virus and killed bacterial vaccines are injected into the body, whereas in the natural disease process, microorganisms enter the body primarily through the mucous membranes of the respiratory and gastrointestinal tracts, where the inflammatory immune response to the challenging microorganism begins.

Because vaccine developers do not fully understand the biological mechanisms involved in the immune response to natural infection or vaccination, the achievement of vaccine induced mucosal (cellular) immunity has been elusive.[34,35] Vaccine developers of preventive and therapeutic vaccines continue to have trouble developing safe and effective vaccines which mimic the complex interplay between innate and adaptive immunities involved in the stimulation of the immune system during the natural disease process. [36]

Newborn infants do not mount a rapid or strong antibody response to vaccination,[37] which is an atypical manipulation of the immune system with lab altered viruses and bacteria. "Babies are born with a very immature cellular immune system," says Lawrence Palevsky, MD, a New York pediatrician and co-founder of the Holistic Pediatric Association. "Childhood viral infectious diseases like measles, mumps and chicken-pox initially stimulate the cellular part of the immune system, which leads to the production of the signs of inflammation – fever, redness, swelling, and mucus. This cellular immune response stimulates the humoral part of the immune system to produce anti-inflammatory chemicals and antibodies that assist in recovery from these illnesses. The natural process helps the cellular and humoral immune systems to mature."[38]

In other words, this natural "exercise" of the immune system can make it stronger and better able to maintain good health. When the immune system does not function normally, as in many children with autism spectrum disorders, it can get "stuck" on inflammation and lead to chronic illness.

Philip Incao, MD, a holistic family-care physician in Colorado maintains that "Physically, health is about balancing acute inflammatory responses to infection, which stimulate one arm of the immune system, and chronic inflammatory responses to infection, which stimulate the other part of the immune system. Overuse of vaccines to suppress all acute, externalizing inflammation early in life can set up the immune system to respond to future stresses and infections by developing chronic, internalizing disease later in life."[39]

If the hygiene hypothesis continues to be confirmed with future evidence, the elimination of most natural experience with infectious disease in early childhood, through mass use of multiple vaccines, may turn out to be instrumental in disrupting the balance of cellular and humoral immunity, thus causing many children to suffer chronic inflammation and chronic illness, including autism. Those children genetically predisposed to inflammatory conditions such as autoimmune disorders may be at special risk.

Autoimmunity Epidemic: Uncontrolled Inflammation

Many scientists are now concluding that persistent inflammation is at the root of most chronic brain and immune system disorders[40,41] and that genetic variations in the population make some individuals genetically vulnerable to inflammatory disease.[42,43] As has been previously mentioned in this book, the epidemic of autism spectrum disorders in American children between 1980 and 2006 was accompanied by major increases in auto-immune disorders.

Because many American children today, including those with autism, have food and environmental allergies, gluten,[44] and/or casein intolerance,[45] inflammatory bowel disorders, asthma and other signs of immune dysfunction, unresolved inflammation may also play an important role in the development and persistence of autism in children. Genetic factors that predispose children to autoimmunity may be very important in the development of autism in some children, as some researchers have found that mothers of autistic children and family members often have a history of autoimmune disorders, such as thyroid disease, rheumatoid arthritis, and other illnesses marked by chronic inflammation.[46]

- *Allergies* in those with autism spectrum disorders are covered in Chapter 3. One study comparing vaccinated to unvaccinated children in the period 1988 to 1994, found that a child who received DPT or tetanus vaccination was 50 percent more likely to experience severe allergic reactions, more than 80 percent more likely to experience sinusitis, and twice as likely to experience asthma, as those children who were not vaccinated. The authors concluded that "asthma and other allergic hypersensitivity reactions and related symptoms may be caused, in part, by the delayed effects of DTP or tetanus vaccination."[47]
- *Diabetes* is an autoimmune disorder that affects the body's ability to utilize sugar, and involves immune cells attacking insulin producing islet cells of the pancreas thus causing chronic inflammation. Statistics show a 17-fold increase in Type I diabetes, from one in 7,100 children in the 1950s[48] to one in 400 now.[49] The development of insulin dependent diabetes mellitus after mumps infection was first reported in the late 1800s.[50] The literature also documents diabetes following the mumps vaccination[51,52] the measles-mumps vaccination,[53] and measles-mumps-rubella vaccination.[54] Juvenile diabetes has been associated with the Hepatitis B vaccine,[55,56] the Hib and MMR vaccines,[57,58] the DPT vaccine,[59] and the rubella vaccine.[60,61] Barthelow Classen, MD, warned in 2000 that mass use of Prevnar vaccine may also be associated with an increase of diabetes in children.[62]
- *Asthma*, an autoimmune disease that involves inflammation of the bronchial tubes, increased four fold from 1979[63] to 2001.[64] Asthma has been associated with receipt of the pertussis vaccine in previously healthy children.[65-68]
- *Juvenile rheumatoid arthritis*, an autoimmune disease that involves inflammation of the joints, was so rare 25 years ago that public health officials did not keep any statistics

on it; it now afflicts 300,000 American children.[69] Both acute and chronic arthritis are associated with both rubella disease and the rubella vaccine.[70]

California neurologist Lawrence Steinman, MD, who investigated the biological mechanisms and genetic factors involved in pertussis vaccine-induced brain inflammation in the 1980s, and is now conducting cutting edge research into the interplay of genes and environment in development of multiple sclerosis and other autoimmune diseases, said in 2003 "We are learning from studies on the experimental autoimmune encephalomyelitis (EAE) model that components of the allergic response are critical in the modulation of Th1 autoimmunity."[71]

Brain Inflammation and Seizures in Autism

For more than 200 years the medical literature has documented inflammation of the brain, known as encephalitis, encephalomyelitis, or encephalopathy. Brain inflammation, ranging from mild to severe, can be caused by both viral and bacterial infections, as well as by the vaccines containing lab altered viruses and bacteria.

Symptoms of brain inflammation may include fever, vomiting, high pitched screaming (cri encephalique) in infants, loss of consciousness, convulsions, and coma which can lead to death or permanent brain dysfunction, including mental retardation, persistent seizure disorders, and developmental delays. Mild brain inflammation can occur with less obvious symptoms but can result in lesser forms of permanent brain dysfunction that includes learning disabilities, ADHD and other mental, emotional and physical delays. If these symptoms sound familiar, it is because they are the very same symptoms that manifest in adverse vaccine reactions.

The first two vaccines used by humans, smallpox and rabies, caused the same kind of brain inflammation and permanent neurological damage as the diseases they were designed to prevent.

- *Smallpox and Smallpox Vaccine* The most feared complication of both smallpox infection and smallpox vaccine, created by British physician Edward Jenner in 1796, was brain inflammation. Jenner's vaccinia virus, used to prevent smallpox in 1796, caused acute disseminated encephalomyelitis (ADEM) within one to six weeks in an estimated one in 5,000 persons.[72]
- *Rabies and Rabies Vaccine* Rabies is a viral disease that takes from 10 days to 12 months to reach the brain. Once it does, however, symptoms are serious, and include excessive motor activity, excitation, agitation, confusion, combativeness, bizarre aberrations of thought, seizures and other central nervous system (CNS) dysfunction. Soon after Pasteur began to inject patients with rabies vaccine in the 1880s, brain inflammation was an obvious side effect. In the early 1930s, virologist Thomas Rivers studied the brain damaging effects of rabies vaccine and provided the first evidence that immune cells can attack the brain when he established the model for EAE.[73] Encephalitis and polyneuritis have been estimated to occur in as many as one in 400 rabies vaccinated individuals.[74]

Seizures are a hallmark of brain inflammation. Convulsions and seizures are among the most common serious complications of vaccine reactions, leading to regression and permanent neurological damage. The whole cell DPT vaccine, given routinely to American children in the late 1940s until the late 1990s, was well known for causing afebrile, medication-resistant seizures. A U.S. study found that one in 875 children suffered a convulsion after receipt of DPT vaccine[75] and a British study found that one in 110,000 children suffered brain inflammation after DPT vaccination.[76] The MMR vaccine, routinely given to American children since the late 1970s, is associated with brain inflammation and the development of seizures between 8 and 14 days after vaccination.[77]

Kanner described convulsions in his autistic patients in the 1950s, and in the early 1970s autism researchers noted a high number of autistic children have "gross EEG abnormalities" and are neurologically handicapped with learning and behavior disorders.[78] Mnukhin and Isaev found a high incidence of epileptic seizures in autistic children in 1975, arguing that autism has an organic, neurological basis,[79] and a year later Ornitz and Ritvo agreed.[80] Today, seizure disorders are estimated to occur in about 25% of cases of autism.[81]

Seizures can be difficult to diagnose, especially if they involve subtle "staring" spells that may not register on routine waking EEG's. A sleep EEG may be required to identify clinically relevant epileptiform activity present only during slow-wave sleep in a subset of children with autism spectrum disorders.[82] In 2005, researchers found that "nearly all children with autism and seizures also showed epileptiform activity on electroencephalograms." Furthermore, supporting the brain damaging potential of uncontrolled seizures, their study showed that "adults with infantile autism without epilepsy, had higher IQ scores than adults with both autism and epilepsy."[83]

Brain inflammation can cause more than seizure disorders. Paralysis, ataxia, abnormal behavior, mental retardation and other kinds of cognitive impairments can also result. In severe cases, the myelin sheath, which encloses nerve fibers, and helps transmit neural impulses, becomes damaged and degenerates, in a process called demyelination, which prevents the body's nervous system from functioning properly.

Viruses and Viral Vaccines

Chapter 3 explains the role of several viruses in autism. The virus that has attracted the most attention is:

- *Measles* Measles virus infection has long been associated with demyelinating disorders.[84-86] Within three weeks of even a mild measles infection, one in 1,000 cases develops encephalomyelitis with symptoms such as fever, headache and drowsiness. Residual brain damage from measles encephalitis ranges from mental regression, to seizure disorders, and includes motor, sensory and movement disorders.[87] Of particular interest to the optometrist is that optic neuritis involving inflammation of the optic nerve can occur in children after both measles disease and measles vaccination[88] Optic neuritis has also been reported after hepatitis B infection and hepatitis B vaccination[89] and influenza and rubella vaccinations.[90,91] A review of the patient's medical history may reveal a recent viral infection or vaccination.

The association between the measles virus and the live virus MMR vaccine, as mentioned previously, was documented by Andrew Wakefield, MD, and 13 other physicians at Royal Free Hospital in London in 1997.[2] They inadvertently stumbled upon the connection between inflammatory bowel disease (IBD) and regressive autism while studying Crohn's disease in children. This pioneering research showed the presence of the measles virus in the guts of children suffering with Crohn's disease and autism.

The mother of one young patient, Rosemary Kessick, urged Wakefield to look for the biological mechanism for simultaneous development of IBD and autism in previously normal children. A commonality in the medical history was that half of the children reported onset of symptoms of IBD and autism following MMR vaccination.

During the course of their investigation, Wakefield and his colleagues discovered that in 1961 Hans Asperger had observed a high rate of gastrointestinal (celiac) disease in those diagnosed with autism. The authors hypothesized that persistent viral infection, either from natural disease or live virus vaccines, could cause chronic inflammation of the bowel, and damage to the central nervous system development in some children. Those interested in the medical explanation for this phenomenon should read the section on intestinal pathology and the opioid excess theory in Chapter 3.

Wakefield et al. emphasized that they had not proven a cause and effect relationship between the MMR vaccine and a non-specific colitis, which they described as "autistic ileal-lymphoid-nodular hyperplasia." Although they simply called for more studies to explore the relationship, their report was immediately met with intense criticism in the U.S. and Europe.

Part of Wakefield's hypothesis was that the combining of three live viruses into one vaccine (MMR) was exposing children to an atypical simultaneous presentation of the three viruses, which in past generations were experienced by children at different times in childhood. In other words, children almost never become infected with measles, mumps and rubella disease at the same time. His suggestion that children receive the three vaccines separately, rather than in the combination MMR vaccine, became the central focus of the anger of the vaccine establishment.

After Wakefield's study was published in the *Lancet,* Neal Halsey, MD, Director of the Institute for Vaccine Safety at Johns Hopkins University and chairman of the AAP Committee on Infectious Diseases, as well as Brent Taylor, a British physician, attempted to discredit Wakefield. Halsey cited "good evidence for genetic predisposition and other factors including intrauterine exposure to rubella, head injuries, and encephalitis as "possible contributing factors."[92] Taylor accused Wakefield of a possible "conflict of interest" because Wakefield was treating autistic children whose parents were considering civil litigation involving an MMR vaccine manufacturer. Taylor presented epidemiological data he claimed disproved Wakefield's findings [93] and was, in turn, criticized by parent groups and independent physicians for publishing biased and methodologically flawed research.

Although Wakefield and his colleagues went on to identify measles viral DNA in the intestines of autistic children,[94] and his findings have been replicated by other researchers, he continues to be attacked by U.S. and British government health officials while being hailed as a hero in the autism community. He founded a research institution, Thoughtful House, in Austin, Texas and has steadfastly stood by his original findings.

Other viruses and viral vaccines including mumps, rubella, varicella, polio, and influenza are also known to cause brain inflammation which may contribute to the "total load" in autism.
- *Mumps* has been known to cause meningitis and encephalitis since the 18th century. Many studies report and document meningitis within three weeks of mumps vaccination,[95] primarily with the Urabe vaccine strain virus. There have also been reports of meningitis after vaccination with the Jeryl Lynn mumps vaccine strain[96] now used in MMR vaccine. Russell and Donald, observed in 1958 that "the clinical resemblance between mumps encephalitis, and the encephalitis which may follow measles, varicella and rubella, and the fact that the histological appearance of perivascular demyelination are common to them all, suggest that they arise from the same pathological process."[97]
- *Rubella* disease is caused by an RNA virus. Although mild in children, it can be transmitted from mother to fetus in utero, and cause enchephalitis and devastating harm to the unborn child, including mental retardation, hearing and vision loss, heart and neuromuscular deformity. In the rubella epidemic that swept the U.S. in 1964, an estimated 20,000 to 30,000 children, whose pregnant mothers were infected with rubella,

were born severely damaged, and a high rate of classic and "partial" autism was observed in those children by Chess in 1971.

In 1977, Chess reported that the rate of autism in children born with congenital rubella from the 1964 epidemic was equivalent to a rate of "412 per 10,000 for the complete syndrome of autism of those with rubella, and 329 for the partial syndrome."[98] The combined rate of 741 per 10,000 of those with rubella and autism, compared to the rate of autism in children without congenital rubella syndrome was estimated in 1966 to be only 2.1 cases of autism per 10,000 children.[99]

Rubella disease and rubella vaccine have also been associated with acute and chronic arthritis.[100,101] In 1991, the IOM published a report which evaluated scientific evidence that rubella vaccine could cause chronic arthritis, and found that the evidence indicates a causal relation between the RA27/3 rubella vaccine and acute arthritis in adult women. That evidence is consistent with a causal relation between rubella vaccine and chronic arthritis.[102]

- *Varicella zoster* virus, which causes chicken pox, is a member of the herpes virus family. A clinical association between varicella zoster and herpes zoster (shingles) has been recognized for more than 100 years. For the majority of children, chicken pox is a mild childhood disease. However, brain inflammation can be a more common serious complication for teenagers and adults. The live virus chicken pox vaccine has also been associated with brain inflammation, including seizures. In 2000, an analysis of the reports made to the government's Vaccine Adverse Events Reporting System (VAERS) revealed one in 33,000 doses of varicella zoster vaccine resulted in a report of a serious health event such as shock, convulsions, encephalitis and death.[103]

- *Poliomyelitis* is caused by an enterovirus. One to two percent of infected individuals develop inflammation of nerve cells of the brain stem and spinal cord. Fewer go on to have residual paralysis or die. Likewise, within one to six months of receiving the live attenuated polio vaccine, complications can occur from persistent vaccine strain polio virus infection resulting in paralysis or death. According to the IOM in 1994, live polio vaccine complications can also trigger Guillain-Barre Syndrome (GBS), which is characterized by muscle weakness, numbness, pain and paralysis caused by inflammation of the myelin sheaths of the peripheral nerves of the limbs and face.[104]

In both cases, the polio virus invades the central nervous system and destroys neurons. By 1999, the only cases of paralytic polio occurring in the US were caused by the live oral polio vaccine (OPV). After parents of children paralyzed by OPV, as well as OPV paralyzed adults lobbied for change, the CDC recommended that all American children receive only the inactivated polio vaccine (IPV). IPV cannot cause polio either in the person vaccinated or in someone who comes in contact with that person's body fluids.

- *Influenza* or the "flu" is an umbrella term that describes thousands of viruses that can cause symptoms such a runny nose, nasal congestion, cough, sore throat, headache, muscle aches, fever, chills and generalized weakness. Only about 20% of all flu-like illness is actually caused by viral influenza. Every year health officials gather information about influenza activity around the world and make an educated guess about which three flu strains to include in the formula for the upcoming year. The flu vaccine only protects against the three specific viruses included in each year's formulation and sometimes the flu vaccine does not contain the flu virus that causes most of the flu in a given flu season. An assessment of the 2003-2004 flu season in the U.S. revealed that only 3-14% of those who got vaccinated were protected against the strain that was prevalent in the U.S. that year.[105]

In 2002, the CDC recommended universal use of flu vaccine annually in all healthy children six months of age and older,[106] even though no long-term safety trials of flu vaccine had ever been conducted including infants and children. Both the killed virus injectable vaccine and the live virus flu vaccine squirted up the nose can cause flu-like symptoms, including fever, fatigue, painful joints and headache. The most frequently reported serious reaction, which usually occurs within two weeks of vaccination, is GBS. The live nasal flu vaccine is not recommended for people with asthma or respiratory disease because it worsened those conditions in clinical trials.[107]

- *Hepatitis B* is a virus that attacks the liver. It can cause such severe joint pain, fatigue and weakness that it is sometimes mistaken for rheumatoid arthritis or lupus. Within weeks of recombinant hepatitis B vaccination, some children and adults experience recurring fevers, severe joint pain,[108-110] optic neuritis,[111] memory loss, muscle weakness, debilitating fatigue and other chronic immune-mediated neurological dysfunction, which can involve demyelination of the brain.[112] In 1996, Italian researchers evaluated infants who suffered seizures and autism following hepatitis B vaccination and concluded that "autoimmune diseases are more frequent in nations where vaccines are widely used" and they identified high risk genetic markers which predispose for autoimmunity following hepatitis B vaccination.[113]

In 2004, British researchers found that hepatitis B vaccination "was associated with a threefold increase in multiple sclerosis within the three years following vaccination."[114] In 2005, a biological mechanism study found evidence for immunological cross-reactivity between hepatitis B surface antigen and myelin mimics[115] and, in 2006, French researchers concluded that hepatitis B vaccine contaminants could trigger an autoimmune process against myelin in some vaccinated subjects causing multiple sclerosis or other central demyelinating disorders.[116]

Bacteria and Bacterial Vaccines

Brain inflammation is not only caused by viruses and viral vaccines, but also by bacteria and bacterial vaccines. Many types of bacteria, some of which are contained in vaccines, such as B pertussis, pneumococcus, haemphilus influenzae B, streptococcus, staphylococcus, meningococcus and tuberculosis, can cause brain inflammation and permanent neurological damage.

- *Pertussis* or whooping cough is a respiratory disease caused by the Bordetella pertussis bacteria. B pertussis bacteria attach themselves to the mucus membranes of the respiratory tract and also release toxins, such as pertussis toxin (PT) and endotoxin, which can cause inflammation in the body, especially brain inflammation. The most common serious complication of both pertussis and pertussis vaccine is brain inflammation leading to varying degrees of permanent brain dysfunction. Pertussis toxin (PT) is one of the most lethal toxins in nature. It is thought to be the main component of B. pertussis bacteria responsible for both stimulating the production of protective antibodies after natural infection or vaccination, as well as for causing brain inflammation during pertussis infection or after injection of pertussis-containing vaccines. Because PT can cross the blood brain barrier when conditions are right, encephalitis has always been the most dreaded complication of both whooping cough[117] and pertussis vaccination.[118,119]

The authors of the National Childhood Encephalopathy Study noted in 1993[120] and IOM confirmed in 1994,[121] that DPT vaccine-induced brain inflammation is associated with a broad range of long term brain dysfunction that affects the physical, social, behavioral and educational outcomes for children. Signs of brain inflammation within seven days of DPT or DTaP vaccination include a high fever, irritability, high pitched screaming, prolonged crying, drowsiness, vomiting, seizures, collapse and unresponsiveness, followed by immediate frank regression or progressive changes in mental, emotional and physical health.[122] [123] Death, or a diagnosis of mental retardation, seizure disorders, learning disabilities, attention deficit disorder, autism and other chronic neurological and health problems often follows.

Since the 1950s, scientists have injected the lethal pertussis toxin into lab animals whenever they want to deliberately induce histamine, serotonin and endotoxin sensitivity[124] or experimental autoimmune encephalomyelitis.[125-127] PT induces lymphocytosis, leukocytosis, stimulates insulin secretion and sensitizes histamine,[128] which is involved in an inflammatory response and CNS and allergic reactions.[129] The newer DTaP vaccine still contains pertussis toxin with the ability to induce brain inflammation which could lead to brain dysfunction or other kinds of chronic inflammatory disease in vulnerable children.

The role of genetic factors in vaccine injury are highlighted in the work of pediatrician Mary Megson, MD, who identified a g-alpha protein defect in some children which makes them vulnerable to pertussis toxin-containing vaccines.[130] Lawrence Steinman also identified genetic susceptibility to pertussis vaccine induced encephalopathy involving genes of the major histocompatibility complex correlating to genetic regulation of antibody response to bovine serum albumin (a cow's milk protein).[131]

The first reports of brain inflammation and chronic brain damage, including death, after pertussis vaccination were published in 1933 by Madsen[132] and in 1947 by Brody,[133] followed by numerous reports during the next 40 years. Finally, after nearly 50 years of evidence in the medical literature, the 1981 National Childhood Encephalopathy Study (NCES) confirmed that the DPT vaccine was causing brain inflammation and permanent brain damage in previously healthy children.[134]

The 1985 book, *DPT: A Shot in the Dark,*[1] examines the history of pertussis and the pertussis vaccine within the larger context of the medical, scientific, legal, social, and political issues involving mass vaccination policies. The book includes more than 100 case histories of DPT vaccine associated brain inflammation and immune system dysfunction. Several of the cases describe children who developed autistic behaviors after DPT vaccination, making it the first published report of an association between autism and vaccination.

Children diagnosed with autism today have much in common with the children described in *A Shot in the Dark,* who reacted neurologically to DPT vaccine in the 1970s and 1980s. Many of the DPT vaccine injury cases in the book revealed children with a personal and/ or family history of allergy, particularly milk allergy. Some had been vaccinated while they were sick with a coinciding viral or bacterial infection. Others were on antibiotics or recently completed antibiotic therapy before vaccination. In addition to neurological damage following DPT vaccination, many were also left with chronic gastrointestinal dysfunction and new allergies, as well as autoimmune disorders such as asthma. A personal or family history of inflammatory autoimmune disorders appeared to outweigh a history of neurological disorders in terms of being a high risk factor for reacting to DPT, although a history of convulsions in the family was also a high risk factor.

In 1996, a child with mental retardation and autistic behaviors was awarded compensation under the National Childhood Vaccine Injury Act despite vigorous protests by federal health officials that there was no proof DPT vaccine caused the autism. The child had been healthy with above average intelligence before he reacted within four hours of his DPT shot at 19 months of age with a convulsion followed by days of fever and screaming. The U.S. Court of Claims made the award, agreeing with the plaintiff's lawyer that autistic behaviors can be the result of brain injury from any cause, including the DPT vaccine.

Fourteen years of lobbying by parents finally resulted in the licensing of a second-generation DTaP vaccine for American babies in 1996. Introduced in Japan in 1981, this purified vaccine reduced the amount of endotoxin and the bioactivity of pertussis toxin through chemical inactivation with formaldehyde and/or gluteraldehyde (both formaldehyde and gluteraldehyde remain residually in the vaccine).[135,136] Because the DTaP vaccine still contains pertussis toxin, (10 - 25 mcg per dose) with varying amounts of bioactivity,[137] it is still capable of inducing brain inflammation. A company producing a genetically engineered DTaP vaccine in the early 1990's, Chiron, explained why chemically inactivated PT will always be a problem: "Genetic detoxification ensures that no active form of the pertussis toxin is present, while chemically detoxified pertussis toxins may revert to toxicity."[138]

In addition to brain inflammation, acellular pertussis vaccine can cause extensive swelling at the site of the injection. Some vaccine researchers think this swelling may be due to a hypersensitivity reaction or be related to DTaP vaccine-induced Th2 type cytokines, Th2 skewing of the immune response and a subsequent delay in Th1 development in some children.[139-141]

Although brain inflammation is thought to occur less frequently with DTaP than with DPT, because DTaP vaccine is associated with the same kind of brain inflammation and other CNS complications as the whole cell DPT vaccine, the same contraindications and precautions that were in force with DPT vaccine are also applicable to DTaP vaccine.[142]

- **Tetanus** bacteria produces several potent toxins which attack blood cells and can cause violent muscle spasms as well as severe damage to the brain. In 1994, the IOM concluded that tetanus vaccine can cause GBS within one to four weeks after vaccination. The tetanus vaccine can also cause brachial neuritis, a neuropathy that usually appears within three weeks of vaccination. Brachial neuritis involves painful nerve inflammation in the arm and shoulder which can progress over a period of many months.
- **Haemphilus influenzae B** (HiB), a type of bacterial meningitis, has a direct effect on the central nervous system, and can cause seizures and profound brain damage. Although reports of demyelination have been reported after children receive HiB vaccine, a causal relationship has not yet been confirmed. HiB vaccine has a high endotoxin content, which could contribute to reactions[143] (see below).
- **Pneumococcal** disease is caused by the bacterium Streptococcus pneumoniae and more than 80 different serotypes exist. Pneumococcus can cause pneumonia, otitis media (inner ear infection), and blood poisoning. One of the most feared complications is meningitis (inflammation of the outer layer of the brain and spinal cord), that can leave adults and children with seizure disorders and other kinds of long term neurological damage. The pneumococcal vaccine for children, called Prevnar, which includes the seven most antibiotic resistant strains of pneumococcus, has been associated with brain inflammation and neurological symptoms, including prolonged crying, general irritability and seizures.[144]
- **Meningococcal** disease is a type of meningitis caused by at least 13 different serotypes of gram negative bacteria. Humans are a natural reservoir for meningococci, and most become immune to the organisms. A small number of individuals, however, develop meningitis that begins with a sudden fever, rash, headache and stiff neck and can progress to pneumonia, organ failure and death. Reported reactions to the vaccine have included headache, fever, stiff neck, disturbances of behavior, and paralysis. In

2005, the FDA and CDC issued an alert that the Menactra vaccine, given to teenagers, is associated with GBS.[145]

Endotoxin in Vaccines

Some vaccines, such as HiB, flu, hepatitis B, meningococcal, DPT and DTaP, contain varying amounts of endotoxin.[146-150] Endotoxin is a lipopolysaccharide that is part of the cell wall of gram negative bacteria that cause infections. When the immune system detects the presence of endotoxins, it produces a defensive inflammatory immune response, including release of cytokines such as histamine, which can induce fever, swelling, diarrhea, collapse, shock and death.[151,152] DPT and other vaccines have long been associated with infant death, including sudden infant death syndrome (SIDS).[153]

Antibiotics kill bacteria rapidly and the dying bacteria release large amounts of endotoxin into the body.[154,155] Veterinary medicine offers evidence that a combined load of endotoxin from infections, bacterial vaccines and other sources can contribute to endotoxin-related shock, death, spontaneous abortion and other reactions.[156,157] The product insert of meningococcal vaccine (Menomune) warns that, "due to the combined endotoxin content, the vaccine should NOT be administered at the same time as whole cell pertussis or whole cell typhoid vaccines."[158]

In 2005, the Medicines Control Council in Britain stated that, "injected endotoxins cause fever and swelling and may, in larger doses, precipitate endotoxic shock that can be life threatening, particularly in infants." The Council recommends that infant vaccines that contain more than five International Units of endotoxin per dose include a warning on the package insert stating that doctors take care when using endotoxin containing vaccine simultaneously with other products containing endotoxins.[159]

In consideration of evidence that significant endotoxin release in the body can cause inflammation, shock, abortion and death, giving multiple bacterial vaccines containing endotoxin to pregnant women and babies, especially if they are sick or taking antibiotics, could increase the risk for serious health consequences.

Vaccine Additives

Few parents know that vaccines contain many potentially toxic additives, including mercury, aluminum, formaldehyde, phenooxyethanol, gluteraldehyde, sodium chloride, monosodium glutamate (MSG), yeast, sodium borate, human and bovine albumin, protein, gelatin and other substances.[160,161] Some are adjuvants, (substances which make the vaccine more potent), and others are preservatives, which keep the vaccine sterile. Vaccine adjuvants and preservatives have the potential on their own to cause immune mediated inflammation leading to brain damage and autoimmunity. In addition, the effects of adventitious agent contaminants from animal and human cell substrates used to make vaccines, such as monkey, kidney, cow, pig and aborted human fetal lung tissue, is unknown at this time.[162,163] (The vaccine manufacturer product inserts included with packages of vaccine contain information on cell substrates.)

Mercury as a Neurotoxin

Chapter 3 includes details about the many environmental sources of mercury. This chapter also contains a synopsis of "Autism: A Unique Form of Mercury Poisioning," which includes several famous historical examples that demonstrate how toxic mercury can be, especially for the nervous systems of the developing fetus and young children.

Today in the U.S., exposure to mercury is primarily from old dental fillings, eating certain kinds of fish and through exposure to the vaccine mercury preservative, thimerosal. Both organic (methyl) and inorganic (ethyl) mercury can kill nerve cells and cause brain damage and immune dysfunction.[164] Thomas Burbacher reported that monkeys who were injected with ethyl mercury in the form of the vaccine mercury preservative, thimerosal, had higher concentrations of mercury in their brains than the monkeys who swallowed methyl mercury.[165] A comparison of total mercury levels in 20 preterm or term infants, both before and after receiving a single thimerosal containing hepatitis B vaccine, found that both groups sustained high levels of mercury in the blood 48 to 72 hours after vaccination, with the highest levels in pre-term infants.[166]

Mercury as Thimerosal

Thimerosal, created by Eli Lilly & Co. in 1928 under the name merthiolate, is an organo-mercurial antiseptic that is used as a preservative, an anti-infective, an antibacterial and a topical antifungal. Thimerosal is 49.6 percent ethyl mercury by weight. In 1930, Eli Lilly conducted a single study on 22 patients seriously ill with meningitis to prove that thimerosal was safe for injection into humans. All died, but their deaths were attributed solely to meningitis and not to any effects of injected thimerosal. Eli Lily then pronounced thimerosal safe for human use.[167]

Thimerosal was added to pertussis vaccine in the 1930s and the DPT vaccine in the 1940s. For more than 50 years, thimerosal was included in certain drugs, cosmetics, eye drops and contact lens solutions, and was a common preservative in multi-dose vials of inactivated bacterial vaccines in an attempt to keep them sterile. Adding thimerosal allows medical personnel to use one vial of vaccine for more than one person, thus reducing the cost. The more expensive single dose vials do not require a preservative to remain sterile. In 1998 the FDA banned thimerosal from most products because of its toxicity and many adverse reaction reports, but allowed it to remain in multi-dose vials of killed bacterial vaccines such as DPT, DTaP, hepatitis B, HIB and flu vaccines.

Thimerosal and Autism

In 1999, the FDA, CDC and Environmental Protection Agency (EPA) directed U.S. vaccine manufacturers to remove thimerosal from all children's vaccines as soon as possible. Their directive was in response to 1997 federal legislation requiring evaluation of mercury content in products, and the subsequent finding that a six-month-old child born in the 1990s would have received a cumulative ethyl mercury exposure in vaccines 187 times greater than the EPA's limit for daily exposure to methyl mercury.[168] The 1999 directive caught the attention of Sallie Bernard and Lyn Redwood, co-founders of SAFEMINDS and co-authors of "Autism: A Novel Form of Mercury Poisoning" (See Chapter 3.)

In October 2001, the IOM published the first formal scientific review of evidence for and against an association between thimerosal and autism. It concluded that there was not enough evidence to prove or disprove the hypothesis that thimerosal containing vaccines cause children to develop autism and other neuro-developmental disorders. However, the Committee recommended erring on the side of caution and removing preservatives containing inorganic mercury from all vaccines and over-the-counter products, in consideration of the strong scientific evidence that exposure to organic mercury harms the developing fetus and human brain.[169]

The 2001 IOM report would be the first and only official admission by the U.S. scientific community that it was biologically plausible for mercury containing vaccines to cause neuro-immune dysfunction leading to autism. What followed was a six year effort on the part of U.S. government health officials and vaccine manufacturers, with the assistance of European officials and vaccine manufacturers, to prove the safety of thimerosal. They quickly published retrospective epidemiological studies denying that mercury containing vaccines have caused autism.

In *Evidence of Harm*[4] and *Deadly Immunity*[5] the authors review evidence for a coverup by government health officials and vaccine manufacturers of data linking autism and thimerosal. They reveal details of a June 2000 conference at Simpsonwood, near Atlanta, Georgia, where top government scientists, national and international health officials and vaccine manufacturers met. The purpose of the meeting was to evaluate potentially alarming data from the CDC's Vaccine Safety Datalink (VSD), which revealed a causal relationship between thimerosal-containing vaccines and autism. A CDC epidemiologist, Tom Verstraeten, had found a statistically significant association between children receiving thimerosal containing vaccines and later development of autism. The group spent most of its time discussing ways to suppress the information that a dramatic increase in the numbers of children with autism and other developmental delays occurred in 1991, immediately after the mercury-containing HIB and hepatitis B vaccines were added to the childhood vaccination schedule-which already included mercury-containing DPT vaccine.

Verstraeten and the CDC finally published the VSD data results in 2003,[170] stating that, "no consistent significant associations were found between thimerosal containing vaccines and neurodevelopmental outcomes." This statement would later be refuted by evidence found by geneticist Mark Geier, MD, PhD, and his son, David Geier, when they further analyzed the VSD and VAERS data. They found that children who received mercury-containing DTaP shots were significantly more like to become autistic than children given mercury-free DTaP shots. [171] [172]

Also in 2003, researchers Karin Nelson and Margaret Bauman,[173] exchanged conflicting reports in the medical literature, with parents of autistic children[174] about whether thimerosal could cause brain damage in children. Two epidemiological studies, funded and conducted by U.S. and Danish researchers affiliated with vaccine manufacturers and/or government health agencies, further muddied the waters as to whether thimerosal could cause autism when they were published in 2003.[175,176] These studies either compared thimerosal exposures and autism rates over time, or used old medical records to compare the health status of children who received mercury containing vaccines versus those who did not. Researchers concluded that autism rates continued to climb in Denmark, even after thimerosal was removed from vaccines, and that the individual risk of autism and other autistic spectrum disorders did not differ significantly between children vaccinated with thimerosal containing vaccines and children vaccinated with thimerosal-free vaccines.

The conclusions of the studies were highly publicized by U.S. health agencies and the media, and strongly criticized by parent groups, including SafeMinds,[177] which maintained that the research was methodologically fatally flawed. Some criticized the emphasis on epidemiological studies which rely on old medical records to determine cause and effect, rather than on scientific research assessing the biological and genetic factors involved in autism. Critics pointed out that:

- Scandinavian children received fewer vaccines with lower amounts of thimerosal, and received those vaccines at different ages, compared to American children
- the studies capriciously excluded or included cases of autism in order to skew the data toward a "no association" finding
- the autism rates in Scandinavia historically have been lower than those in the U.S.
- the biological responses of genetically homogeneous populations in Denmark and Sweden cannot be compared to the genetically diverse population of America

Between 2001 and 2007, independent researchers, some of whom are also parents of children with autism, worked steadily to investigate the biological mechanisms of thimerosal-induced autism at the cellular and molecular level in order to find ways to heal autistic children. Funded by the M.I.N.D. Institute at the University of California at Davis, as well as by some independent advocacy organizations, foundations and individuals, many committed doctors and scientists have investigated how exposure to thimerosal through vaccination can interact with genetic factors, coinciding infections, other vaccines, antibiotics and environmental exposures to disrupt brain and immune function in both animals and humans. Their findings are reviewed in Chapters 5 and 6.

Proposed biological mechanisms for thimerosal-induced autism have focused on mercury containing vaccines and genetic factors interacting to create:

- oxidative stress leading to impaired methylation and lowered levels of cysteine and glutathione[178-180]
- DNA damage and death of brain cells[181-185]
- brain inflammation[186,187]
- autoimmunity and/or genetic susceptibility[188-191]

Despite the mounting evidence from independent researchers that thimerosal contributed to the development of autism in a subset of children who cannot efficiently excrete mercury from the body,[192] at the request of the CDC in 2004, the Institute of Medicine issued a new report on thimerosal and autism.[193] In this report, the IOM Committee totally rejected all clinical, biological mechanism and epidemiological evidence showing a causal relationship between thimerosal containing vaccines and the development of autism and other neuroimmune disorders in children. The Committee went one step further declaring that no more scientific research need be funded into the relationship between vaccines and autism.

Aluminum

Aluminum is a metal which is neurotoxic when it accesses the nervous system[194,195] The biological mechanisms for aluminum-induced toxicity and neuroimmune dysfunction are similar to that of mercury. Chapter 3 includes information about the many surprising sources of aluminum, such as baby formula and personal care products that add to an individual's total load.

Aluminum is also a common adjuvant in many vaccines in the form of aluminum hydroxide, aluminum phosphate or potassium aluminum sulfate (alum). Aluminum adjuvants have been used for decades to boost and extend the effectiveness of vaccines, even though there is limited data on pharmacokinetics and toxicities of aluminum injected into humans.[196] No clinical trials were conducted before aluminum adjuvants were added to vaccines in the mid-twentieth century. Research shows that aluminum containing vaccines and aluminum adjuvants both increase aluminum levels in the brain tissues of lab animals.[197,198] Aluminum adjuvants in vaccines have been associated with motor neuron death in mice[199] and inflammation at the site of vaccine injections in humans associated with macrophagic myofasciitis,[200] causing chronic joint and muscle pain, muscle weakness, fatigue and multiple sclerosis-like symptoms.

Childhood vaccines contain from 170 mcg to 625 mcg of aluminum per dose.[201] Children receiving multiple vaccines on one day (pneumococcal, DTaP, hepatitis B, hepatitis A) could receive as much as 1250 mcg of aluminum. The FDA stated in 2004 that "Patients with impaired kidney function, *including premature neonates*, who receive parenteral [by intravenous or intramuscular injection] levels of aluminum greater than 4 to 5 mcg/kg/day, accumulate aluminum at levels associated with CNS and bone toxicity. Tissue loading may occur at even lower rates of administration."[202]

Aluminum has an affinity for the brain, bones, lung and liver.[203] It can make the blood brain barrier more permeable and cross it, leading to neuron death.[204-207] Symptoms of aluminum poisoning include personality changes, progressive speech disorder, stuttering, apraxia, tremors, myoclonic jerks, seizures, abnormal EEG, psychosis and dementia.[208,209]

Elevated levels of aluminum have been found in the brains of those diagnosed with Alzheimer's disease.[210] Alzheimer's patients suffer from mental regression, memory lapses, personality changes, mood disturbances, agitation, aggression, pacing, changed sleep patterns, appetite disturbances, confusion, depression and dementia.[211] Aluminum has the ability to cause chronic inflammation of the brain, leading to the death of brain cells.[212,213]

Bottom line: Whether or not aluminum exposure through vaccination has contributed to the development of regressive autism in children, especially those who are genetically vulnerable to the toxic effects of aluminum, is still unknown.

The Rest of the Story

Regressive autism is a neuroimmune disorder that is increasing in prevalence, and is associated with increased vaccination during the last half of the 20th and the beginning of the 21st centuries. Although many parents and doctors have hoped that the removal of the mercury preservative, thimerosal, from vaccines would end the epidemic of autism, the evidence presented in this and other chapters of this book suggests that the autism epidemic is about more than mercury. Regressive autism may stem from unresolved inflammation in genetically vulnerable children, caused by use of too many vaccines. Used singly and in combination these vaccinations can cause neuroimmune dysfunction via a variety of biological mechanisms.

Brain Inflammation and Autism

As reviewed in this chapter, for about 200 years the medical literature has shown that neurological and immune system dysfunction caused by infectious diseases are often identical to neurological and immune system dysfunction caused by the vaccines created with those same viruses and bacteria. A host/disease or host/vaccine interaction causes inflammation, which is acute at first, and becomes chronic rather than resolving and leaving the host with good health. In both cases, the end result is unresolved inflammation leading to immune mediated brain dysfunction of varying degrees of severity, which is the same profile many have observed in children with autism spectrum disorders.[214,215]

Researchers have found evidence of chronic inflammation in the brains of patients with autism, particularly in the cerebellum. Autistic brains have been observed to be in "a chronic state of specific cytokine activity." The suggested biological mechanisms responsible for the observed brain inflammation included chronic disease or an external environmental source.[216]

Autoimmunity: the Key to Vaccine Responses

Clearly, viral and bacterial diseases, as well as vaccines containing lab altered viruses and bacteria, have the biological capability of causing immune mediated brain dysfunction leading to autism. Scientists are just beginning to understand which individuals are most vulnerable and why. Autoimmunity appears to be the key, and it runs in families.

In Chapter 3, the authors identified immune system abnormalities as key to autism. The reader is referred back to that chapter for a review of studies related to depressed T-cell response. Some with autism also have defective antibody responses to rubella vaccine.[217] Others have abnormal cell-mediated immune responses to myelin basic protein, a component of brain myelin.[218]

Dr. Vijendra Singh is the name most associated with the presence of auto-antibodies to myelin basic protein in children with autism. The strongest link found in his studies was between measles virus antibodies and antibodies to myelin basic protein (MBP). He hypothesized that "an immunological assault, secondary to a virus infection, occurring pre-natally, post-natally, during infancy, or early childhood, could possibly result in poor myelination or abnormal function of the neuro-axon myelin."[219,220] In 2005, researchers at the M.I.N.D. Institute, UC-Davis, showed that children with autism have an imbalance of the cellular and humoral immune responses. These researchers thus concluded that an autoimmune mechanism may explain a subset of autism.[221]

The medical model of autism described in the 1980s, by Ritvo and Freeman concluded, "The symptoms (of autism) are due to neuropathology which, in turn, may have a variety of etiologies." They observed a high rate of abnormal EEG's, seizures, severe allergies, and significant differences in brain metabolism patterns and brain chemistry in children diagnosed with autism, compared to those who are not autistic.[222]

Autoimmunity and Genetics: It's All in the Family
In 1986, Reed Warren first described immune abnormalities in individuals with autism.[223] In 1998 he and others collected mounting evidence that autism indeed has an immunogenetic basis.[224]

F. Edward Yazbak, MD, provided evidence for a relationship between maternal antibodies and autism in nursing mothers who were re-vaccinated with rubella or MMR vaccine following childbirth. Because many of their children became autistic following MMR vaccination, he concluded that mothers may transfer maternal antibodies to rubella to their babies either transplacentally, or through breast milk. When the babies are vaccinated with MMR, some develop an autoimmune reaction with pre-existing rubella antigen that leads to autistic behaviors.[225]

The familial link between autism and autoimmunity goes beyond the mother. One study reported that when two or more family members had autoimmune disorders, such as rheumatoid arthritis, systemic lupus and connective tissue disorders, the offspring were twice as likely to have autism; those with at least three family members and autoimmune disorders were 5.5 times more likely to have autism; and those whose mothers had autoimmune disorders were 8.8 times more likely to be affected. Researchers concluded that "individuals with autism inherit a genetic predisposition for autoimmunity that, in conjunction with medical triggers or other environmental factors, results in neurologic pathology.[226]

Some autoimmune disorders are associated with genes of the major histo-compatability complex (MHC). The MHC is made up of hundreds of genes, some of which are involved in helping cells of the immune system work together to resist infection and recognize the body's own tissue. Warren, Singh and others, found that abnormalities in the MHC complex occurred more than twice as often in individuals with autism as in those without.[227]

If exposure to viruses, bacteria or chemical toxins damages these genes or abnormally rearranges them, they can cripple the body's defenses against some infections, or cause the immune system to mistakenly attack the body's own tissues. It is this genetic autoimmune mechanism that is involved in diabetes, for example, when the immune system attacks cells in the pancreas. In celiac disease, an autoimmune disorder common in children with autism and developmental delays, chronic inflammation of the small intestine due to gluten intolerance causes diarrhea, constipation, failure to thrive, irritability, emotional withdrawal, mouth ulcers, and seizures, among other symptoms.

Genotoxic Events and Chromosome Damage
Studies in 1978 and 1980 revealed that smallpox vaccination can cause chromosomal damage.[228,229] Decades later, microbiologist Howard Urnovitz, PhD, an expert on adventitious

agent contamination of polio vaccines, found abnormal RNA in the blood of 50 percent of sick Gulf War veterans and none in the age and sex matched healthy non-military controls, [30] indicating that chromosomal change had occurred in the sick veterans.

The RNA found in the sick Gulf War veterans is encoded by genetic material that occurs only in chromosome 22q11.2. This chromosome is uniquely susceptible to genetic rearrangements and mutations. Damage to it has been linked to autoimmune diseases such as juvenile rheumatoid arthritis, thrombocytopenia pupura and multiple myeloma cancer. Pointing out that "genotoxic events" may damage the human chromosome, Urnovitz suggested that when the body is subjected to toxic events such as exposure to viruses, bacteria, drugs, chemicals, or radiation, there appears to be molecular memory. He maintained that the human chromosome may be able to take just so many toxic exposures before it begins to break down. Individuals with certain genotypes may be particularly at risk for sustaining chromosomal damage after exposure to toxic events.

Dr. Urnovitz, criticized the Defense Department in 1995 for administering multiple vaccinations to soldiers heading for the Gulf War. Their vaccines included cholera, live oral polio, typhoid fever, meningitis, pertussis, tetanus, diphtheria, yellow fever, recombinant hepatitis B, influenza and two experimental vaccines, anthrax and botulinium, along with an experimental drug, pryridostigmine bromide. Urnovitz maintained that the multiple vaccinations weakened the soldiers' immune systems, making them more vulnerable to environmental toxins and opportunistic infections encountered in the Gulf War, causing tens of thousands to become chronically ill with "Gulf War Syndrome." These soldiers experienced symptoms such as chronic muscle and joint pain, rashes, headache, disabling fatigue, memory loss, inability to concentrate, personality changes, diarrhea, hair loss, and sleep disturbances.

Whether vaccine injured children, including those who have regressed into autism after vaccination, have sustained chromosomal damage is unknown. Neurosurgeon Russell Blaylock, MD, suggests there might be a link between the biological mechanisms for chronic dysfunction in autism and chronic brain dysfunction in Gulf War syndrome. He points out that both conditions are characterized by overstimulation of the systemic immune system often after repeated vaccinations spaced close together, resulting in chronic activation of brain microglia. He said "both syndromes manifest an impaired immune system, a possible consequence of excessive vaccination itself, neurotoxic vaccine additives (aluminum and mercury), and immune suppressive viruses such as the measles virus."[231]

Vaccines, Politics and Conflict of Interest

Who decides which vaccines should be recommended for universal use on the U.S. Childhood Immunization Schedule? The CDC's 15-member Advisory Committee on Immunization Practices (ACIP) is primarily in charge of setting national vaccine policies, and the AAP usually follows the CDC's lead by issuing similar recommendations.

Between 1999 and 2003, the U.S. House Government Reform Committee, chaired by Congressman Dan Burton (R-IN), examined vaccine safety issues, of the MMR and anthrax vaccines, as well as mercury containing vaccines. Congressman Burton's two grandchildren reacted to vaccines. Danielle Burton Sarkine's newborn daughter almost died after a hepatitis B vaccination, and her healthy 14-month-old son became autistic after being injected with nine different vaccines on the same day. In 2003, the U.S. House Government Reform Committee issued an 84-page report entitled "Mercury in Medicine: Taking Unnecessary Risks."[232]

After September 11, 2001, when the Department of Health and Human Services and Department of Defense persuaded Congress to pass the Homeland Security Act in 2002, pharmaceutical companies lobbied to insert a "thimerosal rider" in the anti-terrorism bill. Parents of vaccine injured children across the country protested the attempt to shield drug companies from liability for vaccine injuries potentially caused by mercury in vaccines. The rider was later removed from the Homeland Security bill.

Drug companies continued their lobbying, and in 2003 (Project Bioshield) and 2005 (Pandemic Flu legislation), Congress voted again to shield drug companies from liability for injuries caused by vaccines. These acts have the potential to force American citizens to use any vaccine, even experimental ones, whenever the Secretary of Health declares a public health "emergency."[233]

Vaccine advisory committees at the FDA and CDC, as well as NIH research funding agencies, have come under criticism for employing individuals with financial ties to vaccine makers. However, conflict of interest concerns are not confined to U.S. public health agencies. Authors of one of the Danish studies, conducted to theoretically put to rest concerns that MMR vaccination might cause autism,[234] did not make two important disclosures:
- that the "Statens Serum Institut," where three of the authors work, is Denmark's largest for-profit vaccine manufacturer
- that four other authors of the research had financial ties to this company. Only one of the eight study authors was not associated with this Institute - the U.S. Centers for Disease Control employs him

Research on Vaccine Safety Holds the Key

Health officials consider a vaccine to be safe if no or very few serious adverse events occur in pre-licensure clinical trials. However, the truth is that most serious adverse events which do occur in clinical trials are dismissed as unassociated with the experimental new vaccine being investigated.[235] When new vaccines are added to the universal use list, very few children have ever received the experimental vaccine in combination with other vaccines, and follow-up of these children is limited to a few days, weeks or months post vaccination. Furthermore, vaccine manufacturers and U.S. federal health agencies have not conducted studies to assess the long-term effects of a vaccination schedule that recommends American children be injected with 48 doses of 14 vaccines by age six, starting at birth, and another dozen doses of vaccines by adolescence.

In order to fully understand the pathological effects on the developing brain and immune system of this kind of vaccination schedule, researchers would have to conduct a prospective, case controlled study comparing completely vaccinated to completely unvaccinated children living in the U.S. They would have to evaluate the children for at least 10 years for all morbidity and mortality outcomes, for pathological changes in immune and brain function at the cellular and molecular levels, and for changes in chromosomal integrity. Within the first five years, differences between the two groups, in terms of biological integrity and rates of autism, learning disabilities, ADHD, asthma, juvenile diabetes and other brain and immune system disorders, would begin to emerge.

In 1991, the committee of IOM appointed physicians examining medical evidence that vaccines cause injury and death, stated, "In the course of its review, the committee encountered many gaps and limitations in knowledge bearing directly or indirectly on the safety of vaccines. These include inadequate understanding of the biologic mechanisms underlying adverse events following natural infection or immunization, insufficient or inconsistent information from case reports and case series, inadequate size or length of follow-up of many population based epidemiologic studies [and] few experimental studies published in relation to the number of epidemiologic studies published."[236]

In 2000, at the National Institutes of Health (NIH), directors of four of the five NIH health agencies and representatives of national parent organizations, whose members have children with autism, discussed public and private autism research efforts and needs. They all agreed that what was most important was determining which children are genetically or otherwise biologically at risk for suffering vaccine complications that could lead to immune and brain damage, including autistic behaviors. Unbiased scientific research into the biological mechanism of vaccine adverse events is necessary in order to develop pathological profiles separating health problems caused by vaccines from those that are not.

In a subsequent letter to DHHS Secretary Donna Shalala, I joined with M.I.N.D. co-founder Rick Rollens and ARI founder Bernard Rimland, PhD, in a call for non-governmental researchers, with no financial ties to vaccine manufacturers or the CDC, to be involved in any government-led investigation into causes for the national autism epidemic. Parent groups suggested a public-private collaborative research effort to fund basic science research into the biological mechanisms of vaccine-induced autism. Since then, government health agencies have made little effort to investigate the biological mechanisms for vaccine-associated autism, especially after the Institute of Medicine declared in 2004 that no more government funds should be expended to investigate the link between vaccines and autism.

We are only in the beginning stages of unraveling all of the biological mechanisms and genetic factors involved in vaccine-induced, neuro-immune dysfunction that can cause autism in some children. Society must make a commitment to exploring how exposure or lack of exposure to viral and bacterial infections and environmental toxins interact with vaccines and genetic factors to increase chronic disease and disability risks for children. The key to the prevention and cure of autism lies with the scientists and doctors with integrity and vision who will conduct the kind of basic science research that will answer the outstanding questions that remain about vaccines and autism. Without the will and funding commitment on the part of Congress and federal health agencies, that forges an equal and collaborative partnership between government and independent researchers, finding the truth will be left to parents and private foundations.

Doctors and Parents: A Matter of Respect

Informed parents, who suspect that their children are genetically at risk for vaccine complications, are challenging the utilitarian rationale adopted by public health officials to justify forced vaccination policies. The idea that everyone has to get vaccinated for the "greater good" and that it is acceptable for some children to be sacrificed for the welfare of the rest, is unacceptable. It is especially inappropriate when one-size-fits-all vaccine policies end up targeting the genetically vulnerable as expendable.

The right to informed consent to any medical procedure that carries a risk of injury or death, including vaccination, is a human right. The right to make an informed, voluntary decision about what you are willing to risk your life or your child's life for is at the very heart of what it means to be free in a democracy that values the life of each individual.

Increasingly, well educated parents are demanding to be equal partners in making health care decisions for their children, even as increasingly defensive pediatricians, unaccustomed to being questioned, are throwing parents out of their practices when they refuse to give their children every government recommended vaccine. According to the Archives of Pediatrics and Adolescent Medicine, more than one-third of pediatricians say they would dismiss a family from their practice for refusing vaccinations.[237] Some doctors post signs in their waiting rooms warning against resisting use of all government recommended vaccines.

Doctors in positions of authority in state health, education and social service systems can, and do, report parents for failing to vaccinate their children according to state laws, and charge parents with child medical neglect. If they persuade a judge to order it, a child can be forced to be vaccinated according to state laws. While not frequent occurrences, such cases happen, especially during contentious divorces involving child custody, and during emergency room visits, when parents are asked if their child's vaccinations are up-to-date. Some hospitals and clinics have a policy that requires the attending physician to make a report to the state social service agency if parents admit the child is unvaccinated and then refuse to immediately vaccinate the child.

Parents who believe their children are at high risk of developing immune or brain system problems following vaccination must be allowed to make informed, voluntary vaccination decisions for their children without facing legal, economic, educational or other sanctions. In his book, *Diagnosis Autism: Now What? 10 Steps to Improve Treatment Outcomes, a Parent-Physician Team Approach,*[238] Lawrence Kaplan, PhD, encourages parents to become educated and then to develop healthy relationships with their doctors. If more medical schools would teach young physicians about the very real risks of vaccination for some individuals, rather than concentrate solely on promoting the benefits of vaccination for the community, physicians would be more open to participating in healthy relationships with parents.

Since *DPT: A Shot in the Dark*[1] was published in 1985, many books about vaccines have been written to further public knowledge about vaccines. In addition to those cited in the references for this chapter, other books include:
* *The Virus and the Vaccine* by Bookchin and Schumacher[239]
* *What Your Doctor May not Tell You about Childhood Vaccinations*, by Stephanie Cave, MD[240]
* *The Vaccine Guide* by Randall Neustaedter, OMD[241]
* *Vaccinations, A Thoughtful Parent's Guide* by Aviva Romm[242]
* *The Vaccine Book: Making the Right Decision for Your Child* by Robert Sears, MD.[243]

Making a Vaccination Decision: Before You Vaccinate, Ask Eight
To minimize vaccine reactions and become an effective partner with a physician in making an educated vaccination decision for a child, following are several steps parents can take if they choose to vaccinate their child:

1. ***Physical Exam*** Ask the doctor to give a child a careful physical exam before each vaccination to determine that the child is in good health and has no illness, especially fever at the time of vaccination. (Make sure the results of the exam are written in your child's medical record so that you have proof of the state of health your child was in before vaccination). Be sure to tell the doctor if the child has recently recovered from an illness or if any other members of the family are ill. Some studies suggest that not only is an individual at increased risk of reacting to a vaccination if there is a coinciding viral or bacterial illness, but also an ill individual may not mount the expected antibody response to the vaccination.

* *Precaution* In an attempt to achieve a 100% vaccination rate in the U.S., the current federal government recommendation is to vaccinate children at every opportunity including emergency room visits or hospitalization. Doctors are being encouraged to screen children for their vaccination status when accompanying parents or

siblings for other services. Health care providers in subspecialty clinics (for example, cancer clinics) are also being encouraged to screen patients for missed vaccinations.

Hospital, clinic or emergency room staff often asks about a child's vaccination status. Parents need not provide them with written proof; a verbal response is satisfactory. However, when questioned closely, and pressured to vaccinate a sick child,   a parent has the right to refuse to give permission if he/she believes vaccination at the time will endanger the child's health or life. Instead, reassure medical personnel that a private pediatrician will be consulted for further guidance about vaccination.

- *Special Precaution* When pregnant women are admitted to a hospital to have a baby, many times while in active labor, the hospital will require that the mother or father sign a paper agreeing to have the baby treated by medical personnel while in the hospital. Signing this paper may also constitute your consent to have your newborn vaccinated with hepatitis B vaccine shortly after birth. Many parents have reported that their newborns have been vaccinated without their knowledge and, when they ask why, they are told they signed a consent form prior to admission agreeing to medical treatment the hospital determined was necessary. Read every consent form carefully before signing. If necessary, write in an exception, such as, "I do not consent to have my child given any vaccinations prior to discharge from the hospital." Bring this to the attention of both the Admitting office and the nursery supervisor and ask to have it printed on the outside of the chart. Some parents take the extra precaution of never leaving the newborn alone with hospital personnel.

2. ***Detailed Medical History*** The examining physician should take and record a detailed medical history of the child and the extended family (parents, grandparents, uncles and cousins) before the child is vaccinated. Be sure to mention if a child or anyone in the family has a history of convulsions or neurologic disease; severe allergies, immune system disorders or a history of reactions to vaccinations. Remember to tell the doctor if a child was born prematurely, had a difficult labor and delivery, is chronically ill or has breathing problems. Most importantly, be sure to include any previous vaccine reactions because a deterioration in health following previous vaccination(s) can greatly increase a child's risk of a serious vaccine reaction leading to permanent disability or death. Do not omit anything in describing previous vaccine reactions. Usually the appointment is too short for the doctor to ask everything, so prior to the appointment take a few minutes and write down a child's medical history, and ask to have a copy placed in the medical record.

3. ***The Timing of Vaccination***   In the past, some European countries have not routinely vaccinated children until three to six months of age. Some doctors maintain that a child's immature immune and neurological systems, which develop most rapidly within the first few years of life, are also most vulnerable to insult in the first few years of life. Others believe that it is important to wait to determine whether a newborn has an underlying neurological or immune system disorder or other undiagnosed health problems before vaccination begins.

Some parents, who have made the decision to vaccinate, are choosing to begin vaccination at a later age and are taking special precautions to keep their unvaccinated children out of daycare or crowds to reduce the risk of exposing their children to adults and other children who may be sick with serious diseases. Many parents, who have decided to either delay vaccination or who have decided not to vaccinate, are consulting health care professionals who specialize in chiropractic, homeopathic, naturopathic, Traditional Chinese Medicine (including acupuncture) and other holistic health care therapies which focus on enhancing the functioning of the immune system and maintaining wellness.

Other parents, however, especially those with children in daycare, are choosing to begin vaccinating early, allowing only one or two different vaccinations to be given simultaneously, rather than four to six or more at a time. Some parents are choosing to space vaccinations further apart so that, if a reaction occurs, no confusion exists about which vaccine may have caused the reaction. These parents also feel more comfortable with allowing four or more months between vaccinations to give the child's immune system extra time to adjust to the viral and bacterial antigens that have been introduced.

Because U.S. federal vaccine policy today allows a one-year old child to be vaccinated with as many as 12 different vaccines on one day, consider whether a child should get just one or two vaccines or many different vaccines on one day. Becoming well informed about options makes parents more comfortable about whatever decision they make.

4. ***On the Day of Vaccination*** Some physicians suggest a child should be given fruit juice or glucose water before and after vaccination to help maintain blood sugar levels. Some medical literature suggests that nutritional deficiencies, such as Vitamin C deficiency, may play a role in reactions to vaccination and some parents supplement their child's diet with vitamin C before vaccination. None of these measures, however, will guarantee that a child will not have a vaccine reaction. Consider a morning appointment for vaccination, in order to have the whole day to observe any reactions to the shot. Vaccine reactions can develop within hours, days or weeks after vaccination, depending upon the vaccine(s) given and it is important to monitor a child for reaction symptoms for longer than 24 hours.

5. ***Check the Vial and Keep Records*** Whenever a child receives a vaccination, check the vaccine vial to confirm it is the type of vaccine you have agreed to give your child and that the expiration date on the vial has not passed. Consider asking for a new, unopened vial of vaccine if you suspect the vial has been stored for some time, or that your child would receive the last dose in the vial. Mercury containing killed bacterial vaccines come in multi-dose vials. The only way to be certain a vaccine is mercury-free is if it is in a single dose vial.

Parents should always ask for a copy of the vaccination record to keep in a file at home. This record should include the type of vaccine, date and lot numbers and name of the vaccine provider.

The National Vaccine Information Center has established guidelines to help parents make informed vaccine decisions. A "yes" to questions one through three is reason to reconsider vaccination carefully. Everyone should be able to answer "yes" to questions four through eight before vaccinating.

1. Is my child sick right now?

2. Has my child had a bad reaction to a vaccination before?

3. Does my child have a personal or family history of:
    o   vaccine reactions
    o   convulsions or neurological disorders
    o   severe allergies
    o   immune system disorders

4. Do I know if my child is at high risk of reacting?

5. Do I know how to identify a vaccine reaction?

6. Do I know how to report a vaccine reaction?

7. Do I know the vaccine manufacturer's name and lot number?

8. Do I know I have a choice?

Know the signs and symptoms of serious infectious diseases, whether you choose to vaccinate or not to vaccinate a child with a particular vaccine or combination of vaccines. Recognition of serious complications of infectious diseases as well as vaccines will help you protect your child's health. Go to NVIC's website at <www.nvic.org> for more information on infectious disease symptoms and vaccine reaction symptoms.

Vaccine Exemptions

In the U.S. vaccine laws are state laws. What is not defined in the U.S. Constitution as a federal activity defaults to the states and public health laws fall into the state activity category. In the U.S. all 50 states have mandatory vaccination laws. The laws are enforced to a greater or lesser degree depending upon how the state law is worded, what kinds of exemptions are allowed, and how the state's health, education and social services agencies implement the law.

Parents should become familiar with the legal requirements for vaccination in their state and understand the difference between a legal requirement and a recommendation. For instance, while federal vaccine policymakers *recommend* that all children be given the MMR (measles-mumps-rubella) shot, some states require only measles and rubella vaccines. In this case, parents have the legal option to vaccinate with only measles and rubella vaccines and not with mumps vaccine.

Some states also offer the option for exemption from vaccination or re-vaccination with documentation that immunity exists. All vaccines only offer temporary immunity, which is why more than one dose and boosters are often required. A blood test from a private laboratory, costing about $55, can determine whether a child has sufficiently high antibody titers to prove existing immunity to a specific disease, such as measles or whooping cough.

Some children have proof of immunity after a single shot, which lasts for many years and others cannot show proof of immunity even after many boosters. Duration of vaccine induced immunity varies from person to person, just as the risk for vaccine reactions varies from person to person.

- **Medical Exemptions** All 50 states allow a medical exemption to vaccination. Proof of medical exemption must take the form of a signed statement by a Medical Doctor (MD) or Doctor of Osteopathy (DO) that the administering of one or more vaccines would be detrimental to the health of an individual. Most doctors follow the AAP and CDC narrowly defined contraindications to vaccination. Some states will accept a private physician's written exemption without question. Other states allow the state health department to review the doctor's exemption and revoke it if health department officials don't think the exemption is justified.

  In recent years, more doctors in private practice are declining to write a medical exemption for a child even when they believe the child is at high risk for suffering vaccine induced brain and immune system dysfunction. Doctors are afraid they will be second-guessed by state health or education officials and harassed for writing medical exemptions that allow a child to attend public school without receiving all CDC recommended vaccines.

- **Religious Exemption** All states allow a religious exemption to vaccination except Mississippi and West Virginia. The religious exemption is intended for people who hold a sincere religious belief opposing vaccination to the extent that if the state forced vaccination, it would be an infringement on their right to exercise their religious beliefs. Some state laws define religious exemptions broadly to include personal religious beliefs, similar to personal philosophical beliefs. Other states require an individual who claims a religious exemption to be a member of a church or state recognized religion with official tenets that prohibit invasive medical procedures such as vaccination. (This kind of language has been ruled unconstitutional when it has been challenged in state Supreme Courts because it forces a citizen to belong to a certain religion in order to have equal protection under the law and violates the separation of church and state.) Some laws require a signed affidavit from the pastor or spiritual advisor of the parent exercising religious exemption that affirms the parents' sincere religious belief about vaccination, while others allow the parent to sign a notarized waiver.

The constitutional right to have and exercise personal religious beliefs about vaccination, whether or not they are based in Christian, Jewish, Muslim or another faith, has been reaffirmed in state high courts and can be defended. The religious exemption is granted based on the First Amendment of the Constitution, which is the right to freely exercise your religion. Because citizens are protected under the First Amendment of the United States, a state must have a "compelling State interest" before this right can be taken away. One "compelling State interest" is the spread of communicable diseases. In state court cases which have set precedent on this issue, the freedom to act according to your own religious belief is subject to reasonable regulation with the justification that it must not threaten the welfare of society as a whole.

In order to legally take a religious exemption to vaccination a family must truly hold personal religious beliefs opposing vaccination, as this belief must be defended in court if the exemption is challenged by state officials. Certain states, such as New York, have been pulling religious exemptions on file or denying religious exemptions after state officials grill parents for hours on the sincerity of their religious beliefs about vaccination. Some of these disputed cases are making their way through the civil court system.

- **Philosophical, Personal and Conscientious Belief Exemption:** The following 18 states allow exemption to vaccination based on philosophical, personal or conscientiously held beliefs: Arizona, Arkansas, California, Colorado, Idaho, Louisiana, Maine, Michigan, Minnesota, New Mexico, North Dakota, Ohio, Oklahoma, Texas, Utah, Vermont, Washington and Wisconsin. In some of these states, individuals must object to all vaccines, not just a particular vaccine in order to use the philosophical or personal belief exemption.

Many state legislators are being urged by federal health officials and medical organizations to revoke the philosophical exemption, as well as the religious exemption, to vaccination. Those who object to vaccination for philosophical or religious reasons should monitor their state legislatures, as public health officials may seek to amend state laws to eliminate these exemptions.

If parents believe a child is at high risk for suffering vaccine induced injury or death, they have the moral right to protect their child from harm. If they choose to selectively vaccinate a child or use no vaccines at all, they should be prepared to hire a lawyer if charged with child medical neglect for failing to vaccinate a child with all state required vaccines. Once more mothers and fathers stand up and demand the right to informed consent to vaccination, pediatricians and government officials will have more incentive to choose to become partners, rather than adversaries, with parents in preventing vaccine reactions.

Looking to the Future

The pharmaceutical industry is currently spending billions of dollars to create more than 200 new vaccines, public health officials and doctors are implementing laws mandating their use, and the Gates Foundation is earmarking billions more to vaccinate all the world's children. Few appear to appreciate the potential harm that could come from the attempt to eliminate all infectious disease with the mass use of multiple vaccines. However, many parents, whose children are casualties of unsafe vaccines and one-size-fits-all vaccine policies, are determined that what happened to their children after vaccination will not be forgotten. For their children and those who are yet to be born, parents of vaccine injured children and the doctors who treat them are asking for the:

- development of screening techniques to identify children at genetic or other biological risk for developing vaccine-induced health problems
- removal of toxic components in vaccines
- re-examination of vaccine licensing standards, especially for new and combination vaccines
- limitation of simultaneously administered vaccines
- re-evaluation of benefits and risks of vaccinating pregnant women
- an end to one-size-fits-all vaccination policies and a tailoring of vaccine policies to the individual
- careful monitoring of children following vaccination for signs of developmental regression so that re-vaccination does not take place
- inclusion of informed consent protections in all vaccination laws, including truthful and complete information about vaccine benefits and risks; less restrictive medical exemptions and respect for religious and conscientious belief exemptions

Take Home Points

- Since the early 1980s, American children have experienced a chronic disease and disability epidemic with a doubling or tripling of the numbers of children suffering from autism and other forms of brain and immune system dysfunction; at the same time, the numbers of doses of vaccines have doubled and vaccination rates have achieved an all time high.
- When children do not naturally experience viral and bacterial infections (flu, chicken pox, etc.) but instead experience repeated atypical manipulation of the immune system through use of multiple vaccines, they can become more vulnerable to immune system dysfunction, including chronic inflammation leading to chronic illness.
- Vaccine induced brain and immune system inflammation and subsequent chronic illness mimics that caused by viral and bacterial infections.
- Children, who are genetically vulnerable to immune mediated chronic inflammation, are particularly at risk for vaccine induced brain/immune system dysfunction, including regressive autism, and the biological mechanisms involved in the type of injury they will suffer are dependent upon the vaccine(s) given and the child's individual genetic profile.
- Additives and contaminants in vaccines can cause harm on their own, and contribute to chronic inflammation that results in brain and immune system dysfunction.
- Those who promote and profit from mandatory use of multiple vaccines (public health agencies, drug companies, medical organizations, IOM) are attempting to minimize the extent and severity of vaccine risks and are persuading Congress to pass legislation removing all liability for vaccine injuries from vaccine manufacturers and providers.

- Parents of vaccine injured children led the discovery of truth about vaccine risks (DPT, OPV, MMR, mercury). They are working with enlightened doctors, who are investigating the biological mechanisms for vaccine induced autism, and are developing alternative therapies and protocols for healing that have helped lessen neuroimmune dysfunction for some autistic children. The healing of vaccine injured autistic children has bolstered the argument that autism has biological, not psychological causes.
- When a medical intervention, such as vaccination, carries of risk of injury or death, informed consent becomes a human right.

A Brave New World

While the global village gets smaller and smaller, public health officials are warning parents that terrible diseases killing children in Africa and other countries are "just a plane ride away." Every day, Americans read and hear media reports about how deadly infectious diseases are and how safe vaccines are, with most reports calling for increased use of vaccines by children and adults and an end to exemptions for those who decide not to vaccinate. At the same time, there are signs that viruses and bacteria, eager to survive, may be outsmarting vaccines as highly vaccinated populations in the U.S. and Europe experience outbreaks of whooping cough,[244] measles[245] and mumps[246] and vaccine strain pneumococcal organisms are replaced with non-vaccine strains causing disease.[247]

Will the microbe hunters promoting mass, mandatory use of an unlimited number of vaccines today make the "Brave New World" of tomorrow truly infection free? If we stay the present course, will mankind be free from infectious disease but crippled by growing epidemics of chronic disease and disability? Or will the microbes that man is trying to eradicate and suppress through mass vaccination evolve into vaccine resistant forms in the same way that mass use of antibiotics put pressure on microbes to evolve into antibiotic resistant forms?

These are critical questions which must be answered without delay. Only then can we take steps to protect the biological integrity of future generations in America and every nation.

References

1. Coulter HL, Fisher BL. DPT: A Shot in the Dark. New York: Harcourt Brace Jovanovich, 1985.

2. Wakefield AJ, Murch SH, Anthony A, Linnell J, et al. Ileal-lymphoid-nodular hyperplasia, non-specific colitis, and pervasive developmental disorder in children. Lancet 1998;351:637-41.

3. Bernard S, Enayati A, Redwood L, Roger H, Binstock T. Autism: A novel form of mercury poisoning. Med Hypotheses 2001 56(4):462-71.

4. Kirby D. Evidence of Harm: Mercury In Vaccines And The Autism Epidemic, A Medical Controversy. New York: St. Martin's Press, 2005.

5. Kennedy RF, Jr. Deadly immunity. Rolling Stone Magazine 2005 Jun 30(977-978:57-66.

6. Coulter HL. Vaccination, Social Violence and Criminality. Berkeley: North Atlantic Books, 1990.

7. Institute of Medicine. Adverse Effects of Pertussis and Rubella Vaccines. Washington, D.C: National Academy Press, 1991.

8. Chess S. Autism in children with congenital rubella. J Autism Childhood Schizophrenia 1971;1:33-47.

9. Gupta S, Aggarwal S, Heads C. Brief Report: Dysregulated immune system in children with autism. J Autism Dev Dis 1996;26(4):439-52.

10. Maugh, II, TH. Changes in the Population of Persons with Autism and Pervasive Developmental Disorders in California's Developmental Services System 1987-1998. Los Angeles Times 1999 Apr 16.

11. Goodwin MS, Campbell W. In a dark mirror. Mental Hygiene 1969;53:550-63.

12. Preblud SR. Some current issues relating to rubella vaccine. J Am Med Assoc 1985;254:253-6.

13. Tingle AJ, Chantler JK, Pot KH, DW Paty, et al.. Postpartum rubella immunization: association with development of prolonged arthritis, neurological sequelae, and chronic rubella viremia. J Infect Dis 1986;152:606-12.

14. Centers for Disease Control. Recommended childhood and adolescent immunization schedule – United States, 2006. Morbidity and Mortality Weekly Report 2006 Jan 6;54:51-2.

15. A User Friendly Vaccine Schedule. www.donaldmiller.com Accessed July 12, 2006)

16. The Jordan Report: 20th Anniversary of Accelerated Developments of Vaccines National Institute of Allergy & Infectious Diseases, National Institutes of Health, 2002.

17. Vaccination Coverage Among Children Entering School -- United States, 2005-06 School Year. Centers for Disease Control. Morbidity and Mortality Weekly Report 2006 Oct 20;55(41);1124-6.

18. Lumen ET, Ching PLYH, Jumaan AO, Seward JF. Uptake of varicella vaccination among young children in the United States: a success story in eliminating racial and ethnic disparities. Pediatr 2006;117:999-1008.

19. Centers for Disease Control. Childhood Immunization Rates Surpass Healthy People 2010 Goal. Morbidity and Mortality Weekly Report 2005 July 26 2005.

20. Surveillance for safety after immunization: vaccine adverse event reporting system (VAERS) – United States. Centers for Disease Control. MMWR 2003 Jan 24;52:1-24.

21. www.hrsa.gov/vaccinecompensation/statistics_report.htm. (Accessed Feb 4, 2008)

22. www.cdc.gov/vaccines/programs/vfc/. (Accessed Feb 4, 2008)

23. Strachen DP. Hay fever, hygiene, and household size. Br Med J 1989:299: 1259-60.

24. www.epa.gov/indicators/roe/html/roeHealthSt.htm. (Accessed Feb 4, 2008)

25. Liu A. Murphy J. Hygiene hypothesis: Fact or fiction? J Allergy Clin Immunol 2003;111,3:471-8.

26. Ball TM, Castro-Rodriguez JA, Griffith KA. Siblings,day-care attendance, and the risk of asthma and wheezing during childhood. NEJM 2000;343:538-43.

27. Ponsonby AL, van der Mei I, Dwyer T, Blizzard L. Exposure to infant siblings during early life and risk of multiple sclerosis. JAMA 2005 Jan 26;293:4.

28. Enriquez R, Addington W, Davis F, Freels S, et al. The relationship between vaccine refusal and self-report of atopic disease in children. J Allergy Clin Immunol 2005 Apr;115:737-44.

29. Olmsted D. The Age of Autism: The Amish anomaly. The Washington Times 2005 Apr 18.

30. Heine H, Lien E. Toll-like receptors and their function in innate and adaptive immunity. Int Arch Allergy Immunol 2003;130:180-92.

31. Park H, Zhaoxia L, Yang XO, Chang SH, et al. A distinct lineage of CD4 T cells regulates tissue inflammation by producing interleukin 17. Nature Immunol 2005;6:1133-41.

32. Vojdani A, Erde J. Regulatory T cells, a potent immunoregulatory target for CAM researchers: the ultimate antagonist (I). Evid Based Complement Alternat Med 2006;3(1):25-30.

33. Rook GA, Zumia A. Gulf war syndrome: is it due to a systemic shift in cytokine balance towards a Th2 profile? The Lancet 1997; 349:1831-3.

34. Thalhamer J, Leitner W, Hammerl P, Brtko J. Designing immune responses with genetic immunization and immunostimulatory dna sequences. Endocrine Regulations 2001;35:143-66.

35. McKenzie BS, Corbett AJ, Johnson S, Brady JL et al. Bypassing luminal barriers, delivery to gut addressin by parenteral targeting elicits local IgA responses.?? Int Immunol 2004;16(11):1613-22.

36. Biragyn A. Defensins – non antibiotic use for vaccine development. Current Protein Peptide Science 6 2005:53-60.

37. Siegrist CA. Neonatal and early life vaccinology. Vaccine 2001;19(25-26):3331-46.

38. Fisher BL. In the Wake of Vaccines. Mothering Magazine 2004 Sept/Oct:44.

39. Fisher BL. Shots in the Dark. The Next City 1999 Summer,4:4.

40. Gorman C, Park A. Inflammation is a secret killer: the surprising link between inflammation and asthma, heart attacks, cancer, Alzheimer's and other diseases. Time Magazine 2004 Feb 23.

41. Wellen KE, Hotamisligil GS. Inflammation, stress and diabetes. J Clin Invest 2005;115:1111-9.

42. Moffatt MF, Cookson W. Genetics of asthma and inflammation: the status. Curr Opin Immunol 1999;11:606-9.

43. Zhong F, McCombs C. An autosomal screen for genes that predispose to celiac disease in the western counties of Ireland. Nature Genetics 1996 ;14:329-33.

44. Pruessner HT. Detecting celiac disease in your patients. Am Fam Physician 1998 Mar.1;57(5).

45. Hidvegi E, Cserhati E, Wahn U, Yamaoka A, et al. Serum immunoglobulin E, IgA, and IgG antibodies to different cow's milk proteins in children with cow's milk allergy: association with prognosis and clinical manifestations. Pediatr Allergy Immunol 2002;13(4):255-61.

46. Sweeten TL, Bowyer SL. Increased prevalence of familial autoimmunity in probands with pervasive developmental disorders. Pediatr 2003;112(5).

47. Hurwitz E., Morgenstern H. Effects of diphtheria-tetanus-pertussis or tetanus vaccination and allergy related respiratory symptoms among children and adolescents in the U.S. J Manipulative Physiol Ther 2000;23:81-90.

48. Palumbo PJ. Diabetes mellitus: incidence, prevalence, survivorship and causes of death in Rochester, Minnesota, 1945-1970. Diabetes 1976;25(7):566-73.

49. National diabetes fact sheet. Centers for Disease Control, 2003.

50. Harris HF. A case of diabetes mellitus quickly following mumps. Boston Med Surg J 1899;55:38.

51. Sinaniotis CA, Daskalopoulou E, Lapatsanis P, Doxiadis S. Diabetes mellitus after mumps vaccination (letter). Arch Disease Childhood 1975;50:749-50.

52. Otten A., Helmke K, Willems, WR, R Brockhaus, et al. Mumps, mumps vaccination, islet cell antibodies, and the first manifestations of diabetes mellitus type 1. Behring Institute Mittelungen 1984;75:83-8.

53. Quast U, Hennessen W. Vaccine induced mumps-like diseases. Developments in Biological Standardization 1979 ;43:269-72.

54. Taranger J, Wilholm BE. The low number of reported adverse effects after vaccination against measles, mumps, rubella. Lakartidningen 1987;84:948-50.

55. Poutasi K. Immunisation and diabetes (letter). NZ Med J 1996;109:283.

56. Classen JB. Childhood immunization and diabetes mellitus (letter). NZ Med J 1996;109:95.

57. Classen JB, Classen DC. Association between type 1 diabetes and Hib vaccine, causal relation likely. Brit Med J 1999;319:1133.

58. Classen DC, Classen JB. The timing of pediatric immunization and the risk of insulin-dependent diabetes mellitus. Infectious Diseases in Clinical Practice 1997;6:449-54.

59. Champsaur HF, Bottazzo GF, Bertrams J, Assan R, et al. Virologic, immunologic, and genetic factors in insulin-dependent diabetes mellitus. J Pediatri 1982;100:15-20.

60. Menser MA, Forrest JM, Bransby-Lancet RD Rubella infection and diabetes mellitus. Lancet 1978;1:57-60.

61. Rubenstein P, Walker ME, Fedun B, Witt ME, et al. The HLA system in congenital rubella patients with and without diabetes. Diabetes 1982;31:1088-91.

62. Classen B. Public Comment. Vaccines & Related Biological Products Advisory Committee Meeting, FDA. November 5, 1999.

63. Mannino DM, Homa DM, Pertowski CA, Ashizawa A, et al. Surveillance for asthma: United States, 1960-1995. Morbidity and Mortality Weekly Report 47(SS-1) 1988 Apr 14.

64. Bloom B, Cohen RA, Vickerie JL, Wondimu EA. Summary health statistics for U.S. children: national health interview survey, 2001. National Center for Health Statistics, Vital and Health Statistics Series 10: 2003 Nov:216.

65. Koeng E. Zur pertussisimpfung und ihre gegenindikationen. Helvetica Pediatrica Acta 1953;8:90-8.

66. Halpern SR, Halpern D. Reactions from DPT immunization and its relationship to allergic children. J Pediatr 1955;47:60-7.

67. Hopper JM. Illness after whooping cough vaccination. Medical Officer 1961 Oct 20:241-4.

68. Hannik CA. Major reactions after DPT-polio vaccination in the Netherlands. International Symposium on Pertussis, Bilthoven. Symposium Series on Immunobiological Standardization 13. Basel, Munchen, New York: Karger 1969:161-70.

69. Arthritis Foundation. www.arthritis.org. (Accessed Feb 4, 2008)

70. Adverse Effects of Pertussis and Rubella Vaccines. Institute of Medicine. Washington, D.C: National Academy Press, 1991.

71. Steinman L. Optic neuritis: a new variant of experimental encephalomyelitis, a durable model for all seasons, now and in its seventieth year. J Experimental Med 2003;197(9):1065-71.

72. Adams JM, Brown WJ, Eberle ED, Vorhy A. Neuromyelitis optica: severe demyelination occurring years after primary smallpox vaccination. Presented at the 3rd National Symposium of Neuropathology, Bucharest, September 20-22, 1972.

73. Rivers TM, Sprunt DH, Berry GP Observations on attempts to produce acute disseminated encephalomyelitis in monkeys. J Exp. Med. 1933;58:39-53.

74. Hemachudha T, Griffen DE, Giffels JJ, Johnson RT, et al. Myelin basic protein as an encephalitogen in encephalomyelitis and polyneuritis following rabies vaccination. NEJM 1987;316:369-74.

75. Cody CL, Baraff LJ, Cherry JD, Marcy SM, et al. Nature and rates of adverse reactions associated with DTP and DT immunizations in infants and children. Pediatr 1981;68:650-60.

76. Alderslade R., Bellman MH, Rawson NSB, Ross EM, et al. The National Childhood Encephalopathy Study: a report on 1000 cases of serious neurological disorders in infants and young children from the NCES

research team. In: *Whooping Cough: Reports from the Committee on the Safety of Medicines and the Joint Committee on Vaccination and Immunisation*. Department of Health and Social Security, London: Her Majesty's Stationery Office. 1981.

77. Weibel RE, Casserta V, Benor DE, Evans G. *Acute encephalopathy followed by permanent brain injury or death associated with further attenuated measles vaccines: a review of claims submitted to the national vaccine injury compensation program*. Pediatr 1998 Mar;101(3):383-7.

78. Demeyer JK, Barton S, DeMyer WE, Norton JA, et al. *Prognosis in autism: a follow-up study*. J Autism Childhood Schizophrenia 1973;3:199-246.

79. Mnukhin SS, Isaev DN. *On the organic nature of some forms of schizoid or autistic psychopathy*. J Autism Childhood Schizophrenia 1975;5:99-108.

80. Ornitz Em, Ritvo E. *The syndrome of autism: a critical review*. AJ Psychiatry 1976;133:609-21.

81. Tuchman RF, Rapin I. *Regression in pervasive developmental disorders: seizures and epileptiform electro-encephalogram correlates*. Pediatr 1997;99:560-66.

82. Lewine JD, Andrews R, Chez, M, Patil AA, et al. *Magnetoencephalographic patterns of epileptiform activity in children with regressive autism spectrum disorders*. Pediatr 1999;104(3):558-59.

83. Gabis L, Pomeroy J and Andriola MR. *Autism and epilepsy: cause, consequence, comorbidity, or coincidence?* Epilepsy and Behavior 2005;7:652-56.

84. Lidin-Janson G, Strannegard O. *Two cases of Guillain-Barre syndrome and encephalitis after measles*. British Med J 1972;2:572.

85. Grose C, Spigland I. *Guillain-Barre syndrome following administration of live measles vaccine*. Am J Med 1976;60:441-3.

86. Schneck SA. *Vaccination with measles and central nervous system disease, Part 2*. Neurol 1968;18:79-82.

87. Weibel RE, Caserta V, Benor DE, Evans G. *Acute encephalopathy followed by permanent brain injury or death associated with further attenuated measles vaccines: a review of claims submitted to the national vaccine injury compensation program*. Pediatr 1998;101:383-7.

88. Riikonen R.*The role of infection and vaccination in the genesis of optic neuritis and multiple sclerosis in children*. Acta Neurol Scand 1989;80:425-31.

89. Albitar S, Bourgeon B, Genin R, Fen-Chong M et al. *Bilateral retrobulbar optic neuritis with hepatitis B vaccination*. Nephrol Dial Transplant 1997;12(10):2169-70.

90. Hull TP, Bates JH. *Optic neuritis after influenza vaccination*. Am J Ophthalmol 1997;124(5):703-04.

91. Kline L, Margulies SL, Oh SJ. *Optic neuritis and myelitis following rubella vaccination*. Arch Neurol 1982;39:443-44.

92. Halsey NA, Hyman SL. *Measles-Mumps-Rubella Vaccine and Autistic Spectrum Disorder. Report from the New Challenges in Childhood Immunizations Conference convened in Oak Brook, Illinois, June 12-13, 2000*. Pediatr 2001;107.

93. Taylor B, Miller E, Farrington CP, Petropoulos M-C, et al. *Autism and measles, mumps, and rubella vaccine: no epidemiological evidence for a causal association*. The Lancet 1999 June 12;353:2026-29.

94. Uhlmann V, Martin CM, Sheils, O Pilkington L, et al. *Potential viral pathogenic mechanism for new variant inflammatory bowel disease*. Molecl Pathol 2002;55:84-90.

95. Brown Eg, Furesz, Dimock K, Yarosh W, et al. *Nucleotide sequence analysis of Urabe mumps vaccine strain that caused meningitis in vaccine recipients*. Vaccine 1991;9:840-42.

96. Ehrengut W, Zastrow K. *Complications after preventive mumps vaccination in West Germany (including multiple preventive vaccinations)*. Monatsschr Kinderheilkd 1989;137(7):398-402.

97. Russell R, Donald JC. *The neurological complications of mumps*. British Med J 1958;27-30.

98. Chess S. *Follow up report on autism in congenital rubella*. J Autism 1977;1:69-81.

99. Lotter V. *Epidemiology of autistic conditions in young children*. Soc Psychiatr 1966;1:124-37.

100. Merck & Co., Inc. *MMR II (Measles, mumps and rubella virus vaccine live) Product Information Isert*, 2003.

101. Tingle AJ, Yang T. *Prospective immunological assessment of arthritis induced by rubella vaccine*. Infect Immun 1983 40(1):22-8.

102. *Adverse Effects of Pertussis and Rubella Vaccines*. Institute of Medicine. Washington, DC: National Academy Press, 1991.

103. Wise RP, Salive ME, Braun MM, Mootrey GT, et al. *Postlicensure safety surveillance for varicella vaccine*. JAMA 2000;284(10):1271-9.

104. *Adverse Events Associated with Childhood Vaccines: Evidence Bearing on Causality*. Institute of Medicine, Washington, DC: National Academy Press, 1994.

105. Centers for Disease Control. Preliminary assessment of the effectiveness of the 2003-2004 inactivated influenza vaccine – Colorado. Morbidity and Mortality Weekly Report 2004 Jan 16.

106. Prevention and control of influenza: recommendations of the advisory committee on immunization practices (ACIP). Centers for Disease Control. Morbidity and Mortality Weekly Report 2002 Apr 12.

107. Medimmune Vaccines, Inc. Influenza virus vaccine live, intranasal (fluMist). 2006-2007 Formula. Package Insert, May 2006.

108. Pope JE, Stevens A, Howson W, Bell DA. The development of rheumatoid arthritis after recombinant hepatitis B vaccination. Rheumatol 1999;7:1636.

109. Grezard P, Chefai M, Philippot V. Cutaneous lupus erythematosus and buccal aphthosis after hepatitis B vaccination in a 6-year old child. Ann Dermatol Venereol 1996;123(10):657-9.

110. Sibilia J, Maillefert JF. Vaccination and rheumatoid arthritis: induction of rheumatoid arthritis by vaccination against hepatitis B – myth or reality? Ann Rheumatic Dis 2002;61:575-6.

111. Stewart O, Chang B, Bradbury J. Simultaneous administration of hepatitis B and polio vaccines associated with bilateral optic neuritis. Br J Ophthalmol 1999;83:1194.

112. Tourbah A, Gout O, Liblau R, Lyon-Caen O, et al. Encephalitis after hepatitis B vaccination. Neurol 1999;53:396.

113. Montinari M, Favoino B, Roberto A. Diagnostic role of immunogenetics in post-vaccine diseases of the CNS: preliminary results. Medit J Surg Med 1996;4:69-72.

114. Hernan MA, Jick SS, Olek MJ, Jick H Recombinant hepatitis B vaccine and the risk of multiple sclerosis. Neurology 2004;63:838-42.

115. Bogdanos DP, Smith H, Ma Y, Baum H, et al. A study of molecular mimicry and immunological cross-reactivity between hepatitis B surface antigen and myelin mimics. Clin Dev Immunol 2005;3:217-24.

116. Comenage Y, Girard M. Multiple sclerosis and hepatitis B vaccination: Adding the credibility of molecular biology to an unusual level of clinical and epidemiological evidence. Med Hypothesis 2006;66:84-6.

117. Lurie LA, Levy S. Personality changes and behavior disorders of children following pertussis. JAMA 1942;120:890-4.

118. Byers RK, Moll PC. Encephalopathies following prophylactic pertussis vaccination. Pediatr 1948;1:437-57.

119. Menkes JH, Kinsbourne M. Neuropediatr 1990;21:171-6.

120. Madge N. Diamond J, Miller D, Ross E, et al. The National Childhood Encephalopathy Study: A 10-year follow-up. A report of the medical, social, behavioral, and educational outcomes after serious, acute neurological illness in early childhood. Dev Med Child Neurol 1993;68:35:1-118.

121. DPT Vaccine and Chronic Nervous Dysfunction: A New Analysis. Institute of Medicine. Washington, DC: National Academy Press, 1994.

122. Strom J. Further experience of reactions, especially of a cerebral nature, in conjunction with triple vaccination: a study based on vaccinations in Sweden 1959-1965. Bristish Med J 1967 Nov 11;4(5575):320-23.

123. Kuhlenkampff M., Schwartzman JS, Wilson, J. Neurological complications of pertussis inoculation. Arch Dis Child 1974;49:46-9.

124. Kind LS. The altered reactivity of mice after inoculation with bordetella pertussis vaccine. Bacteriol Rev 1958;22:173-82.

125. Mitsuzawa E, Yasuda T. Experimental allergic encephalitis (EAE) in mice: histological studies on EAE induced by myelin basic protein, and role of pertussis vaccine. Jpn J Exp Med 1976;46:205-12.

126. Kallen B, Nilsson O. Effect of bordetella pertussis vaccine on experimental autoimmune encephalomyelitis in rats. Int Arch Allergy Appl Immunol 1986;80:95-9.

127. Steinman L, Sriram S, Adelman N, Zamvil S, et al. Murine model for pertussis vaccine encephalopathy: linkage to H-2. Nature 1982;299:738-40.

128. Gupta RK, Sharma SB, Ahuja S, Saxena SN. Glutaraldehyde inactivated pertussis vaccine: a less histamine sensitizing vaccine. J Biol Stand 1987;15:159-64.

129. Hofstetter HH, Shive CL, Fortshuber TG. Pertussis toxin modulates the immune response to neuroantigens injected in incomplete Freund's adjuvant: induction of Th1 cells and experimental autoimmune encephalomyelitis in the presence of high frequencies of Th2 cells. J Immunol 2002;169:117-25.

130. Megson M. Testimony, U.S. House Committee on Government Reform. April 6, 2000.

131. Steinman L, Weiss A, Adelman N, Lim M, et al. Pertussis toxin required for pertussis vaccine encephalopathy. Proc National Academy of Sciences 1985 Dec 15;82:8733-6.

132. Madsen T. Vaccination against whooping cough. JAMA 1933;101:187-8.

133. Brody M. Neurologic complications following the administration of pertussis vaccine. Brooklyn Hospital J 1947;5:107-13.

134. Miller DL, Ross EM, Aldershade R, Bellman MH, et al. Pertussis immunization and serious acute neurological illness in children. Brit Med J 1981;282:1595-9.

135. GlaxoSmithKline Biologicals. Infanrix. Dipththeria and tetanus toxoids and acellular pertussis vaccine adsorbed product information insert, 2003.

136. Sanofi Pasteur. DAPTACEL (Diphtheria and tetanus toxoids and accelular pertussis vaccine adsorbed) product information insert, 2003.

137. Report: Working group on the standardization and control of pertussis vaccines. World Health Organization 2003 May 6-7.

138. Business Wire. Chiron Biocine genetically engineered acellular pertussis vaccine proves superior to currently licensed vaccine. July 13, 1995. www.highbeam.com. (Accessed Feb 4, 2008)

139. Mielcarek N, Debrie AS, Raze D, Bertout J et al. Live attenuated B. pertussis as a single-dose nasal vaccine against whooping cough. Public Library of Science Pathogens 2006 Jul;2:7.

140. Ausiello CM, Urbani F. Vaccine and antigen-dependent type 1 and type 2 cytokine induction after primary vaccination of infants with whole-cell or acellular pertussis vaccine. Infect Immunol 1997 Jun;65:2168-74.

141. Robbins JB, Schneerson R, Trollfors B. The diphtheria and petussis components of diphtheria-tetanus-toxoids-pertussis vaccine should be genetically inactivated mutant toxins. J Infect Dis 2005 Jan 1;191: 81-8.

142. Centers for Disease Control. Pertussis vaccination: use of acellular pertussis recommendations of the advisory committee on immunization practices. MMWR 46(RR-7) 1997 Mar 28:1-25.

143. Ochiai M, Kataoka M. Endotoxin content in haemophilus influenza type b vaccine. Jpn J Infect Dis 2004;57:58-9.

144. Wise RP, Iskander J, Pratt RD, Campbell S, et al. Postlicensure safety surveillance for 7-valent pneumococcal conjugate vaccine. JAMA 2004;292:1702-10.

145. FDA. FDA and CDC issue alert on Menactra meningococcal vaccine and Guillain Barre syndrome. FDA News 2005 Sept 30.

146. Geier M., Stanbro H, Merril CR. Endotoxins in commercial vaccines. Applied Environmental   Microbiol 1978;38(3):445-8.

147. Ochiai M, Kataoka M Toyoizumi H, Kamachi K et al. Evaluation of endotoxin content of diphtheria-tetanus-acellular pertussis combined (DTaP) vaccines that interfere with the bacterial endotoxin test. Vaccine 2003 May 16;21(17):1862-6.

148. Levandowski RA. Influenza vaccine production. Presentation prepared for Institute of Medicine Immunization Safety Review. 2003 Mar 13. www.iom.edu (Accessed Feb 4, 2008)

149. Vaccine Weekly. Limulus amoebocyte lysate assay detects endotoxin in hepatitis B virus vaccine. Vaccine Safety 2005 Nov 9.

150. Peltola H, Kayhty H, Kuronen T, Haque N, et al. Meningococcus group A vaccine in children three months to five years of age. Adverse reactions and immunogenicity related to endotoxin content and molecular weight of the polysaccharide. J Pediatr 1978;92:818-22.

151. Todar K. Mechanisms of bacterial pathogenicity: endotoxins. Todar's Online Textbook of Bacteriology. http://textbookofbacteriology.net/endotoxin.html, 2002.

152. Hinshaw LB, Emerson JR. A comparative study of the hemodynamic actions of histamine and endotoxin. Am J Physiol 1962 ;203:600-06.

153. Torch WC. Diphtheria-pertussis-tetanus (DPT) immunization: a potential cause of the sudden infant death syndrome (SIDS)) (abstract). American Academy of Neurology, 34th Annual Meeting, April 25-May 1, 1982. Neurol 1982;32.

154. Prins JM, Sander JH. Clinical relevance of antibiotic-induced endotoxin release. Antimircrob Agents Chemother 1994 ;8(6):1211-18.

155. Lamp KC, Rybak MJ. Influence of antibiotic and E-5 monolonal immunoglobulin M interactions on endotoxin release from Escherichia coli and Psuedomonas aeruginosa. Antimicrob Agents Chemother 1996;40:247-52.

156. Hollis LC. Vets hear new concepts on endotoxins in cattle. Kansas State Vet Qtrly 2003 Summer;6.

157. Voss LJ, Bolton DPG. Endotoxin effects on markers of autonomic nervous system function in the piglet: implication for SIDS. Biol Neonate 2004;86:39-47.

158. Sanofi Pasteur. Menomune A/C/Y/W-135 meningococcal polysaccharide vaccine product information insert, 2003.

159. Medicines Control Council. Draft guidelines on simultaneous use of vaccines containing endotoxins in infants. Gov Gazette 2005 Oct 28;28(28150).

160. Gupta RK, Relyveld EH. Adverse reactions after injection of adsorbed diphtheria-pertussis-tetanus (DPT) vaccine are not due only to pertussis organisms or pertussis components in the vaccine. Vaccine 1991 Oct;9:699-702.

161. Moghaddam A, Olszewska W, Wang B, Tregoning JS, et al. A potential molecular mechanism for hypersensitivity caused by formalin-inactivated vaccines. Nat Med 2006;12:905-07.

162. Robertson JS. Strategy for adventitious agent assays. Dev Biol Stand 1996;88:37-40.

163. FDA Center for Biologics Evaluation and Research. Vaccines and Biological Products Advisory Committee Meeting Transcript (on designer cell substrates, risk for residual DNA, adventitious agent contamination of vaccine). May 16, 2001. www.fda.gov (Accessed Feb 4, 2008)

164. www.epa.gov/ttn/atw/hlthef/mercury.html (EPA - Mercury Compounds). (Accessed Feb 4, 2008)

165. Burbacher TM, Shen DD, Liberato N, Grant KS, et al. Comparison of blood and brain mercury levels in infant monkeys exposed to methylmercury or vaccines containing thimerosal. Environmental Health Perspectives 2005 Aug;113(8):1015-21.

166. Stajich GV, Lopez GP, Harry, SW, Sexson, WR. Iatrogenic exposure to mercury after hepatitis B vaccination in preterm infants. J Pediatr 2000;136(5):679-81.

167. Jamieson WA, Powell HM. Merthiolate as a preservative for biological products. Am J Hyg 1931;14:218-14.

168. Centers for Disease Control and Prevention. Notice to Readers: Thimerosal in Vaccines: A Joint Statement of the American Academy of Pediatrics and the Public Health Service. Morbidity and Mortality Weekly Report 1999;48:563-65.

169. Immunization safety review: thimerosal containing vaccines and neurodevelopmental disorders. Institute of Medicine. Washington, DC: National Academy Press, 2001.

170. Verstraeten T, Davis RL, DeStefano F, Lieu TA, et al. Safety of thimerosal-containing vaccines: a two-phased study of computerized health maintenance organization databases. Pediatr 2003;112(5):1039-48.

171. Geier, DA, Geier MR. Neurodevelopmental disorders following thimoersal-containing childhood immunizations: a follow-up analysis. Int J Toxicol 2004;23:369-76.

172. Geier DA, Geier MR. A two-phased population epidemiological study of the safety of thimerosal-containing vaccines: a follow-up analysis. Med Sci Monit 2005;11:160-70.

173. Nelson KB, Bauman ML. Thimerosal and Autism? Pediatr 2003;111:674-9.

174. Blaxill MF, Redwood L, Bernard S. Med Hypothesis 2004;62:788-94.

175. Madsen KM, Lauritsen MB, Pedersen CB, Thorsen P, et al. Thimerosal and the occurrence of autism: negative ecological evidence from Danish population-based data. Pediatr 2003;112:604-6.

176. Hviid A, Stellfeld M. Association between thimerosal-containing vaccine and autism. JAMA 2003;290: 1763-66.

177. Blaxill M. Danish Thimerosal-Autism Study in Pediatrics: Misleading and Uninformative on Autism-Mercury Link. Sept. 2, 2003. www.safeminds.org (Accessed Feb 4, 2008)

178. James SJ, Slikker W, Melnyk S, New E et al. Thimerosal neurotoxicity is associated with glutathione depletion: protection with glutathione precursors. Neurotoxicity 2005;26:1-8.

179. Mutkus L, Aschner JL, Syversen T, Shanker G, et al. In vitro uptake of glutamate in GLAST-and GLT-1-transfected mutant CHO-K-1 cells is inhibited by the ethylmercury-containing preservative thimerosal. Biol Trace Elem Res 2005;105:71-86.

180. Waly M, Olteanu H. Activation of methionine synthase by insulin-like growth factor-1 and dopamine: a target for neurodevelopmental toxins and thimerosal. Mol Psychiatr 2004;9:644.

181. Makani S, Gollapudi S. Biochemical and molecular basis of thimerosal induced apoptosis in T cells: a major role of mitochondrial pathway. Genes Immun 2002;3:270-8.

182. Baskin DS, Hop N, Didenko V Thimerosal induces DNA breaks, caspase-3 activation, membrane damage, and cell death in cultured human neurons and fibroblasts. Toxicol Sci 2003;74:361-8.

183. Humphrey ML, Cole MP, Pendergrass JC, Kiningham, KK. Mitochondrial mediated thimerosal-induced apoptosis in a human neuroblastoma cell line (SK-N-SH). Neurotoxicol 2005;26:407-16.

184. Parran DK, Barker A, M Ehrich. Effects of thimerosal on NGF signal transduction and cell death in neuroblastoma cells. Toxicol Sci 2005;86:132-40.

185. Herdman ML, Marcelo A, Huang Y, Niles RM, et al. Thimerosal induces apoptosis in a neuroblastoma model via the cJun N-terminal kinase pathway. Toxicol Sci 2006;92:246-53.

186. Vargas DL, Nascimbene C, Krishnan C, Zimmerman AW. Neuroglial activation and neuroinflammation in the brain of patients with autism. Ann Neurol 2004;57:67-81.

187. Herbert MR. Autism: a brain disorder, or a disorder that affects the brain? Clin Neuropsychiatr 2005;2:354-79.

188. Hornig M, Chian D, Lipkin WI. Neurotoxic effects of postnatal thimerosal are mouse strain dependent. Mol Psychiatr 2004;9(9):833-45.

189. Havarinasab S, Hultman P. Organic mercury compounds and autoimmunity. Autoimmun Rev 2005;4:270-5.

190. Haley BE. Mercury toxicity: genetic susceptibility and synergistic effects. Med Veritas 2005;2:535-42.

191. Goth SR, Chu RA, Gregg JP, Cherednichenko G, et al. Uncoupling of ATP-mediated calcium signaling and dysregulated interleukin-6, secretion in dendritic cells by nanomolar thimerosal. Environmental Health Perspectives 2006 Jul;114:1083-91.

192. Holmes A. Toxic metal clue to autism. New Scientist 2003 Jun 18.

193. Immunization Safety Review: Vaccines and Autism. Institute of Medicine. Washington, DC: National Academy Press, 2004.

194. Alfrey AC, LeGendre GR, Kaehny WD. The dialysis encephalopathy syndrome: possible aluminum intoxication. NEJM 1976;294:184-8.

195. Yokel RA. The toxicology of aluminum in the brain: a review. Neurotoxicol 2000;21:813-28.

196. Eickhoff TC, Myers M. Conference Report Workshop Summary: aluminum in vaccines. Vaccine 20, Suppl 2002;13:S 1-4.

197. Redhead K, Quinlan GJ. Aluminum-adjuvanted vaccines transiently increase aluminum levels in murine brain tissue. Pharmacol Toxicol 1992;70:278-80.

198. Sahin G, Varol I, Temizer A. Determination of aluminum levels in the kidney, liver and brain of mice treated with aluminum hydroxide. Biol Trace Elem Res 1994;41:129-35.

199. Petrik MS, Wong MC, Tabata RC, Garry RF, et al. Aluminum adjuvant linked to Gulf War illness induces motor neuron death in mice. Neuromolecular Med 2007;1:83-100.

200. Gherardi RK, Coquet M, Cherin P, Belec L, et al. Macrophagic myofasciitis lesions assess long-term persistence of vaccine-derived aluminum hydroxide in muscle. Brain 2001;124:1821-31.

201. www.chop.edu/consumer/index.jsp (Search vaccine adjuvants) (Accessed Feb 4, 2008)

202. Code of Federal Regulations. FDA. Food Drug and Cosmetic Act (Title 21). Subpart G 201.323: 2004. Aluminum in large and small volume parenterals used in total parenteral nutrition. Appendix A to Part 201.

203. Alfrey AC, LeGendre GR, Kaehny WD. The dialysis encephalopathy syndrome. NEJM 1976;294:184-8.

204. Banks WA, Kastin AJ. Aluminum-induced neurotoxicity: alterations in membrane function at the blood-brain barrier. Neurosci Biobehav Rev 1989;13:47-53.

205. Suarez-Fernandez MB, Soldado AB, Sanz-Medel A, Vega JA et al. Aluminum-induced degeneration of astrocytes occurs via apoptosis and results in neuronal death. Brain Res 1999;835:125-36.

206. Johnson VJ, Sharma RP. Aluminum disrupts the pro-inflammatory cytokine/neurotrophin balance in primary brain rotation-mediated aggregate cultures: possible role in neurodegeneration. Neurotoxicol 2002;24:261-8.

207. Griffioen KJ, Ghribi O, Fox N, Savory J, et al. Aluminum maltolate-induced toxicity in NT2 cells occurs through apoptosis and includes cytochrome c release. Neurotoxicol 2004;25:859-67.

208. Parkinson IS, Ward MK, Kerr DNS. Dialysis encephalopathy, bone disease and anaemia: the aluminum intoxication syndrome during regular haemodialysis. J Clin Pathol 1981;34:1285-94.

209. Aluminum overload and toxicity in chronic kidney disease. Clinical Practice Guidelines. National Kidney Foundation. www.kidney.org Accessed September 24, 2006.

210. Krishnan SS, McLachlan DR, Krishnan B, Fenton SSA, et al. Aluminum toxicity to the brain. Sci Total Environ 1988 ;71:59-64.

211. Forester BP, Oxman TE. Measures to assess the non-cognitive symptoms of dementia in the primary care setting. J Clin Psychiatry 2003;5:158-63.

212. Campbell A, Bondy SC. Aluminum induced oxidative events and its relation to inflammation: a role for the metal in Alzheimer's disease. Cell Mol Biol 2000;46:721-30.

213. Campbell A. Inflammation, neurodegenerative diseases, and environmental exposures. Ann NY Acad Sci 2004;1035:117-32.

214. Jyonouchi H, Geng L, Ruby A, Zimmerman-Bier B. Dysregulated innate immune responses in young children with autism spectrum disorders: their relationship to gastrointestinal symptoms and dietary intervention. Neuropsychobiol 2005;51:77-85.

215. Blaylock RL. The central role of excitotoxicity in autism spectrum disorders. JAMA 2003;6:10-22.

216. Vargas DL, Nascimbene C, Krishnan C, Zimmerman AW et al. Neuroglial activation and neuroinflammation in the brain of patients with autism. Annals of Neurology, 57, 1:2004, 67-81.

217. Stubbs EG. Autistic children exhibit undetectable hemaglutinin-inhibition antibody titers despite previous rubella vaccination. J Autism 1976;6:269-274.

218. Weitzman A, Weisman R, Szekely GA, Wijsenbeek H, Livni E. Abnormal immune response to brain tissue antigen in the syndrome of autism. Am J Psychiatr 1982;139):1462-65.

219. Singh VK, Warren RP, Odell JD, Warren, L, et al. Antibodies to myelin basic protein in children with autistic behavior. Brain Behav Immun 1993;7:97-103.

220. Singh VK, Sheren XL, Yang VD. Serological association of measles virus and human herpesvirus-6 with brain autoantibodies in autism. Clin Immunol Immunopathol 1998;89:105-08.

221. Goth SR, Chu RA, Gregg JP, Cherednichenko G, Pessah IN. Uncoupling of ATP-mediated Calcium Signaling and Dysregulated IL-6 Secretion in Dendritic Cells by Nanomolar Thimerosal. Envir.Health Perspectives 2006;114:1083-91.

222. Ritvo ER, Freeman BJ. A medical model of autism: etiology, pathology and treatment. Pedaitr Ann 1984;13:298-305.

223. Warren RP, Margaretten N, Pace N, Foster A. Immune abnormalities in patients with autism. J Autism Dev Dis 1986;16:189-97.

224. Burger RA, Warren RP. Possible immunogenetic basis for autism. Mental Retardation and Developmental Disabilities Res Rev 1998;4:137-41.

225. Yazbak FE, Lang-Radosh KL.. Adverse outcomes associated with postpartum rubella or MMR vaccine. Med Sentinel 2001;6:95-9.

226. Comi AM, Zimmerman AW, Frye VH, Law PA, Peeden JN. Familial clustering of autoimmune disorders and evaluation of medical risk factors in autism. J Child Neurol 1999;14:388-94.

227. Warren RP, Singh VK, Cole P, Odell J D, et al. Increased frequency of the null allele at the complement C4b locus in autism. Clin Exp Immunol 1991;83:438-40.

228. Knuutila S, Maki-Paakkanen J, Kahkonen M, Hokkanen E. An increased frequency of chromosomal changes and SCE's in cultured blood lymphocytes of 12 subjects vaccinated against smallpox.Human Genetics 1978 Feb 23;41:89-96.

229. Kucerova M, Polivkova Z, Matousek V. Chromosomal aberrations and SCE in lymphocytes of children revaccinated against smallpox. Mutation Res 1980;143:271-74.

230. Urnovitz HB, Tuite JJ, Higashida JM, Murphy WH. RNA's in the sera of Persian Gulf War veterans have segments homologous to chromosome 22q11.2. Clin Diag Lab Immunol 1999;6:330-35.

231. Blaylock RL. Chronic microglial activation and excitotoxicity secondary to excessive immune stimulation: possible factors in Gulf War syndrome and autism. J Am Phys Surg 2004;9:46-51.

232. Mercury in Medicine. 2003 "Mercury in Medicine." May, 2003. www.generationrescue.org Accessed October 23, 2006.

233. Barbara Loe Fisher. Letter to Col. Robert P. Kadlec, M.D. (USAF,ret.), Staff Director, Subcommittee on Bioterrorism and Public Health Preparedness, U.S. Senate, Nov. 15, 2005. www.nvic.org (homepage: Liability Shield Given to Pharma). Accessed October 19, 2006.

234. Madsen KM, Hviid M, Vestergaard M, Schendel D, et al. A population based study of measles, mumps and rubella vaccination and autism. NEJM 2002;347:1477-82.

235. Merck's Gardasil Vaccine Not Proven Safe for Little Girls. NVIC. Press Release, June 27, 2006. www.nvic. org Accessed October 27, 2006.

236. Stratton K, Gable A, Shetly P, McCormick M, eds. Immunization Safety Review: Measles, Mumps, Rubella, Vaccine and Autism. Institute of Medicine, Washington, DC, 1991.

237. Flanagan-Klygis EA, Sharp L, Frader JE. Dismissing the family who refuses vaccines. Arch Pediatr Adolesc Med 2005;159:929-34.

238. Kaplan L. Diagnosis Autism: Now What? Steps to Improve Treatment Outcomes. Chicago:Etham Books, 2005.

239. Bookchin D, Schumacher J. The Virus and the Vaccine: The True Story of a Cancer-causing Monkey Virus, Contaminated Polio Vaccine, and the Millions of Americans Exposed. New York: St. Martin's Press, 2004.

240. Cave S, Mitchell D. What Your Doctor May Not Tell You About Children's Vaccinations. New York: Warner Books, 2001.

241. Neustaedter R. The Vaccine Guide: Risks and Benefits for Children and Adults. Berkeley, CA: North Atlantic Books, 2002.

242. Romm AJ. Vaccinations: A Thoughtful Parent's Guide. Rochester, VT: Healing Arts Press, 2001.

243. Sears R. The Vaccine Book: Making to Right Decision for Your Child. Boston: Little Brown, Inc., 2007.

244. Sheldon T. Dutch doctors warn parents over whooping cough vaccine. British Med J 2004 Aug;329:28.

245. Barrero PR, Zandomeni RO, Mistchenko AS Measles virus circulation in Argentina: 1991-1999. Arch Virol 2001;146:815-23.

246. Gemmill IM. Mumps vaccine: is it time to re-evaluate our approach? CMAJ 2006 29 Aug;175:491-92.

247. Porat N, Barkai G, Jacobs MR, Trefler R, Dagan R. Four antibiotic-resistant Streptococcus pneumoniae clones unrelated to the pneumococcal conjugate vaccine serotypes, including 2 new serotypes causing acute otitis media in sourhern Israel. J Inf Dis 2004;189:385-92.

Chapter 5
A Biomedical Approach
to Autism Spectrum Disorders

Kelly Dorfman, MS, and Patricia S. Lemer, MEd

In Chapter 3 the authors enumerated the many risk factors that accumulate to raise an individual's total load. As load factors increase, the likelihood of an autism spectrum diagnosis increases. Total load theory not only contributes to understanding the causes of autism, it also leads to the road to recovery. "Peeling the onion" to systematically remove individual components of the total load improves outcomes. Each therapy or intervention that alleviates a risk factor lessens the load, freeing up the body's energy for physiological, cognitive, sensory, language, and social-emotional development to take place.

This chapter focuses on interventions that boost the depressed immune system, clean up and heal the damaged gastrointestinal system, enhance neurological and metabolic function, and remove the toxins from the body. In order to determine the level of immune system dysfunction for an individual child, an extensive medical and developmental history is essential. Refer to Chapter 2 for what a thorough history includes. Identifying all toxic exposures sometimes requires relentless questioning. Laboratory testing, important for establishing baselines, and essential for determining a treatment plan in complicated cases, is outlined in Chapter 3.

Why should an optometrist or any other professional treating those on the autism spectrum become familiar with biomedical treatments? Because when a patient is balanced biochemically, clinical outcomes improve. Children who are not responding to vision or other therapies may be malnourished, immune compromised or toxic. Correcting underlying biochemical problems permits a patient's body to be fully available and able to make maximum use of any therapy.

An optometrist referred a child for nutritional counseling who had made little progress in vision therapy. The child's visual system was operating five years below age level, and was getting worse despite intervention. After removing sugar from the diet, visual functioning jumped one year in one month, with the same therapy program. The parents thought the optometrist was brilliant.

Most practitioners utilizing a biomedical approach rely on blood, urine, stool, hair and saliva tests, even though laboratory testing can be costly and sometimes not covered by insurance. If cost is a factor, or a patient chooses not to do testing, many practitioners initially recommend some simple, non-invasive interventions that work with a majority of patients, and that any optometrist or family can try to improve the biochemical environment. Most start with dietary modification and basic nutritional supplementation.

Strategies covered in this chapter are:

Dietary modification, including the gluten-free and casein-free (GF/CF) diet, the allergy-elimination diet, the Feingold diet, the soy-free diet, the specific carbohydrate diet (SCD), the yeast-free diet, and the body ecology diet (BED)

Nutritional supplementation, including vitamins, minerals, enzymes, probiotics, cognitive enhancers

Detoxification *techniques*, including chelation and a far infared sauna.

Remove the Bad Stuff through Dietary Modification

Dr. Jacqueline McCandless, author of *Children with Starving Brains,*[1] and the grandmother of a girl with autism, believes that putting those with autism on a strict diet is the number one thing that kids with autism need to heal. "When I first started working with kids, I had two groups of parents. One, those parents who were very conscientious, and obeyed everything they had to do: they took away the wheat, they took away the milk, they took away the soy, and finally they took away the sugar. These kids were starting to get well, and well, and well. I had another group where the parents were resistant. They couldn't believe that a little bit of sugar would hurt, or a little bit of bread, or a cookie here and there. And those kids would constantly keep getting yeast infections, clostridia infections, have regressions, over and over."[2] McCandless finally refused to work with any parent who was unwilling to be strict with the diet. The basic diet Dr. McCandless and others often start with is the gluten-free, casein-free (GF/CF) diet.

Gluten-free, casein-free diet Studies show that removal of gluten and casein from the diet can make a marked and often immediate difference in many children on the autism spectrum.[3-5] In clinical practice, approximately one third of children with autism improve dramatically, and sometimes no longer qualify for the diagnosis. Another third show improvement in secondary symptoms, such as poor sleep and perseverative behavior, although the diagnosis of autism remains.

If recommending this diet, parents must understand that, while full compliance is desirable, it is not necessary in order for a child to improve. Because gluten and casein masquerade under many names, avoiding every food containing gluten and/or casein may be difficult at first. In most cases, avoiding the major offenders will be adequate as a start. Stricter adherence comes with practice and after seeing small gains.

The best candidates for the GF/CF diet are children who:
• are already eat a limited diet of mostly gluten and casein containing foods
• get sick easily and/or have chronically loose stools
• have a history of ear infections and/or colic and/or
• have poor eye contact and are difficult to engage

Many other diets have proven successful in autism and AD(H)D. Some of the most popular are:

Allergy Elimination diet Doris Rapp was one of the first to show the benefit of eliminating certain foods in children with attention, behavior and learning problems. Parents report an increase in the understanding and use of language, improved eye contact, and more relatedness.[6] Recall the classic study on ear infections cited in Chapter 3 that showed the elimination of ear infections and chronic fluid in 86% of children when parents removed allergic foods.[7] The problematic foods in this study were milk, wheat, corn, eggs, soy and chocolate. When these are eliminated from the diet, ear infections cleared, and adults saw improvement in other aspects of health and function, as well.

Feingold diet In the 1970's, Dr. Benjamin Feingold, from the Kaiser-Permanente Medical Center in San Francisco, was concerned about the behavior of children in his pediatric practice. He noticed that some became hyperactive after ingesting aspirin (salicylic acid) and specific food products. He developed and wrote about a diet free of artificial colors, flavors, additives and naturally occurring salicylates.[8]

Recent research supports implementation of the Feingold diet for some children with autism, due to their impaired detoxification capacities.[9] The liver breaks down salicylates using drug detoxification pathways. Youngsters on the autistic spectrum are now known to have increased oxidative stress and impaired methylation and transsulfuration capacity. Methylation and sulfation are two biochemical processes utilized in the second stage of detoxification. As a result, salicylates in the diet may cause irritability and hyperactivity because the body cannot metabolize them properly.[10]

Feingold's legacy is the Feingold Association of the United States (FAUS). For a small yearly fee parents can purchase an extensive booklet that shows by brand what products are acceptable and those that are not. The organization has evaluated every product in most grocery stores and publishes a list of "acceptable" and "unacceptable" products. Parents use the food list to shop and can thus avoid having to read every label. This list is kept up-to-date with monthly addenda as new products come on the market and old ones are modified. To learn more go to <www.feingold.org >.

Soy-free diet Clinical evidence suggests that soy may also bother some children who react to casein. The chemical structure of the soy protein is similar to casein and a cross sensitivity may exist in up to 50% of those who react to dairy products. Therefore, it is inadvisable to substitute soy milk for cow's milk during elimination trials. For an extensive treatise on the controversies concerning the use of soy in human diets, read *The Whole Soy Story* by Kayla Daniels.[11]

Specific Carbohydrate diet (SCD) The goal of the SCD is to stop the vicious cycle of malabsorption and microbe overgrowth by removing the preferred foods and microbes: disaccharide sugars and starch. The SCD goes a step further than the GF/CF diet by prohibiting all complex carbohydrates, (grains and starch) and white sugar (sucrose). This diet allows only the simple carbohydrates found in fruits because simple carbohydrates do not need to be broken down in order to be absorbed. Partially digested complex carbohydrates sit in the intestines and provide a breeding ground for yeast and bacteria. By-products from fungus and "bad" bacteria irritate the gut lining causing inflammation.

The SCD starts with an introductory plan, consisting of proteins and a limited selection of "specific" carbohydrates including fruits, honey, properly-prepared yogurt and certain vegetables and nuts. All fruits and vegetables must be peeled, seeded and cooked in order to make them more easily digested. Nuts, seeds, raw fruits and certain vegetables, such as salad greens, carrots, celery, and onions are not allowed at this stage, but are introduced later, after diarrhea is under control. All cereal grains are strictly and absolutely forbidden. This step usually lasts about a week or two.

To thoroughly understand and implement the SCD, read *Breaking the Vicious Cycle*[12] by Elaine Gottschall. This SCD "bible" details the progression of allowed foods as well as providing many delicious recipes. SCD websites abound. Go online to: <www.scdrecipe.com>, <www.pecanbread.com>, <www.breakingtheviciouscycle.com> and <www.scdiet.org>.

Yeast-free diet Recall the findings of Dr. William Shaw (see Chapter 3), who found that children with a diagnosis of autism had extremely high levels of yeast by-products in their urine.[13] Because of his ground-breaking work, the yeast free diet has become a staple of biochemical intervention for autism. Yeasts and fungi are common organisms that live in all of us. When an individual consumes too much sugar, or the immune system is weak, the yeast population can grow aggressively. Yeasts manufacture waste products that can be toxic or irritating. Symptoms of yeast overgrowth are mood swings, itching, especially around the genitals or anus, excessive gas, bloating, putrid smelling stools, fuzzy thinking and crankiness.

Because sugar is the food of yeast, restricting sugar is an important component of dietary modification. Yeasts ferment sugars into alcohol, leaving a child acting drunk, hung over, unfocused or hyperactive.[14] More than 100 recognized substances are described as sugars,[15] These include, but are not limited to, sucrose, turbinado, honey, fructose, barley malt, rice or yinnie syrup, dextrose, sorbitol, xylitol, aspartame, mannitol, and lactose. Fruit juice is one of the most common and over-looked sources of sugar. Many children consume up to a quart of juice each day. Fruit juices should be diluted and limited to one cup. Apple and grape juice both contain salicylates, so these products give susceptible children a double dose of potential poisons.

Limiting yeast-containing foods to prevent further introduction of yeast is useful, although may not be sufficient. Patients must also take supplements containing good bacteria called probiotics to displace the yeast, and in severe cases, take anti-fungal substances to kill the yeast. Natural yeast killers, such as oregano oil, garlic, olive leaf extract and other herb combinations, work in mild cases. Stubborn cases require drugs available only by prescription, such as Nystatin, Diflucan and Nizoral. Use these products along with the yeast free diet.

The most usual improvements noted with anti-fungals are increased focus and concentration and diminished bowel symptoms. Other improvements may include more frequent and clearer vocalizations, less spinning, a decrease in aggressive or self-abusive behavior like head-banging, better sleep patterns, increased socialization and improved eye contact. Antifungal therapy is least effective with individuals who have normal or marginally elevated yeast metabolites.

Body ecology diet (BED) Since 2003, many with autism and related disorders have shown rapid and remarkable improvement on the BED, developed by nutritional consultant Donna Gates. The BED both heals the gut by reestablishing colonies of good gut flora, and nourishes it with nutritious foods to allow organ systems to rebuild. This diet is compatible with both the GF/CF and Specific Carbohydrate diets. It fights chronic yeast infections, by combining the best of Western and Eastern tenets, adding guidelines to improve the health of those on these favorite programs.

The BED strives to increase the intake of whole, unrefined foods, using the following principles:
- Eat copious amounts of root and leafy green vegetables
- Eat animal foods and sugars in very small quantities
- Practice regular bowel cleansing
- Combine protein with fruits and vegetables in a given meal, but not with carbohydrates

Want to know more? Read *The Body Ecology Diet* by Donna Gates.[16]

The Low Oxalate Diet Susan Owens, a researcher who discovered that Epsom salt baths can help many with poor detoxification pathways, noted that the urine of children with autism is much higher in oxalates than normal. Oxalate and oxalic acid are compounds occurring in many common fruits, vegetables, nuts and other foods, including berries, spinach, beets, peanuts, pecans, almonds, cashews and chocolate. They are also a product of metabolism. Oxalates are not found in meat or fish.

Given her findings, Owens has proposed a "low oxalate diet" for those on the autism spectrum with high urine markers. The low oxalate diet removes many nutritious foods and non-animal protein sources, further restricting an already limited diet. What remains is mostly meat and "white" items, with limited nutritional value.

The authors believe that this diet is an example of applying reductionist thinking to autism. If scientists were to develop diets to reduce the chemical input of every substance found to be high in a segment of children with autism, they would be treating numbers on lab tests, not the larger imbalances and toxicities responsible for causing this epidemic. Instead of recommending a nutritionally insufficient diet to avoid possibly faulty pathways, we should be asking why certain children cannot properly metabolize oxalate-containing foods. While some parents report improvement in speech, motor skills, sleep and cognition on this limited diet, use it with considerable caution.

General Dietary Guidelines

While special diets most certainly can help many children on the autism spectrum, the key to a strong, healthy immune system for all children is optimal nutrition. A diet based on a balanced variety of unrefined, unprocessed, fat, protein and carbohydrate sources is the goal. Unprocessed foods are less likely to cause problems than those with additives. Try to include beans, fresh fruits and vegetables, nuts and seeds. Be sure to have at least 10 grams of protein for breakfast to facilitate learning.

Drink water, which is a better choice than fruit juice as a beverage for most children, because it has no sugar, salicylates or allergens. Make sure the water is good quality. Tap water may contribute to the toxic load because it may contain chlorine, fluoride, aluminum, lead, and even parasites. Chlorine reacts with organic matter to spawn cancer-producing substances such as chloroform.[17] Fluoride is a neurotoxin that increases the possibility that the water will leach heavy metals from cookware and foods.[18] Elevated aluminum and lead from old plumbing and city water supplies are often overlooked as possible causes of hyperactivity, violent behavior and subtle learning disabilities.[19,20]

Picky Eating

Most kids with developmental delays are picky eaters. They thus cannot obtain all the nutrients their bodies need through the foods they eat. When picky eaters with autism spectrum disorders move to a "special diet" such as one of the above, they choose primarily processed foods. Though the BED and SCD are far more nutritious than a GF/CF diet, because they do not allow processed grains, even these diets can fall short due to poor absorption and limited variety.

One reason so many children with autism have eating issues is because of immature development of their nervous systems. Poor functioning of the primitive nervous system can lead to sensory integration issues, such as an aversion to tastes, textures or smells, thus making eating habits even worse. Some youngsters reject foods they have never tasted just by looking at or smelling them.

Nobody knows exactly what a child is experiencing when he/she refuses to eat any vegetables or will only eat chicken nuggets from a particular restaurant. The visual system clearly plays a role. Parents report that the smallest change in packaging or the slightest shift in color can cause a picky eater to abandon a previously well loved food choice. See Chapter 7 for ideas regarding how to deal with the sensory issues involved in picky eating.

How can you tell if a child you are working with is well nourished? A degree in nutrition or medicine is not required.

A well nourished child	*A poorly nourished child*
Has good coloring	Has a pasty complexion/yellow or grey pallor
Is well most of the time	Has three or more illnesses a year
Is interested in a variety of foods	Has severely restricted eating habits
Has fairly consistent responses to therapy	Is erratic and unpredictable
Has clear eyes	Has dull eyes
Has good breath	Has sour or bad breath

If a child looks unhealthy, he probably is. Consider working with a practitioner who specializes in dietary intervention to improve vision therapy. The best outcomes emerge when the entire family becomes involved.

Optimize Nutrition by Adding the Good Stuff

The use of therapeutic nutrients is becoming increasingly accepted, especially for children with behavioral and developmental problems. These youngsters need more nutrients than typical children do because they have a combination of poor absorption, long-standing self-restricted diets, impaired ability to detoxify environmental chemicals and pollutants, and/or inherited nutrient deficiencies.

A logical step in closing the nutritional gap between what a child eats and what the body needs is the therapeutic use of supplements. Unfortunately, many commercial vitamins for children may be low in important trace minerals, and they often contain colors, flavors, preservatives and fillers, to which children on the autism spectrum sometimes react negatively. Therefore, look carefully at the entire content of a supplement before recommending it.

Essential fatty acids (EFAs) EFAs are a crucial part of the structure of the nervous system which is 60-70% fat. EFAs must be ingested, because the body cannot produce them. Unfortunately, the traditional American diet is low in EFAs. Furthermore, non-essential fatty acids, such as the hydrogenated vegetable oils used to make margarine, and to fry fast food are high in trans fatty acids. These "bad fats" may affect neuronal fluidity by virtue of a different chemical structure, when compared to the biologically preferred cis fatty acids. They have the potential to interfere with a child's ability to make use of the marginal amounts of EFAs a child consumes.[21]

Two types of EFAs are important in autism: omega-3 and omega 6. The pattern in children with autism is usually a deficiency of omega-3 fatty acids, with elevations of arachidonic acid (an omega 6 fat) and trans fatty acids.

Omega-3 is essential for development, as it increases cell membrane fluidity. Almost all kids have deficiencies in omega-3 fats, because they do not eat fish or seaweed. Even though many ingest some omega-6 fats, found in dairy products, nuts and seeds, omega-6 can also be deficient, especially if a child eats too many hydrogenated fats.

Optometrists must be vigilant concerning essential fatty acids, because the omega 3 fat, docosahexaenoic acid (DHA) enhances visual performance in infants and young children.[22-24] Babies have a limited ability to make DHA, and are dependent upon its addition to infant formula, or in their mothers' diets, if they are breastfeeding.[25] DHA supplementation can even help older children with developmental coordination disorder. In the famous Oxford University study, children age five to 12 given DHA showed significant improvement in reading, spelling and behavior.[26]

Symptoms of essential fatty acids deficiency are hair loss, dry or peeling skin, eczema, fatigue, aggression, dry brittle hair, eating disorders, excessive or diminished thirst, gallstones, growth impairment, immune deficiency, hyperactivity, and impaired wound healing. Essential fatty acids can be deficient due to inadequate dietary intake, chronic diarrhea, loose stools, inadequate production of pancreatic enzymes, or inadequate production or secretion of bile or bile salts.

Fortunately, supplementing fish oil no longer requires holding your nose, as many products now make this supplement palatable. Omega 3 fats come in flavored capsules, liquids and pudding-like pastes. Essential fats are fragile, and when overprocessed or exposed to air, they become rancid and can be harmful. Refrigeration can slow deterioration.

Minerals Minerals are important nutrients, as vitamins, proteins, enzymes, amino acids, fats, and carbohydrates all require minerals for activity. Mineral deficiencies are very common in children who eat high carbohydrate diets and processed foods. Balance is the key. A shortage or overabundance of just one mineral can throw off many bodily functions.[27]

Zinc (Zn) Zinc is a necessary ingredient for at least 25 enzymes involved in digestion and metabolism. Zinc deficiency is associated with growth retardation, impaired development of bone and cartilage, poor wound healing, hair loss, night blindness, impaired immune function and delayed sexual maturation. Zinc is important to the eyes because it is present in high concentration in the ocular tissue (especially the retina and choroids) and is a cofactor for vitamin A.[28] Zinc levels are often low in picky eaters because this mineral is mostly found in meat and nuts, not in a "white" diet of French fries, crackers and breads. Excessive zinc intake is rare, and may cause copper deficiency and certain anemias.

Adequate zinc protects against adverse effects from heavy metals, including lead, cadmium, and copper. Zinc can help normalize the sense of taste and may aid in acceptance of "new" foods during diet adjustment trials. If children demonstrate weak night vision, poor eye contact or slow adaptation between light and dark, consider recommending 15- 20 mg of chelated zinc along with vitamin A.

Calcium (Ca) Calcium is the most abundant mineral in the body. Children on dairy-free diets require calcium supplements. Adequate calcium enhances detoxification as it neutralizes excess aluminum.[29] Individuals with calcium deficiency may be irritable, hyperactive, sleep-disturbed, inattentive, have stomach and muscle cramps and tingling in arms and legs. Though dark green vegetables and almonds contain calcium, in practice children rarely eat enough of these foods to cover their calcium needs without supplementation.

The recommended amount of calcium for children age one to ten is 800-1000 milligrams (mg) per day. Contrary to popular belief, calcium need does not rise dramatically during childhood because the requirements in the early years are already high, due to rapid bone growth.

Calcium must be properly balanced with magnesium.[30] Magnesium also improves calcium absorption, and can cause loose stools. A general consideration for ages two to four is 100-200 mg of magnesium, and for ages five and up, 200-300 mg along with the calcium.

Some forms of calcium are easier for the body to use, and therefore provide more benefit. The most absorbable forms of calcium are calcium citrate, calcium hydroxyapatite, and protein-bound calcium such as calcium chelate and gluconate. Calcium citrate is arguably absorbed the best. Use it in small amounts mixed with other forms of calcium for young children, because it is very acidic and in large quantities can cause mouth sores. Not recommended is calcium carbonate (oyster shell), a poorly absorbed and inexpensive, but popular form of calcium that is the main ingredient in "Tums."

Calcium can be taken as pills, powder, liquids, or chewables. Children often reject powder and chewable forms because their texture is chalky. If a child will accept ground-up pills or a powder, look for one that contains several forms of calcium mixed together. Divide the 800-1000 mg dose between two meals or snacks for maximum absorption.

Liquids are usually the most successful way to supplement calcium in children who have difficulty swallowing. Unfortunately, the best absorbed commercially prepared liquid contains artificial sweeteners. Custom formulas are an option that require preparation by a compounding pharmacy with a prescription from a licensed health care provider. However, they have a limited shelf life, lasting a maximum of two months in the refrigerator. They can be shipped without refrigeration, however.

A pharmacist can make up a liquid calcium supplement using the following generic formula: 300 mg calcium gluconate, 300 mg calcium hydroxyapatite, 300 mg calcium chelate, and 400 international units of Vitamin D per day. 100-300 mg chelated magnesium can also be added, depending upon age. Ask the pharmacist which natural flavor bases are available. Sugar, maple syrup or stevia can be used to sweeten the mixture, or it can just be mixed in distilled water. If using a water-based formula, put it in one to two ounces of juice, so the child will accept it. Make sure the child drinks of all the juice. Give this liquid in two divided doses.

Magnesium (Mg) Magnesium, the eighth most plentiful element on the planet, and the fourth most abundant mineral in the body, is essential for over 300 biochemical bodily reactions, many of which have gone awry in individuals with autism, attention issues and other developmental delays.[31] Mg is the single most important mineral for maintaining proper electrical balance and facilitating smooth metabolism in the cells. One of the major roles of magnesium is stabilizing cell membranes.

The health status of the digestive system and the kidneys significantly influence Mg status. Mg is absorbed in the intestines and then transported through the blood to cells and tissues.

Signs of magnesium deficiency include constipation, hypersensitivity to loud and high-pitched sounds, irritability, muscle cramps and twitches, cold hands and feet, insomnia, carbohydrate cravings, numbness and tingling, and the inability to inhale deeply. Mg deficiency is most likely in those who eat many processed foods, over-cook foods and drink soft water. Deficiencies can develop when Mg elimination is increased by taking many medications, like diuretics, birth control pills, corticosteroids and anti-psychotics, because these products, as well as alcohol, caffeine and sugar, leach Mg. Colicky babies may also be magnesium deficient because their stressed hormones trigger the excretion of greater than normal levels of Mg in their urine.

Foods high in Mg are avocados, beans, molasses, almonds, Brazil nuts, cashews, pumpkin and sunflower seeds, whole grains, fish, kiwis, and leafy greens, especially spinach. Buy organic. Supplement Mg as Mg citrate and Mg glycinate, two of the best absorbed forms. Recommended daily allowance (RDA) is four mg of Mg daily per pound of body weight (e.g., 160 mg for a 40-pound child). Read labels carefully, always looking for the number of milligrams of *elemental* Mg in the tablet or capsule.

See further on in this chapter, and in Appendix A in the next chapter, articles about the beneficial effects of supplemental magnesium given along with vitamin B6 to improve its absorption in individuals with autism. In the late 1960s, Dr. Bernard Rimland started collecting data on this subject, which is indisputable today.[32]

Mg metabolism has a quirk: if Mg levels are low enough to cause symptoms, the deficiency can cause the body to lose its ability to use what it takes in orally. Only a third to a half of dietary Mg is absorbed into the body. Furthermore, the gut has a low tolerance for Mg; diarrhea is often the outcome before sufficient amounts can be ingested. Bypassing the digestive tract can solve this problem by supplementing Mg transdermally, using bath salts or creams.

Susan Owens has shown the benefits of Epsom salts, which are magnesium sulfate. Pour one cup of Epsom salts into a tub of warm water, soaking for approximately 30 minutes per day. Epsom salts can help both with magnesium supplementation *and* sulfur levels in the blood, which may aid detoxification. All salts tend to dry and become "powdery" on the skin, which may limit absorption. Mg chloride bath flakes are hydroscopic, meaning they attract water, thus staying wet on the skin, where they are more likely to be absorbed.[33]

Other Minerals Selenium, chromium, manganese and other trace minerals are also important as supplements for many children, because levels tend to be low in refined diets. These minerals are often included for children on biomedical programs by using a general mineral product to support general development. Selenium, an antioxidant, is particularly beneficial for youngsters who have had significant exposure to toxic elements. Chromium is involved in the synthesis of EFAs. Diets high in sugar can deplete chromium. Manganese plays a role in activating numerous enzymes.[27 (p.14-16)]

Vitamins

Nutritionists and others have used vitamins to increase immunity and cognitive function for many years. Both deficiencies and toxic levels can contribute to poor learning and aberrant behavior. The supplements used therapeutically most often are combinations of vitamin A, B complex, C, and E, along with aforementioned minerals, such as zinc, chromium, selenium and calcium.

Vitamin A – In the late 1990s, Mary Megson, MD, a developmental pediatrician in Richmond, VA, became interested in the fact that many of the children in her practice regressed following a vaccine. Her theory is that some vaccines may act as an "off switch" to genetically weakened receptors for the processing of language, vision and perception. She has found that natural vitamin A switches these receptors back on in many children.

Megson's findings are vitally important to the optometrist, as she sees autism as a biological, perception-deficit problem. Many of the visual issues in autism improve with vitamin A supplementation. Here is what she says about the visual system in autism:

> *Probably one of the most profound things I have discovered is how children with autism "see" their world. Once you understand it, then you begin to realize that the way the children look at you and the world around them makes perfect sense, given the way their eyes function. These children live in a "magic-eye puzzle."*

> *A blocked pathway has caused the rods in their eyes to not function correctly thus affecting their vision, so they can't see like most people do. They must compensate for the rod dysfunction the best way they can. They "see" the world around them as though it's in a 3-D box. They have such a limited visual field that everything*

that doesn't fit in their box blurs and is perceived as color and shape alone. And, the most incredible thing is that they actually have to piece together each "box" that they see in order to see a complete shape.

So, in order to live and perceive the world outside of their limited "box," they have to organize it according to color and shape. That's why the children "melt down" when objects are moved or when you clean up their lines or piles of toys sorted by color. They have to work so hard to perceive their world that it frightens and overwhelms them when the world as they are able to see it changes. It also explains why the children are known to organize things so carefully. It's the only way they can "see" their world. This is a visual perception problem! When you say, "look at me, look at me," they really are. But they have to look at you sideways. They turn their eye so that the light reflected from your face lands on the edge of the fovea or the lateral retina where they have some rod function. The fovea is the area in the back of the eye where the cones are closest together. That's the only way they can "see" you. When you force their pupil to appear to focus on you, you are actually forcing them to look away from you because their "best vision" is off to one side.

When taking vitamin A as cod liver oil, rod function improves. One of the first effects we see is the disappearance of the "sideways glance" that the children are known for. The sideways glance is a biological adaptation, given how their vision pathway has been blocked. The body always tries to adapt the best way it can. So, this way of looking at things is "normal" for the child with autism. As rod function improves, they look right at you and can really see you! They move back from and become less interested in TV and videos. Until "the box" expands, the only place they always hear the right language for what they are looking at is to set "the box" (i.e. TV, video, computer). As vision improves, their ability to see and hear the right language for what they are looking at improves.[34]

Megson's preferred source of vitamin A is a tried and true remedy that grandma used: cod liver oil. Vitamin A in the cod liver oil slowly, steadily, improves language and social issues while simultaneously healing the body. This source of vitamin A turns on T-cells, which are important in immune system protection. T-cells remember exposures to foreign proteins, viruses and bacteria when the immune system is working correctly. Turned on immune cells return to the point of initial exposure, often the gut wall, and create inflammation. Vitamin A heals mucous secreting glands that line the gastrointestinal tract and secrete IgA, the protein the body makes to fight ear, throat respiratory and gastrointestinal infections. It also helps the immune system to remember those infections so they don't recur.[35]

Megson recommends checking both vitamin A and D levels before beginning cod liver oil, with a recheck after two months. Levels must be monitored closely. Some children have very low vitamin A levels, while others do not. Regardless of the child's vitamin A level, a natural form of vitamin A is absolutely critical for the molecules to attach to the receptors in the brain controlling vision and language. Dosages must not exceed the normal recommended daily allowance of vitamins A and D for a child's age.

B Vitamins – The B vitamins are coenzymes that play a role in energy production, as well as for healthy nerves, hair, skin, eyes, liver and mouth. They are also crucial in maintaining good muscle tone in the gastrointestinal tract. While usually taken together as a team, individual B vitamins are sometimes supplemented for specific purposes. Children with autism spectrum disorders can take B vitamin supplements containing up to 50 mg of vitamin B-1 and B-2, with the other Bs provided in balance. Watch for irritability, the most common side effect of taking too many Bs.

B6 - According to Dr. Bernard Rimland of the Autism Research Institute, the scientific literature supports no biological treatment for autism more strongly than the use of high dosage vitamin B6, preferably given along with magnesium. See Chapter 6 for a list of over 20 studies, published since 1965, showing conclusively that high dose vitamin B6 confers many benefits to about 50% of those with autism. None of the studies of B6 in autism has reported any significant adverse effects, nor would any significant adverse effects be expected. While B6/magnesium is not a cure, for many with autism, it has often made a very significant difference.

B12 - Chronic gut inflammation, toxicity, and vegetarian diets can all contribute to low levels of Vitamin B12. Dr. James Neubrander in Edison, NJ pioneered injections of concentrated vitamin B12 in the form of pure methylcobalamin, for children with autism spectrum disorders. He recommends up to 55 mcg/kg twice a week. Injections, unlike oral B12, bypass the impaired gut and directly feed the nervous system. Methylcobalamin is the active form of vitamin B-12, and is better utilized than other commercially available forms.

Jacqueline McCandless believes that combining folinic acid with methylcobalamin, and sometimes TMG, is probably one of the best things that we can do for all of our spectrum kids. This treatment is especially suited to those with a history of vaccination with thimerosal containing vaccines, autistic enterocolitis and chronic loose stools. When combined with folic acid, B12 participates in the complicated steps of detoxification by facilitating the methylation processes important for creating optimum metabolic balance. Then, the body can eventually detoxify itself. [1] (p. 275)

Vitamin C - Vitamin C is an extremely safe water soluble antioxidant which is immensely beneficial to the brain and body in a multitude of ways. Its potential for preventing and treating autism has barely been touched.[36] For children under 18, use 250-1000 mg per day, or in higher doses to protect against illness. Diarrhea occurs before the body can absorb too much, so toxicity is not a concern.

Vitamin E - Many health care practitioners add vitamin E to nutritional programs for autism to aid in detoxification, because it is an important fat soluble antioxidant. Since cell membranes are basically a lipid (fat) bilayer, vitamin E is important for protecting membrane integrity. It also helps the mitochondria clean up debris for more efficient energy production. Take as mixed tocopherols, 200-400 IU.

Dimethylglycine (DMG) and Trimethylglycine (TMG) - DMG has been shown to improve language, although it can increase self-stimulatory behavior. Dr. Rimland has followed the use of this substance in autism for over 25 years and has found it to be non-toxic and potentially helpful. TMG, a related substance, has been added recently to the autism vitamin arsenal as a methyl group donor to improve detoxification pathways. Folic acid sometimes acts as an antidote to the irritability caused by DMG or TMG.

Secretin

Secretin is a gut neuropeptide produced by the stomach that aids in regulating gastric function, and is also intimately involved in many activities of the brain, including the production and utilization of the neurotransmitter serotonin.[37] Secretin enhances intestinal fluid production, which, in turn allows the normal metabolism of protein. The end products are formed stools and a rise in blood serotonin levels that stimulate the production of other neurotransmitters, leading to increased attention, language production and socialization.[38]

In the late 1990s Victoria Beck, the mother of a boy with autism, requested an upper GI procedure to find the cause of her son's severe diarrhea and gut pain. Immediately following the procedure, which included an infusion of secretin, her son, who had not spoken in months, startled everyone by speaking coherently. Many were hopeful that by replenishing secretion in those with autism, language delays and difficulties with relatedness could be reversed. While the initial excitement around secretin has decreased in recent years, some doctors are still using it as a part of a "heal the gut" protocol.

The Autism Research Institute (ARI) has gathered anecdotal evidence from parents of thousands of children with autism who have taken secretin. Most reports are positive with parents reporting improvements in eye contact, interest in the environment, better sleep patterns and accelerated language development.[39] About 5-10% of the children had negative reactions, such as hyperactivity and aggressiveness, and a very small number of documented cases had grand mal seizures.[40] The vast majority received secretin by IV injection; a few had transdermal application or sublingual drops.

Research does not support the efficacy of secretin in autism.[41] In 2004, the Repligen Corporation, the manufacturer of porcine secretin released the long-awaited preliminary results of its Phase III study of secretin efficacy in autism. To the surprise and dismay of many, the results, though incomplete were negative. The negative report contrasted sharply with a great deal of very positive earlier data from the company. Dr. Rimland believes that the study did not properly screen participants to identify the subgroup of potential "responders."[42]

Mary Megson, encouraged by the reported action of secretin in her patients, proposes using very low doses of a prescription medication called Bethanechol, approved for reflux in children in the 1970s. Bethanechol mirrors the effects of secretin by addressing the problems in the gut. In some children, it seems to "jump start" the process, by stimulating the blocked pathway. Bethanechol does not cross the blood brain barrier; it stimulates blocked pathways in the hippocampus through gut to brain connections.

Megson sometimes uses Bethanechol by mouth, only after a child has been on cod liver oil for at least two months, thus giving the gut receptors a chance to heal and reconnect. In some children, cod liver oil alone is enough to reconnect those blocked pathways. Other children may need something more. She always administers the first dose of Bethanechol in her office, observing a patient for an hour, noting any allergic sensitivity or reaction. Bethanechol is contra-indicated for children who are ill or have active asthma, as it may increase mucous secretions in the airway. Atropine is a direct antidote to Bethanechol.[43]

Miscellaneous Supplements
Digestive enzymes, probiotics, choline compounds, and various other plant-based supplements often work synergistically in combination with vitamins and minerals, for the treatment of hyperactivity and autistic-like symptoms. Anti-fungals can also be helpful, and are included in the Defeat Autism Now! chapter.

Digestive enzymes – Health care professionals use digestive enzymes extensively in the biomedical treatment of autism because a substantial subgroup of children has chronic digestive disturbances. When the gut lining is irritated or inflamed, the body has a reduced capacity to produce and utilize digestive enzymes. Vaccinations, the aggressive use of antibiotics, prematurity and environmental toxins are all suspect as contributors to digestive pathology. Common digestive symptoms include chronic loose stools, excessive gas and bloating, unusually putrid bowel movements, pain, poor eating habits and reflux.

Adding supplemental enzymes sometimes helps the gut break down food so it is absorbed better, and does not become fodder for yeast and unhelpful bacteria. Properly digested food is also less aggravating to the immune system and may reduce food reactions. Two companies specialize in digestive enzymes for children: Kirkman at <www.kirkmanlabs.com> and Houston Nutraceuticals at <www.houstonni.com>.

Probiotics - Pro-biotics, meaning "in support of life," are a class of supplements made up of many different organisms with names such as lactobacillus acidophilus. Healthy people should have a pound or more of good bacteria growing in their bodies. Adding these good bacteria to the gut is critical for healing the gut lining in those with intestinal symptoms, because they produce the raw materials needed to mend injured guts. Like worms are to soil, probioitics process fiber found in food, and produce short chain fatty acids needed for repair.

Probiotics line both the interior and exterior surfaces of the body and serve as sentries that:
* protect the body against infection[44]
* reduce diarrhea[45]
* prevent young children from developing allergies
* re-establish intestinal integrity[46]

Various companies sell different proprietary blends of "bugs." Finding the right combination of good bacteria is like finding the right plants for your garden. Brand A may work well for one person and do nothing for the next. If one type does not help, try increasing the dose or moving to a different brand. Use two or more brands together to increase the chances of getting the right mix. Look for ones that contain billions (not millions) of organisms, such as Culturelle, Threelac, and MegaFlora. Keep probiotics refrigerated, as most organisms quickly die when exposed to high temperatures.

Grapeseed or pine bark extract is a non-toxic, water-soluble antioxidant that is a non-prescription alternative for improving focus, memory, fine motor skills and eye contact. It is sometimes sold under the patented names Pycnogenol or OPC complex. The active ingredient is a type of bioflavonoid called proanthocyandin. OPC complex, unlike many antioxidants, crosses the blood brain barrier. Empirical evidence suggests grapeseed extract may affect the part of the brain responsible for fine motor skills.

Choline Compounds - Choline is an amino acid essential for brain development,[47] found in eggs, fish and soybeans. A lack of choline early in life can permanently limit brain capacity for learning. In 1998, the National Academy of Science recognized choline, and established a daily requirement of 425-550 mg. Adding it as a supplement can improve structural integrity and signaling ability of the nerve cell membranes.[48]

Several forms of choline, including ***phosphatidylcholine*** and ***Dimethylaminoethanol*** (DMAE), a relative of choline, are beneficial in autism, as they are building blocks for the neurotransmitter ***acetylcholine***. Acetylcholine, abundant in both the cerebral cortex and cerebellum, is involved in the cognitive processes controlled by these parts of the brain, such as memory, motor planning, problem solving, organization, rational thinking, balance and movement. Children with motor issues and low arousal may benefit from an increase in acetylcholine availability.

Choline as *phosphatidylcholine* is absorbed directly into cell membranes and regulates permeability. Preliminary empirical data from clinical practice suggests phosphatidyl-choline may increase complex language. Phosphatidylcholine, available as both capsules and in liquid form, is given in doses of 1-3 grams.

Dimethylaminoethanol (DMAE), unlike some forms of choline, readily crosses the brain-blood barrier. It directly increases the generation of acetylcholine. DMAE can increase muscle tension. It thus works best for children whose prevailing problems are spaciness and poor organizational skills, and least well in those children who have high muscle tension, sleep disturbances or agitation, rather than distractibility. Dosing range is 50 -200 mg for children. As with all supplements, stop DMAE immediately if irritability occurs.

Transfer Factors - Transfer factors (TF) are naturally occurring molecules that contain our immune history. They are made by white blood cells which travel to the maturing mammary glands and release the donor's immune history into the maturing mammary tissues. As the newborn nurses he receives his mother's immune history via her immune factors, hence the name. If one thinks of vitamins and minerals as the bricks and mortar that build immune system cells, transfer factors are the blueprints that determine were the brick will be placed.

Hugh Fudenberg, MD, is the researcher usually associated with transfer factors. In a group of 22 children with autism, 15 of whom had become autistic following an MMR vaccine, all but one responded positively to TF, with ten regaining sufficient skills to enter mainstream schools. After discontinuing treatment, some showed regression, but none returned to their prior baseline levels.[49] In another study, 88 children who used TF at the recommended doses for at least 6 months were compared to a matched sample. The TF group had a 74% reduction in illness and an 86% reduction in antibiotic use.[50]

Start with one 200 mg capsule, and work up to as high as 2,000 mg a day, gradually increasing over the first month. Do not combine with digestive enzymes. Parents report improved health and mental focus during the first six months of supplementation.

Drs. Kenneth Bock and Jeff Bradstreet, very well-respected Defeat Autism Now! doctors, both include Transfer Factors as part of their treatment protocols to boost the immune system in patients with autism. For more information read *Transfer Factor: Natural Immune Booster*[50] by William Hennen, and visit <www.transferfactorinstitute.com>.

DETOXIFICATION
If autism is indeed a "unique form of mercury poisoning," and tests of children with autism also show high levels of aluminum, lead, pesticides, preservatives, solvents and other pollutants (see Chapter 3), then ridding the body of these and other toxins is impera-tive. Proving that a particular child has toxic levels of a specific poison is extremely difficult, however, even in clear cases of overexposure, such as mercury loading from vaccinations.

Identifying Children Who are Toxic
Until recently, measuring accurate levels of toxicity via laboratory testing has been elusive. Blood levels do not yield answers, because metals are stored in fat tissue, not blood. Now tests can identify molecular damage in blood and urine that only toxins can cause, by measuring the presence of porphyrins, a chemical ring structure that the body uses to make hemoglobin. It is the "heme" of hemoglobin. Hemoglobin is a porphyrin ring with iron in the middle. Because of the presence of iron, blood, which contains hemoglobin, is red.

Mercury and other toxins interfere with the production of porphyrin at specific places on the ring. Scientists believe mercury interferes at the fifth and sixth step, The result is malformed or incompletely formed porphyrin that the body excretes because it cannot use it to build hemoglobin. Other toxins disrupt production at other junctures, resulting in the elevation of different porphyrins.

The urine test detects specific incomplete, unusable porphyrins discarded before the disrupted step, such as pentacarboxy porphyrin (5-CP) and coproporphyrin (4-CP), which denote the presence of mercury. Have you ever noticed that some children with delays appear unusually pale? That's because a defect in hemoglobin production from either inadequate iron or poor porphyrin genesis gives them pasty complexions.

In the United States, Lab Corp and Quest Laboratories offer tests measuring porphyrins in plasma and urine. Both domestic labs have limited experience with the test, and do not report all of the by-products. Laboratoire Philippe Auguste in France has broader experience with the testing, and provides clear results. Patients can send a urine sample via air mail; the test takes about 10 days to process. Go to <www.labbio.net> for more information.

Health care professionals have found many inventive ways to detoxify. For a comprehensive overview of removing heavy metals, read Chapter 7 in *Children with Starving Brains*, by Jacqueline McCandless[1] and a published interview with McCandless in *Medical Veritas* Journal.[2]

Chelation Physicians embracing a biomedical approach have looked to lead removal for a model to rid the body of all metals. The process is called "chelation," derived from the Greek word for "claw," describing the chemical binding of metal ions. Alternatives for chelation include nutritional programs under the guidance of health care practitioners and drug-based chelation, directed by physicians.

Every mineral taken into the body, whether essential or toxic, must be bound to another substance, because raw minerals are unstable. This instability is noted by the little 2+ often written after a mineral. (Calcium noted as "Ca2+" or lead as "Pb2+".) Calcium, lead, magnesium, mercury and some others have two unpaired electrons, indicated by the 2+. These 2 "unmarried" electrons are so desperate to find mates that almost any molecule short two electrons will do. Chelating agents are such molecules.

The heaviest, and generally most toxic metals such as mercury, lead, nickel and cadmium, are the most "eligible." They bond to chelating agents first. The resulting "chelated" minerals are stabilized minerals. For example, chelated calcium, sold as a supplement, is a well absorbed, stabilized form of calcium that does not remove calcium.

Preparing the Body for Chelation

Before attempting to remove bad metals, make sure that a child is eating sufficient protein, because heavy metals are not excreted well when the diet is low in protein. A child eating only starches, such as waffles and French fries, is not ready for chelation. Children age three to four require a minimum of 25 grams daily, while those five and up require 30 grams. They also need a minimum of three to four servings per day of fruits and vegetables, not including juice, as fruits and vegetables contain the phyto-nutrients and natural antioxidants that support the body's detoxification pathways.

Prior to chelation add a basic multi-vitamin such as Kirkman's New and Improved Super NuThera with P5P (www.kirkmanlabs.com) or New Beginnings' Basic Nutrients Plus (www.nbnus.com) to the nutritional mix. Some mineral overlap with the recommended comprehensive mineral supplementation is inevitable, because most children's nutrients contain small amounts of many minerals, though not enough to support chelation.

Add extra nutrients even if balancing the basic diet is successful. The poorer the diet, the more nutrients a child needs, whether or not chelation is down the road. Heavy metal excretion depletes minerals and antioxidants. Thus, safe detoxification requires extra nutrients. A sample base nutrient program for a child over three includes:
- Vitamin C - 250-500 mg
- Vitamin E - 200-400 IU as mixed tocopherols
- A comprehensive mineral supplement containing 30 mg of zinc, 100-200 mcg of selenium, and 2-5 mg of manganese., such as Minerall, from Kirkman or Basic Nutrients Plus from New Beginnings Nutritionals.
- Essential Fatty Acids (EFAs) - 1 tsp. from mercury-free fish oil or flaxseed oil
- Methyl B-12 - 1,000 mcg
- Trimethylglycine (TMG) - 300-500 mg
- Folinic acid- 800 mcg
- Lipoceutical glutathione (see below) - ¼- tsp. twice per day

Add nutrients one at a time, three days apart. Monitor reactions, the most common of which is irritability. Using the above supportive nutrition program along with chlorella, METAL FREE™ (see below), or other over-the-counter metal removal agents alone will promote slow detoxification in most children.

Balancing the bowels is also a must before starting chelation, because heavy metals are partially excreted through the stool. Use dietary modification and nutritional supplementation to get the bowels functioning properly, as well as to heal the gut, and strengthen immunity. A good nutrient program naturally encourages detoxification and gentle heavy metal displacement, even if chelating agents are not used. These measures alone often "jump start" the body's natural methylation and sulphation mechanisms.

Supporting Chelation Nutritionally
Children also need additional nutritional support once chelation programs have begun, in order to balance and increase good nutrients. During chelation, individuals must continue a diet rich in antioxidants, the primary job of which is to alleviate oxidative stress, because many symptoms caused by metal toxicity are from the proliferation of oxidative free radicals. Children who are vaccine injured are at an increased risk for gut problems when detoxing if they are not taking sufficient therapeutic doses of antioxidants. Any safe heavy metal removal program should have free radical protection, and include supplements of antioxidants such as vitamins A, C and E, selenium, alpha-lipoic acid, and the most important antioxidant of all: glutathione.

Glutathione (GSH) is a peptide, composed of three amino acids: cysteine, glycine and glutamic acid: the basic building blocks of protein. The antioxidant part of GSH comes from the sulfur section of the L-cysteine. In chemistry, the electron donating sulfur group (-SH) is called thiol. To detoxify mercury, arsenic, lead and cadmium, GSH provides a thiol group that binds to metals and other poisons. The body then excretes a metal-cysteine mixture.

The body's glutathione level determines how many toxins it absorbs. Individuals with high levels of toxicity have used up their body's natural glutathione. When GSH levels are low, the body accepts more heavy metals. Adequate levels of GSH are necessary for many aspects of immune function. Low levels impair immunity, which leads to frequent infection. The body's poor response to infection causes inflammation and oxidative stress, which, in turn, lowers glutathione. A vicious cycle perpetuates when the body has inadequate glutathione to offset oxidative stress, further reducing immunity, and allowing opportunistic infections (like yeasts and parasites) to proliferate. As glutathione levels rise, the body is better able to excrete poisons.[1 (p.255-256)]

The body makes about half the glutathione it needs. The cofactors for incorporating cysteine into GSH are methyl vitamin B-12, folinic acid and trimethylglycine (TMG). These allow the body to produce more glutathione and absorb it better.

Once the body produces GSH, it works as an antioxidant only in its active form, confusingly referred to as reduced-L-glutathione (GSH). When GSH gives away its electron, it becomes inactive oxidized glutathione (GSSG). Vitamin C converts the inactive oxidized GSSG back to its active version. Therefore, NAC, vitamin B-12, folinic acid, TMG and vitamin C are all important nutrients for increasing and maintaining healthy glutathione levels, by giving the body the raw materials.

Dr. Jill James and her colleagues are some of the major proponents of supplementing GSH in combination with methyl B12 for detoxification of heavy metals in those with autism spectrum disorders. Those in their landmark study showed both improved speech and levels of cognition.[10] Children with suspected vaccine damage and heavy metal exposure are prime candidates. Infants and toddlers with colic, diarrhea or constipation are more likely to have low GSH, and thus be at risk to environmental exposures.

While initially doctors prescribed oral GSH, taking GSH by mouth is less popular now because it is poorly absorbed. Intravenous GSH is both successful and expensive, although using needles with children who have sensory problems can be challenging.

Essential Glutathione™, which surrounds the glutathione with fat droplets called liposomes is the delivery method of choice for most children. Preliminary studies suggest that liposomes optimize absorption by protecting the GSH from oxidation. Essential Glutathione™ is available without prescription from Wellness Pharmacy (800-227-2627). The cost is $50 for a bottle containing 12 teaspoons. Give ¼ tsp. twice daily per 30 pounds of body weight, always starting with a smaller dose in sensitive children. Ongoing feedback from parents is available at <www.wellnesshealth.com>.

Chelation Options

Doctors are still looking for the best chelation methods. Originally, children with autism took strong chelators orally. Oral chelation has lost favor, due to gut symptoms and reports of developmental regression. Presently, those practicing chelation prefer transdermal and intravenous delivery systems, both of which bypass the gut. These methods require meticulous medical monitoring, and not all families can afford or access this level of care. Health care professionals fall into two schools of thought regarding chelation: slow and fast.

"Slow" chelation programs may be preferable for children who are already progressing well with their therapy programs, and whose laboratory tests show high metal levels. A slow program protects the body from violent withdrawal reactions by taking more time; progress may not be noticeable on a day-to-day basis. Youngsters often become better regulated and more responsive to therapy; language often improves more rapidly. An occasional child shows dramatic developmental gains. While every child undergoing chelation should be monitored, slow chelation can be followed by a nurse or nutritionist trained in detoxification techniques, as well as by a physician. A home based program is not a substitute for appropriate, individual medical care.

Slow chelation uses natural over-the-counter agents including the proteins glycine, methionine, cysteine, histidine, glutathione and taurine. Substances found in food-based agents like cilantro, chlorella (algae), garlic, and sodium alginate also assist in the mobilization of metals. This section concentrates on two with good records of safety and efficacy.

Chlorella - Extracted from algae, chlorella contains vast amounts of chlorophyll, nature's own detoxification agent. Sun Chlorella™, available as both a powder and tablets, is considered one of the purest forms, free of metals and other toxins. Downside: the powdered drink looks, smells and tastes like pond water, and the tablets could be difficult to swallow. Dose at four pellets or one packet of Sun Chlorella™ twice per day for children over three.

METAL-FREE™- This complex nutritional chelating agent contains chlorella, as well as glycine, algae, hyaluronic acid, alpha lipoic acid and other nutrients, in a liquid base that can be sprayed into the mouth or taken as drops. Start with one spray (or 4 drops) under the tongue for one week, and then two sprays the second week, up to a dose of 4 sprays (16 drops). Take at least an hour away from food, such as before bed. If a child becomes cranky or agitated, decrease the dose. METAL-FREE™ is available from <www.bodyhealth.com> or by calling 877-804-3258.

Zeolite - Deposits of alkaline ash-alumino-salicates that are formed when volcanoes erupt are called zeolites. The wind carries the ash, which mixes with salt water, and results in the formation of natural zeolites. Aluminum and silica form stable, three dimensional honeycomb structures with different compositions, depending on temperature, geographic location and other environmental factors.

One of the members of the zeolite group of minerals is called clinoptilolite. Clinoptilolite is the form used medically, and has a ratio of silica to aluminum of 4 to 1. The channels in the zeolite provide large surface areas that can absorb ions and gas molecules.[51]

The silicon building block of zeolite is electrically neutral, while the aluminum molecule carries a negative charge. These multiple charge sites created by aluminum attract positively charged minerals (called cations), such as calcium, iron, cadmium, mercury, nickel and arsenic. Positive ions attracted to the zeolite switch places with positively charged toxins (like pesticides). Zeolite can also trap free radicals.[52]

While zeolite is available in powder and liquid form, liquefying zeolite may change the chemical structure, allowing the release of aluminum into the body. All studies to date use the powdered form. A new study with children on the autistic spectrum is underway using liquid zeolite. To learn about it go to <www.zeoliteautismstudy.com>. Zeolite in powder or encapsulated powder is available from <www.zeohealth.com>.

"Fast" is the method of choice when time is of the essence for young children with the potential for developing permanent delays. High heavy metal toxicity levels and little developmental progress may also justify an aggressive approach in older individuals. "Fast" chelation MUST be done under a doctor's supervision and with close medical monitoring. Few doctors are experienced in this treatment, so the cost is high and will likely involve travel.

The "fast" school argues that metals, particularly mercury, should be removed as quickly as possible, because less aggressive methods allow mercury to float around and possibly settle into other tissues before being excreted. Fast chelation uses strong chelators, such as the prescription drugs, Dimercaptosuccinic acid (DMSA) and Dimercaptopropane sulfonate (DMPS) which bind strongly to heavy metals; both can be hard on the kidneys.

DMSA is the primary chelator used by DAN! practitioners. Refer to Chapter 6 in the section entitled "Detoxify the Body" by Dr. Jon Pangborn for more information about DMSA.

Transdermal thiamine tetrahydrofurfuryl disulfide (TTFD) is a synthetic version of allithaimine, a naturally occurring substance found in garlic. Dr. Derrick Lonsdale believes that TTFD has three sulfur-related mechanisms that benefit children with autism spectrum disorders.[53] While few doctors are using this drug anymore, it is still included in the Defeat Autism Now! protocol. Available from Coastal Compounding Pharmacy (912-354-5188), TTFD is a prescription item.

Ethylenediamine tetra-acetic acid (EDTA) is a synthetic amino acid with a strong binding affinity to calcium and lead. Traditionally, it has been used orally for lead poisoning; however, it can remove many metallic ions.[54] In an attempt to find more effective treatment agents for increasing numbers of heavy metal poisoned kids, doctors are using EDTA experimentally both orally and by IV.

DMPS- Another good chelator of mercury is DMPS, which must be used "off-label" on children. In 1994, Rashid Buttar, a North Carolina physician, developed a transdermal (TD) version of DMPS for his son with autism. Dr. Buttar has many enthusiastic followers who credit his product for safe removal of mercury from the bodies of their children.

TD-DMPS® is a highly stable and oxidation resistant lotion that is rubbed into the skin. Its unique formulation, covalently conjugated with amino acids, permits the greatest level of assimilability into the body. The result is a generally well-tolerated, highly efficacious version of the original chelator.

Laboratory testing is mandatory to insure patient safety and to document mobilization of mercury. Doctors administer daily vitamins and other nutritional supplements to detoxify and heal the GI tract, as are needed, according to the results of pre-chelation lab tests. To avoid mineral depletion, many physicians start an aggressive two- week mineral repletion program *prior* to initiating treatment with TD-DMPS®. Health care practitioners can order TD-DMPS® from Advanced Medical Therapeutics (AMT) Pharmacy (866-828-8203).

Because chelation protocols are rapidly changing and evolving, details of all the different programs cannot be listed here. Chelation need not be intimidating. Start with a safe, good quality nutrient regimen, whether or not a child has had heavy metal exposure. Contact a health care practitioner with chelation experience to help sort the possibilities and choose the best program for an individual child.

Infrared sauna- One of the safest ways to detoxify heavy metals and balance the body's pH is by using a sauna. A far infrared sauna duplicates the same frequencies as normal body heat. Far infrared heat rays penetrates the body to a depth of 1.5 to 2 inches. The body's tissues selectively absorb these rays as water in the cells reacts in a process called "resonant absorption," which causes toxins to be released into the blood stream. These toxins are then excreted in sweat, feces, and urine. Because no chemicals are added, and the heat forces the use of sweat as the major mode of toxin elimination, this method puts less stress on the kidneys and liver.

Saunas are available for two, three or four persons; the best are poplar, which unlike cedar, redwood, spruce or pine, does not outgas any chemicals. Some are equipped with stereo speakers. A great source is High Tech Health at 800-794-5355 or <www.hightechhealth.com>. Mention this book to receive a discount. High Tech Health will also make a donation to Developmental Delay Resources (DDR) upon purchase.

Hyperbaric Oxygen - The "new kid on the block," not easily categorized into any section of this chapter, is hyperbaric oxygen therapy (HBOT), a powerful treatment previously proven efficacious for those who have had drowning accidents, stroke and other brain injuries. Some physicians are now using it for individuals diagnosed with autism spectrum disorders. Patients of all ages are entirely enclosed in a chamber in which they breathe oxygen at a pressure of more than one atmosphere. Both the enclosed chamber and the pressure are necessary for HBOT. Treatments last one to two hours. Forty to 60 sessions are often necessary to see significant benefit.

Pressurized oxygen has tremendous healing capabilities. HBOT delivers oxygen deep into the tissues of the body where it attacks and kills yeasts and anaerobic (oxygen-hating) bacteria, with a short-lived die-off that is not hard on the liver. Reported outcomes include improved speech and language, attention, concentration, and a reduction in hyperactivity.

Drs. Dan Rossignol, Elizabeth Mumper and others performed a preliminary study in 2006 using HBOT with 18 children diagnosed with autism. Pre- and post-testing showed improvements in aberrant behavior, social responsiveness and other areas. Informal observations showed significant changes in communication, motivation, mannerisms, sensory and cognitive awareness and overall health.[56]

While the application of this treatment to those with autism shows promise, more research is necessary. For more information about HBOT and practitioners using this treatment go to <www.hbotusa.org>.

CONCLUSIONS

Autism is treatable. Addressing the underlying biological issues in autism can often result in profound changes in behavior and learning. While the earlier treatment starts, the better, even adults can show positive benefits. Improving and/or restricting the diet are the first and best strategies parents can use to start their children toward recovery.

Nutrition can be viewed from two perspectives. One: what is missing in the diet that can help the healing process? Two: what is being consumed that is getting in the way of recovery? Once we stop food intake that inflames the gut and irritates the nervous system, we give those with autism spectrum disorders the nutrients required to feed their starving brains. We can then begin correcting their impaired detoxification systems and remove toxins.

We have learned ways of chelating the heavy metals from their bodies with mild agents that aid detoxification such as METAL-FREE™, to more serious and safe chelation agents such as DMSA and DMPS in an effective and non-invasive transdermal form. This broad-spectrum bio-medical approach is now bringing great improvement, and even recovery, to unprecedented numbers of children.[2]

References

1. McCandless J. *Children with starving brains*, 2nd ed. Putney, VT: Bramble Books, 2005.

2. Arranga E. McCandless J, Small T. *Interview with Dr. Jaquelyn McCandless concerning medical evaluation/treatment for autism spectrum disorder. Reprint of Autism One Radio interview.* Medical Veritas 2005;2:456-64.

3. Reichelt KL, Ekrem J, Scott H. *Gluten, milk proteins and autism: Dietary intervention effects on behavior and peptide secretion.* J Applied Nutrition 1990;42(1):1-11, .

4. Knivsberg AM, Reichelt KL, Nodland, M. *Reports on dietary intervention in autistic disorders.* Nutritional Neurosci 2001;4:25-37.

5. Shattock P, Whiteley P. *How dietary intervention could ameliorate the symptoms of autism.* The Pharmaceutical J 2001 Jul 7;267:7155.

6. Rapp D. *Is this your child?* New York, NY: Quill Books, 1991:122-31.

7. Nsouli TM. *The role of food allergy in serious otitis media.* Ann Allergy 1991;66:91.

8. Feingold B. *Why your child is hyperactive.* New York, NY: Random House, 1975.

9. James SJ, Cutler P, Melnyk S, Jernigan S, et al. *Metabolic biomarkers of increased oxidative stress and impaired methylation capacity in children with autism.* Am J Clin Nutr 2004;80:1611-7.

10. James SJ. *Impaired transsulfuration and oxidative stress in autistic children: Improvement with targeted nutritional intervention.* Self published, 2004.

11. Daniels K. *The Whole Soy Story: The dark side of america's favorite health food.* Washington, DC: New Trends Publishing, 2005.

12. Gottschall, E. *Breaking the vicious cycle: intestinal health through diet.* Baltimore, Ontario, Canada: The Kirkton Press, 2004.

13. Shaw W, Kassen E, Chaves E. *Increased excretion of analogs of Krebs cycle metabolites and arabinose in two brothers with autistic features.* Clin Chem 1995:41:1094-104.

14. Crook WG. *Help for the hyperactive child.* Jackson, TN: Professional Books, 1991:170-4.

15. Braly J. *Dr. Braly's food allergy and nutrition revolution.* New Canaan, CT: 1992:241.

16. Gates D. *The body ecology diet*, 9th ed. Juno Beach, FL: Healthful Communications, 2006.

17. Morris RD, Audet AM, Angelillo IF, Chalmers TC et al. *Chlorination, chlorination by-products, and cancer: a meta-analysis.* A J PubHealth 1992;82:955-63.

18. Tennakone K, Wickramanayake S. *Aluminum leaching from cooking utensils.* Nature 1987;325:270-2.

19. Howard JMH. *Clinical import of small increases in serum aluminum.* Clin Chem 1984;30:1722-23.

20. Guillete EA. *Examining childhood development in contaminated urban settings.* Environ Health Persp Supp 2000 Jun;108(S3).

21. Schmidt MA. *Smart fats: how dietary fats and oils affect mental, physical and emotional intelligence.* Berkeley, CA: Frog, Ltd, 1997:85-98.

22. Agostoni C, Trojan S, Bellu R, Riva, E, et al. *Neurodevelopmental quotient of healthy term infants at 4 months and feeding practice: the role of long-chain polyunsaturated fatty acids.* Pediatr Res 1995 Aug;38:262-6.

23. Desci T, Koletzko B. *N-3 fatty acids and pregnancy outcomes.* Curr Opin Clin Nutr Metab Care 2005;8:161-6.

24. Neuringer M, Connon WE, Lin DS, Barstad L, et al. *Biochemical and functional effects of prenatal and postnatal omega 3 fatty acid deficiency on retina and brain in rhesus monkeys.* Proc Natl Acad Sci USA 1986;83):4021-5.

25. Auestad N, Scott DT, Janowsky JS, Montalto MB, et al. *Visual, cognitive and language assessments at 39 months: a follow-up study of children fed formulas containing long-chain polyunsaturated fatty acids to one year of age.* Pediatr 2003;112:177-83.

26. Richardson AJ, Montgomery P. *The Oxford-Durham study: a randomized, controlled trial of dietary supplementation with fatty acids in children with developmental coordination disorder.* Pediatr 2005;115:1360-6.

27. Dunne LJ. *Nutritional Almanac, 5th edition.* New York: McGraw Hill, 2002:10.

28. Grahn BH, Paterson PG, Gottschall-Pass KT, Zhang Z. *Zinc and the eye.* Am Coll Nutr 2001;20:106-18.

29. www.tetrachemicals.com *The importance of calcium.* (Accessed October 28, 2006)

30. Smith LH. *Hyperkids.* Santa Monica, CA: Shaw/Spelling Assoc, 1990.

31. Durlach J. Clinical aspects of chronic magnesium deficiency. In: Seelig MS, ed. Magnesium in health and disease. New York: Spectrum Publications, 1980.

32. Martineua J, Barthelemy C, Lelord G, Longterm effects of combined vitamin B-6-magnesium administration in an autistic child. Biol Psychiatr 1986;21:511-8.

33. Owens SC. Understanding the sulfur system. Defeat Autism Now! 2003 Conference Proceedings. Philadelphia PA, May, 2003:65-76.

34. Megson M. The biological basis for perceptual deficits in autism. www.megson.com (Accessed June 10, 2006)

35. www.megson.com (Accessed June 10, 2006)

36. Rimland B. Vitamin C in the prevention and treatment of autism. Autism Res Rev International 1998;12:2-3.

37. Ng SS, Yung WH, Chow BK. Secretin as a neuropeptide. Molecular Neurobiol 2002;26:97-107.

38. Koves K, Kausz M, Reser D, Horvath K. What may be the anatomical basis that secretin can improve the mental functions in autism? Regulatory Peptides 2002;109:167-72.

39. Horvath K, Stefanatos G, Sokolski KN, Wachtel R, et al. Improved social and language skills after secretin administration in patients with autistic spectrum disorders. J Assoc Academ Minority Physicians 1998;9:9-15.

40. Rimland B. Secretin update: March 1999. Autism Res Rev International 1999;13:1.

41. Conglio SJ, Lewis JD, Lang C, Burns TG, et al. A randomized double-blind, placebo-controlled trial of single dose intravenous secretin as treatment for children with autism. JPediatr 2001;138:649-55.

42. Rimland B. Secretin: The controversy continues. Autism Res Rev International 2004;18:1,3.

43. www.megson.com (Accessed 11/25/05)

44. Anand SK Rao LK. Antibacterial activity associated with bifidobacterium bifidum. Cultured Dairy Products J 1984 Nov:6-8.

45. Isolauri E, Juntunen M, Rautanen T, Sillanaukee P, et al. A human Lactobacillus strain (Lactobacillus casei sp strain GG) promotes recovery from acute diarrhea in children. Pediatr 1991;88:1.

46. Majamaa H, Isolauri E. Probiotics: A novel approach in the management of food allergy. J Allergy Clin Immunol 1997;99:179-85.

47. Zeisel SH. Nutritional importance of choline for brain development. J Am Coll Nutr 2004;23(6):621S-626S.Wurtman RJ, Zeisel SH. Alzheimer's disease: a report of progress. Brain choline: Its sources and effects on the synthesis and release of acetylcholine. Aging 1982.

48. Fudenberg HH. Dialyzable lymphocyte extract (DLyE) in infantile onset autism: a pilot study. Biother 1996;9(1-3):143-7.

49. Markowitz DM. Quiet victories: a journey towards health and wellness : A quarterly newsletter. www.shirleys-wellness-cafe.com (Accessed October 28, 2006)

50. Hennen W. Transfer factor: natural immune booster. Orem, UT: Woodland Publishing, 1998.

51. Peiper H. Zeolite. Sheffield, MA:Safe Goods Publishing, 2006.

52. Ramos AJ, Fink-Gremmels J, Hernandez E. Prevention of toxic effects of mycotoxins by means of nonnutritive absorbent compounds. J Food Protections 1996;59:631-41.

53. Lonsdale D, Shamberger RJ, Audhya T. Treatment of autism spectrum children with thiamine tetrahydrofurfuryl disulfide: A pilot study. Neuroendocrinology Letters 2002 Aug;23:4.

54. Cranton EM, Frackelton JP. Scientific rationale for EDTA chelation therapy: mechanism of action, A textbook on chelation therapy, 2nd ed. Charlottesville, VA: Hampton Roads Publishing, 2001.

55. Neubauer RA, Walker M. Hyperbaric oxygen therapy. Garden City Park, NY: Avery Publishing Group, 1998.

56. Hyperbaric oxygen therapy improves symptoms in autistic children. <www.icdrc.org/rossignol> Accessed October 31, 2006.

Chapter 6
The Defeat Autism Now!
Movement

PART 1
The History of the Autism Research Institute and
the Defeat Autism Now! Project
Bernard Rimland, PhD

My Introduction to Autism

It all began with the birth of my autistic son in 1956. Mark was a screaming, implacable infant who resisted being cuddled and struggled against being picked up. He also struggled against being put down. Our pediatrician, Dr. Black, who had been in practice for 35 years, had never seen nor heard of a child like Mark.

Neither Dr. Black nor I, who at that time was three years post-PhD, psychology, had seen or heard of "autism." It was not until Mark was two years old that my wife remembered reading about children who looked through people rather than at them, and who accurately repeated radio commercials and nursery rhymes but did not engage in communicative speech. I found her dusty box of old college texts and there, five years after I had earned a PhD as a research psychologist, saw the word "autism" for the first time. Today autism is an all-too-familiar word-even to high-school students.

Autism as an Incurable "Psychological" Disorder

Starting with the several references cited in my wife's old text, I began to read everything I could find on the subject of autism. I was appalled to learn that it was uniformly believed, and presented as an established fact in every textbook, that autism was an emotional (psychological) disorder. The only treatment recommendations were psychoanalysis or other forms of psychotherapy for both the mother and the child. The mother was required to acknowledge her guilt and confess that she hated the child and wished it had never been born. The child, in so-called "play therapy," was provided with a paper or clay image of a woman (his mother) and was encouraged to tear it to bits, thus expressing his hostility toward his mother who the psychotherapists were positive had caused his autism. There were a few drugs that were also used with autistic children, but then, as now, the idea was not to treat the autism, but to slow the children down enough to make life tolerable for those who must deal with them.

I decided to read what I could find on the subject of autism, not only to learn what might be done to help Mark, but also to try to understand on what basis the psychiatrists had decided that mothers were to blame for their children's autism. After four years I had devoured everything, including translations of foreign language articles. I learned that, despite the supreme arrogance with which the authorities proclaimed the mothers were to blame, I could find no shred of scientific evidence for such a belief.

A Psychologist Objects and Becomes an Expert

I wrote a book entitled, *Infantile Autism: The Syndrome and its Implications for a Neural Theory of Behavior*, which won the Century Award in 1964. This publication resulted, as I had intended, in the destruction of the "psychogenic hypothesis" that autism was an emotional disorder caused by bad mothering. Instead, I successfully argued that researchers must search for biological causes of autism.

Overnight I became the world authority on autism. I received many invitations to speak at universities and medical schools, as well as untold numbers of letters and phone calls from parents and research scientists interested in exploring the ideas presented in my book.

Autism Research Institute is Born

In 1965 I founded the Autism Society of America (ASA) to provide a nationwide forum for informing parents about new and important developments in the field of autism. Two years later I founded the Autism Research Institute (ARI) as a center for collecting, analyzing and disseminating research on possible causes and efficacious treatments. Since its establishment in 1967, the Autism Research Institute has had, as a major priority, the tracking of promising treatments for autism. Intensive study of the scientific literature, and analysis of case reports from literally thousands of parents of autistic children, convinced me that much can be done to help the children. Founding the ASA and ARI were expressions then, as now, of my lack of confidence in most of the professionals who deal with autism.

The Vaccine-Autism Connection

In the mid-1960s I began to suspect a link between the DPT vaccination and. More recently, I repeatedly heard a similar story, this time related to the measles/mumps/rubella (MMR) vaccine. As the number of vaccines given infants has increased, the number of parents reporting vaccine-related deterioration has skyrocketed. The reader is referred to Chapter 4 to learn more about the vaccine-autism connection.

Vitamins not Drugs

One of the first letters I received after my book was published came from a mother in Canada who was experimenting with high doses of certain vitamins in the treatment of her autistic child. It seemed to me to be a rather crazy idea, but she was reporting good results. The Canadian mother sent me a letter that she had received from her own mother who was a nurse in a psychiatric hospital in Saskatoon.

The grandmother's letter observed that two sophisticated young psychiatrists, Drs. Abram Hoffer and Humphry Osmond (who later became my friends and colleagues) were experimenting with large doses of vitamin B3 on their adult schizophrenic patients. She wrote that she and other psychiatric nurses and staff members could see remarkable improvement in patients who were treated with "megavitamin" B3. The improvement was clearly better than that seen in the patients being treated by the other psychiatrists who used only drugs. Nevertheless, to the surprise and disappointment of the nursing staff, the traditional psychiatrists refused to see that megavitamin treatments were in fact effective.

It did not surprise me that these same doctors who had shown a lack of intellectual integrity by falsely blaming the mothers for causing autism (on the basis of no data) would also be reluctant to examine the efficacy of treatments. Hoffer and Osmond published a number of scientific, controlled double- and triple-blind studies supporting their initial findings. It made no difference to the great majority of establishment psychiatrists who were, and still are, hooked on drug treatments.

Progress in the acceptance of useful medical interventions is painfully slow. It is not uncommon for a safe and effective treatment to be available for decades before it is widely implemented. Hoffer's and Osmond's discovery in the early 1950s that vitamin B3 confers major benefits to adults with acute-onset schizophrenia is still largely ignored by the psychiatric establishment. Another more recent example is the use of small amounts of folic acid, a very safe B vitamin, as a means of preventing severe birth defects. It is estimated that over 25,000 cases of mental retardation could have been prevented in the U.S. if widespread use of folic acid supplements had been recommended when the discovery was first announced in the 1960s, rather than 30 years later, in the 1990s. There are a multitude of similar examples.

Over a period of several years I began to hear from mothers, all over the country, that they were, on their own, trying high doses of vitamins on their autistic children, and that certain vitamins, especially vitamin B6, seemed to help. There was so much consistency in these reports that I decided to conduct a large-scale study of several of the most promising vitamins. In the late 1960s I undertook a study, based on several hundred autistic children whose parents had contacted me seeking help and advice.

Finding Quality Vitamins

The first problem was to find flavored vitamins, since some of the vitamins of interest, especially B6 and B3, are very bitter. I wrote to 24 vitamin manufacturers asking if they would be willing to make flavored vitamins for a study we were planning on autistic children. Twenty-two of the 24 companies did not reply. One of the two who replied simply said, "Not interested." The other company, Kirkman Labs of Portland, Oregon, said, "Certainly, we'll be glad to help. Just tell us what you need." A very welcome and very important letter! Remember, in those days, the late 60s, autism was extremely rare-probably only one or two children per 10,000, and almost no one had even heard the term "autism."

Kirkman Labs worked diligently with us for many months, sending us sample after sample of tablets flavored to mask the taste of B3 and B6, so they would be palatable to autistic children. Kirkman did this at its own expense, which must have been considerable. Without them we would have failed. As a parent and as a researcher, I will forever be grateful to Kirkman which continues to manufacture vitamins and other products tailored to the needs of autistic children.

Research Proves Parents Right: Vitamins Work

The results of my first study were quite positive, especially for vitamin B6. At the time of this writing I am aware of 22 studies of vitamin B6 use in autistic children, conducted by researchers in seven countries, and all studies but one (with only nine subjects) showed positive results. (See Appendix A for a list of these and other studies.) Adding magnesium to the B6 has repeatedly been found to be essential for best results. Eleven of the studies have been double blind, placebo-controlled studies. Nevertheless, a great many articles and textbooks representing the views of the medical establishment still continue to say that vitamin therapy for autism has not been proven, or that it is unsafe. Both contentions are false just as their view that autism was caused by bad mothering was false.

As the years went on, I continued to find that the parents, especially the mothers, were remarkably observant about factors that appeared to cause their children's behavior to worsen. They were also extremely effective at identifying treatments that were helpful to their autistic children.

Data Collection: Parents Report on Treatment Effects

For too many years, autism research was largely confined to describing symptoms or precisely pinpointing affected brain areas. Physicians continuously try various psychiatric drugs, developed for other diseases, searching for a reduction of symptoms. Even with limited goals, progress has been far from encouraging. Drugs, apart from their harmful side effects, have absorbed far too many research funds, time and attention. Autism has never been caused by a deficiency of Ritalin or Risperdal.

Since the 1960s thousands of parents of autistic children have provided informal feedback through letters, phone calls and personal conversations. I eventually developed a questionnaire, still used today, for newly diagnosed families to complete. In 1967 the Autism

Research Institute began formal surveys on the effects of various drugs and supplements. I later began to collect information about the effects of milk and wheat on children's behavior, since many parents reported that their children thrived on a casein-free and/or gluten-free diet. I eventually added other diets and interventions to the checklist. Parents report on whether they think their children got worse, better or had no change. The results, compiled over 37 years, show how over 25,000 children have responded. This table is included as Figure 2 in Chapter 1 of this book. As the table shows very clearly, the nutritional supplements and special diets are far safer treatment options and far more likely to be helpful than any drug.

Defeat Autism Now! "Think Tanks" and Conferences

Over the years, I had had many conversations about autism with two colleagues, Sidney Baker, MD, and Jon Pangborn, PhD. Drs. Baker and Pangborn have worked together to understand the biochemistry of autism since the early 1980s. Each has made a contribution to this chapter.

Dr. Baker, a graduate of and former faculty member of the Yale Medical School, is former director of the Gesell Institute of Human Development. He has extensive training and experience in pediatrics, allergy, immunology, neurology, biochemistry and computer science. Dr. Pangborn is a fellow of the American Institute of Chemists and Certified Clinical Nutritionist, and also the father of an autistic son. Now a private consultant, Pangborn was formerly president of Doctor's Data, a major medical laboratory, and very probably has studied more biochemical workups of autistic patients than anyone.

In mid-1994 Baker, Pangborn and I decided to organize an autism think-tank in Dallas in January 1995 to "Defeat Autism Now!" We invited approximately 30 competent and open-minded physicians and scientists from the U.S. and Europe, who shared our ideas. All had special expertise in autism research and treatment. Psychiatry, neurology, immunology, allergy, biochemistry, genetics and gastro-enterology were among the fields represented. A number of attendees were, like Jon Pangborn and me, parents of autistic children. The purpose of the gathering was to identify safe treatments for which there was credible evidence of efficacy. Once these efficacious treatments were identified, an attempt would be made to find why they work, so their benefits could be increased.

Our first gathering was a great success. There was a cordial meeting of the minds and a very rapid consensus among the participants, most of whom had never met before, as to the most useful approaches to treatment. Drs. Baker and Pangborn have planned nine subsequent Defeat Autism Now! Think tanks, ranging in duration from a day to a weekend, which include leading physicians and researchers in autism and related fields. Think tanks precede Defeat Autism Now! Conferences, which are open to both parents of children with autism and the professionals who serve them. From 1995 to 2000, Defeat Autism Now! conferences were held annually, and increased to twice a year since 2001, because of heightened interest.

Defeat Autism Now! conferences have produced a worldwide network of physicians who employ rational, scientifically sound approaches to the diagnosis and treatment of autism, and who regard psychoactive drugs as their last choice, not their first. A list of these doctors is available on the ARI website at <www.AutismResearchInstitute.com>.

The Defeat Autism Now! Protocol

Participants at the original Defeat Autism Now! conference agreed that one of the major priorities should be the publication of a document representing the best ideas and practices of those in attendance. "Biomedical Assessment Options for Children with Autism and

Related Problems" (often referred to as the Defeat Autism Now! Clinical Options Manual the Consensus Report or the Defeat Autism Now! Protocol) was first published in February 1996, and updated several times since.[1]

The Defeat Autism Now! Clinical Options Manual is written for:
- Physicians and other health care professionals who wish to apply state-of-the-art medical knowledge and technology to the process of diagnosing and treating their autistic patients. Optometrists and others can order it online from <www.AutismResearchInstitute.com>, by writing to ARI at 4182 Adams Avenue, San Diego, CA 92116, or by fax at 619-563-6840. *Editor's Note:* Since writing this chapter, Drs. Baker and Pangborn have updated and re-named their manual. Its title is now *Autism: Effective Biomedical Treatments*. Published in 2005, it supercedes previous concensus reports.
- Parents of autistic children to take to their child's physician to encourage him/her to follow the steps outlined therein.

Those parents who believe (correctly, I think, in most cases) that vaccines have played a causal role in their child's autism will need medical support in the detoxification of mercury and other heavy metals. The ARI "Mercury Detoxification Consensus Report," the product of the mercury detoxification think-tank, is available free online, for that purpose. It can be extremely helpful in understanding and implementing the detoxification process.

Finding a Defeat Autism Now! Doctor
Parents obviously need to find a well-qualified Defeat Autism Now! doctor. Despite the efforts of the Defeat Autism Now! team to educate health care practitioners around the world, there are still too few well-qualified physicians, nurses and nutritionists. Often their first available appointment is many months away; some are so busy with their present case-load that they cannot even see any new patients.

What To Do While Waiting
What should you suggest if your patients can't get a timely doctor's appointment? Do exactly what I have been recommending to parents for over three decades: Place the child on high dose vitamin B6 and magnesium, and on dimethylglycine (DMG), for a trial period of at least six weeks, and see if these very safe non-prescription nutritional supplements will help. Also, try placing the child on the gluten-free, casein-free (GFCF) diet for at least several months, again on a trial basis, while waiting for the results of the lab tests recommended by the Defeat Autism Now! protocol.

Parents often ask me if they should start all of these treatment approaches at once. That is debatable. Scientific research studies try only one treatment at a time, so as not to confuse the effect of treatment X with treatment Y. Many parents choose this approach so they can better understand the effects of each intervention on the child.

On the other hand, kids are not scientific experiments. Most parents feel that their primary job is to help their children as much and as quickly as possible, not publish the results in a professional journal; time is of the essence. They will thus try several interventions, such as B6/magnesium, DMG, and the GFCF diet, simultaneously. I support this approach: "Help the child first, worry later about exactly what it is that's helping the child."

There's no way to know if these interventions will help a child without trying them; every child is unique. But after almost four decades of research, I am very confident that B6, magnesium, DMG, and a GF/CF diet will help a large percentage of children, and will harm none of them.

Keep Confidential and Good Records

Before undertaking any treatments I recommend that parents:

Complete a baseline Autism Treatment Evaluation Checklist (ATEC), and then repeat it periodically, perhaps every two to four weeks, to keep track of any behavioral changes. The ATEC is a simple, one-page means of evaluating the effect of various interventions on a child.

Refrain from mentioning new interventions to anyone working with the child, including teachers, therapists, babysitters, relatives and neighbors. Very often, within a few days, someone will notice increased progress. Keeping trials of new interventions unknown to those in the child's environment provides an invaluable opportunity to benefit from unbiased observations. Each child thus becomes, in effect, a subject in a double blind "mini-study."

Wearing Two Hats: Physicians as Parents of Children with Autism

One of the consequences of the huge upsurge in autism during the past decade has been that many physicians find themselves to be parents or grandparents of children with autism. Two psychiatrists, both mothers of autistic sons, recently commented to me that, "It is one thing to be looking in the Physicians Desk Reference for a drug for another mother's child. When it is for your own child, you see the same words with very different eyes."

Many of these one or two physician families first explored conventional medicine's approaches, and after finding them ineffective, joined the ranks of Defeat Autism Now! doctors. Dr. Jaquelyn McCandless, a board certified psychiatrist and neurologist, is a case in point. She was about to retire when her 14th grandchild, Chelsey, was diagnosed as autistic. After diligent research, she adopted the Defeat Autism Now! approach. Her story is told in *Children With Starving Brains*, now considered the "bible" to understanding a biomedical approach to diagnosing and treating autism.

Parents continue to discover treatments that are much more effective and safer than the drugs for their autistic children. Videotapes of Autism Research Institute-sponsored panel presentations entitled "Physicians Who Have Successfully Treated Their Own Autistic Children" are available from ARI. Some of their stories and those of others not in the medical fields are documented in *Treating Autism: Parent Stories of Hope and Success*, published by ARI in 2003. In this book, educated, sophisticated parents tell tales of watching their children disappear into the world of autism and then gradually recover.

Autism is Treatable!

After the publication of *Treating Autism*, I launched my newest endeavor: the "Autism is Treatable" campaign. Unfortunately, most doctors still view autism as hopeless, and refuse to recommend biomedical treatments, even when there are strong research findings behind them. ARI is prepared to meet with the media at any time to share the stories of some of the remarkable families who refused to give up on their children and have recovered them.

What Happened to Mark?

Oh yes! You are wondering about my son Mark, who we were told to institutionalize and forget at age five, who was still in diapers at seven, and who did not ask or answer a question until age eight. Mark began to improve dramatically when we started behavior modification and vitamin B6 with magnesium. Later, dimethylglycine (DMG) also helped greatly.

Mark is now 47 and is still on megadoses of B6 and magnesium. He lives at home with his parents, attends a day program for mentally disabled adults, takes the city bus to his program and makes daily visits to art galleries and coffee shops in the neighborhood. We discovered at age 22 that Mark was a remarkably talented artist. He has been interviewed about his art on NBC, CBS, CNN, and PBS. (He confided to the CBS interviewer, "I like being famous.") He did the illustrations for his sister Helen Landalf's children's book, *The Secret Night World of Cats*, and had the pleasure of meeting with Dustin Hoffman, as Hoffman prepared for his role in "Rain Man." My wife and I are proud of Mark, not such a bad outcome, after all!

APPENDIX A

Vitamin B6/magnesium, DMG and other supplements have been the topic of many editorials I have written for the *Autism Research Review International (ARRI)* since 1987. The following pages, covering such topics as research findings, safety, dosages, etc., are available from the ARRI:

Title	Date
Vitamin B6 and Magnesium in the Treatment of Autism	1987, Vol. 1, No.4
Candida-Caused Autism?	1988, Vol. 2, No.2
Dimethylglycine (DMG): A Nontoxic Metabolite and Autism	1990, Vol. 4, No.2
Vitamin B6 vs. Fenfluramine: A Case Study in Medical Bias	1991, Vol. 5, No.1
Vitamin B6 in Autism: The Safety Issue	1996, Vol. 10, No.3
Our Children: Victims of Both Autism and Dogma	1997, Vol. 11, No.3
What is the Right 'Dosage' of Vitamin B6, DMG and Others	1997, Vol. 11, No.4
Vitamin C in the Prevention and Treatment of Autism	1998, Vol. 12, No.2
The Most Airtight Study in Psychiatry? Vitamin B6 in Autism	2000, Vol. 14, No.3
Controlling Self-Injurious and Assaultive Behavior in Autism	2001, Vol. 15, No.4

PART 2
Autism Intervention Priorities and Schedule According to the
A Consensus Report of the Defeat Autism Now!
Scientific Effort
Contributor: Jon Pangborn, PhD

Editor's note: This material is compiled from personal communications and published work of Jon Pangborn, PhD, and Sidney Baker, MD. Please be aware that autism treatment is a rapidly evolving field and new and better treatment options are everyone's goal. The 2005 edition of *Autism: Effective Biomedical Treatments* and the 2007 supplement, co-authored by Sidney Baker, MD, and Jon Pangborn, PhD, suggest a series of biomedical options for intervention in autism. I, Patricia Lemer, editor, have condensed the content into a task-schedule format that helps health professionals, including optometrists, understand how Defeat Autism Now! doctors are treating autism.

Defeat Autism Now! clinicians recommend doing these procedures sequentially. Doing treatments concurrently can lead to disappointment and to confusion between disease symptoms and effects of intervention. If the sequence is not adhered to, it is frequently necessary to return to and re-focus on a particular area. This occurrence is common with treatments for intestinal dysbiosis, or yeast overgrowth, a particular "pesky" problem in autism. Doctors and patients must be patient, not discouraged, when regression occurs. The order of interventions suggested by Defeat Autism Now! is in Table 6-1.

Table 6-1 Recommended Tests and Treatments
• Diagnosis of autism
• Prerequisite tests
• Clean up diet
• Casein avoidance trial
• Use digestive enzymes & basic nutritional supplements
• Gluten avoidance trial
• Evaluate for intestinal dysbiosis
• Treat bacterial dysbiosis
• Treat yeast/fungal dysbiosis
• Provide immune support and anti-viral measures
• Add more nutritional supplements
• Detoxify the body
• Sulfur supplements
• Metabolic fine-tuning
• Sensory, educational and other therapies

This schedule may not be appropriate for all cases of autism, and one should not suppose that positive outcomes will always result when following it. Each person with autism is an individual with unique metabolic and immunologic capabilities and faults. When in doubt, treat the individual, not the autism, because autism occurs coincidentally with many different disorders, and is not just one homogenous entity. Nevertheless, experience has shown that following this schedule has a higher chance of success than do random interventions, "magic bullet" therapies, or starting with advanced interventions, such as detoxification, before correcting underlying nutritional problems and digestion.

1. Confirm Autism Diagnosis

Get an objective diagnosis of autism from a qualified professional. This diagnosis assures that once symptoms begin to alleviate, the autism diagnosis will not be questioned. It may also lead to more direct and effective treatment, should the condition be one of the unusual, but many "inherited" metabolic disorders that can feature autism among other problems.

2. Run Pre-requisite Testing

Do a series of preliminary tests. Include both laboratory and sensory evaluations. Testing could indicate the presence of conditions that feature the symptomology of autism, or a metabolic disease that has autistic manifestations. The tests marked with an asterisk* should always be done if they are available and the family can afford them. Others are optional and should be done at the discretion of the doctor(s) making the diagnosis. This list is not intended to exclude any additional tests that a doctor or medical consultant recommends or suggests.

> *Vision and hearing tests, including auditory and visual processing
> *Blood chemistry, CBC and thyroid markers
> *Urinalysis
> *PKU screen if not done during infancy
> *Tests for celiac disease or gluten enteropathy
> Amino acid analysis
> Organic acid analysis
> Serum iron and ferritin determination
> Urine uric acid, 24-hour or ratioed to creatinine
> EEG, CAT scans and MRI for abnormal brain structure/function or Landau-Kleffner syndrome (acquired epilepsy)
> Chromosome or DNA studies for Fragile X, Rett syndrome, and other genetic disorders that may feature autism. (Such tests may also be performed after doing the nutritional and bio-medical tasks that follow - see item 14.)

3. Clean up the Diet

Adjust the diet, including all medications, to restrict intake of sugar and food additives, including artificial colors, flavors, and preservatives. Many people with autism show intolerance to blue food dye. Exclude all foods that show as problematic on the baseline testing.

4. Casein Avoidance Trial

Remove any products that contain casein for at least 30 days. Casein is a dairy protein that occurs naturally in milk, ice cream, yogurt, cheese, and is added to many processed foods. Some find phasing out casein-containing foods over a week or two easier than going "cold-turkey." The 30-day period does not start until avoidance is complete, however.

Begin by replacing favorite casein-containing foods with casein-free substitutes. Many companies now make dairy-free products. *Special Diets for Special Kids, Volumes I & II* by Lisa Lewis have recipes for dairy-free versions of everything from macaroni and cheese to pizza.

Withdrawal from dairy products is rarely voluntary, because casein is known to be addictive. Incomplete digestion can result in morphine-like reactions in the brain by producing opiate-acting peptides, called casomorphins. Some children have withdrawal symptoms, including irritability and worsened behaviors. Activated charcoal can reduce these symptoms if taken between doses of nutritional supplements or medications. If no worsening or improvement in symptoms is noted after 30 days, do a deliberate challenge meal of several casein-containing foods and observe. If the child does not respond negatively, casein is unlikely to be a contributing factor in the child's autism. See item 6 below for laboratory testing that can confirm the need for casein avoidance.

5. Use Digestive Enzymes and Basic Nutritional Supplements

Digestive enzymes are secreted along the gastro-intestinal tract in a healthy digestive system. Their purpose is to break down food into particles that can be readily absorbed and assimilated in the body. Many children on the autism spectrum have reduced digestive enzymes, and they benefit from taking enzyme supplements. Symptoms of the need for digestive enzymes include abdominal pain, bloating, gas, reflux, diarrhea and constipation. Laboratory tests showing deficiencies of essential nutrients would be consistent with need for digestive aids.

After day 10, but before day 20 of the 30-day casein avoidance trial, introduce digestive enzymes with Dipeptidyl peptidase-IV (DPP-IV) activity. DPP-IV can assist in the digestion of casomorphin peptides. Proceed gradually at first, one capsule or half a capsule for young children with breakfast, then add lunch and last add dinner. Eventually give enzymes with all meals and snacks, with the number of capsules depending upon the size of the meal. Children should take enzymes at the start of the meal.

Recent clinical studies have shown that many autistic children also have difficulty digesting complex sugars – disaccharides and polysaccharides. These sugars are abundant in many vegetables and grains. Digestive aid supplements that contain disaccharidase enzymes, such as lactase, maltase, isomaltase and sucrase, can be very beneficial.

Continued use of digestive enzymes may be beneficial whether or not casein is a contributing factor. Use is recommended indefinitely, even if gluten is excluded from the diet, because avoidance is often imperfect, and offending peptides can have long-lasting effects. Digestive enzymes have far-reaching benefits, as they also aide in breaking down fats and carbohydrates, and they will increase tolerance for "new" or substituted foods in the diet.

Some basic nutritional supplements can be beneficial at this stage. Certainly, calcium will be needed if dairy foods are eliminated. Also usually beneficial at this time are: vitamin B6 with magnesium, vitamin C, melatonin, taurine, zinc, and vitamin A.

Dr. Rimland's previous article in this chapter details the use of vitamin B6 and C. Melatonin is a sleep aide for those for whom this is an issue. Zinc can help normalize the sense of taste and may aid in acceptance of "new" foods during diet adjustment trials. Zinc is often low, while copper may be high in blood cells on lab testing. For convenience, patients may prefer using proprietary supplement combination blends especially designed for autism, such as Brainchild, D-Plex, Super Nu-Thera, Thera-Response and Spectrum Complete. Avoid adding amino acids, other than taurine, sulfur nutrients, or strong detoxing nutrients yet in the intervention process.

6. Gluten Avoidance Trial

After the 30-day casein avoidance trial, all gluten should be eliminated for at least 60 days, while continuing digestive enzymes, basic nutritional supplements and activated charcoal, if necessary. Continue casein avoidance if child appears to benefit. Again, consider going slowly; do not begin counting days until avoidance is complete. Gluten is a protein in most grains, including wheat, oats, rye, barley, kamut, spelt and triticale. It can produce gluteomorphins when digestion is incomplete. Fortunately, gluten-free flours, breads, cakes, crackers and other products are now readily available.

After 60 days, do a deliberate challenge meal of several gluten-containing foods and observe. If the child does not respond negatively, gluten is unlikely to be a contributing factor in the child's autism.

If a family is in doubt about casein or gluten avoidance, immunologic tests can aid decision-making. Blood IgG levels for casein and gluten can be indicative of immunologic intolerance, but are not foolproof for overall tolerance. "Food allergy tests" can be used to determine if rotation of food type, is advisable in addition to certain dietary exclusions. Laboratories that offer these tests are listed in *Autism: Effective Biomedical Treatments Report.*[1]

7. Evaluate for Intestinal Dysbiosis

In-depth laboratory testing can be used to determine appropriate intestinal therapies. Most patients with autism have intestinal dysbiosis, a state where bad flora disrupt the delicate balance in the gut. These flora can have harmful effects due to putrefication and fermentation of waste material. In addition, they can cause or worsen gut inflammation and leakage of toxins into the bloodstream.

Defeat Autism Now! suggests the following diagnostic tests to evaluate intestinal dysbiosis:
* Comprehensive stool analysis, including measures of digestive function, bacteriology, and mycology
* Intestinal permeability analysis, a urine test that involves ingestion of two sugars, one of which is not supposed to be absorbed in the gut
* Urine organic acids analysis that include dysbiosis markers which are produced by offending gut flora
* Endoscopic examination for ileal-lymphoid hyperplasia by a gastroenterologist

Empirical trials of antibiotic and antifungal medications can be carried out, because the lab tests are not perfect, and sometimes produce false negative results. Baker and Pangborn's book[1] discusses specific medications for this purpose. Many individuals with autism experience increased sensitivity to yeast/fungi, whether gut levels are normal or excessive.

After a period of dysbiotic control, repeat testing is recommended, especially if undesirable symptoms re-appear.

8. Treat Bacterial Dysbiosis

Once analytical testing is complete, and the family chooses to treat bacterial dysbiosis, start by controlling the most easily managed dysbiotic flora, bad bacteria and parasites. Use anti-bacterials, including medicinal and herbal agents, such as Uva ursi, berberine and perhaps grapefruit seed extract. After bacteria are under control, periodic or maintenance doses of herbals that keep bacterial flora in check may be beneficial. Probiotics such as Lactobacillus and Bifidus also are essential to restore and maintain intestinal balance.

9. Treat Yeast/Fungal Dysbiosis

Confront this problem after treatment for bacterial dysbiosis with the use of anti-fungals. The book describes both over-the-counter and prescription products that have anti-fungal activity. Patients will need a doctor's help with medicinal anti-fungals like Nystatin or Diflucan. Some children gain benefit from herbals and nutrients such as capryllic acid, garlic, and a friendly yeast called Saccharomyces boulardii. These are also used as adjuncts to the prescription products and for maintenance after the gut is under control.

Defeat Autism Now! doctors usually start anti-fungals gradually with a low dose and ramping up. If using Nystatin, a week of pre-treatment with capryllic acid at one capsule for two days, then two capsules/day for the rest of the week is recommended. Many strains of yeast are now unaffected by Nystatin, and other more potent medicinals are often needed.

One of the side effects of anti-fungals is "die off." When a yeast or fungal cell dies, its cell wall ruptures, releasing the contents of the cell into the gut. This "die off" can cause severe reactions, such as headaches, increased hyperactivity, attention deficits, transient worsening of autistic traits, irritability and aggressive/destructive behavior. These symptoms usually cease shortly after the offending organisms are gone. If die-off produces severe symptoms, it may be necessary to discontinue the prescriptive anti-fungal medications for a week or two, and use only the gentler herbals such as capryllic acid, along with activated charcoal, and then reintroduce the prescriptives. If the patient is taking activated charcoal, it must be given between doses of all medications, as it will absorb whatever it comes into contact with.

Bowel regularity (movements once or twice a day) is important in combating dysbiosis. Irregular elimination or constipation contributes to continued dysbiosis. Increasing vitamin C and/or magnesium supplements often helps to stimulate the bowel movements.

Many patients experience re-infection; then the gut stabilizes. Digestive enzymes, adherence to diet and probiotics, along with maintenance doses of caprillic acid and garlic are helpful, and perhaps necessary, in these cases.

10. Provide Immune Support and Antiviral Measures

Measuring a titer using a blood sample assesses the body's viral response. Some children with autism have high blood titers, suggesting that their bodies are still fighting the virus. If the autistic individual has abnormal viral titers, then a physician experienced in these matters or an immunologist or virologist should be consulted.

Recent Defeat Autism Now! investigations speculate that nucleotide metabolism impairments in autism may be altering immune and cellular response, so that viruses and other infections are problematic. In addition, some infections, especially measles, may not run their normal courses, instead, they may become fixed in certain cells, where they inhibit cell functions.

Some Defeat Autism Now! doctors are using prescription, therapeutic anti-virals, although there is no consensus about this practice yet. In addition to anti-viral medications, some also use a course of herbal anti-virals (turmeric and milk thistle) and flavonoids. Also possibly helpful in combating viral infections are Vitamin A and cod liver oil, casein-free colostrums, and transfer factor.

Some of these substances may effect sulfation, a process that is often impaired in autistics. Sulfation is the process of attaching sulfate to molecules of the body tissues in order to give them a certain function or to allow excretion. Health care practitioners must weigh the benefit gained in using such herbals against a possible detrimental effect on already impaired sulfation. Those interested in this topic are referred to the *Autism: Effective Biomedical Treatments*[1] for further details.

11. Add More Nutritional Supplements

Once the gastrointestinal tract is working properly, it is time to introduce and gauge the response to more advanced nutritional supplements. Baker and Pangborn recommend waiting for a period of stable or constant behavior rather than a time of change for the introduction of a new, possibly beneficial nutrient. The body may need a nutrient or biochemical agent, but react badly to it solely due to malabsorption and the presence of dysbiotic flora.

Supplements should always be phased in one at a time, except for vitamin B6 and magnesium, which are used together. (You can use magnesium without B6, but not B6 without magnesium.)

Some nutrients, such as zinc, vitamin C, calcium, magnesium and B6 often are introduced during earlier intervention steps to improve behavior. If an autistic individual has not yet tried them, now is the time. Parents should keep careful records or a supplement diary. Good records help with future comparisons and decisions.

Optometrists should refer to *Autism: Effective Biomedical Treatments* and the 2007 supplement for detailed information on all nutritional tests. Doctors must order nutritional analyses, including amino acid analysis, if the patient uses an exclusionary diet. The tests, of course, should be done following dietary intervention, to insure adequacy of essential nutrients.

In addition, blood, urine and hair analyses can be used for assessing mineral status. Plasma or urine amino acid analysis, vitamin assays and blood cell fatty acid analyses can also be of assistance.

Supplements to be considered at this stage include those that might be sub-normal after dietary changes, per the laboratory tests.

- Vitamin E may help as an antioxidant
- Minerals such as molybdenum, manganese and selenium may need bolstering
- Amino acids, especially lysine are needed
- Glutamine can help with gut healing

Other advanced supplements include di-methylglycine (DMG) or tri-methylglycine (TMG) or betaine, creatine, methyl-cobalamin, L-carnitine and maybe glutathione (GSH). Methyl-cobalamin is administered by injection; the best protocol is from James Neubrander, MD.[3] GSH can be administered orally, trans-dermally, or intravenously. Depletion of active, reduced GSH and oxidant stress is documented in autism. Use of these supplements in autism is taught at Defeat Autism Now! conferences by experienced clinicians.

Parents sometimes report issues with use of nutritional supplements. Reasons can be obscure, complicated, or just unknown. Here are some clues to the most common problems:

Symptoms worsen
Possible cause #1: Bacterial dysbiosis is still a problem and some degree of malabsorption is present.

Solution: Check for IgE- and IgG-mediated food allergies, if this has not already been done. Allergenic foods may those that are incompletely digested. Maldigestion leads to a food supply of dysbiotic flora, which can do mischief with nutritional supplements. The amino acids that are most troublesome in the presence of malabsorption are phenylalanine, tryptophan, tyrosine and glutamine. When carried into the bowel, these amino acids can foster the growth of dysbiotic organisms, which can develop into toxic substances.

Possible cause #2: Fungal or yeast dysbiosis is still a problem.

Solution: Recheck for yeast in the stool, or yeast markers in the urine. Make sure that you are using a maintenance dose of capryllic acid or other yeast control nutrients. Perhaps you skipped ahead to the next step, detoxification, and used a sulfur-containing agent, like DMSA, which exacerbates yeast problems. The amino acids and other nutrients that are most troublesome in the presence of yeast dysbiosis are cystine, cysteine, N-acetylcysteine, lipoic acid, and possibly oral glutathione.

Possible cause #3: The patient has vitamin B 12 deficiency and is intolerant to folate.

Solution: Try methylcobalamin or di- or tri-methylglycine.

New symptoms appear
If a nutrient produces regression, severe reactivity, or a reaction that lasts more than three to four days, discontinue it immediately. Try it again at a later date or forget it.

12. Detoxify the Body

The body detoxifies various foreign chemicals using different processes. Detoxifcation processes that can be dysfunctional in autism include methylation, sulfation, glutathione conjugation, acetylation and glucuronidation. Several of the previous steps begin the detoxification process. Avoiding casein and gluten allows the body to rid itself of casomorphins and gluteomorphins. Clearing the gut rids it of toxins, as well. The next step is to address other toxins.

Elevated mercury, antimony, tin, aluminum, arsenic and lead levels are most common in autism. Mercury, for example, is escorted out of the cells by glutathione. If glutathione is inadequate, as is the case in many individuals with autism, chelating agents must be used to remove toxic elements, including mercury, arsenic and antimony. This treatment must be carefully managed by an experienced Defeat Autism Now! doctor or toxicologist.

Further specialized laboratory testing, such as blood cell element or urine analysis following provocation with a chelating agent, can be very helpful in determining whether a patient shows evidence of heavy metal burden. Hair and urine tests can also be useful to monitor progress during detoxification therapy. However, hair is not indicative of mercury burden in autism before detoxification treatment begins.

Several detoxification agents are showing success with patients on the autism spectrum:

Dimercaptosuccinic acid (DMSA) is the primary substance most Defeat Autism Now! practitioners are using to remove mercury and other heavy metals from the bodies of children with autism. The FDA approved DMSA, also known as Chemet, for lead removal in 1988. Its safety in children is documented and researched. DMSA binds to certain metals in the bloodstream and allows them to be excreted in the urine.

A one-day trial of DMSA may be tried under medical supervision. If the DMSA trial yields excessive levels of toxic elements, then a course of DMSA therapy could be extremely helpful. If DMSA therapy is warranted, adjunct nutritional therapy, along with a continuation of anti-fungal, anti-yeast nutrients is essential.

Some patients can show regression during detoxification with DMSA because circulation of the toxins may increase. According to parent responses on the ARI questionnaire, a majority show benefit, using chelation therapy. The most common result is increase in speech output during chelation.

Dimercaptopropane sulfonic acid (DMPS) is under review by Defeat Autism Now! clinicians and researchers for use as a chelating agent in autism. It is not FDA approved, but is allowed and may be provided by some pharmacies.

13. Sulfur Supplements

The majority of children with autism are low in sulfur-enhancing nutrients, and most benefit from nutrients such as glutathione (GSH) and N-acetylcysteine (NAC).[4] All serve to enhance metallothionein (MT) formation, among their many functions in the body. However, all are culture media for the yeast candida. Health care providers should emphatically avoid using them in individuals with unresolved intestinal dysbiosis problems, especially early on in the intervention.

MT's functions include limiting copper uptake through the intestinal mucosa. Those interested in MT are directed to the research of Dr. William Walsh at the Pfeiffer Treatment Center in Naperville, IL. He found that those with autism demonstrated low MT and high copper/low zinc levels.[5]

14. Do Metabolic Fine Tuning

The vast majority of individuals with autism demonstrate no severe genetic abnormalities or acute metabolic faults. A small minority, however, have abnormal biochemical conditions that feature autism as one of its manifestations. The following rare conditions can be ruled out with genetic and other laboratory tests: tuberous sclerosis, neurofibromatosis, adenylosuccinate lyase deficiency, phenylketonuria (PKU), fragile X, Rett, Angelmann, Prader-Willi, and other genetic disorders. If health care practitioners suspect any of these conditions, refer the patient to a competent genetic specialist.

> *Editors note:* Dominic Maino, OD, has written extensively about vision issues in genetic syndromes. See his *Diagnosis and Management of Special Populations,* published by OEP.

Autism in those individuals without frank metabolic faults may be a result of acquired disorders in the molecules required for cellular perception and response. Interestingly, the cells that are primarily affected are the cells of the nervous system (neurons), immune cells (lymphocytes), and the secretory cells of the gastrointestinal tract. The dire consequences include disordered sensory perceptions, poor social responsivity, lowered immune function, and poor disgestion of casein, gluten, carbohydrates and fats.

Individuals with sub-clinical metabolic faults or simple phenotypical variants develop autism when toxic and immunological insults overload. This subject is covered in Chapter 3, "Total Load Theory." The preceding 13 steps work on the problems layer by layer. The ultimate pay-off is faster learning, improved sociability and breakthroughs in language development.

15. Add Sensory, Educational and Other Therapies

One important objective of the above interventions is to make special education and adjunct therapies work better and more quickly. If cellular perception and response are unburdened from impaired biochemistry, toxic elements, xenobiotic and infectious toxins and exorphin peptides, then sensory output can be transformed into understanding and action. Adjunct therapies are thus essential to help children's development catch up. Occupational and physical therapists with expertise in sensory integration training, special educators and, of course, optometrists become important team members.

Anyone interested in patients with autism should attend a Defeat Autism Now! conference. They are held twice a year, once on the east coast and once on the west coast. At every conference Defeat Autism Now! clinicians teach about the latest research.

To see the conference schedule, go to <www.DefeatAutismNow.com>.
Updates on the latest findings by the Defeat Autism Now! researchers can be found at <www.autism.com>.

PART 3

Individuality in Autism Spectrum Disorders-Points to Consider
Sidney MacDonald Baker, MD

Editor's note: This article is excerpted from one originally appearing in the Defeat Autism Now! Conference Syllabus, Spring 2003. For a complete and updated discussion of "Individuality" please refer to Section 1 in *Autism: Effective Biomedical Treatments* by Pangborn and Baker, published by The Autism Research Institute in 2005.

1. The cause of symptoms in all those diagnosed with "autism" is not the same.

In the present epidemic of autism, one would think that all participants in the epidemic "have the same thing," just as would be the case for chicken pox, in which there is "one cause." The concept is not as neat as the term "epidemic" implies. Children with autism vary markedly,

2. While those with autism are, by definition, similar, their responses to treatments are not the same.

Even though all patients diagnosed with autism fulfill the diagnostic criteria for problems in socialization, communication and behavior, and their lab results are similar, neither diagnosis nor lab test results is predictive of response to treatment. Children show a paradoxical diversity of response to treatments such as gluten- and casein- free diet, anti-fungal therapy, supplementing nutrients or other accessory nutritional factors. The paradox is a departure from the usual medical expectation that diagnostic labels or, especially, lab results predict response to treatment.

3. Parental choices of treatments for their child's autism are usually influenced by pre-conceived professional opinions.

Many medical pioneers were burned in the crucible of their critics' disaffection. Practitioners and parents must not get caught in that kind of crossfire when making decisions about what therapies to try. Everyone must work as a team in relating diet to behavior, the potential for gut abnormalities to produce systemic problems, the safety of immunizations, the effectiveness of nutritional pharmacology, the dangers of mercury toxicity, or whether medical treatment should be directed at the disease or the individual.

4. An evolving consensus of parents, practitioners and researchers since 1995 agrees on the following points:

- Autism is a biomedical problem in which biomedical treatments enhance the therapeutic effects of sensory, educational, and other therapies;
- A web of factors combine to cause autistic symptoms in genetically pre-disposed children, but the epidemic is not caused by genetics per se;
- The key causes of autism have to do with metabolic quirks, toxic and infectious factors whose interconnections are responsible in different children for a wide range of problems including autism, attention problems, asthma, inflammatory bowel disorders and other conditions that have become more prevalent in recent decades;
- A biochemical nexus affecting certain cell signaling compounds (purines) appears to lie at the core of the congenital or acquired pathology of these kids. This chemistry, involves dysfunction in single carbon transfer (methylation), sulfation, and purine chemistry in ways that interconnect the digestive, immune and neurological systems.

- Defects in purine chemistry are present in all of the known biochemical syndromes featuring autistic symptoms. The strong implication of his observation is that children caught in the current epidemic are likely to have a similar involvement. Abnormalities in the chemistry of folic acid, sulfation, detoxification, and uric acid, as well as treatment benefits from DMG, vitamin B12, reduced glutathione and other sulfur-bearing molecules require that we learn more about this chemistry in children on the autism spectrum.

5. In the previous article, Dr. Pangborn outlined a sequence of steps that parents and practitioners can consider for a child on the spectrum.

Clinicians must remember that these steps do not treat "autism." They are designed to treat each child individually, for whom there is no sure pre-determined recipe. Treatment is an iterative process of tailoring, so that the best time to discuss whether any (safe) treatment would be good is about three weeks after a child has tried it. It important to emphasize that the scheme Dr. Pangborn presents is just a way of thinking.

6. The sequence of treatments for every child with autism must begin with cleaning up the diet and the gut, which, of course, is never "clean," even in the sense we are using here.

Each Defeat Autism Now! clinician approaches his or her patients with some version of this scheme, and each child responds with his or her version of benefits, reactions, miracles or disappointments. Five, 10, or 20 years from now we will have a better understanding of how to pick the winners in the therapeutic contest, but right now parents who do not want to wait for the full scientific ripening of these options can have confidence that this general approach has a high benefit-to-risk ratio in most children.

7. Be skeptical of all "out-of-the-can" remedies or "programs" for all children with autism.

Because each child reached the diagnosis of autism from a unique sequence of events, no "one-size-fits-all" program is appropriate for everyone.

8. "Have I done everything I can for this child?" is the question that comes up and haunts me every time I see a child.

At the end of the day practitioners must confront that question. You as optometrists may be able to answer it only after you understand the Defeat Autism Now! method, recommend extensive lab tests and therapeutic trials. If you try to answer this question at each step of the way, you might lose your focus. I thus recommend that you can refocus by remembering that all you need to decide today is what to do next.

References

1. *Pangborn JB, Baker SM. Autism: Effective Biomedical Treatments. San Diego, CA: Autism Research Institute, 2005.*

2. *Lewis L. Special Diets for Special Kids. Arlington, TX: Future Horizons, 1998.*

3. *Lewis L. Special Diets for Special Kids II. Arlington, TX: Future Horizons, 2001*

4. *Neubrander J.Biochemical Context and Clinical Use of Vitamin B12. Defeat Autism Now! 2003 Conference Proceedings, Philadelphia, PA, May, 2003:103-17.*

5. *Owens SC. Understanding the Sulfur System. Defeat Autism Now! 2003 Conference Proceedings, Philadelphia PA, May, 2003:65-76.*

6. *Walsh W, Usman A, Tarpey , Kelly T. Metallothionein and Autism, 2nd ed. Pfeiffer Treatment Center, Naperville, IL 2002.*

Chapter 7
Sensory-Based Approaches Including
the Role of the Occupational Therapist

Patricia S. Lemer, M. Ed.

Introduction

Clinicians have long recognized sensory issues in autism. Both Bernard Rimland and Edward Ornitz observed and described these problems in the 1960s.[1, 2] As a young girl visiting her relatives' farm, Temple Grandin, PhD enjoyed the deep pressure of the machine used to hold cattle for branding. This early experience resulted in her invention of the Squeeze Machine (see later in this chapter.) She also describes her hearing sensitivities: certain noises that "sounded like a dentist drill going through my ears."[3]

In the 1970s Carl Delacato was the first to propose that the sensory abnormalities of those with autism were treatable.[4] Since then, practitioners from a variety of disciplines have designed numerous programs for remediating all types of sensory issues. This chapter includes treatments primarily for problems with touch, pressure, movement and balance. Vision therapy is covered in Chapter 9, and sound therapies in Chapter 10.

The Case for Collaboration

Occupational therapists (OTs) are the most likely profession to treat sensory problems in autism, although other professionals have designed sensory-based approaches. Developmental optometrists (ODs) and OTs "adopted a whole person, integrated, functional approach to treatment long before it was even vaguely fashionable."[5] Both professionals recognize the importance of vision and movement in development. Optometry stresses the role of vision as primary and movement skills as foundational. Occupational therapy focuses on movement and balance, viewing vision as one of the most important sensory systems.

Few would argue that occupational therapists benefit from an understanding of vision development and how vision deficits can interfere with function. Many OTs collaborate with optometrists. Most find that lenses, prisms and vision therapy complement occupational therapy by treating underlying dysfunctions of the visual system. They see positive changes in tone, posture, movement, visual-motor, visual-spatial, visual-perceptual and cognitive function that cannot be attributed to their therapy alone. Likewise, optometrists can benefit from learning about the work of occupational therapists whose sensory-based therapy focuses on tactile and proprioceptive awareness, kinesthesia, vestibular function and motor planning that can positively affect ocular control, visual-motor integration and visual-perception.

In 1990,[6] and again in 1999,[7] Lynn Hellerstein, OD, FCOVD and Beth Fishman, OTR, wrote about the synergistic relationship that can develop between behavioral ODs and OTs. Workshops on OT/OD collaboration have spawned numerous OT/OD pairs whose collaborative work may be familiar to the reader. There are few areas of application more suited to these alliances than autism and related disorders.

In order to fully understand what goes wrong sensorily in AD(H)D, LD, PDD and autism, the reader is referred to several publications that cover this topic in depth. During the beginning of the autism epidemic, the American Occupational Therapy Association (AOTA) published a compendium on treating sensory issues in autism for OTs. *Autism: A Comprehensive Occupational Therapy Approach*[8] provides excellent information about both autism and occupational therapy, and how the two intersect through the lifespan.

Understanding the Nature of Sensory Integration with Diverse Populations,[9] *Exploring the Spectrum of Autism* and *Pervasive Developmental Disorders: Intervention Strategies*[10] and *Autism: A Sensorimotor Approach to Management*,[11] are also excellent resources. Two other publications, *Sensory Perceptual Issues in Autism and Asperger Syndrome*[12], and *Asperger Syndrome and Sensory Issues*[13] both focus on explaining the unusual sensory perceptions present in autism to the public. All of these books provide extensive explanations of theory and techniques, and the intention of this chapter is not to repeat the information they contain.

The Seven Sensory Systems

A review of the seven sensory systems, tactile, proprioceptive, vestibular, visual, auditory, gustatory and olfactory, and how they work, is necessary to understand the nature of sensory issues in autism spectrum disorders. When an individual has a sensory experience, receptors or specialized cells throughout the body deliver messages to the central nervous system. As these messages travel along neural pathways, different parts of the brain compare, combine and interpret the sensory experiences, storing them for future reference.[10]

Efficient foundational sensory skills, especially in the tactile and vestibular systems, are not only essential for sustaining attention, understanding and using language and for social interaction, but for all aspects of vision. *Tactile processing* is especially important in connecting to others emotionally, and in participating in social situations. Sitting at circle time, standing in line, and negotiating moving bodies on the playground can involve human contact that is intermittent and unpredictable. For the child with autism who experiences tactile sensitivity, and who has difficulty reading cues that tell him what to expect next, these situations are likely to create anxiety and discomfort.[14]

Veteran occupational therapist Josephine Moore describes the importance of the vestibulo-oculo-cervical (VOC) triad.[15] According to Moore, the vestibular and proprioceptive systems work together to provide information about the body's position in space. The vestibular system detects the position and movement of the head relative to gravity, while proprioception allows the brain to interpret sensations from the tendons, muscles and joints. Thus, receptors in the neck orient the head according to the demands of the task, coordinating movements of eyes, head and body.[16]

While all senses are important, the *vestibular system* is of particular interest because of the close neural relationship between it and the visual system. Some of the visual disturbances in those with autism spectrum disorders relate to the interactions between these two systems. Sometimes called the "balance system," the vestibular system is located in the inner ear, where it receives signals from the labyrinths, which regulate eye position when the head moves.

Many children with autism spectrum disorders appear to have under-developed vestibular systems. A baby's vestibular system is one of the first systems to myelinate in utero.[17] The mother's movements stimulate vestibular development in the fetus. Confining a mother with a high-risk pregnancy to bed-rest during the third trimester of pregnancy could result in a baby being born with an under-developed vestibular system. Furthermore, repeated ear infections can also disturb its function.

Normalizing vestibular function is crucial for a child's development to proceed in a predictable, efficient fashion. Physiologically, the vestibular system is connected to the digestive tract, language center of the brain, the limbic system and to the muscles of the eyes. A well-functioning vestibular system will thus contribute to healthy digestion, the emergence of receptive and expressive communication, emotional bonding, and visual focus, all areas of concern in individuals with autism. Consider what happens when an adult lifts a baby off the ground playfully, holds the child overhead, smiles and babbles at him. A child with a well-functioning vestibular system returns the smile, makes eye contact, babbles back, and in some cases, throws up! What an amazing system it is!

Including vestibular stimulation activities as part of the daily routine of a child on the autism spectrum can be extremely powerful. Working against gravity on suspended equipment could result in secondary gains in the crucial areas of digestion, visual function, including eye contact, communication and socialization.

A review of the literature on the relationship between vestibular function and vision showed that children who received therapy in both areas made the best progress. While vestibular intervention alone improved balance, sensory integration and socialization, adding visual therapy and including the use of lenses and prisms also improved binocular function.[18]

Senses Discriminate and Protect

Each of the sensory systems has two functions: discrimination and protection. Discrimination provides information about details, texture, temperature, shape and size. Accurate discrimination allows a person to use objects appropriately. The protective function keeps people from danger. Table 7-1 shows possible offenders in the environment which could trip a protective response from those with autism spectrum disorders.

Table 7-1. Frequent Environmental Offenders from which Hypersensitive Individuals Seek Protection
(Copyright , The HANDLE Institute; reprinted with permission)

Clothing on themselves
- Stiff tags
- Stiff fibers (e.g., jeans)
- Seams in socks
- Waistbands & belts
- Jewelry
- Hairbands
- Synthetic fibers

Odors
- Paints, varnishes, glues
- Room fresheners
- Cologne, perfumes, after-shave
- Hairspray, gels, etc
- Clothes that have been dry-cleaned
- Fabric softeners applied in the dryer
- Orange peel, banana peel
- Synthetics (e.g., plastic food packaging)
- Fatty foods (e.g.,broiled chops)
- Extremely sweet odors
- Extreme or unexpected body odors

Body-in-Space Sensations
- Light contact with seat, ground, other slightly tipped/irregular surfaces
- Swivel chairs
- Open areas behind one's back
- Close quarters
- Remaining seated while others move past

Clothing on others
- Synthetic fibers
- Intricate patterns
- Metallic look
- Reflecting accessories (e.g.,sequins, watches)
- Noise makers (e.g., bangle jangle bracelets, watch alarms)

Lighting
- Fluorescent lights
- Halogen lights
- Strobe lights
- Flickering sunlight (e.g., through leaves, blinds)
- Severe contrast (e.g., stage productions)
- Lighted mirrors
- Reflective materials
- Certain colors (e.g., yellow-orange)
- Color contrasts (e.g., black/red)
- White paper (esp. glossy magazines)
- LCD signboards
- Automobile lights at night or in the rain
- Automobile lights in white tiled tunnels

Sounds
- Unexpected loud sounds
- High-pitched sounds
- Deeply resonating sounds
- Disharmonious sounds
- Background conversation

When the nervous system interprets a stimulus as potentially harmful, it triggers a "flight or fright" response both internally (rapid heart rate) and externally (sweating or running away.) These responses are typically viewed by others as "aberrant behavior." Judith Bluestone of the HANDLE (**H**olistic **A**pproach to **N**euro**D**evelopmental and **L**earning **E**fficiency) Institute suggests that instead, we view behaviors as communication, rather than as symptoms to be masked or controlled.[19]

Sensory Integration

The late A. Jean Ayres, PhD, an occupational therapist who made it her life's work to understand and treat sensory issues, is the name that is almost always associated with the term "sensory integration." Beginning in the 1960s, Dr. Ayres systematically investigated the nature of how the brain processes sensory information so that it can be used for learning, emotions and behavior. Ayres defined *sensory integration* as "the organization of sensory input for use."[20] "Sensory integration is a neurobiological process that forms the foundation for adaptive responses to challenges imposed by the environment and learning. Sensory integration theory considers the dynamic interactions between a person's abilities/disabilities and the environment."[21]

In 2004, approximately two dozen people practicing and teaching about sensory integration worldwide, including former co-workers and students of Dr. Ayres, who are now among the leading experts in the field, gathered in California for an International Networking Meeting. At this meeting these individuals founded an organizational body to promote and protect Ayres' theory and it's applications in practice: the Sensory Integration Global Network (SIGN). In collaboration with Ayres' nephew, Brian Erwin, the successor trustee to the Jean Ayres Trust, who trademarked the term *Ayres Sensory Integration*®, they established guidelines for anyone wishing to carry forth with Dr. Ayres work.

Ayres Sensory Integration® includes the theory, assessment, patterns of dysfunction and intervention concepts, principles and techniques articulated by Dr Ayres and applied by therapists trained in this approach worldwide. A summary of the main components of *Ayres Sensory Integration*® is available on the SIGN website at <www.siglobalnetwork.org>.

Sensory Integration Dysfunction and Sensory Processing Disorder

All behaviors are a result of the processing of one or more of the seven senses. If any sense is inefficient in any of the above areas, the integration process can be disrupted and dysfunction occurs. In the past, the term for this outcome has been sensory integration dysfunction, often abbreviated SID. However, because of the possibility of confusing it with the unrelated disorder Sudden Infant Death Syndrome (SIDS), the term was changed informally among those in the field to dysfunction in sensory integration, or DSI.

According to the SIGN website, the most common patterns of sensory integration dysfunction include: visual perception deficits; visual motor deficits; visual construction and praxis deficits (visuodyspraxia); tactile discrimination deficits; vestibular processing deficits; proprioceptive processing deficits and poor body scheme; bilateral integration and sequencing deficits including poor postural control (bilateral integration and sequencing); somatosensory-based dyspraxia (somatodyspraxia), language-based dyspraxia (dyspraxia on verbal command), sensory sensitivities especially tactile defensiveness and gravitational insecurity.

Sensory integration dysfunction that demonstrates motor incoordination, fine and gross motor delays, deficits in balance or poor praxis is often included in the diagnostic category of Developmental Coordination Disorder. Patterns of sensory integration dysfunction that include unusual over-, under- or fluctuating responses to sensation may be included in deficits such as Regulatory Disorder or Sensory Processing Disorders.[22]

Recently, a small group of those in the field, led by sensory integration researcher Lucy Jane Miller, PhD, OTR, has suggested yet different terminology, sensory processing disorder, or SPD, as an umbrella term encompassing sensory modulation disorder, sensory-based motor disorder, and sensory perception/discrimination disorder. The long-term goal of this movement is to include SPD in a revision of the *Diagnostic and Statistical Manual of Mental Disorders* (DSM)[23] due out in 2012. Ayres followers are split on the use of this new nosology, comparing the movement to the one described in Chapter 1 regarding AD(H)D. In fact, a November, 2007 article in *Time* asked, "Is SPD the Next Attention Deficit Disorder?"[24] To learn more about SPD, go to the website of Miller's SPD Network at <www.spdfoundation.net>.

Sensory Integration and Autism

Ayres recognized in the 1970's that many children on the autistic spectrum have a significant number of symptoms of sensory integration dysfunction.[17] She noticed that the sensory issues of those with autism occurred primarily in the areas of touch and movement, and were either in "registration," or in "modulation," their ability to exert consistent behavioral control over the sensory stimulus. She speculated that children with autism fell into one of two categories. The first includes those who are under- (hypo-) reactive to stimulation, and seek sensory experiences; the second includes those who are over- (hyper-) reactive to tactile and vestibular sensations, and show defensive behaviors. Ayres further proposed that the abilities of those in both categories to register and modulate sensory stimuli varied from time to time and in different environments.[25]

Research supports Ayres' theory, and suggests that these inconsistent responses are due to either high thresholds for sensory input (hypo-) or sensory defensiveness (hyper-).[26] Psychiatrist Stanley Greenspan, MD and psychologist Serena Wieder, PhD found that 95% of 200 children with autism in their study exhibited sensory modulation difficulties.[27] Australian psychologist Jan Piek and her colleagues found that deficits in sensory integration contribute to problems in motor coordination and visual perception in students with autism spectrum disorders.[28] Another study of eight boys with autism, compared to eight controls, found that those with ASD had sensory issues that contributed to balance issues. Furthermore, these boys were over-dependent upon their visual skills to maintain balance. [29]

Both hypo- and hyper-reactions, not only to touch and movement, but also to sound, smell, taste, and of course, vision, are the hallmarks of autistic behavior. Table 7-2 shows typical behaviors of those on the autism spectrum classified by sense and whether they represent hypo- or hyper-reactivity.

Table 7-2. Autistic Behaviors Resulting from Hyper- and Hypo-Reactivity to Each Sense

SENSE	HYPER-REACTIVITY	HYPO-REACTIVITY
HEARING	Covers ears Dislikes haircuts	Attracted to sounds Likes vibrations
TOUCH	Avoids messy foods Ticklish Picky about clothing Won't walk on grass or sand	Ignores food on face Self-injurious behavior Touches everything High pain tolerance
TASTE & SMELL	Gags at new foods Reacts to odors Picky eater	Prefers spicy foods Smells clothing, self Mouths objects
VISION	Blinks excessively Covers eyes Picks up specks of dust Poor eye contact	Poor focus Lacks awareness Fascinated by reflections Flicks fingers by eyes
VESTIBULAR/ PROPRIOCEPTIVE	Fearful of movement Gets car-sick Fear of being upside-down	Seeks spinning Wiggles and squirms Rocks back & forth

Inappropriate reactions to the hundreds of sensations from foods, clothing and all aspects of the environment, such as flinching when touched, tuning out, hiding under the furniture, and covering eyes and ears, are the results of sensory "overload." All of these responses interfere with development and can cause further problems with eating, dressing, bonding, learning and just "being." On a cognitive level, those with autism have significant difficulty with higher level sensory processing tasks such as organization, because these activities depend upon giving meaning to their world using efficient sensory integration. With extreme sensory overload, one or more of the sensory systems eventually shuts down." [12]

In Chapter 2, Dr. Randy Schulman notes that patients with AD(H)D, LD, PDD and autism present with a multitude of sensory-driven behaviors upon which their diagnoses are based. Their varying degrees of motor, sensory-motor and sensory integrative difficulties both affect and are affected by vision. It is helpful for the optometrist to have a global understanding of the relationship between each of the sensory systems and vision.

Dysfunction in any part of the vestibulo-oculo-cervical (VOC) triad disrupts function in the others, resulting in compromised adaptive responses to environmental demands. Why is this important in autism? Because many children with autism spectrum disorders experience gravitational insecurity, resulting in significant feelings of anxiety and fear in response to vestibular-proprioceptive stimulation, such as being tilted back in a chair or simply walking on uneven surfaces. If the secondary emotional responses are treated without addressing the probable underlying sensory causes, further incidents are inevitable.

While sensory-seeking and sensory-avoidance behaviors are frequently interpreted by behaviorists as problematic, and in need of being extinguished, those taking a developmental perspective recognize that these and all behaviors are adaptive responses that serve a purpose. Primitive, self-stimulatory activities, such as rocking, flicking fingers in front of the eyes, or fondling a favorite blanket, are calming for some, and alerting for others, depending on the degree and nature of an individual's unique combinations of sensitivities. Whatever the reason, sensory difficulties lead to a variety of functional skill deficits in communication, social interaction, learning, and the development of appropriate visual skills.

Ayres' sensory integration theory stresses that the body's ability to process and interpret information coming in through touch, movement, balance and body position lays the foundations for motor development. Thus, if processing of sensory input is aberrant, motor skills will be delayed. Research shows that gross, fine and visual-motor deficits are common in children with autism spectrum disorders.[30] One report found motor problems, including low muscle tone, motor planning problems and other issues in over 80% of their cases of autism.[31] Some researchers are suggesting that an analysis of movement skills in the first few days of life holds clues to diagnosing autism early. Videos of all 17 children later diagnosed as autistic showed persistent asymmetries in lying, righting, crawling and sitting before the age of six months.[32]

Praxis and Dyspraxia in Autism

Praxis is one of the outcomes of motor, sensory and sensory-motor integration all working efficiently. Simply defined as "the ability to do,"[33] Ayres writes that praxis refers to a process underlying the planning and execution of novel and complex motor patterns and sequences.[34] Praxis involves timing, sequencing, initiating, transitioning and ideation.

A dysfunction in praxis, or "dyspraxia," is becoming more widely recognized as one of the critical functional deficits in autism spectrum disorders.[14] While motor planning issues certainly present problems in isolation, their dramatic effect on functional skills cannot be under-estimated. Dyspraxia could account for a number of the symptoms of autism, with social-emotional development, especially inter-personal relatedness, language development and symbolic play reported to be the areas most affected.[35] Turn-taking, the pragmatics of language and reading social cues most certainly involve timing, sequencing and ideation.

Motor Planning Progresses from the "Bottom-Up" and the "Inside Out"

Good organizational skills and appropriate social interaction are two results of efficient motor planning. When motor development progresses smoothly, a child gains control over his/her body in the following order: lower body, upper body, shoulders and neck, upper arm, lower arm, hands, fingers. At the same time, head control develops, moving first along with the upper body, then independently, and the eyes move first with the upper body, head, and finally on their own. The ability to move parts independently depends upon the stability of the larger muscles and body parts.

Picture a one-year-old child beginning to walk with a wide-based gait, arms raised for balance and stability. As lower limbs strengthen and the trunk becomes more stable, arms drop to the sides. At first a child is unable to both walk and hold something in her hand. Eventually, as the trunk stabilizes, walking becomes more automatic, and the hands and arms can perform actions without fear of falling. As the upper body strengthens, the arms and hands then become more coordinated.

Watch a three-year-old paint at an easel. The legs are positioned in a wide stance, the brush is held in a fisted grasp, and the movement is with the whole arm. Usually the eyes are not focused on the easel; if they are, they are looking at the finished product, not the active painting. Eventually, as the upper arm stabilizes, the grasp improves, and the standing posture narrows and is more flexible.

As motor development continues to take place, a child can sit comfortably at a table to write or draw, with upper body held strong and not collapsed,. Both sides of the body begin to work together as two eyes and two hands coordinate, one to execute, and one to support the task at hand. The shoulders are still, an elbow may rest on the table, and the joints of the fingers work independently to engage the writing implement.

At any point in this sequence, if the demands for production exceed motor and visual maturity, or if a reflex has not integrated, the child's body must physically compensate, and aberrant postures will emerge. A teacher may observe a child slumping at the desk, wrapping her foot around the leg of the table, laying her head on an arm to write, or demonstrating other symptoms indicative of the lack of motor and visual readiness.

Likewise with the eyes and body. Many young children with autism "look" with their whole bodies. Ask them to follow a moving object, and observe that they move not only their eyes, but heads and trunks, as well. Rather than insist that they keep their bodies still, suggest intervention activities that strengthen the upper body and allow the head, and eventually the eyes to work alone. Children who read with head and body movements across the page are not ready to read. Until two eyes can work together in concert and eye movements are smooth, reading instruction is contra-indicated.

Uneven or spotty development (such as low tone and poor motor control) can result in skipped important developmental steps over time (such as poor eating or omitted crawling). Parents, teachers and therapists must be patient and focus on improving these lower level skills rather than moving prematurely to higher skill levels. Pushing academics prematurely can result in diagnosed learning disabilities, attentional issues or autistic-like behavior later on.

A review of the occupational therapy literature on autism uncovered no reference to the connection between praxis and vision. Optometrists who wish to collaborate with OTs working with patients on the autism spectrum must educate occupational therapists about the relationship between vision and early movement dysfunction, crawling abnormalities and motor delays. An early developmental optometric evaluation and visual intervention can most certainly improve overall motor function, and heavily impact upon the many functional skills affected by dyspraxia.

Piaget's Developmental Hierarchy

Many developmental optometrists turn to the seminal work of Jean Piaget[36] to understand that motor and visual development take place in tandem, in a predictable hierarchy. First comes the **Motor stage**, during which individuals move primarily without purpose, as the receptors for touch, proprioception, balance, vision and hearing are maturing. As tone heightens, sensory integration takes place, and movement becomes more directed.

The **Motor-Visual stage** follows next. For months, the typical infant's and toddler's movements take the eyes along for a ride, as the brain learns to control the upper and lower body. The eyes process what they see wherever they are directed. Many children with autism spectrum disorders, regardless of age, are still at this stage. They often wander aimlessly around their classrooms, finding themselves somehow in the block corner, where they may line up blocks. When an adult offers crayons or markers to children at this stage, they scribble, sometimes not even looking at their hands or what they are drawing. They possibly start out with an idea of drawing a person, and end up with a tree, as their motor skills over-ride their visualization abilities.

Next comes the **Visual-Motor stage**. Progressing to this level is a major hurdle in development. Vision now directs movement. Instead of moving purposelessly through space, children at a visual-motor stage take inventory of the space around them, find a target, and move toward it. Movement and drawing become purposeful. They see the block corner, recall the tower they built yesterday, and race there to re-experience that pleasure it gave them. They take the crayon and draw a person, one body part at a time. The motor and emotional experience have now become one.

The last step is the **Visual stage**. At this level, people no longer need the actual bodily movements for experience; rather they can "move" in their mind's eye. A child at this stage tells her mother, prior to going to school, that when she arrives, she will go right to block corner to make a tower. Her sensory, motor, visual and emotional brains have memory of the experience and want to have it again. This step is the beginning of the ability to plan, organize, conceptualize, ideate: all results of the senses and motor abilities integrating efficiently.

An in-depth evaluation of all sensory functions adds to the overall knowledge about a patient and to the optometrist's ability to assist in both the diagnosis and treatment of visual dysfunction in the autistic patient. The next section gives an overview of both formal and informal options for assessing the efficiency of individual sensory systems and how well they work together.

Evaluation of Sensory Issues

Occupational therapy evaluations can include both formal and informal assessments of sensory processing, motor planning, kinesthesia, muscle strength and tone, motor control, attention to task, visual perception and visual-motor integration.[37] Those on the autism spectrum experience difficulties in many or all of these areas. Therapists also depend upon their clinical observations, which are especially helpful with this population.

Evaluating sensory processing is an on-going process, as behaviors change day-to-day and in different settings with varying demands and people. Information should be gathered at home and school, from teachers and parents, and from any other setting where the child can be observed, to assure a most complete history and observation of sensory responses. For those on the severe end of the spectrum, whose behaviors are the most challenging, informal assessments, questionnaires and checklists yield more information than formal testing, because of limited compliance to demands. Sensory evaluations are measuring many of the areas with which these children have the most difficulty.

Some occupational therapists have developed forms for taking sensory histories, as well as checklists and questionnaires to evaluate the sensory functioning of those on the autism spectrum. A popular informal instrument available to them is **Questions to Guide Classroom Observations** by Kientz and Miller. [38] Teachers respond to a series of 38 questions about the child, a specific task, the physical environment, as well as the social and cultural context. This questionnaire is most commonly used to informally guide teachers and therapists on how to improve a child's performance at school. It is especially helpful in identifying environmental issues such as noises from heating and air conditioning, difficulties with lighting or **excessive visual stimulation**. Altering any of these factors can improve a student's potential for success.

Another popular instrument for use with this population is the **Sensory Profile** by Dunn.[39] Using a Likert scale, caregivers rate a child's responsivity to 125 items. Information is categorized into six domains of sensory processing (auditory, **visual**, vestibular, tactile, multi-sensory and oral), five domains of modulation, and three domains of behavioral outcomes. Modulation information relates to tone, body position, activity level, and visual input affecting emotional responses and activity level. Based on a comparison to a standardized sample of over 1000 children ages five to ten, a report of a child's sensory processing is classified as "typical," "probably atypical," or "definitely atypical."

Studies are ongoing using the **Sensory Profile** for both making a differential diagnosis and for remediation recommendations. One study found that this instrument was able to discriminate among those with pervasive developmental disorders, attention deficits and those who were not disabled with 90% accuracy.[40] The **Sensory Profile** is also excellent for monitoring progress and adapting intervention techniques.

The newest informal assessment tool is the **Sensory Processing Measure (SPM)**, published by Western Psychological Services (WPS).[41] Available in three forms for *home, classroom,* and the *school environment*, this comprehensive instrument makes it possible to obtain a complete picture of sensory functioning for children age five through 12. Future plans include expansion to include both pre-school and secondary school students.

A child's parent or home-based care provider completes the 75 item *Home Form*, and the primary classroom teacher fills in the *Main Classroom Form* (62 items). Adjunct school personnel complete the *School Environments Form* (10 to 15 items per environment) to assess sensory processing in six environments: during Art, Music, Physical Education, Recess/playground, in the cafeteria, and on the school bus. Because it solicits input from school staff members who are not typically involved in assessment – the art teacher and school bus driver, for example – the *School Environments Form* serves a team-building function. It educates school personnel about sensory processing disorders and uses their observations to obtain a more comprehensive picture of the child.

The *School Environments Form* is provided on an unlimited-use CD, and each environment has its own rating sheet, which can be printed and distributed to raters as needed. Each rater can complete his or her 15-item rating sheet (10 items for the School Bus setting) in under 5 minutes. Each rating sheet is interpreted using a cutoff score for the environment to which it applies. Scores at or above the cutoff point indicate that the child is experiencing an unusually high number of sensory processing problems in a given environment. The *School Environments Form* is always administered in conjunction with the *Main Classroom Form*; it cannot be used alone.

Each form requires about 15-20 minutes, and yields eight parallel standard scores in

- Social participation
- Vision
- Hearing
- Touch
- Body awareness (proprioception)
- Balance and motion (vestibular function)
- Planning and ideas (praxis)
- Total sensory systems

Scores for each scale fall into one of three interpretive ranges: "Typical", "Some Problems", or "Definite Dysfunction". Within each sense, the **SPM** offers descriptive clinical information on processing vulnerabilities, including under- and over-responsiveness, sensory-seeking behavior, and perceptual problems. In addition, for the first time, an Environment Difference score permits direct comparison of the child's sensory functioning at home and at school. While the scales on the *Home* and *Main Classroom Forms* are identical, the items themselves are specific to each environment. Individual item responses reveal how sensory difficulties manifest in these two different settings.

The *SPM* is a psychometrically sound, comprehensive, and clinically rich new addition to sensory assessment. Studies in the Manual document that the **SPM** differentiates typical children from those with clinical disorders. However, its use in autism is not yet established.

If a child is able to comply with the demands of standardized testing, most OTs administer a formal measure. Formal tests, coupled with the examiner's clinical observations, can elicit a great deal of information about a child's response to sensory stimulation, posture, balance, coordination, and movement activities. These reactions are compared to norms established for the child's age. After carefully analyzing data and putting them in the context of the child's home and school environments, the therapist can make recommendations.

The standardized instrument of choice is the **Sensory Integration and Praxis Test (SIPT)**.[42] Specially trained and certified occupational or physical therapists can conduct a formal evaluation using this test, which can serve to establish a baseline of functioning in each of the sensory systems. The **SIPT** is an extremely comprehensive measure, which has norms for age four through eight. It consists of 17 subtests measuring **space visualization**, **figure-ground perception**, standing/walking balance, **design copying**, postural praxis, bilateral motor coordination, praxis on verbal command, constructional praxis, **post-rotary nystagmus**, motor accuracy, sequencing praxis, oral praxis, manual form perception, kinesthesia, finger indentification, graphesthesia and localization of tactile stimuli. Those subtests which elicit information about vision are in boldface type. It is clear that OTs are collecting data that can be very useful to the optometrist.

In a study by Parham and others[43] all of the subtests of the **SIPT** discriminated significantly between children who were developing typically and those with high-functioning autism. Those with autism demonstrated significant difficulties in praxis, bilateral integration, sequencing, and some aspects of vestibular function.

For children who are outside the norms of the **SIPT**, or who cannot comply with standardization procedures, occupational therapists observe spontaneous play with toys and equipment, coordination, tone, laterality, goal orientation, and initiation of actions in the same fashion as recommended for the optometrist in Chapter 2. These clinical observations are sometimes as or more valuable than the test results.

When collaborating with an occupational therapist on a child with AD(H)D or autism, the optometrist is encouraged to obtain copies of any testing results, or better yet, on at least one occasion, observe the administration of the **SIPT**. It would also be illuminating for the OT to watch the optometrist in the examination of the common patient.

Intervention

An individual who spent her professional life applying sensory integration theory to patients with autism and other developmental disabilities is the late Lorna Jean King, OTR/L, FAOTA, founder and Director of the Children's Center for Neurodevelopmental Studies in Glendale, AZ. Beginning with just one student in 1978, this model center has served thousands of children age three through 22, who are treated by various therapists utilizing sensory integration techniques. To learn more about King's legacy go to <www.thechildrenscenteraz.org>.

Sensory integration based occupational therapy consists of guided activities that challenge and enhance the body's ability to respond appropriately to one or more sense. Certification is required for those performing evaluations, but not to do sensory integration therapy. Therapists use controlled tactile, proprioceptive or vestibular input to elicit the simplest adaptive responses. Some activities are aimed at improving the processing of an individual sense, while others facilitate components of praxis, such as initiation, sequencing, bilateral coordination, timing, and imitation.

At first the child participates in simple, safe and purposeful sensory activities, such as swinging, receiving deep pressure under pillows and being touched with a soft cloth. Eventually, with gentle guidance, the patient might tolerate increasingly stimulating activities such as merry-go-rounds, hair brushing and new foods. Soon a child recognizes that swinging on the playground fulfills the same sensory need as running in circles, and chooses a socially appropriate, rather than an inappropriate activity independently. As efficient, organized responses occur more frequently and become more consistent, they ultimately heighten a child's ability to pay attention, relate, sit still, organize language, and focus.[14]

Therapy does not focus on the training of specific skills, because then the body does not learn how to adapt to future similar activities, but rather just how to do that single task. A variety of equipment is necessary. Table 7-3 shows some of the tools occupational therapists use to normalize each system.

Table 7-3 Occupational Therapy Tools for Normalizing Sensory Processsing

Auditory	Whistles, musical instruments, CDs, environmental sounds
Tactile	Stretch fabrics, including lycra & spandex; fingerpaints, play dough, ball pits
Taste & Smell	Salty, sweet, sour, crunchy foods; aromatherapy oils
Visual	Slant boards
Vestibular	Hammocks, swings, slings, scooters, teeter-totters, gliders, skates, bikes, rockers
Proprioceptive	Weighted vests, blankets, ankle and wrist weights, seat cushions, beanbag chairs

Most occupational therapists integrate some auditory input during therapy for those with sound sensitivities. While this can beneficial for those with mild problems, many on the severe end of the spectrum require the intensity of one of the auditory therapies described in Chapter 10.

A review of the literature yielded only a single study on outcomes of Ayres sensory integration-based occupational therapy on four children with autism spectrum diagnoses. This study designed to evaluate whether or not sensory integration therapy was better than play therapy in helping with the behavior of children with autism. The authors found no change in the children's behavior immediately following sensory integration therapy.[44]

Anyone interested in sensory integration therapy should make it a point to observe treatment sessions by a number of different therapists. OT styles differ as markedly as those of behavioral optometrists. Some work very intuitively, while others have more structured therapy agendas.

Special Programs

A number of occupational therapists have developed packaged programs that address the sensory needs of their patients. While not specifically for those on the autism spectrum, those are very adaptable for those with attention deficits and learning disabilities, as well as those with high-functioning autism. Teachers and parents can take courses, learn these tried and true techniques and integrate them at home and at school. Two which are particularly good are the *Alert Program for Self-Regulation*, also known as "How Does Your Engine Run?"[45] and the *Tool Chest for Teachers, Parents and Students.*[46]

The Alert Program Mary Sue Williams and Sherry Shellenberger, the occupational therapist authors of the Alert program designed it to empower students to learn how to regulate their own arousal systems. By comparing the body to a car, kids rev up their engines for active times of day, such as recess, and bring down the tachometer for re-entering the classroom for reading. The techniques can also be used to prepare for anxiety-producing situations, such as going to the doctor and over-stimulating environments such as restaurants and shopping malls. In their newest book, *Take Five! Staying Alert at Home and School,*[47] these innovative therapists provide a myriad of activities for the hypo- and hyper-sensitive child in five areas: touch, movement, vision, audition, and oral-motor. Some of these activities are appropriate for in-office use to maximize an exam or enhance therapy. The manual also includes an extremely valuable check-list for adults with sensory issues.

Tool Chest Diana Henry, the occupational therapist who designed the Tool Chest handbooks and DVDs offers many activities for home and school. Her focus is on mitigating undesirable behaviors by addressing their sensory roots. She travels around the United States giving workshops for school systems. Her techniques are worth seeing if she is ever in your area. Go to her website at <www.ateachabout.com> to see her schedule.

Sensory Learning A unique program, which does not come from an occupational therapist, is the Sensory Learning Institute, founded in 1997 by Mary Bolles, a mother who was seeking help for her son. Not speaking at age three, Jason was exhibiting behaviors consistent with children on the autism spectrum. Mary discovered that combining three individual modalities (visual, auditory and vestibular) into one multi-sensory experience provided the positive results she'd been seeking for Jason.

This intervention targets students at both ends of the autism spectrum. Based on an evaluation of an individual's auditory, visual and vestibular function, computer assisted technology prescribes an individualized remediation program. The visual component uses syntonics: colored lights that pulse on and off about six times per minute. The vestibular stimulation is delivered on a motion table that rotates in various planes. The auditory part uses headphones that contain modulated music.

About 15 Sensory Learning Program centers nationwide, provide clients with two 30-minute sessions each day for 12 consecutive days, including weekends and holidays. Each session is an individual sensory experience simultaneously engaging visual, auditory and vestibular systems to work in an integrated way. The repetitive sensory activation of each session builds on the session before. After 12 days of sessions, the individual returns home with a portable light instrument to continue the program, with a 20-minute session each morning and evening for the next 18 days. Several Sensory Learning Centers are under the direction of optometrists. For more information on Sensory Learning and locations of centers, go to <www.sensorylearning.com>.

HANDLE is another non-occupational therapy-based program that treats the sensory issues in autism along with the accompanying nutritional and digestive problems. An acronym for the **H**olistic **A**pproach to **N**euro**D**evelopment and **L**earning **E**fficiency, the concept for this approach grew out of founder Judith Bluestone's need to understand and heal her own challenges.

Since 1994 the HANDLE Institute in Seattle, Washington, has certified hundreds of trainers across the United States, in Israel, the United Kingdom, South Africa and Australia. Thousands of individuals have benefited from HANDLE training for learning disabilities, attention deficits, autism, PDD, dyspraxia, language disorders, Tourette syndrome and a plethora of perceptual and behavioral disorders.

Strengthening the vestibular system, enhancing muscle tone and increasing differentiation are the goals of HANDLE. These are all accomplished through deceptively simplistic activities that are sensitive to the client's physical and social-emotional needs. Small, measured doses of specific activities are incorporated into daily activities in the home or in a daycare/school setting. Therapy time typically requires approximately a half hour, preferably interspersed throughout the day. Some of the more frequently suggested activities involve:

* drinking from a crazy straw
* playing follow-the-leader with a flashlight
* rhythmic ball bouncing
* copying designs by feel alone
* catching a suspended ball
* stepping through a hula hoop "maze"

For more information on HANDLE, read *The Fabric of Autism: Weaving the Threads into a Cogent Theory*[48] and visit <www.handle.org>.

In *Asperger Syndrome and Sensory Issues*,[10] the authors include over 25 pages of behaviors, such as "has rituals," "won't eat certain foods," and "poor eye contact" with possible sensory interpretations and suggested interventions. This section of the book is worth having as a reference for parents to help them understand the role of touch, movement, vision and the other senses in the aberrant behavior they see in their kids.

The Squeeze Machine

Dr. Temple Grandin, probably the most well-known and successful adult with autism, invented the squeeze machine. As a child she regularly visited a relative's farm where she was attracted to the machine used to restrain cows while they were branded. She loved the deep pressure the machine provided her body, and found that it calmed her and decreased her severe tactile defensiveness. This life-changing experience led to her career as the world's authority on livestock handling equipment.

Today, families of children with autism can purchase a prototype she designed, available for use in homes and schools from the Therafin Corporation at <www.therafin.com>. The Squeeze Machine allows the individual to control the amount of and need for pressure. According to the website, "this ingenious system is used for deep touch stimulation and produces a calming effect on hyperactive and autistic individuals."

Sensory Connections to Other Problems in Autism

Sleep disturbances, picky eating, and toilet training, three of the most problematic issues in autism spectrum disorders, all have sensory connections. Parents frequently call upon the occupational therapist to intervene in these troublesome areas.

Sleep Children at both ends of the spectrum have difficulties falling asleep, staying asleep and waking up. Professionals in the field attribute these difficulties to sensory regulatory issues. Physical therapist Debra Dickson and occupational therapist Anne Buckley-Rein conceived a sleep hygiene program called SANE. The SANE approach facilitates change through restorative **S**leep, **A**ctivities to reduce stress, balanced **N**utrition, and nurturing **E**nvironments.

The SANE program begins 30 minutes before lights out.

- **Establish a set bedtime** - 7:30 pm for preschoolers and 8:30 pm for school-age.
- **Banish TV, computer or video games for at least one hour before bedtime** - These tend to rev up, rather than calm down, young minds.
- **Provide a calming and soothing warm bath for about 15 minutes, followed by a deep towel massage to arms, legs, back, hands and feet** - Add Epsom salts for detox and calming. Speak quietly and soothingly. Put on pajamas and get straight into bed. (This is important because the body temperature drops after coming out of the bath, just as it does in the first stage of sleep- so the body is already "gearing down.")
- **Read one short story and turn the lights out.** Accept no excuses for more.
- **Offer protein and B vitamins**, especially at breakfast and lunch to achieve a deep restorative sleep 12 hours later. Diets high in sugar and other stimulants (chocolate, caffeine) will inhibit sleep. Save these treats for special occasions; never eat them after 4 pm. Check also for side effects of medications which very often interfere with sleep cycles.
- **Adjust the energy flow in children's bedrooms**, according to feng shui principles. For children who need lights on to fall asleep, get a dimmer switch and turn lights all the way out, once they are asleep. Any light on in the night will stimulate the pineal gland and inhibit production of sleep hormone.
- **Use music** with a 60 beat per minute tempo to calm to body and mind and regulate the child who is out of balance. Try two great CDs: "Baby Go To Sleep" (birth to 7) and "The Surf" (all ages). Played throughout the night on repeat mode the music enhances regulation of the sleep cycles.

Buckley-Rein and Dickson contend that following their routine at the same time every night, results in significant changes in 1-2 weeks.[49]

Picky eating The nutritional issues in autism are covered in Chapter 5. Nutritional deficiencies often begin as early as in the preemie nursery with a combination of sensory and oral motor issues. Tubes taped to the faces of tiny babies produce sensitivities on the lips and face. Babies can emerge from the infant intensive care unit (ICU) with tactile defensiveness, low tone, or hypo-sensitivity in the very areas responsible for their survival. Nursing from a breast or a bottle may be difficult. As feeding becomes a challenge, infants and mothers become anxious. The train has just left the station for a possible lifetime of eating disorders.

Occupational and speech-language therapists recognize that oral motor difficulties affect both eating and speaking. Therapists in both fields address oral motor problems. Some hospitals have "feeding clinics" featuring a multi-disciplinary team of oral motor specialists and nutritionists. Without early, expert oral motor therapy, many infants are destined to become picky eaters.

While many teams have developed protocols for oral motor deficiencies, Theresa Szypulski has conceived one specifically addressing oral motor deficiencies in autism, which she calls Interactive Oral Sensory-Motor (IOSM).[50] She believes that dyspraxia and sensory deficits are primary. First she does an assessment of the child's oral sensory seeking/avoiding behaviors and oral motor capabilities and tolerances. Next, she gently guides oral sensory input at the child's comfort level and ability, keeping the stimulation pleasurable. She then regulates the level of input while engaging the client in a "teachable moment" designed to shape communication behaviors, including eye contact and vocalizations. At the same time she mediates undesirable and socially inappropriate behaviors, replacing them with more acceptable ones.

Kelly Dorfman, a nutritionist in suburban Washington, DC, and co-founder of Developmental Delay Resources (DDR),[51] is an expert on picky eating. Her approach focuses on the nutritional and oral motor deficits, as well as on the psycho-emotional and behavioral issues in picky eating.

She believes that children with autism, especially those with significant sensory issues, refuse food because this is one way they can control their surroundings in order to lessen their anxiety. Dorfman notes four factors which contribute to picky eating:

- Sensory misreading in the mouth or poor oral-motor skills
- Nutritional deficiencies
- Weak digestive function
- Drug side effects

Oral-motor problems are the shared expertise of OTs and speech-language pathologists. Families of picky eaters must seek out an oral motor expert to facilitate better eating. Chapter 5 covers both nutritional deficiencies and weak digestive function in those with autism spectrum disorders, and methods of alleviating both. Decreased appetite is one of the many side effects of prescription drugs. Before assuming that a child is not hungry, consider lowering the dosage of medications with this reaction. Parents often must choose between the problematic behavior without a drug and a different behavior or symptom caused by a drug. For that reason alone, over-the-counter supplements may be preferable.[52]

To encourage children to eat better, Dorfman recommends that parents stay focused on healthy eating without forcing. Positive changes take place when parents take charge of their own behavior. Because children are so closely linked to their parents, when adults change, kids must also change their responses. Psychotherapists insist that you cannot change another person, but you can affect the dynamics of any relationship by changing yourself.

Dorfman lists four steps in approaching picky eating.

Step 1- Work on one food at a time. A new food everyday is overwhelming. Pick one item that would improve the diet. If a child already eats ice cream and milk, pudding is not qualitatively better. Consider fruits, vegetables or protein foods (like small pieces of chicken). These foods are often missing in the diets of fussy eaters.

Choose a version of the food close in texture to other foods the child eats. Kids preferring soft creamy foods might handle applesauce or pureed chicken soup. For those drawn to crunch try peeled cucumbers or thinly sliced apple. Also consider foods the child liked in the past but no longer eats.

Step 2- Give a child a small "job." Learning to eat well is a job. Children should be told ahead of time that their job is to learn to eat healthy foods like Elmo, Thomas the Tank Engine or some other figure they like. Their "job" is a doable task, such as taking one bite or in extreme cases, picking up the food. Encourage them to help you select the food by giving them several choices.

Step 3- Acknowledge only positive behavior. Most fussy eaters will refuse both when asked to chose between pears and carrots. If this occurs say, "I see you need help deciding, so I will pick this time. You can choose next time." The child can then see that lack of cooperation changes nothing.

Food appearing at dinner (a better time than the morning) is another opportunity for the child to see if resistance works. Keep discussion about the "job" to a minimum. If the task is accomplished, stay warm and connected. Act like you knew he could do it all along. If the child refuses or throws a fit, briefly make sure he is safe and walk away. Say you will return when he calms down.

If the job is unfinished, become unavailable for anything else the child wants until it is. Put off watching TV, reading a story, playing computer games or going to the park until the job is done. Don't threaten; say "when, then." When you are finished eating, then we can read a story. If a child wanders around all evening without eating the food, simply comment that tomorrow you will be working on the job again.

Step 4- If you lose your temper, take a time out. Teach children that cooperating works. After a long day, even when it is challenging, stay calm when they are frustrated and misbehaving. When you reach your limits, give yourself a time out. Forcing a child into "time-out" rewards bad conduct with increased interaction. A child needs a parent to stay calm, so he can get calm.

Dorfman believes that focusing on positive attempts at eating, youngsters learn to get attention by cooperating. With consistent application of this principle, even the most finicky eater can expand his palate.[53]

Toilet Training Toilet training is one of the most elusive milestones for many families working with children on the autism spectrum. Sensing that the bladder or intestine is full and acting upon it requires a high level of sensory integration. When children with autism are calm, they may be able to feel the sensations that they need to urinate or defecate, but if they experience sensory overload they may not be able to feel that urge. Thus, sometimes these kids can use the toilet correctly, while at other times they will not.

Dr. Temple Grandin believes that severe sensory processing problems play a large role in toileting issues. Some children may like to flush the toilet repeatedly as pleasurable sensory stimulation. For others with severe hearing sensitivities, the sound of the toilet flushing may hurt their ears or simply terrify them.

Grandin states two major causes of toilet training problems in children with autism: they are either afraid of the toilet or they do not know what they are supposed to do. Sometimes the highly sensitive child can learn to use a potty chair located a short distance from the frightening toilet. Most need to see someone else use the toilet in order to learn.[54]

Several excellent references enumerate management strategies for toilet training the child with autism. A chapter is devoted to this subject in *Autism: A Sensorimotor Approach to Management*.[55] *Toilet Training for Individuals with Autism and Related Disorders*[56] is a complete book on the subject. Both focus first on habit training and determining readiness, then on sensory strategies and generalizing to unfamiliar environments. Readers interested in this subject should consult these excellent resources.

Conclusion

Sensory issues in autism often are responsible for behaviors that are unacceptable. Instead of trying to extinguish them, therapists taking a sensory approach evaluate behaviors, always looking for possible underlying sensory causes. Once it is determined which senses are hyper-reactive, and which may be hypo-responsive, an intervention program can be designed to normalize sensory processing, and thus normalize behavior.

Occupational therapists and others have put together innovative programs that can help those with autism spectrum disorders. Developmental optometrists and occupational therapists have worked together for years co-treating patients with visual and motor problems. The patient with autism offers another opportunity for mutually beneficial collaboration. Sensory integration theory and practice includes vision, and patients on both ends of the autism spectrum have sensory issues that affect and are affected by vision. Both evaluation and treatment options offer each profession a chance to grow in knowledge and experience. The patient who works with both optometrists and professionals who focus on resolving the sensory issues inherent in the autism diagnosis will inevitably have the best prospects for maximal performance.

References

1. Rimland B. Infantile Autism: The syndrome and its Implications for a Neural Therapy of Behavior. New York: Appleton Century Crofts, 1964.

2. Ornitz EM. Disorders of perception common to early infantile autism and schizophrenia. Comprehensive Psychiatr 1969; 10: 259-74.

3. www.brainyquote.com (Accessed January 28, 2008)

4. Delacato C. The Ultimate Stranger: The Autistic Child. Novato, CA: Academic Therapy Publications,. 1974.

5. Cool SJ. Occupational therapy and functional optometry: an interaction whose time has come? Sensory Integration Special Interest Newsletter, AOTA 1987; 10:1-6.

6. Hellerstein LF, Fishman B. Vision therapy and occupational therapy: an integrated approach. J Behav Optom 1990; 1(5): 122-6.

7. Hellerstein LF, Fishman B. Collaboration between occupational therapists and optometrists. J Behav Optom 1999; 10(6):147-52.

8. Miller-Kuhaneck H. ed, Autism, A Comprehensive Occupational Therapy Approach, Bethesda, MD: AOTA Press, 2004.

9. Smith Roley S, Blanche EI, Schaaf RC, eds. Understanding the Nature of Sensory Integration in Diverse Populations. Tucson, AZ: Therapy Skill Builders, 2001.

10. Murray-Slutsky C, Paris BA. Exploring the Spectrum of Autism and Pervasive Developmental Disorders: Intervention Strategires. San Antonio, TX: Therapy Skill Builders, 2000.

11. Huebner RA, ed. Autism: A Sensorimotor Approach to Management. Gaithersburg, MD: Aspen Publishers, 2001.

12. Bogdashina O. Sensory Perceptual Issues in Autism and Asperger Syndrome. Different Sensory Experiences, Different Perceptual Worlds. London: Jessica Kingsley Publishers, 2003.

13. Myles BS, Cook KT, Miller N. et al. Asperger Syndrome and Sensory Issues.. Shawnee Mission, KS: Autism Asperger Publishing Co., 2000.

14. Mailloux Z. Sensory integrative principles in intervention with children with autistic disorder. In Smith Roley S, Blanche EI, Schaaf RC, eds. Understanding the Nature of Sensory Integration in Diverse Populations. Tucson, AZ: Therapy Skill Builders 2001, 365-84.

15. Moore JC. The Functional Components of the Nervous System: Part I. Sensory Integration Qrly 1994; 22:1-7.

16. Kawar M. Oculomotor Control: An Integral Part of Sensory Integration. In Bundy AC, Lane SJ, Murray E, eds. Sensory Integration: Theory and Practice, 2nd ed. Philadelphia, PA: FA Davis Company, 2002.

17. Ayres AJ. Sensory Integration and Learning Disorders. Los Angeles: Western Psychological Services, 1972: 113-29.

18. Solan HA, Shelley-Tremblay J, Larson S. Vestibular function, sensory integration and balance anomalies: a brief literature review. Optom Vis Dev 2007; 38:1-5.

19. Bluestone J. *The Foundations of HANDLE.* www.handle.org Accessed December 27, 2007.

20. Ayres AJ. *Sensory Integration and the Child.* Los Angeles: Western Psychological Services, 1979: 184.

21. Spitzer S, Smith Roley S. *Sensory integration revisited: a philosophy of practice.* In Smith Roley S, Blanche EI, Schaaf RC, eds. *Understanding the Nature of Sensory Integration in Diverse Populations.* Tucson, AZ: Therapy Skill Builders 2001, 5.

22. www.siglobalnet.net (Accessed January 30, 2008)

23. American Psychiatric Association. *Diagnostic and Statistical Manual of Mental Disorders, Fourth Edition (DSM-IV)* Washington, DC: American Psychiatric Association, 2000.

24. Wallis C. *The next attention deficit disorder?* Time November 29, 2007:

25. Ayres AJ. *Hyper-responsivity to touch and vestibular stimuli as a predictor of positive response to sensory integration procedures in autistic children.* Am J Occup Ther 1980; 34: 375-86.

26. Baranek GT, Foster LG, Berkson G. *Tactile defensiveness and stereotyped behaviors.* Am J Occup Ther 1997; 51:91-5.

27. Greenspan SI, Wieder S. *Developmental patterns and outcomes in infants and children with disorders in relating and communicating: A chart review of 200 cases of children with autistic spectrum diagnoses.* J Dev Learn Dis 1997; 1:87-142.

28. Piek JP, Dyck, M.J. *Sensory-motor deficits in children with developmental coordination disorder, attention deficit hyperactivity disorder and autistic disorder.* Hum Movement Sci 2004; 23, 475-88.

29. Molloy CA, Kietrich KN, Bhattacharya A. *Postural stability in children with autism spectrum disorder.* J Aut Dev Dis 2003; 33(6):643-52.

30. Jones V, Prior, M. *Motor imitation abilities and neurological signs in autistic children.* J Aut Dev Dis 1985, 15:37-46.

31. Case-Smith J, Miller, H. *Occupational therapy with children with pervasive developmental disorders.* Am J Occup Ther 1999; 53:506-13.

32. Teitelbaum P, Teitelbaum O, Nye N, Fryman J, Maurer R. *Movement analysis in infancy may be useful for early diagnosis of autism.* Proc. Natl. Acad. Sci USA 1998; 95:13982-7.

33. Trecker A. *Play and Praxis in Children with an Autism Spectrum Disorder.* In Miller-Kuhaneck H, ed. *Autism, A Comprehensive Occupational Therapy Approach* 2nd ed Bethesda, MD: AOTA Press, 2004.

34. Ayres AJ. *Developmental Dyspraxia and Adult Onset Apraxia.* Torrance, CA: Sensory Integration International, 1985.

35. Rogers SJ, Bennetto L, McEvoy R et. al. *Imitation and pantomine in high functioning adolescents with autism spectrum disorders.* Child. Dev 1996; 67:2060-73.

36. Suchoff IB. *Cognitive Development: Piaget's Theory.* Santa Ana, CA: Optometric Extension Program; 1978.

37. Hessellund K, Nutto J. *Understanding Occupational Therapy's Role in Sensory Integration.* In: Barber A, ed. *Vision and Sensory Integration,* Santa Ana, CA: Optometric Extension Program, 1999.

38. Kientz MA, Miller H. *Classroom evaluation of the child with autism.* School System Special Interest Section Qtly 1999, 6(1):1-4.

39. Dunn W. *The Sensory Profile.* San Antonio, TX: The Psychological Corporation, 1999.

40. Ermer J, Dunn W. *The Sensory Profile: A discriminant analysis of children with and without disabilities.* Am J Occup Ther 1998; 52:283-90.

41. Miller-Kuhaneck H, Henry D, Glennon TJ, Parham D, Ecker CL. *The Sensory Processing Measure.* Los Angeles, CA. Western Psychological Services, 2007.

42. Ayres AJ. *Sensory Integration and Praxis Test.* Los Angeles, CA: Western Psychological Services, 1989.

43. Parham D, Mailloux Z, Smith Roley S. *Sensory processing and praxis in high functioning children with autism.* Paper presented at Research 2000, Feb 4-5, 2000, Redondo Beach, CA.

44. Watling R., Dietz J. .*Immediate effect of Ayres's sensory integration-based occupational therapy intervention on children with autism spectrum disorders.* Amer J Occup Ther 2007: 61(5): 574-83.

45. Williams MS, Shellenberger S. *How Does Your Engine Run? A Leaders' Guide to the Alert Program for Sensory Regulation.* Albuquerque, NM: Therapy Works, 1996.

46. Henry D. *Tool Chest for Teachers, Parents and Students.* Youngtown, AZ: Henry OT Services, 1999.

47. Williams MS, Shellenberger S. *Take Five! Staying Alert at Home and School.* Albuquerque, NM: Therapy Works, 2001.

48. Bluestone J. *The Fabric of Autism: Weaving the Threads into a Cogent Theory.* Seattle, WA: The HANDLE Institute 2004.

49. Buckley-Rein A, Dickson D. *The SANE approach to sleep.* New Dev Winter 2002-2003; 8(2):6.

50. Szypulski TA. Oral sensory-motor therapy as a portal to interaction in autism. *New Dev* Fall 2003;9(1):4.

51. www.devdelay.org or 800-297-0944.

52. Dorfman K. The picky eater, *New Dev* 1999 Spring; 4(4): 6.

53. Dorfman K. Picky eater part 2 *New Dev* 2002 Fall; 8(1): 7.

54. http://www.autism.org/temple/faq.html (Accessed January 28, 2008)

55. Leone EF, Rogers SL. Sensory applications for sleep and toilet training. In Huebner RA., ed. *Autism: A Sensorimotor Approach to Management.* Gaithersburg, MD: Aspen Publishers, 2001: 355-63.

56. Wheeler M. *Toilet Training for Individuals with Autism and Related Disorders: A Comprehensive Guide for Parents and Teachers,* Arlington, TX: Future Horizons, 2001.

Chapter 8
Primitive Reflexes and
Autism Spectrum Disorders

Patricia S. Lemer, MEd, NCC
Contributing authors:
Samuel Berne, OD, FCOVD, FCSO
Carol Marusich, OD, FCOVD
Brendan O'Hara

Have you ever watched a baby startle, grasp at an adult's hand, or turn his head toward an out-stretched arm? These behaviors are the result of primitive "survival" reflexes. Termed "survival," primitive reflexes protect the fetus in utero, assist in the birthing process, and help the newborn learn and develop outside the safe confines of its mother's womb.

What are Primitive Reflexes?

Primitive reflexes are involuntary, stereotyped movements that an infant makes in response to a stimulus. Babies are born with many reflexes, which emerge sequentially during the first weeks of fetal development. Primitive reflexes account for most of the movement patterns during the first few months of life. Visually, they help infants to focus on and identify what they see in front of them; to coordinate the eyes to work together; and to develop accommodation and depth perception. Neurologically, primitive reflexes provide infants with learning experiences that build the foundation for all motor and cognitive skills.

Primitive reflexes originate in the brainstem, the earliest part of the brain to develop. The brainstem directs them without involvement of the higher, more recently evolved cerebral cortex. One section of the brainstem, the Reticular Activating System (RAS), responsible for arousal and muscle tone, has been implicated in Attention Deficit Disorder.[1] Any load factors, especially birth trauma and vaccines can harm the RAS. The result is impaired attention, concentration and tone.

Ideally, primitive reflexes have a limited life span of six to 12 months. They emerge at a predictable time of development to assist in moving the baby from motorically helpless to ambulatory. As each fulfills its function, it integrates just as a more advanced postural reflex, controlled by the cortex, emerges. The higher brain centers know reflexively how to integrate primitive reflexes so that the postural reflexes can move the baby through the appropriate steps of growth and development.

When primitive reflexes linger in the brainstem, they can interfere with development in the cerebellum. Unintegrated reflexes can thus impede normal sensory and motor development because the brainstem interferes with cortical processing.

What do Reflexes have to do with Learning and Behavior?

Moving the body intentionally helps lay the foundations for learning and controlled behavior. As primitive reflexes integrate and postural reflexes emerge, a baby begins to move. The developing child gradually acquires intentional muscle control in the eyes, mouth, limbs, hands and feet. This control allows the child to move eyes independently and together, to shape the mouth to make sounds and chew, to crawl, walk, and to write legibly. The sequential integration of primitive reflexes and emergence of postural reflexes is responsible for all later learning and behavior.

Any of the factors comprising the "total load" can interfere with reflex emergence or integration. Optometrist Carol Marusich believes that impediments can be pre- peri- or post-natal.[2] A traumatic birth, prematurity, health issues, and lack of opportunity can all contribute to problems with reflexes. Many occupational therapists and other professionals working in the field of motor development believe that some of today's societal practices are interfering with the natural emergence of reflexes. Recommending that babies sleep only on their backs to prevent sudden infant death syndrome (SIDS), for instance, denies them of opportunities to use their hands to bear weight and to connect the hands with the eyes to crawl. Specialists are thus having to prescribe '"tummy time" for babies whose development lags.

"Tummy time" is essential for an infant to learn midline awareness and bilateral integration. Children with limited tummy time experience problems with later learning tasks that require crossing the midline, such as writing.

In the developmental sequence, the next step for the infant who is on her tummy is to push up into a sitting position. Transitioning to sitting helps develop muscle tone and arousal, as well as proper head and neck control, both prerequisites to later oculomotor control and binocularity. In experiencing this important developmental transition, the infant is also learning neurological flexibility, going from a disorienting experience to a reorienting experience – a critical phase in overall mind-body control. The strength of an infant's head and neck control also reflect the level of vestibular development. Optometrists should thus observe head and neck control as a part of any infant visual evaluation.

Problems arise when primitive reflexes are weak, early, late or retained,[3] because then they interfere with both motor and vision development. If a baby misses steps in motor development or acquires unusual motor patterns, resultant movements are neither smooth nor coordinated. When muscles obey an unconscious reflex instead of responding to intention, skills cannot become automatic. Eye movements might be poor, and an individual could have difficulty shifting from nearpoint to distance. Only when primitive reflexes emerge strongly and integrate to be replaced by postural reflexes, can a baby gradually gain control of both the body and visual skills. He/she can then achieve the right balance between automatic and intentional learning and behavior.

Academic learning depends upon the automatization of basic skills at a physical level. If a child fails to develop automatic motor control, a teacher might observe such symptoms as poor concentration, distractibility, reversals in reading and writing, mis-articulations, poor impulse control, trouble reading body language or unsatisfactory peer relationships, all despite good intelligence. Without addressing the underlying neuro-developmental problem, smooth growth is unlikely.

An Historical View of Reflexes

According to Sally Goddard, the earliest reference to the word "reflex" can be traced to a seventeenth century medical physiologist, Thomas Willis. Willis used the terms "motus reflexus" and "reflexion" to describe how "spirits" in the nerves reflected back to the muscles. Today's model dates back only to the 1960s, and focuses on the relationship between the presence of unintegrated reflexes and the motor, sensory-motor and vision problems seen in autism spectrum disorders.[4]

Twentieth century research was undertaken mostly by occupational therapists.[5] In a 1976 study, Dr. Miriam Bender, a pioneer in learning disabilities (LD), found that 75% of those diagnosed with LD had a retained symmetric tonic neck reflex (STNR).[6] O'Dell and Cook, psychologists who co-founded and directed a center in Indianapolis continuing Dr.

Bender's work, found a retained STNR to be a significant factor in a group of children with ADD and AD(H)D. All improved markedly when the STNR was integrated as a result of a specific movement program.[7] Bein-Wierzbinski used an infra-red computerized eye tracking machine to show that the STNR was a factor in a group of children with eye tracking problems.[8] Later, Pavlides found that a high percentage of children with learning disabilities omitted stages of crawling and creeping in infancy, which is consistent with a retained STNR.[9]

Of all the reflexes, the symmetric tonic neck reflex (STNR) can be one of the most troublesome, interfering with visual function in those on both the mild and severe ends of the spectrum. See the sections that follow on the STNR for more details on this important reflex.

What Do Primitive Reflexes Have to Do with Autism Spectrum Disorders?

Most individuals on the autism spectrum still retain some primitive reflexes. The interference of reflexes with the development of complex motor skills most probably accounts for some of their odd movement and behavior patterns. Any child whose body fails to gain full control over primitive reflexes develops in what Goddard calls a reflexive "no man's land" where some of the primitive reflexes remain present and the postural reflexes cannot develop fully. These children, who have enormous difficulty with voluntary movement patterns, are eventually labeled "dyspraxic" or "apraxic" in addition to being given labels on the autism spectrum.

In a 1998 study of home videotapes of 17 infants later diagnosed with autism,[10] Philip Teitelbaum, PhD. observed atypical ways of rolling over, sitting up, crawling, and walking in all subjects. Every child demonstrated at least one movement disturbance by six months of age. The subjects had difficulty turning over, supporting themselves to crawl, and struggled to move forward by resting weight on their elbows or forearms, digging in their toes and lifting their rumps. Some pulled themselves along with one arm beneath the torso, while attempting to crawl with the free arm. Others crawled atypically, with one leg moving and the other leg dragging behind. Most were late in walking.

A follow-up study in 2002[11] suggested that unintegrated reflexes were at the root of the movement disturbances in Teitelbaum's subjects, especially those later diagnosed with Asperger syndrome. Consistent with a total load approach, Teitelbaum has suggested movement analysis of infants as a means for early identification of those who might become autistic. Is it possible that a reflex remediation program could have prevented autism in these infants?

Brendan O'Hara, an Australian expert on movement in learning, believes that identifying and integrating retained reflexes in women before they become pregnant, or even during pregnancy, can reduce reflex issues in their unborn babies. While not "genetic," these neurological pathways move from generation to generation without intervention.[12]

Sally Goddard and her husband Peter Blythe have emerged as the premier researchers in the relationship between reflexes, learning and behavior. They use "Neuro-Developmental Delay (NDD)" as an umbrella term which includes most of the diagnoses in the autism spectrum. The Institute for Neuro-Physiological Psychology (INPP), in Chester, England, which they direct, attracts practitioners from around the world to training courses, workshops and an annual spring conference. To learn more go to <www.inpp.org.uk>.

INPP researchers have identified over 100 primitive reflexes. The most common ones discussed in the literature are the amphibian, asymmetrical tonic neck, babinski, fear paralysis, head-righting, moro, palmar, plantar, rooting, spinal gallant, tonic labyrinthine, suckling, symmetrical tonic neck, and vestibular. While each of these has a purpose in development, this chapter focuses on only five. Those interested in learning more are urged to consult one of the primary references.

Table 8-1 lists the five primitive reflexes that most affect development, their lifespan, purpose and potential hazards of retention.

Table 8-1 Primitive Reflexes that Most Affect Development in Autism Spectrum Disorders				
Name of Reflex	Emerges at	Integrated by	Purpose	Lack of Integration Can Cause Problems with
Moro Reflex	9 weeks in utero	2-4 months	Survival; also known as "startle reflex"	Balance and coordination, visual-motor processing
Tonic Labyrinthine Reflex	16 weeks in utero	6 weeks to 3 years. Most by 4 months	Integrates head with neck to work against gravity	Balance, tone, visual-motor processing
Spinal Galant Reflex	20 weeks in utero	9 months	Assists body through birth canal. Enables response to sound vibration in utero	Bladder control, attention, concentration, short-term memory
Asymmetrical Tonic Neck Reflex	18 weeks in utero	6 months	Assists body through birth canal. Coordinates 2 sides of the body	Crawling, walking, skipping, balance, laterality, convergence
Symmetrical Tonic Neck Reflex	6-9 months	9-11 months	Assists in rising up on hands & knees	Creeping, crawling, crossing the midline, focusing, reading, writing

The next section provides a description of each reflex. The information combines writings of optometrists Samuel Berne and Carol Marusich, Sally Goddard (Blythe), Director of the Institute for Neuro-Physiological Psychology (INPP), in Chester, England and Brendan O'Hara. For an in depth view of Dr. Berne's approach, read his book *Without Ritalin: A Natural Approach to ADD*,[13] watch his DVD entitled "A.D.D. to Autism: Reaching Your Child's Potential Naturally"[14] and go to <www.newattention.net>.

Marusich observes that in the process of typical development, reflexes emerge in a distinct pattern from full flexion and extension such as in the Moro and TLR, to reflexes which involve individual movements. Examples are

- the Spinal Galant, which involves homolateral flexion and extension of body and head on one side only
- the ATNR, which involves homolateral flexion of the body on one side with homolateral extension of the body and head flexion on the opposite side
- the STNR, which involves upper body flexion with lower body extension or the opposite

The emergence of the later reflexes involve movement patterns which "break up" earlier patterns, causing movements out of the full flexion or extension postures. As these reflexes emerge, the infant gains experience with individual movement patterns outside of the earlier reflex movement patterns. It is her belief that this movement experience is key in the integration of movement patterns through which the infant can experience and learn voluntary movement control.

Marusich has lectured extensively on this subject. Readers can obtain an audiotape of the presentation she gave at the 2002 COVD annual meeting from <www.instatapes.com> or watch her DVD, "Integration of Primitive Motor Reflexes: Why Should I Care?"[2]

Goddard's work is published as *Reflexes, Learning and Behavior*[4] and *The Well Balanced Child: Movement and Early Learning.*[15] All are available from OEP. To learn more about O'Hara go to <www.movementandlearning.com.au>.

The Moro Reflex

The Moro Reflex is the earliest to emerge in utero. It facilitates the first "breath of life," opening the windpipe if there is a threat of suffocation. Maturing into the adult "startle" reflex, the Moro is an involuntary response to threat. Its role is as a survival mechanism in the first months of life.

The Moro is composed of a series of rapid movements of the arms upward and away from the body, accompanied by rapid inhalation and a startle response. It is a "fight or flight" response to threat which immediately alerts the sympathetic nervous system to danger. Blood pressure rises, stress hormones are released, the skin reddens, and an emotional outburst, such as tears or anger results. A Moro Reflex may be triggered by a loud noise, a change in head position, light or touch. When it emerges on time, and becomes integrated appropriately, it forms a strong foundation for future life experiences.

An unintegrated Moro Reflex keeps an individual in a survival mode, and can cause hyper-sensitivity to sound, light, movement or altered position, so that the person is always "on alert." Individuals on both ends of the spectrum can demonstrate Moro Reflex problems. The energy depleting mode of constantly fighting perceived danger leaves scanty reserves for other bodily processes such as digestion and respiration, let alone development and learning.

Many visual abnormalities are indicative of a poorly integrated Moro Reflex. Marusich includes
- poor pupillary response to light
- oculomotor problems
- difficulty with attention to detail
- accommodative dysfunction
- Streff syndrome[2]

Berne also relates late integration of the Moro Reflex to biochemical and nutritional imbalances, which lead to lowered immunity and allergies, resulting in ear and throat infections. Sound familiar?

O'Hara splits the Moro into three parts: physical, auditory and visual. He tests each individually. Visually, an unintegrated Moro can result in difficulties with fixation as well as visual-motor problems.

Symptoms of an unintegrated Moro Reflex
- experiencing the world as too bright and too loud
- difficulty in social situations
- motion sickness
- poor balance
- tight and inflexible muscles
- need to be "in control"
- problems with visual fixation, excessive blinking, poor eye contact

Testing for the Moro Reflex
Physical: Have the child lie on his/her back with two pillows behind the head. Kneeling behind the child, hold the head and move it around, feeling for tension in the neck. Then, gently pick up the head and drop it three inches before catching it. An alternative is to have the person stand or sit. Then lean back or tilt the chair back, while you support him from behind. "Drop" him a few inches, and watch for a response. *Auditory*: Say "boo" or drop a noisy object, such as keys, unexpectedly, and look for a startle. *Visual*: Bring the palm of the hand close to the person's face very quickly. Look for repeated blinking.

The Moro Reflex is positive
- if there is tension in the neck
- you hear a sharp inhalation
- the person blinks excessively or giggles
- arms and fingers fan out
- the face flushes red
- the subject reports anxiety or "a funny feeling" in the stomach

The Tonic Labyrinthine Reflex (TLR)
The Tonic Labyrinthine Reflex (TLR) also develops in utero and provides an infant with a primitive way of responding to gravity. Vertical movement of the head forward and backward causes the arms and legs to flex or extend, depending upon which way the head is moved. This is a "tonic" reflex, meaning that it influences muscle tone throughout the body.

Continuous flexion and extension help the newborn eventually straighten out from the flexed in-utero posture and to develop head control and balance. The TLR assists the young child in head-righting; head control is essential for eye control, as both operate from the vestibule-ocular reflex arc. Brendan O'Hara calls the TLR the "you can't put me in the car seat" reflex.

An infant on its belly works against gravity as soon as it lifts up its head using the neck muscles. Once this movement becomes automatic, sometime about six weeks of age, integration of the Tonic Labyrinthine Reflex begins. This is another reason why "tummy time" is so important. If the TLR fails to integrate, it will constantly "trip" the vestibular system and its interaction with the other senses.

When head control is lacking, visual function also suffers. Vision will be affected by poor balance, and balance will be affected by faulty visual processing. Lacking a secure point of reference in space, the child with an unintegrated TLR could experience difficulties with understanding spatial relationships. As the child tries to walk, he will not be able to acquire true gravitational security, as the head throws off his center of balance.[2] Older children who cannot maintain an upright position for extended periods of time may also have an unintegrated TLR. A lingering TLR thus has wide-reaching ramifications, interfering with all activities that depend upon balance, muscle tone, and visual-motor processing.

Symptoms of an unintegrated TLR
- poor stamina
- gravitational insecurity
- slumped posture
- low tone
- sitting with leg wrapped around the chair
- fear of heights
- poor depth perception
- figure/ground problems
- toe walking
- motion sickness
- convergence insufficiency

Testing for the TLR
Have the child lie on his/her stomach, with arms out to the side like airplane wings, at 45 to 60 degrees, palms down, legs straight, and toes pointed. On the count of three, simultaneously lift head, arms, and legs straight up, as if flying. While the child is posed, ask questions to observe if he/she can talk and think while holding the position. Young children should be able to hold for at least 10 seconds; children over age six for up to 20 seconds.

The TLR is positive if the
- child is holding his/her breath
- body, arms or legs shake or rock from side to side
- child cannot hold the head up
- legs bend or thighs remain on the floor

The Spinal Galant Reflex
The Spinal Galant Reflex emerges about mid-term in pregnancy. This reflex is elicited by placing a hand under the baby's tummy, suspending it in the air, then stroking the skin on one side of the back along the spine from shoulder to hip. The baby's trunk and hips should swing towards the side of the stimulus, as a result of the contraction of the abdominal and other muscles.

Research indicates that pre-natally, the Spinal Galant enables the fetus to hear and feel sound vibrations in the aquatic environment in the womb.[4] At birth, it serves to help the baby work its way down the birth canal during labor.

If the Spinal Galant Reflex lingers beyond the neonatal period, it can interfere with bladder control, resulting in bedwetting after successful toilet-training. When the reflex competes with the child's attention and short-term memory, the child may appear distracted and need to be in constant motion.

Symptoms of an unintegrated Spinal Galant Reflex
- fidgeting, squirming, difficulty sitting still
- preference for loose-fitting clothing
- poor concentration and/or short-term memory
- bed wetting
- hip rotation and/or curvature of the spine

Testing for the Spinal Galant
Have the child get up on hands and knees as if crawling. Feet should be straight and toes flat; back and legs should be parallel to the floor, like a table; arms and thighs are parallel to each other. Knees and wrists are at 90 degrees; elbows are not locked. Lift shirt and lower

pants slightly. Run a blunt pen lightly up and down each side of the spine. Look for any contraction or movement. Next, press hard with a finger, like shiatsu, on either side of the spine. Again, look for any contraction or movement.

The Spinal Galant is positive if you observe
* curling of the toes when the child assumes the position
* a movement or contraction of the hip on either side of the spine, toward the stimulated side, with or without pressure
* arching of the back

The Asymmetrical Tonic Neck Reflex (ATNR)
The ATNR also develops about halfway through the pregnancy, in utero. Most parents are familiar with this reflex, which is fully present at birth. Movement of the baby's head to one side elicits extension of the arm and leg on the same side, and flexion of the arm and leg on the opposite side. During uterine life the ATNR facilitates continuous motion, thus stimulating the vestibular system and developing muscle tone.

At birth, the ATNR coordinates with the Spinal Galant Reflex in moving the baby through birth canal. While the Spinal Galant moves the baby along, the ATNR helps the infant "unscrew" itself to get out. This twisting movement is the first experience of the infant in coordinating both sides of the body. Babies born by either forceps delivery or Cesarean section did not have the opportunity to use the ATNR. Deprived of the twisting action of the birth process, which provides necessary early bilateral integration imperative for the development of crawling, walking and cross lateral skipping, they are at risk having an unintegrated ATNR. Results of this deprivation can include problems with balance, confusion crossing the midline and mixed laterality.

An unintegrated ATNR can also have an adverse effect upon visual tracking. Children with unintegrated ATNRs often have trouble with bilateral activities such as using hands together for throwing, catching or writing. Every time they "keep their eye on the ball," the arm on the same side extends. The only way to throw accurately is to not keep the eye on the ball, thus allowing the elbow to bend in preparation for the throw. Likewise, every time they look at the pencil when writing, the arm extends slightly. Looking away causes the arm to flex. The back-and-forth motion on the pencil results in poor penmanship. To counteract this reflex, children with unintegrated ATNRs often look away as they write, viewing their pencils out of the corners of their eyes.[16]

The quadratus lumborum muscle, one of the muscles that runs down the lower back along the posterior abdominal wall, is associated with this reflex. Adults with lower back pain should undergo testing for a retained ATNR and work with ATNR integration activities.[17]

Symptoms of an Unintegrated ATNR
* left-right confusions
* homolateral skipping
* poor ball skills
* difficulty crossing the midline
* poor balance
* skipping words when reading
* illegible handwriting
* convergence insufficiency.
* classic case of a child labeled AD(H)D

Testing for the ATNR

Svetlana Masgutova recommends this quick check.[17] Have the person lie on his/her back. Stretch and relax each leg. Check the length of legs, noting any discrepancy. Turn the head to one side and recheck leg lengths compared to each other, noting any differences from first measurement. Turn head to the other side. Re-measure.

The ATNR is positive if

Leg length changes from initial measurement with head turned in either or both directions. What this finding means is that the neck, torso and legs are connected neurologically. In other words, there is an inability to isolate and differentiate each part: a mature and desirable response.

Alternative check

Ask the child get down onto the floor on hands and knees, with weight forward over both arms and elbows facing backwards. Roll up any sleeves so you can observe the arms. Get onto the floor next to the child, and gently guide the head from side to side, holding it on each side for five seconds. Place your hand on the child's shoulder and feel whether the movement is easy or restricted. Observe the shoulders and back.

The ATNR is positive if

- arms bow or elbows face out as child assumes the position
- you feel any restriction in the head or neck
- elbows buckle
- shoulders and/or back move or shiver

The Symmetrical Tonic Neck Reflex (STNR)

The STNR has an extremely short lifespan, emerging between six and nine months of life and integrating between nine and eleven months. This short-lived reflex is one of the most pesky, however, having the potential to interfere with many aspects of development. O'Dell and Cook, disciples of Dr. Miriam Bender, have written an entire book on the STNR[18] in which they suggest a relationship between a retained STNR and

- academic issues such as reading, writing, mathematics, spelling, art and music; athletic problems in basketball, football, golf, hockey, soccer, skiing, swimming, tennis, volleyball, and wrestling
- difficulties in public settings such as doctors' offices, beauty salons, restaurants, church, and sporting events; as well as
- psychological consequences such as poor peer relationships, low self esteem, frustration, avoidance, aggression and inflexibility

A major purpose of the STNR is to help the infant to defy gravity to get up on hands and knees and creep, then crawl. When a child is on all fours, flexion of the head causes the arms to bend and legs extend; extension of the head, on the other hand, causes the arms to straighten and the legs to flex. Children who retain the STNR rarely crawl on hands and knees; they scoot, shuffle along or "bear walk" on their hands alone. If they do crawl, they do so in an unsynchronized, unusual fashion, with rotated hands, locked elbows and raised feet.

Creeping and crawling are essential movement patterns for sensory development. The vestibular, proprioceptive and visual systems connect for the first time through creeping. Without going through this stage, babies end up with a poorly developed sense of balance, poor understanding of spatial relationships and poor depth perception.

The motions of creeping and crawling train the eyes to cross the midline of the body. Blythe suggests that the STNR serves to complete a developmentally appropriate sequence of natural vision training. Bending the legs as a result of head extension encourages an infant to fixate at a distance. Bending the arms in response to flexion automatically brings the child's focus back to near, thus developmentally "training" accommodation. Accommodation difficulties can thus be a result of an unintegrated STNR.

As the infant shifts weight from one hand to another, the eyes begin to focus from one side to the other. This learned skill is later necessary for reading, so that the eyes move across the page smoothly, without losing their place.

Dr. Billye Ann Cheatum, an adaptive physical education teacher for over 30 years and Professor at Texas Women's University, believes that one of the most significant difficulties for children with an unintegrated STNR is restricted bilateral movements.[16] The lingering STNR causes a child's legs to make the opposite movement of the neck and arms. If the neck flexes, so do the arms, while the legs extend. When the neck extends, so do the arms, while the legs flex. This bilateral movement of the STNR affects writing. Every movement of the head causes flexion and extension of the arms, making control of the wrist and fingers virtually impossible.

Students with unintegrated STNRs can be clumsy, messy eaters, poor at ball sports, demonstrate a slumping posture, and have difficulty coordinating eye and hand. They may be unable to use one arm without some associated movement in the other. Oppositional arm movements, such as marching, zipping and twisting off caps can also be problematic.

Another interesting symptom associated with an unintegrated STNR is the tendency to sit in the "W" position, a behavior often observed in children with attention deficits, learning disabilities, PDD and autism. O'Hara believes that W-sitters process the world slowly because they cannot distinguish whether their own bodies or the world is moving. They sit and watch, unable to move forward, lowering their center of gravity to improve their balance and feel more secure.[19]

Of all the reflexes, the STNR could be considered the reflex of most interest to the optometrist. Given the hierarchy of development, however, the earlier developing reflexes deserve a careful look before concentrating on this one.

Symptoms of a unintegrated STNR
- clumsiness
- poor posture, especially when sitting
- problems with vertical tracking
- accommodation difficulties
- difficulty copying from the board
- sitting in a "W" position on the floor
- poor eye-hand coordination
- poor or slow copying
- difficulty learning to swim

Testing for the STNR
Seat the child in a comfortable chair or put him/her in a crawling position with weight forward over both arms. Bend the head toward the chest and note extension and flexion of arms and legs. Then, pull the head back and observe again.

The STNR is positive if you observe
- bowed arms
- elbows facing out
- restricted head movement
- the head drop
- tremors in the body
- tense shoulders or arms
- weight shift away from arms, so that child falls back onto haunches
- arms moving in the same direction as the head, and legs moving in the opposite direction of head and arms

A Reflex Integration Program
A number of pioneers in the field, including Arnold Gesell, Carl Delacato, Glenn Doman, Temple Fay, Catherina Johanneson-Alvegard, Peter Blythe, and others, invented techniques in the 1960s to remediate aberrant reflexes in children on the less severe end of the spectrum. These students were diagnosed with "minimal brain dysfunction," (the predecessor of attention deficit disorder), learning disabilities, dyslexia and a plethora of other "disorders."[4]

Today's practitioners, including Berne, Blythe, Cheatum, O'Hara, Lena and Thorkild Rasmussen and others have developed specific protocols of movement activities designed to integrate each of the reflexes. A reflex integration program is based on the premise that it is possible to replicate missed stages of development by returning to the missed movement patterns and teaching them to the body through replication. This "patterning" gives the brain a second chance to develop critical neural connections which were omitted or incompletely developed during the first year of life.[4]

As reflexes integrate, the body shifts its attention away from basic motor development to more advanced motor and cognitive development. Learning occurs when physical skills such as balance and coordination of the top/bottom, left/right and front/back of the body all become automatic. This reciprocal interweaving is vital in the development of orientation.[20]

If a child does not develop automatic motor control early on, later behaviors such as reversals in writing and reading, poor attention and clumsiness could show up.[21] Although an individual may have good potential, strong abilities may not be realized until the motor delays are addressed. An inherent part of addressing general developmental delays is integrating the reflexes.

Berne recommends completing the primitive reflex integration program in the this order
- Moro Reflex
- Tonic Labyrinthine Reflex (TLR)
- Spinal Galant Reflex (SG)
- Asymmetrical Tonic Neck Reflex (ATNR)
- Symmetrical Tonic Neck Reflex (STNR)

He finds that the STNR often emerges when working on the ATNR, while the ATNR is frequently the hardest reflex to integrate.

O'Hara uses his background in kinesiology and muscle tests to determine which reflex to work on first, asking the body which one it needs. His experience is the same as Berne's, with the Moro often showing up first, and the integration of the ATNR assisting in integrating the STNR.

Based on the premise that reflexes emerge form full flexion and extension to more individual movements, stated earlier in this chapter, Marusich's integration program differs.

She does not work "one reflex at a time," since that approach does not allow the patient to take advantage of natural movement patterns of established reflexes to develop and learn freedom of movement. Instead, she recommends activities that encourage movement from one reflex posture, through other reflex postures, into voluntary movement patterns and back into the reflex posture as part of therapy. These multiple reflex movement patterns that use the reflex postures as a foundation for voluntary movement are the basis for her intervention program. This approach has been very successful for her patients, allowing them to integrate their movements more quickly than had been previously thought possible.

What Is A Reflex Integration Program?

A reflex integration program consists of specific physical, stereotyped movements practiced a few times a day. Berne recommends working on one reflex at a time, with a retest of that reflex after one to two months. If the reflex has been integrated, then move on to the next reflex. If not, continue with the same one for a while longer. In general, reflex exercises should change about every month or two.

A reflex integration program can precede or be a part of a general vision therapy program or a separate motor development program. Marusich states that if primitive reflexes are interfering with the development of isolated eye and head movements, then optometrists must address them in the treatment hierarchy. Modulating reflexes integrates them and opens pathways for righting reactions and equilibrium responses.[2] One Dutch vision therapist found that delaying vision therapy for at least six months to work on reflex integration either eliminated the need for or decreased the time of traditional oculo-motor and visual perceptual training.[4 (p.111)]

Moro Reflex Integration Program
Starfish (Berne) or Fetal Fling (Marusich)

1. Sit on a bean bag or straight chair with pillows behind the back so that patient is inclined about 45 degrees.

2. Open arms and legs out in full extension, inhaling while moving the limbs out. As the limbs move out, the head moves backwards. Hold five seconds.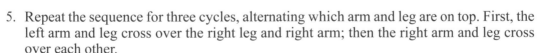

3. While exhaling, move the arms and legs simultaneously in towards each other in full flexion, until the body is in a fetal position with arms and legs on the chest. As the limbs move inward, the head moves forwards. Hold five seconds.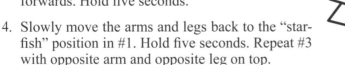

4. Slowly move the arms and legs back to the "starfish" position in #1. Hold five seconds. Repeat #3 with opposite arm and opposite leg on top.

5. Repeat the sequence for three cycles, alternating which arm and leg are on top. First, the left arm and leg cross over the right leg and right arm; then the right arm and leg cross over each other.

6. All movements should feel safe and be relaxed. When a retained Moro Reflex is very obvious, the integration experience can be very intense for the patient. If someone has trouble sitting in the beanbag or on the chair, or becomes dizzy or nauseous, substitute the next exercise, which is also appropriate for lower functioning individuals.

Prayer Pose (Berne)

1. Lie on the back with legs bent and feet pulled up close to the buttocks.

2. Arch the back, pushing the stomach toward the ceiling, while pressing the hands together and inhaling.

3. Hold the breath until the face becomes red.

4. Release the breath quickly and abruptly, while returning the back to the floor.

5. Repeat three times.

The key is in the release. Holding the breath and pressing the hands together activates the sympathetic nervous system. Releasing and letting go stimulates the parasympathetic nervous system. Creating a balance between the two is important.

O'Hara offers activities to integrate each of the three parts of the Moro Reflex.[22]

Arching Cat (Physical Moro)

1. Get on all fours.

2. While inhaling, gently lower the stomach and spine towards the floor, starting with the base of the spine (the sacrum), and finishing by raising the head. Perform the movement as a wave through the spine. The back becomes concave.

3. While exhaling, gently raise the spine, starting again with the base of the spine (the sacrum). Lifting one vertebra at a time, stretch the spine upwards and contract the abdomen. The "wave" movement finishes with the lowering of the head.

4. Repeat sequence three or four times. Make sure that each movement starts from the sacrum at the base of the spine.

©2004 Brendan O'Hara

5. Do "Arching Cat" also with 2 or 3 handheld bean-bags (preferably 100% cotton, 4"x4" and one third filled) on the back to increase awareness of the spine. Using beanbags creates a new environment in which the body can experience movement.

Palming (Visual Moro)

Cover the eyes gently with the palms of the hands. Relax the eyes and feel the warmth. Hold the hands in this position for 1-3 minutes or longer, but only as long as feels comfortable. Palming relaxes and takes the stress out of using vision, allowing the eyes to open to the wonder and beauty of the world.

©2004 Brendan O'Hara

Energy to Ears (Auditory Moro)

Place hands close to, but not on the ears. Hold them there for a minute or two, feeling the warmth.

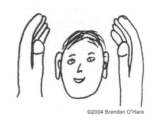

Note: Someone else can hold his/her hands over eyes and ears for Visual and Auditory Moro.

According to O'Hara, the above three activities enhance vision as well as the development, integration and maturation of the kinesthetic sense and the auditory system.

Tonic Labyrinth Reflex (TLR) Integration Program

The purpose of the following activities is to integrate the cervical and lumbar spines.

Flying (Berne)

1. Lie on floor on the stomach with legs straight out behind, arms bent, in front of face, with thumbs touching.

2. Lift the arms, head, and upper body as high as possible, while fully relaxing the lower body. Feel the tension in the lower back. Hold thumbs about an inch off the floor, with visual focus on the thumbs.

3. Keeping left thumb still in front, move the right thumb to the right as far as possible so that it straightens out at the end of the arc, while turning the head to follow the movement of the thumb with the eyes.

4. Bring the right arm and head back to the starting position so that the two thumbs are again touching.

5. Repeat the same procedure to the left. Each side should take about 30 seconds out and back.

6. Slowly lower the thumbs, head and upper body to a relaxed position. Hold 5-10 seconds.

7. Repeat for 3 cycles.

Remember to keep breathing during this activity. Do not bend the knees. Maintain the same distance from the nose while moving each thumb; Move head as far as possible in each direction before fully extending the arm. To view the exact movements, watch Berne's DVD.[14]

A variation on "Flying" from Brendan O'Hara:

TLR Airplane

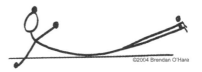

1. Lie on floor on the stomach with legs straight out behind and arms out to the side with palms down.

2. Have someone place beanbags on the top of the head, on the heels, and on the backs of the hands.

3. Gently arch back by lifting legs, arms and head simultaneously.

4. Hold for 10-15 seconds.

5. Return to floor gently.

6. Repeat 3 times. Wonderful for whole body/vision integration.

O'Hara recommends using the lemniscate (∞), also known as the infinity sign or "figure 8," in many imaginative ways to enhance binocularity, spatial awareness, reading fluency and a host of other visual skills.[19 (p 34)]

The following "figure 8" activities are excellent in assisting the integration of all the extrinsic eye muscles and neck muscles.

1. Sitting or standing, follow the ∞ with eyes alone, keeping the head still. Start at the center, move upwards and outwards, in each direction, moving smoothly and at a slow, steady pace.

2. Follow the ∞ with eyes and finger together, keeping head still. One hand, then the other and then both together.

3. Imagine having a pen at the end of your nose and "draw" around the ∞.

O'Hara also recommends various types of "Active 8s" for integrating the TLR.[23]

TLR 8's – Foot Goes Out and In, in time with the Hand

This activity integrates the upper and lower halves, and the left and right sides of the body, for the integration of movement and vision.

1. Stand straight, holding beanbag in the left hand at the navel. Move beanbag up and to the left as if tracing the ∞, while moving the left foot out and in, in time with the beanbag as it sweeps one half of the ∞.

2. Left hand passes beanbag to the right hand at navel.

2004 Brendan O'Hara

3. Complete the ∞ by moving the beanbag up and out to the right side, and back to home base at the navel. The right foot moves out and in, in time with the beanbag.

4. Repeat many times.

Saucer Spin (Cheatum and Hammond)

1. Lie on cushion which has been placed on a snow saucer on a smooth floor. Designate the boundaries of the saucer with chalk or tape.

2. While the child's arms and legs are extended, spin the saucer five to 10 times in one direction, then again in the opposite direction. Some children can spin themselves; others need an adult to spin them.

During this activity, the pull of gravity on the inner ear triggers the TLR; the activity also serves to develop muscle strength and endurance, allowing the child to hold the head and limbs against the gravity's pull.[18]

Cheatum believes that the TLR should also be integrated in a supine position. For this she suggests

Horizontal Mountain Climbing (for ages eight and older)

1. Tie a 15-foot cord to the end of a scooter board.

2. Lie on a scooter board on the back, with the head at the end where the rope is tied.

3. Securely tie the cord to a stable object, such as a piece of furniture, two to three feet off the ground; lay the unused cord straight.

4. Pull head up off the scooter board, grasp the cord and pull the length of the cord, hand over hand as if climbing.

The Spinal Galant (SG) Reflex Integration Program
Angels in the Snow (Berne)

1. Lie on the back with feet together, legs straight and arms at the side.

2. Very slowly and simultaneously, start to move the arms and legs out like a jumping jack, while keeping all limbs on the floor. The arms should be fully stretched, and the hands should touch each other just as the legs reach their widest position.

3. Slowly bring arms and legs back to the starting position.

4. Do three angels to complete the reflex program.

5. This activity is done very slowly and intentionally. Each angel in the snow should last at least one minute. Patients should heighten awareness of their breathing, and the positions of all limbs while performing the exercise. The arms and legs must move at the same speed both out and in. If a child cannot coordinate both arms and legs together, the upper body and lower body can do the exercise separately.

Twitching Tigers - *Spinal Twist (O'Hara)*

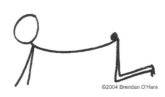

1. Get on hands and knees. Place beanbags on each hip and on sacrum.

2. Look over one shoulder, observing the beanbags; the movement is to bring the shoulders and hips together, one side and then the other, i.e., right shoulder to right hip, and left shoulder to left hip. Arms remain strong, neither stiff nor locked.

3. Repeat on other side.

The "Spinal Twist" is an excellent activity for reducing bedwetting and to help the "wiggle-worm" sit still.

Malkuth 8's (O'Hara)

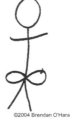

This exercise integrates the flow of the electro-magnetic energy field in the lower body.

Do Malkuth 8's standing with knees slightly bent.

In Front:

1. Hold a beanbag in both hands in front of the pubic bone.

2. The right hand takes the beanbag and begins tracing an imaginary lemniscate (∞) by sweeping up and out to the right, down and around and back up to the pubic bone;

3. Pass the beanbag here from the right hand to the left hand which continues the sweep up and out to the left, down and around and back to the pubic bone. One cycle is completed.

4. Do many cycles.

Out Back:

Repeat the activity behind the body with the sacrum as the center point of the lemniscate.

Do a) with hips still, b) with hips gently swaying with the flow of the leminscate, and c) with hips swaying opposite to the flow of the lemniscate.

190

O'Hara says that "Spinal Twist," "Malkuth 8s," and "Arching Cat," all stabilize the spine and make it more flexible. A strong, flexible spine is an essential component of efficient vision. The intentional movements of these integration activities "rock" the sphenoid bone, to which 10 of the 12 extrinsic muscles (six to each eye) that direct the eyes are attached. Rocking the sphenoid bone releases the sacrum, thereby increasing the flow of cerebro-spinal fluid, and synchronizing the movement of all of the cranial bones with breathing. Results include improved concentration, memory, bladder control and an overall healthier spine.

Asymmetrical Tonic Neck Reflex (ATNR) Integration Program

Activities that integrate the ATNR create situations in which an individual must turn the head in one direction and the arms and legs in the opposite direction. Watching the head position in these exercises is crucial for integrating the ATNR. O'Hara says that these activities assist the integration of the left and right hemispheres of the brain, thus enhancing one's ability to work at and to cross the midline.

ATNR Integration (Berne) – Can be done actively or passively

1. Lie face down with head turned to the left and palms down.

2. Slowly pull up and bend left arm and then leg close to the body.

3. Lift and turn head slowly to the right.

4. Slowly straighten bent leg and arm.

5. Pause for 5-10 seconds.

6. Slowly pull up and bend right arm and leg close to the body.

7. Turn head to left.

8. Pause. One cycle is complete.

9. Repeat two more full cycles.

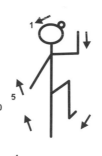
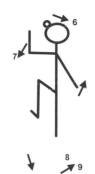

ATNR Eyes (O'Hara)

(O'Hara says he learned this exercise from Dr. Adrian Cornale, a behavioral optometrist in New South Wales, Australia. O'Hara simply added the beanbag.)

1. Standing with beanbag in left hand, move beanbag to the left side at shoulder level, turning head to follow movement. Right hand waits with fingers resting on the right clavicle.

2. Left hand returns to the midline and gives the beanbag to the right hand at the sternum.

3. Complete the cycle with right hand taking the beanbag to the right at shoulder level etc., with head and eyes tracking the beanbag.

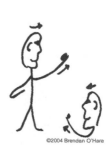
©2004 Brendan O'Hara

4. Repeat cycle 15-20 times.

5. Repeat cycle 15-20 times with head turning (and eyes looking) in the opposite direction from the beanbag. Eyes focus on the beanbag only when it moves from hand to hand at the sternum, which, of course, is at the laterality midline.

ATNR Eyes and Knees (O'Hara)
– For older subjects

Do same exercise as above, adding knee: raise the opposite knee to the hand holding the beanbag. Complete this activity standing and prone with head movements, eyes alone, and eyes opposite from hand movement.

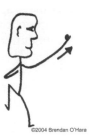

©2004 Brendan O'Hara

Lazy Bubble Blowing (Cheatum and Hammond)
– For younger children

1. Lie on back with bubble-blowing solution in shallow bowl to the side at waist level.

2. Child takes bubble blowing wand, looks and turns toward solution, dips in wand, turns forward and blows bubbles through large hoop that has been placed by his face on the same side as the bubble solution.

Passing Pennies Down the Line (Cheatum) – Great group activity

1. Group members lie on their backs, side by side, an arm's width apart.

2. Place a plate with 10-20 pennies next to the first child, an empty plate between each of the children, and at the end of the line.

3. The first person picks up a penny from the plate, passes it from hand to hand, and then deposits it on the empty plate without turning his head.

4. The next person picks up the penny and repeats the process.

5. Continue until all pennies have made it to the end of the line.

6. Repeat, moving pennies in the opposite direction, again without turning the head.

Cheatum and Hammond recommend doing this activity with teams to see which one can complete it the fastest.

Symmetrical Tonic Neck Reflex (STNR) Integration Program
STNR Integration (Berne)

1. Get down on the floor on hands and knees. Arms are bent.

2. Slowly lower the head, while straightening the arms and inhaling through the nose, so that the forehead touches the ground, while at the same time leaning back on haunches. Come forward as far as possible, keeping the arms stretched out straight.

3. Then move backwards toward the starting position, picking the head up, while exhaling through the mouth, still keeping the arms straight.

4. Continuously move back and forth for 3 minutes, completing 18-25 cycles. Remain aware of body position and breathing while moving.

Quiet Tigers (O'Hara)[29]

1. Get down on hands and knees.

2. Pile 1-4 beanbags on head.

3. *Rock and sway* forwards, backwards and sideways, balancing beanbags.

4. Do with eyes open, eyes closed and with eyes blinking.

5. Add beanbags to back and hips.

6. *Rock* forwards and backwards, balancing beanbags. Quietly roar like a tiger with mouth wide open.

7. *Head moves* – Nod head gently forwards, backwards, left and right, balancing a single beanbag without dropping it.

8. *Still and rocking* – Balancing beanbags on head, back and hips. Draw a ∞ on a notebook size paper, and place on the floor in front of you. Trace around the ∞ with both eyes. When tracing around the lemicsate, always start in the middle; move forwards and out. Balance on one hand, and trace the ∞ with the free hand. Change hands. Trace ∞ with a "nose pencil."

O'Hara loves Quiet Tigers for all young children. Why? Because it

- replicates the actions of a baby before it crawls
- integrates the STNR
- develops the vestibular system and balance
- introduces the body to defying gravity using its own strength
- requires and increases strength in the limbs, spine, muscles and ligaments
- develops binocular vision
- coordinates balance, vision and movement

Bear-Walk Soccer Drill (Cheatum and Hammond)

1. Set up cones in a line at 2-3 foot intervals, so that participants can zigzag through the course.

2. Bend over with hands on the floor, legs extended straight out behind and head on a 10" soccer ball.

3. Tap the ball with the head through the course. Time each child and observe that times lessen as skills improve.

This activity takes practice. If a child cannot inhibit the STNR, he will collapse onto his head as he tries to push the ball forward, and his arms flex simultaneously with the head's flexion toward the chest.

Safe and Sound[24] by Eve Kodiak (Reprinted with permission from author)

Brain Gym consultant Eve Kodiak has designed wonderful song-games to integrate various reflexes. This one can be done with or without the CD that accompanies her book. It is specifically for integrating the STNR. Eve says "Just get down on all sixes (arms, elbows and knees) and rock!

>Rocking on my knees and elbows
>Looking at the ground.
>Rocking on my knees and elbows
>Feeling safe and sound.
>Heads up!
>
>Press my palms into the ground
>Straighten arms and look around.
>Sky and trees and birds and bees
>All flying, swirling round!
>
>I want to see, I want to be
>As tall as any bird or tree.
>Pressing down, swing back, let go
>I'm sitting on my knees!
>I'm sitting up, I'm sitting up
>I'm balanced on my knees!
>Drop my head and slide my elbows
>Down on to the ground.
>Rocking on my knees and elbows
>Feeling safe and sound
>Feeling safe and sound.

O'Dell and Cook devote two chapters to integrating the STNR.[20] Their program, lasting about eight months, consists of specific crawling exercises for 15 minutes a day, five days a week. They believe that any adult or child over five years of age, who has an immature STNR, can benefit.

Two other practitioners deserve mention under the subject of "reflex integration." Veteran Washington, DC, optometrist Harry Wachs has been working with children on the autism spectrum for over 50 years. He was way ahead of his time when he co-wrote _Thinking Goes to School_[25] 30 years ago with Piagetian psychologist Hans Furth. Still in print, this classic contains almost 200 therapeutic activities pairing vision with every other sense. Chapter 6 on "General Movement Thinking" includes several games which focus on reflex integration.

Dr. Svetlana Masgutova is a Russian psychologist who has melded her knowledge of educational kinesiology (Brain Gym), child development and movement theory to create the "Masgutova Method of Neuro-Sensory Motor and Reflex Integration" She teaches world-wide, frequently in the United States and Canada. She holds a therapeutic international camp bi-annually in Poland for children with autism, ADD, ADHD and dyslexia, as well as with cerebral palsy and other neurological involvement. To see her schedule, and to learn about this remarkable woman, go to <www.masgutovamethod.com>.

Summary and Conclusion

The primitive survival reflexes originate in the brainstem, and are automatic movements that help babies be born and newborns integrate the overwhelming amount of stimuli they receive once they leave the mother's womb. Primitive reflexes provide babies with learning experiences that act as a foundation for more complex muscle movements. The purpose of these primitive reflexes is to help infants to

- learn where they are in space
- localize objects around them
- use both eyes together
- focus
- develop depth perception

As babies develop, higher brain centers inhibit the primitive reflexes so that more advanced movement patterns, called postural reflexes, emerge. The visual system is intimately involved in the transition from primitive reflexes to postural reflexes and the cortical control of movement patterns.

Reflexes integrate in a sequential fashion from three to eleven months. If these reflexes are weak, early, or linger past six to 12 months post-natally, they can interfere with cortical processing and impede normal development. Visual problems at a later age can often be attributed to weakness or lingering of one or more of the primitive reflexes. Aberrant reflexes can cause babies to become "developmentally delayed," and then practitioners label them as having one of the disabilities on the autism spectrum.

By completing simple, quick, pleasurable motor activities several times daily for a month or two, children on the autism spectrum can remove neurological impediments to development. Their bodies and brains can then concentrate on interacting with their external, rather than internal environments to learn, interact and grow.

References

1. *ADD/AD(H)D: Reticular Activating System. www.NewIdeas.net/adhd/neurology (Accessed January 14, 2008)*

2. *Marusich CE. DVD: Integration of primitive motor reflexes: why should I care? Santa Ana, CA, Optometric Extension Program, 2002.*

3. *O'Hara B. The primitive and postural reflexes and their effect on our physical, mental and emotional development. In: The Heart & Science of Energy Healing. 30th National Touch for Health Kinesiology Conference Manual, Durham, NC, July, 2005:8-9.*

4. *Goddard S. Reflexes, Learning and Behavior. Eugene, OR: Fern Ridge Press, 2005.*

5. *Rider B. Relationship of postural reflexes to learning disabilities. Am J Occupat Ther 1972;26(5):239-3.*

6. *Bender ML. Bender-Perdue reflex test. San Rafael, CA: Academic Therapy Publications, 1976.*

7. *O'Dell N, Cook P. Stopping Hyperactivity-A New Solution. Garden City Park, NY: Avery Publishing Co., 1996.*

8. *Bein-Wierzbinski W. Persistent primitive reflexes in elementary school children: effects on oculomotor function and visual perception. Paper presented at the 13th European conference on neurodevelopmental delay in children with specific learning difficulties. Chester, England, 2001.*

9. *Pavlides O. Miles T. Dyslexia Research And its Application to Education. Chichester, England: Wiley Publications, 1987.*

10. *Teitelbaum P, Teitelbaum O, Nye J, Fryman J, Maurer R. Movement analysis in infancy may be useful for early diagnosis of autism. Proc Natl Acad Sci Nov 1998;95:13982-7.*

11. *Teitelbaum P, Teitelbaum O, Fryman J, Maurer R. Reflexes gone astray in autism in infancy. J Dev Learn Dis 2002;6:15-22.*

12. *Brendan O'Hara interview. July 17, 2005. by Patricia Lemer. www.devdelay.org. (Accessed January 18, 2008)*

13. *Berne SA. Without Ritalin: A Natural Approach to ADD. New York, NY. Keats Publishing, 2002.*

14. Berne SA. *ADD to Autism: Reaching Your Child's Potential Naturally.* Santa Fe, NM: Color Stone Press, 2005.

15. Blythe SG. *The Well Balanced Child: Movement and Early Learning.* United Kingdom: Hawthorn Press, 2004.

16. Cheatum BA, Hammond AA. *Physical Activities for Improving Children's Learning and Behavior.* Champaign, IL: Human Kinetics, 2000:71.

17. Masgutova S. *Intergration of Dynamic and Postural Reflexes into Whole Body Movement System.* Moscow, Ascension Educational Institute of Psychological and Edu-K Assistance, 1998.

18. O'Dell N, Cook P. *Stopping ADHD: A Unique and Proven Drug-free Program for Treating ADHD in Children and Adults.* New York: Avery Publishing Co., 2004.

19. O'Hara B. *Movement and Learning: Wombat and His Mates Songbook.* Victoria, Australia: The F# Music Company, 2003:37.

20. Sutton A. *Building a visual space world. OEP Curriculum II* 1984;1:47-78.

21. Blythe SG. *Neurological dysfunction as a significant factor in children with dyslexia. J Behav Opt om* 2001;12:145.

22. O'Hara B. *Primitive and postural reflexes: digeridoo and beanbags. Workshop Manual,* Durham, NC, July, 2005.

23. O'Hara B. *Movement and Learning: The Children's Songbook.* Victoria, Australia: The F# Music Company, 2004:31.

24. Kodiak E. *Rappin' on the Reflexes: A Guide to Integrating the Senses Through Music and Movement.* Temple, NH: Sound Intelligence Production, 2005:37-40.

25. Furth H. Wachs, H. *Thinking Goes to School: Piaget's Theory in Practice.* New York: Oxford University Press,1975.

Chapter 9
Vision Therapy for Those
on the Autism Spectrum

Contributing authors:
Melvin Kaplan, OD
Randy Schulman, MS, OD, FCOVD

Introduction

In Chapter 2, Dr. Randy Schulman details guidelines for examining patients with autism spectrum diagnoses. Clearly, optometrists have much to offer individuals with attention deficits, learning disabilities, pervasive developmental disorders and autism. Vision therapy (VT) is a major piece of the autism puzzle, and often necessary for helping individuals on both ends of the autism spectrum reach their full potential.

This chapter is directed primarily to the behavioral optometrist who is looking to learn more about working with patients on the autism spectrum. It contains many terms that may be unfamiliar to the lay person. Parents, educators, therapists, physicians, counselors or others not familiar with vision therapy, may wish to consult additional references for the basics of vision. Some good resources are <www.ocp.org>, <www.children-special-needs.org>, <www.pavevision.org>, <www.covd.org/od/autism>, <www.vision3d.org> and <www.visiontherapy.org>.

Vision Treatment Overview

Schulman believes that vision therapy for those with autism spectrum diagnoses cannot start too young. The success rate is high with early therapy. If a child has not seen a behavioral optometrist prior to an autism diagnosis, he/she should make an appointment immediately thereafter.

Most children do not outgrow delays in visual development without intervention. They may adapt to their inefficient visual systems, but the problems do not go away; and in the meantime, they struggle unnecessarily. Because vision impacts on so many other areas, improving visual function also leads to improvement in areas such as language development and social-emotional skills.

Vision therapy for those with autism typically takes place in the office on a weekly basis. If therapy starts young, even kids with significant visual delays can catch up. Without early therapy, some show limited improvement in visual skills 12 to 18 months later. Typically, vision therapy lasts for from three to nine months, or sometimes years.

One-on-one treatment is essential, at first, especially for those under the age of five and for older patients at the more severe end of the spectrum. A well-conceived home-based therapy program supplements and reinforces office-based activities. Five minutes several times a day may be the maximum that a child can sustain initially. Ultimately 20 to 30 minutes at a time may be attained. Compliance for home vision therapy (VT) activities may be very difficult for those with significant vision and behavioral issues, requiring more emphasis on office-based therapy. For children with minimum involvement, a home program is more likely to succeed.

The primary goal of vision therapy (VT) for persons on the autism spectrum is to help them give meaning to what they see. Although individuals with autism are not "blind" in the traditional sense of the word, many have such poor vision that their behavior is similar to that of a blind person. The mother of a daughter with autism eloquently describes how poorly she used her vision at a young age:

> *Elizabeth was not blind... At 18 months old she flipped the pages of her picture books. What did she see? Did her mind integrate the reds and browns and blacks and blues and greys into a kitten or a car?... If a car pulled up within three feet of where she was playing, she would not look at it. A dog ran past. She seemed to register nothing. She was over three before she looked up and saw a bird.*[1]

Setting the Stage for Vision Therapy

Adapting the office environment is as important for therapy as it is for the vision examination. The same sensory factors that can impact upon evaluation results such as lighting, sounds, smells, colors and temperature, can also influence the success of therapy. Optometrists should be cognizant of sensory issues and possible "overload." Modifications include:

- **Lighting** make sure it is not too bright, has no glare, is adjustable
- **Sounds** minimize noise and distractions from other patients, copy machines, cell phones, computers, printers, lighting, heating, air conditioning, vision therapy equipment
- **Smells** suggest that patients do not wear perfumes or scents
- **Temperature** is adjustable
- **Colors** minimize clothing with patterns and bright colors, jewelry that shines of glitters
- **Space** allow ample "personal" space for each patient to avoid inadvertent personal contact

Some optometrists suggest the following common sense guidelines for working with patients on the autism spectrum:

- Sit next to the person not across from him/her
- Work at eye level to make for ease of communication
- Use a patient's strengths to help remediate weaknesses
- Watch tone, pace and volume of the voice
- Keep instructions simple and short; break tasks down into small steps
- Make sure tasks have obvious beginnings and endings
- Offer choices between two acceptable tasks
- Reinforce task completion
- Make it clear who is in charge, preventing disruptive behaviors to escalate
- Positively reinforce good behavior and note unacceptable behavior immediately

Involving a parent, caregiver, therapist, or other adults who know the patient well, can be extremely advantageous. Having a familiar adult in the room often puts the patient with autism at ease. If, at any time, the adult is distracting, politely ask him/her to leave. Occasionally an adult intervenes in an attempt to help the optometrist understand what a patient is trying to communicate. Although this well-meaning behavior can disrupt vision therapy activities, that outcome is rare.

Day-to-day and week-to-week, patients with autism have their ups and downs. Expect occasional meltdowns that could be related, for instance, to something that happened on the way to therapy. Have a flexible, but structured plan that allows you to deal with what the individual is able to do that day. With a good plan in place, patients with autism change and progress continuously.

The optometrist should schedule progress evaluations about every eight to 12 sessions, both to evaluate visual skills and to review improvements in activities of daily living. Ask specifically about what the patient can do more easily now than in the past. Set new goals. Look at the need to change lens prescriptions, as well as to reduce the need for therapeutic lenses, as a result of improved visual functioning. Some patients decrease their needs quickly, others gradually.

Managing Difficult Behaviors

The first session with a patient diagnosed with autism can be quite difficult. A child with autism may feel uncomfortable and apprehensive in the unfamiliar surroundings and with challenges coming to his already dysfunctional visual system. Dr. Schulman recommends the following:

- *Be patient*, following the child's lead, rather than programming the therapy activities. For instance, if a child wants to touch, let him touch, but only when he uses the therapy glasses. One of her patients, Jack, loves her packing chips. For the first four sessions, he spent most of the 45 minutes in a box with the chips, first, with an adult putting +0.50 flippers, or base in, out, up, and down prism flippers in front of his eyes. Finally, he accepted therapy glasses.

- *Be consistent* because many individuals with autism have difficulty with change.

- *Be disciplined* but flexible in the therapy room, keeping the demands simple and the reinforcements positive. For example, say "first glasses, then bubbles." When you speak this way, a child understands cause and effect, allowing you to get more done in the session. However, this method may not work when you are trying to interfere with a very shaky visual system. One of the best ways to break a tantrum is to dim the lights or even flicker them on and off quickly. You can also try red, yellow, blue or green filters over a child's eyes, or if available, displayed from an overhead projector. Or, if a child likes touch, deep pressure or movement, try rolling him/her on the floor, bouncing him on a ball, or spinning him in a chair to give needed sensory input.

Schulman recalls a four-year-old girl who threw several tantrums during each of the first three or four sessions, if asked to do anything but look in the mirror. She either threw herself on the floor kicking, or crawled under a chair. Every time she looked in the mirror she shook her head from side to side and sang in a high pitched voice. Between peeks in the mirror, she ran back and forth from one window to another, looking down at her feet, while still shaking her head.

Dr. Schulman persisted with this child, following her around the room with different lenses and prisms, refusing to let her look in the mirror without glasses. Although she was really upset, she finally accepted Polaroids, which allowed her to see both eyes in the mirror, only if she was binocular. After taking home a pair of loaner glasses, in the next session, she put on yoked prisms (see next section) without complaint. Her behavioral transition took almost eight sessions, but then she was ready for more traditional therapy.

Working with difficult behaviors can be exhausting; however, the rewards are worth it. Watching a child progress from being totally uncooperative in the first few sessions, to sitting down at a table and putting on glasses without complaining just one month later, is truly amazing.

Hierarchy of Treatment Techniques

Visual treatment for those with autism, just like biomedical and other sensory treatments, is based on the assumption that every patient is unique, and is entitled to an individualized approach. Optometrists must put aside any preconceptions about the course and outcome of therapy; changes occur at different rates for patients with the same diagnosis. For instance, for some, eye contact may improve quickly, while for others it may increase gradually. However, in general, the process of learning to use vision efficiently may take longer and be slower for those with autism than with patients who have other diagnoses.

The following sections detail a sequential treatment plan that is applicable to most patients on the autism spectrum. A combination of lenses, prisms and vision therapy activities is often the best treatment for individuals with numerous developmental delays, including autism spectrum disorders.

Begin with some form of pleasurable, developmentally appropriate, simple visual-motor activity. Ball play, puzzles or tracking will all be very difficult until the visual system is stimulated in a new way, resulting in redirected visual attention and awareness. A good starting activity is putting blocks into a container. Move the container around to various positions, and hand the blocks to the child from many different angles, requiring him/her to make fixations. Do not let go of the block until the child looks.

If possible, have the child do this and other activities wearing lenses. If he/she refuses, simply hold flippers over the child's eyes. Some kids won't let you get any lens near them for awhile, and it takes a very long time to just engage them. In really difficult cases where the child has such significant tactile issues that prevent tolerating the frame on the face, consider sending a loaner frame home, just for the purpose of having the child get used to the feel of something on his/her face. Surprisingly enough, these kids can make real progress, as just having the frame on the face can give the child a sense of central and peripheral viewing and can make a positive difference.

Attempt to rotate yoked prisms or use separate glasses with base up, down, right, and left and again note changes. Sometimes no changes of note occur initially; just creating the change in visual input often allows for changes outside the therapy room, however. Parents occasionally report that right after the initial session, the child appeared upset or tired, but the next day was much happier, made more eye contact and decreased visual stimulatory behaviors. On average, four to eight visits are necessary for the child to acclimate to the routine in the therapy room, and to begin to really respond to the lenses, prisms and activities presented.

Start with simple activities while applying single lenses and prisms, including red/green glasses. Red/green glasses stimulate and develop general visual and spatial awareness and enhance central/peripheral awareness.

Next move to lenses, which can be used along with yoked prisms to visually direct movement. Eventually, the patient will be ready for more traditional vision therapy activities for developing binocular visual skills and visual information processing. At each level, patients should experience a variety of activities. Those with autism are uncanny about gravitating toward those activities which benefit them at the time.

Sometimes a patient accepts a lens prescription immediately. If not, the authors recommend waiting a few therapy sessions, and watching the rate at which an individual is progressing, before prescribing glasses. Waiting allows the optometrist to see what lens or prism a patient responds to most consistently.

Visual Arousal Activities
Inherent in those with autism diagnoses are attention issues which produce varying levels of visual arousal, session to session and even within a session. The optometrist thus cannot make assumptions about a patient's attention levels in general, but rather must meet a patient at his/her level at any given time.

Begin vision therapy with simple, gentle visual arousal activities, the purpose of which is to eliminate any tendencies to use only one eye, and to develop and stimulate binocularity and spatial awareness. Improving these visual skills will improve both the consistency and frequency of eye contact and a child's social skills.

Optometrists recommend including peripheral awareness activities using red/green glasses, which stimulate the ambient visual system. These lenses improve patients' abilities to visually direct themselves. Move from gross to fine motor activities. Next, stimulate the central visual system, with activities using vectograms, lens flippers, a trampoline and the fixator with letter naming charts, and lastly, the computer.

The following activities using red/green glasses are beneficial for those at both ends of the autism spectrum.

- *Angels in the snow* – Have patient lie on his/her back on the carpet, and look at an overhead light through the glasses while making arm and leg movements. Initially, moving the patient's body physically may be necessary. Consult Etta Rowley's *Integrating Mind, Brain and Body*[2] for a hierarchy of simplified movement activities to do for lower functioning patients that eventually lead them into a good bilateral "angel in the snow."

- *White balloons* –
  a. Have patient hand tap and kick white balloons.
  b. Next use a piece of white PCV tubing, a white plastic rolling pin or other white object as a bat to "bat" the balloon.
  c. Make a "Marsden" ball using a white balloon.
  d. Play volleyball with a white balloon.

- *Miner's tag* – Have the patient wear a Miner's light (available from REI) on his/her head. Turn the lights off in the room. As the patient moves the head, increasing awareness of the light's movement will occur. In time, the patient will understand that light movements correlate with head movements.

- *Flashlight tag* – Both the patient and the visual coach have a flashlight. The therapist shines a light on the wall; the patient follows with his/her light. Keep the task very simple at first, slowly increasing demands as the patient becomes more proficient.

- *Ball games* – Play with a white kick ball, volleyball, soccer ball, Kooshball, Nerf ball, and any other kinds of balls.

- *Bowling* – Bowl, using a white bowling ball and white bowling pins. Use white styrofoam cups if bowling pins are unavailable.

- *Marsden ball* – Suspend a white ball.
  a. Have patient hit the ball with his/her hands
  b. Have patient bunt the ball with white PCV tubing or a white plastic rolling pin.

- *Rotating tachistoscope* – Have patient follow light on wall with a laser light or flashlight.

- *Overhead projector* – Have patient do the following:
  a. Make finger shadows on projected light on the wall
  b. Using magnetic letters, stand in front of an overhead with hands hidden from view, have patient move the letters while fixating on the screen.
  c. Using an overhead transparency, draw on it while fixating on the screen.

- *Bean bag games* – Using white beanbags, play catch, toss them into cans, and play tic tac toe.

- *Play hockey* on white marker board with white ping pong ball.

- *Parquetry blocks* – Play matching and stacking games.

- *White pegboard* – Match patterns.

- *Lebarge Electro Therapist/ or Wayne Sequencer*
  a. Push buttons left to right
  b. Work top to bottom
  c. Follow patterns

- *Lite Brite* – Using any pegs, clear pegs, only red and green pegs,
  a. Make any pattern
  b. Follow given pattern

- *Light board* – Write

- *Sports rotator* – Track while on a balance board

- *Marker board* – Using a black pen to run a white race car through mazes.

Performance Glasses

Behavioral optometrists frequently prescribe performance glasses with relatively low powered lenses to "jump start" visual information for specific tasks and activities that involve concentrated focalized visual jobs such as reading, writing, or computer activities. Lenses to aid performance are prescribed to heighten discernment over a larger viewing field. By reducing visual crowding, such as small text, the lenses improve visual selection and often smooth out reading and writing. Most of all, they reduce adverse stress and help a patient improve awareness, comprehension, and insight.

These lenses are behavioral in nature, and often produce extraordinary changes for individuals on the autism spectrum. They can make performance easier and more sustained, increase ease and comfort, and allow more efficient productivity, thus improving achievement by allowing the patient to respond more quickly, accurately and spontaneously to what he sees. The types of changes performance lenses produce are more frequently observed by others rather than by the patient, especially younger children. When patients use performance glasses, as prescribed, they are powerful tools to brighten a patient's life by improved vision understanding.

Single-Prism Lenses

All lenses in glasses are prisms, in that they displace light. Optometrists, ophthalmologists and oculists use single-prism lenses in glasses to correct ocular muscle imbalances. Single-prism lenses address focal vision: a patient's ability to identify objects – the "What is it?" function. Single-prism lenses are typically worn for the rest of a person's life, once prescribed, because they are compensatory. For the optometrist, single-prism lenses are an intervention that addresses the "software" of the visual system.[3]

Prism lenses have a thick edge at the base and a thinner edge at the apex. The lenses deflect the light rays differently at the top and the bottom, forcing the brain to make interpretations about where the body is in space. Prisms are available in various magnitudes from "weak" to "strong," which are measured in diopters. The optometrist can change a patient's perception by altering both the magnitude and the direction of the prism.

Although behavioral optometrists have used lenses for many years, the use of prism lenses for behavioral and learning problems goes back only to the 1970s. At that time, optometric pioneers Drs. Bruce Wolff, Richard Apell and John Streff began using these tools along with vision therapy at the Gesell Institute in New Haven, CT.

Yoked Prisms

Dr. Melvin Kaplan, considered by many to be one of the top experts on using prisms for those with autism, and many other optometrists, use special prism lenses called yoked prisms not to compensate for a mechanical defect, but rather to alter a patient's perceived reality. Kaplan calls this an application for "a software problem."[3] (p. 34)

Kaplan and Stephen Edelson, PhD of the Autism Research Institute completed a double-blind crossover study in which they divided a group of 20 students with autism, and used yoked prisms on one-half, and a placebo on the others. Those wearing prism lenses showed a decrease in behavior problems after two months, compared to those wearing placebo lenses.[5]

When the prisms' bases face in the same direction in both eyes, they are called "yoked." Designed to alter neural organization, yoked prisms are powerful tools that can have a dramatic impact on the lives of those with autism. Yoked prisms address a patient's ability to organize space and create a coherent body schema – the "Where is it?" and "Where am I?" functions. These lenses are used therapeutically to change the neuromotor processing of the brain; after rehabilitation occurs, they are no longer needed.[3] (p. 81)

Yoked prisms can cause the environment to appear to be shifted up, down, left or right. Objects may thus appear closer, farther away or sloped. Table 9-1 shows the effects of yoked prisms.

Table 9-1 Effects of Yoked Prism Lenses				
	Base up	**Base down**	**Base right**	**Base left**
Space shift	Affects rotation around the horizontal axis. Downhill & closer	Affects rotation around the horizontal axis. Uphill & farther	Affects rotation around the vertical axis, and to the left	Affects rotation around the vertical axis, and to the right
*Center of gravity	Forward greater than backward	Backward greater than forward	Rotate right	Rotate left
* Posture	On heels	On toes	To right	To left
Causes changes in	Organization	Organization	Orientation	Orientation

* If a person goes into the "feeling" of the prism rather than reacts against it, the response to the prism might be opposite. Because each person reacts differently, try all combinations.

When a patient is looking at an object and a prism is interposed, a reorientation of the eye to a new position in space is needed for the patient to continue looking at the object. As the eyes re-orient, the motor system adjusts, sending information to the brain, which comprehends that the individual must adapt himself to this new position in space. This readjustment causes a reorganization of the motor and sensory data in the cortex. In time, and with vision therapy, this reorganization becomes permanent.[3] (p. 47)

Success in making the shift in motor orientation occurs not simply because the eye muscles change in alignment, but also because the brain matches the visual information, while at the same time connecting vision, the motor components of vision, the vestibular process, the kinesthetic process, and proprioception. The prisms thus serve to establish balance among all the senses.[4]

The Story of Rickie

Dr. Melvin Kaplan began using yoked prisms in 1972, to reduce the symptoms of learning disabilities, anxiety and motion sickness, when few others were doing so. He was particularly interested in the effects of yoked prisms on the visual-vestibular feedback loop. Kaplan compares this loop to the telephone, in that "incoming" and "outgoing" calls move from one sensory system to another. Visual input affects vestibular function, and vestibular input affects visual function. Using prisms to stabilize eye movements also results in decreased motion sickness and anxiety.

Kaplan's interest in anxiety reduction using prism lenses soon reached the psychiatric community, as disorders previously labeled as "emotional" improved markedly when he addressed underlying vision deficits. One of his most dramatic cases, and one that permanently altered the course of his work was Rickie, the daughter of a prominent psychiatrist. At age 13, she developed symptoms of schizophrenia, requiring hospitalization. After 10 years of attempts at medications, electroshock treatments and psychotherapy failed to cure her, she found her way to Kaplan's office.

Upon examination, Rickie, a beautiful and intelligent young girl, acted like a frightened animal. Kaplan found severely impaired visual processing skills, including tunnel vision, lack of binocularity and lack of depth perception. Her history showed visual dysfunction at age three, which continued with significant learning disabilities. Eventually, Rickie's highly stressed-out visual system collapsed, and relapsed into a psychiatrically diagnosed state.

Rickie completed a year of intensive vision therapy combined with nutritional support and counseling. According to Kaplan, the results were amazing: Rickie blossomed. She gradually gained independence, returned to school, trained as a practical nurse, married and had several children.[3] (p.37-41)

Rickie's father, Frederic Flach. MD, and Dr. Kaplan later collaborated on several projects. Their research revealed that two-thirds of psychiatric patients suffer from some form of visual dysfunction. Nearly 85% of patients with severe, chronic "mental" illness exhibited marked impairments in spatial organization. Those with the most severe visual problems exhibited the highest levels of social withdrawal, academic failure and employment difficulties.[6]

Yoked Prisms to Enhance Learning and Behavior

Yoked prisms exaggerate the effects of moving when a patient walks and/or turns his/her head and/or eyes. Wearing yoked prisms of greater than 5 diopters and as much as 10-15 diopters during movement activities, causes significant disruption of a patient's visual processing. Yoked prisms stimulate spatial awareness, redirect visual focus, increase visual attention and facilitate visual change, all by working on the ambient or peripheral visual system. Most importantly, yoked prisms can make those who have tuned out their visual surroundings begin to notice their environment, thus leading to generally increased attention and awareness.

Kaplan believes that patients with autism have spent much of their lives developing strategies such as eye turns, postural warps and self-stimulating behaviors, to compensate for their visual deficits. By the time they reach an optometrist, these behaviors are habitual and ingrained. His experience is that the behavioral changes resulting from the alteration of perception caused by yoked prisms are often instantaneous and dramatic. Prism lenses instantly create a new visual world in which their adaptive mechanisms are no longer necessary or relevant. As a result, these patients rapidly begin to use previously suppressed visual processing abilities in order to make sense out of their altered environment.[3] One vision therapist Dr. Torgerson knows called 15 diopter yoked prisms a "wake up call."

Kaplan finds it effective to start with disruptive yoked prisms that actually make a patient see the world as more, not less chaotic. This strategy forces the severely withdrawn patient to abandon his/her coping mechanisms, leaving no option but to pay attention to the environment. Using high-magnitude yoked prisms, typically 15-20 diopters, forces an immediate reorganization of the neuromotor system to meet the newly transformed demands.[3(p.82)]

Initially, optometrists should take a gentle, cautious approach when using prisms. Used carelessly, they can cause an individual with autism to experience nausea and visual overload, and then shut down and retreat.

Yoked Prisms as a Visual Probe

In Chapter 2, Dr. Schulman wrote about probing with yoked prisms as part of the evaluation procedure. This exercise should be repeated once vision therapy begins, as well. Torgerson recommends observing the quality of walking, sitting down, ball playing, ascending and descending stairs and any/all movements and posture first without prisms. Ask the patient to walk approximately 10 feet and then sit down in a chair that is facing him/her, so that he/she must turn around. Play catch with a Koosh or suspended ball. Also, observe the patient complete some fine motor activities, such as tracing and cutting along a line, including any activity that the patient finds difficult, such as tying shoes.

Then introduce yoked prisms, one by one, in each orientation, base up, down, left and right. Schulman recommends starting with low amounts of plus and/or prism, probing to find the right amount. If the child is an exotrope, or has hyperactive behavior, try +0.50 along with varying amounts of base-in prism, typically from 1/2 to 2 diopters, noting any changes in attention or awareness.

By changing a patient's visual space with yoked prisms, the optometrist can watch how an individual with autism manages visual space. Typically, most re-orient their gaze, looking at images from a new position in space when wearing prism lenses. The optometrist must watch carefully, making acute observations of the patient's postural adaptations and compensations, noting any increase or decrease in visually directed movement, and visual awareness. Note differences with each orientation.

Repeat the same activities with 10 or 15 prism diopter yoked prisms in all four positions. Again, observe the outcomes, noting any further postural changes and ease and/or difficulty in visually directed movements and visual awareness.

With higher functioning patients, Kaplan uses the results of the Van Orden Star[7] at nearpoint to determine which yoked prisms to use for a patient. The interested reader should consult his book, *Seeing Through New Eyes*[3(p183-196)] for a very detailed description of how to use this tool to enhance the visual analysis and apply lenses. Two clinical pearls he offers is that
- When apices are above the line, base-down prism is indicated
- If apices are below the line, use base-up

For the many patients with autism who are unable to perform the Van Orden Star, however, Kaplan says there is no universal formula for selecting the "right" prisms. Lens selection is a combination of experience mixed with trial and error.

Yoked Prisms for Visual Redirection

As a child learns to use his/her eyes more efficiently, move to visually-directed tasks. Like red/green glasses, yoked prisms can be used with any visually directed movement activity such as the walking rail, ball play, the Marsden ball, bean bag toss, pegboard rotator, LeBarge Electro Therapist, or eye-hand saccadic fixator. Move from gross motor activities to fine motor ones, such as completing mazes or putting pegs in a rotating board. Integrate vision with other senses so that as vision changes, activities are not overwhelming. Activities are as endless as your imagination. Remember: increased visual awareness and visually directed movement are the goals.

A sample activity: Ask a patient to attempt the walking rail wearing first 10 yoked prism base down, then base up. Note how difficult it is for him/her to direct body movements. Is the patient "feeling" the rail for where to put the foot or using vision to direct and guide movements? Look for exaggerations such as flailing of arms; which orientation appears easier? Can the patient voice an opinion about which prism is "better?" Repeat with base right and left, making same observations. Note speed of adaptation with each change of the prism orientation. For non-verbal patients, look at postural and performance changes with different strength prisms.

Dr. Schulman recalls a patient who "hugged" the wall on his right side. When wearing +0.50D base left and then base right lenses, he staightened up and navigated down the center of the hallway.

Educating the Patient about Yoked Prisms
The optometrist should make time during the consultation to educate patients and their caretakers about yoked prisms. Explain the difference between "compensatory" lenses and "therapeutic" lenses. The most important message is that these lenses are going to create changes in how the brain interprets the information the eyes send it. This reorganization and reorientation may feel "different" and maybe even "uncomfortable" for awhile, but after a short time, the eyes will not have to work so hard and the brain will become accustomed to its new way of interpreting the environment. When the eyes lead the mind, a person functions well; when the mind leads the eyes, performance of any kind is difficult.

Explain that after awhile, (you are not sure how long), these therapeutic lenses will no longer be necessary. Further vision training will help the brain work more efficiently to make use of vision, which will, in turn enhance other aspects of function.[3 (99-101)]

Vision Therapy
Kaplan states that, "while yoked prism lenses play a vital role in the treatment process, it is critical to realize that prism lenses are only a first step in a program of visual management. Generally, it takes months (or in some cases more than a year) for patients to obtain full, permanent benefits from prism lenses and vision therapy."[3 (p.46)]

Once a patient is mostly cooperative, vision therapy can progress to the next step, where the goal is working on specific visual skills. Activities should vary and be individualized for each child. The authors agree that the most effective vision therapist recognizes the developmental level and perceptual style of each patient. Everyone with visual deficits adapts differently; optometrists must treat the individual, not the test findings.[3 (p.47)] As optometrists gain experience working with patients on the autism spectrum, they will learn how to "read" the patient and interpret their symptoms with an increasing degree of skill.

Schulman cautions that the optometrist must recognize the level at which the patient is functioning developmentally, working all the time toward moving skills close to an age appropriate level. For instance, a goal for a five-year-old child could be to sustain a pursuit in any field of gaze for more than a second, rather than for an extended period of time.

Monocular work is important for those with autism, according to Schulman, but it may be difficult because some kids can be resistant to patches, due to tactile defensiveness on the face. Once they adapt to the tactility of glasses, however, they may be less resistant to tape patches. Circular tape patches over therapy glasses work very well for pursuits or fixation work. Kaplan does not use monocular training as he believes it interferes with reorganization of the neural process.

Again, start at the child's developmental level and build up from there, making sure to keep activities interesting. Puppets are a great tool. Try moving the puppet in circles and telling the child to touch its nose when you say "Go!" Kids love having their own puppets. Have a child's puppet kiss your puppet as you move it from position to position.

Another great activity is flashlight tag for pursuits. Shine the light on many different positions on the wall or floor and ask the child to touch or step on your light. Move the light slowly on the floor, giving the child adequate time to be successful. If the child is old enough, he/she can also have a flashlight to play tag with your light. Using a Marsden ball, supine, sitting or standing, is another good tracking activity; alternatively, have the child just watch the ball or play catch with it.

Accommodative work can be done with flippers or with the flashlight. Try using flippers while the child attempts a puzzle or plays a stacking game. Shine the flashlight onto a picture on the wall and then ask the child to point to the same picture in a book. Ask a child to shine the light on a picture on the wall and then throw a ball at the same picture on the floor. Be creative, always recognizing the patient's developmental level, and never making the task too demanding.

For binocular work, again use prism flippers or prism glasses and anaglyphs or Polaroids at the patient's level. Anaglyphs with red and green markers are great for mazes or drawings. Present red, green and yellow mega blocks, and start building with them. Schulman has patients wear red and green anaglyphs with the saccadic fixator and the Marsden ball, which is looped with red and green pipe cleaners. She also asks a child to toss black and red checkers in a bucket while calling out the color, or throwing them in separate containers, one for each color, alternating which side the colors are on, to make the task more challenging. The anaglyph work is particularly helpful in the older children and even adults with autism and attention deficits who have made such adaptations as a suppression or strabismus. As with any activity, begin where they can be successful, constantly encouraging them with frequent praise and understanding.

Strabismus in Autism Spectrum Disorders

In Chapter 2, Dr. Schulman cited the research showing that about half of those with autism spectrum disorder diagnoses evidence an eye turn, technically called a "strabismus." This statistic is astounding when compared to only four percent of the population in general with this problem.

An ophthalmologist typically treats a strabismus surgically, possibly creating a cosmetically "straight" eye, but many times the two eyes don't work together as a team. According to Kaplan, reliance upon surgery as "the only answer to a strabismus" is based upon the belief that lost neural connections cannot regenerate. Follow-up treatment with patching is often recommended to heighten awareness in the lazy eye. Neither the cause of the strabismus nor getting the eyes to work together to achieve binocularity and resultant depth perception are addressed.

Leonard Press, OD, FCOVD, wrote a Topical Review of Strabismus in the March, 1991 issue of the *Journal of Optometric Vision Development (JOVD)*.[8] Some of his conclusions after reviewing over 200 research papers include the following:
• The classification and documentation of the age of onset of strabismus has strong clinical implications in deciding when to intervene and in the nature of the intervention.

- Even cases successfully managed by early surgery are at 50% risk of developing accommodative esotropia which will require accommodative therapy.[9]
- The overall success rate for achieving some level of binocular vision with surgery in infantile strabismus is only 22%; the cosmetic success rate is 63%.[10]
- Taking a conservative approach yields better results. Success rates of binocularity from surgery done age 4 months to 2 years has a 27% success rate; 2 years to 4 years, a 20% success rate; greater than 4 years, a 32% success rate.[11]
- The commonality of successful cases reported in optometric literature includes the application of binasal occlusion and low plus lenses.[12]

Although this review is not current, procedures have not changed markedly, and most optometrists believe that vision therapy has a better opportunity for success. They draw that conclusion because optometrists, especially those with post-graduate training in vision therapy techniques, view the strabismus not as an "eyeball" problem, but rather as a brain dysfunction.

According to Brenda Heinke Montecalvo, OD, "a strabismus is a motor-sensory misalignment caused by an infant's unconscious choice for survival."[13] A strabismus is sometimes seen after a traumatic birth, an infection, a high fever, surgery, heavy metal toxicity, sensory deprivation, or any assault on the growing nervous system. According to Kaplan, infants are born with neither an esotropia (a strabismus with an inward turning eye) nor an exotropia (one where the eye turns out). He thus concludes that a strabismus does not stem from a structural deficit of the eye, but is rather an unconscious adaptive response to neural dysfunction.[3 (p.126)]

How a Strabismus Affects Learning and Behavior
In strabismus, one eye accurately aims at the object of regard, while the other eye misses it by aiming above, below or to the left or right of it. Double vision (diplopia) then results. The misalignment may be constant or intermittent, and thus not always noticeable. Disorganization and confusion follow as the brain struggles to integrate competing messages.

In order to minimize the disorganization and confusion, sometimes the unconscious mind adapts to strabismus by suppressing signals from the faulty aiming eye. Eventually, visual suppression may lead to amblyopia or "lazy eye," in which the nerves that transport and interpret visual information lose some of their ability. The result is poor vision in one eye, due to an interference in the neurological interpretive mechanism.

In many instances the reduced vision cannot be corrected with glasses or surgery. *With the eyes functioning at less than 100% efficiency, any sustained visual activity such as reading may require extra effort and strain.* As in strabismus, the only obvious sign of amblyopia may be an eye turn. However, some people with amblyopia may turn their heads to see certain things or close one eye when reading.[14]

According to Kaplan, the body and brain's adaptations to a strabismus are wide-ranging. The strabismic individual experiences three basic losses, which overlap:
- Loss of control of the environment and of the self in relationship to the environment
- Loss of mobility
- Limitation of the range and variety of visual concepts

All of the above losses are a result of the eyes not working together as a team. Without perception occurring as an end-product of a dynamic process involving the use and integration of ALL sensory receptors, including the eyes, the best outcome that a strabismic individual can attain the construct of space, not the true perception of space.[3 (p.126)]

Since a good number of the eye's neural fibers bring information to the body's balance system, it follows that a person's sense of where he is in space is compromised if these fibers deliver inaccurate information. A child who is disoriented in space experiences himself and his environment as unstable and unpredictable. He may grow increasingly inward, become belligerent or demonstrate sensory defensiveness. Because space perception also affects movement, language development, social skills, reading, writing, mathematics, and many untold other areas, these end-product skills all suffer, as well. Strabismic behavior, like mercury poisoning (see Chapter 3), has very, very similar symptoms as autism.

Vision Therapy for Strabismus in the Patient with Autism

Strabismus and amblyopia always require attention. Neither do these conditions go away untreated; nor do children outgrow them. Surgery may cosmetically straighten the eyes, but usually does not improve visual function, especially without pre- and post-surgical vision therapy. Patching the non-amblyopic eye to force the amblyopic eye to see is also of limited value as the sole treatment. For a complete overview of strabismus, the lay reader is encouraged to go to <www.strabismus.org>.

Kaplan cites the work of physiologists David Hubel and Torsten Wiesel, who won a Nobel Prize for their work on visual input to the brain, who concluded that patching eventually leads to the elimination of those visual cells that respond to both eyes simultaneously, eventually leading an individual to attend to the input of only one eye at a time.[3 (p. 130)]

Delve into the tool chest of the behavioral optometrist, take out those lenses, red/green glasses, yoked prisms and vision therapy and motor activities to teach the eyes, body and brain to work together. Kaplan starts by creating binocular diplopia, which overrides the need for suppression (the reason the eye turned in the first place) by applying red/green 3-D glasses behind 20 diopter prisms: right lens base-up, left lens base-down. With lenses in place direct the child to follow a ball hung at chest level, three feet in front. The child will see two balls: one red and one green. Depending on the child's developmental level, the child can point to or hit one of the balls with his/her hand or a stick.

The goal is to recode how the brain interprets the new information in the new visual spatial framework. As the patient's mind recognizes the difference between the "old" way of processing and the "new" way, neural pathways develop that result in higher level visual performance. By laying down new neural pathways, therapies of this type is far superior to patching or surgery that do not improve, and may, in fact impair visual processing.[3 (p.131-2)]

Kaplan's book offers many, many innovative therapy approaches for patients with orientation and spatial organizational issues using a combination of yoked prisms, anaglyphs, hanging objects, dowels, a metronome and more. Readers are urged to consult his book for these extremely valuable techniques.

Breathing

What does breathing have to do with vision? Normal breathing reduces tension and releases energy that allows us to pay attention to the environment. According to Kaplan, a high percentage of patients on the autism spectrum exhibit dysfunctional breathing patterns. Their inability to integrate movement and breathing stresses their muscles, their nervous systems and reduces attention. This tension, in turn, impairs vision, leading to mismatches in how the brain interprets where things are relative to where they appear to be.

Some symptoms of breathing issues in those with autism spectrum disorders:
• Poor blowing skills, such as with candles on a cake, bubbles or with a musical instrument
• Yawning and/or sighing in an attempt to get more oxygen
• Rocking, which compensates for lack of synergistic neural control of the eyes, head and body

- Holding of the breath when giving effort to motor and visual activities, as well as reading and writing
- Hypervenilation related to fear and anxiety[3] (p. 10-163)

Because constraints on breathing affect every aspect of performance, Kaplan believes that an effective vision therapy program must incorporate remediation of inappropriate breathing patterns. He relies on other experts who influenced him: Carola Speads, Dr. Moshe Feldenkrais and F.M. Alexander.

Speads, one of the world's leading teachers of relaxed, efficient breathing for over 80 years died in 1999 at almost 99 years of age. For more about her and her methods, go to <www.breathing.com>. Feldenkrais, an Israeli scientist, physicist and engineer, who devoted his life's work to increasing self-awareness through movement, developed a group of techniques, which take together are known as the Feldenkrais Method. This simple and practical method improves movement, balance and coordination. Therapists of all types use the Feldenkrais Method today throughout the world. For more information and to find a certified teacher, go to <www.feldenkrais.org>. F.M. Alexander was a Shakespearean actor who developed breathing techniques to restore his voice by improving balance and coordination. Although his methods are over 100 years old, they are still practiced by many, including some optometrists. Information about this method is at <www.alexandertechnique.com>.

Incorporating Breathing into Vision Therapy

Kaplan has combined the techniques and philosophies of these innovators to create learning experiences that allow his patients to become aware of and overcome the breathing difficulties that interfere with their visual processing. He uses tissues, bubbles, whistles, straws and ping pong balls to make breathing more efficient. He has also invented several techniques using a three-foot-long dowel, both seated and standing. Very specific breathing patterns elicit a marked relaxation response that eventually leads to increased awareness of the environment. In his therapy program he follows a developmental sequence, moving from postural awareness to movement awareness, to the sensory integration of moving with hearing and seeing. Again, refer to his book to learn specific techniques.

Breathing properly is an inherent part of reflex integration and Educational Kinesiology, as well. Read about the importance of the breath in these therapies for those on the autism spectrum in Chapters 8 and 13 respectively. Therapists from many disciplines recognize that natural and spontaneous breathing brings increased amounts of oxygen, and thus energy, to the cells and the brain. The result: improved movement, language, vision, cognition, learning and behavior.

Progress Evaluations

Dr. Schulman recommends progress evaluations after every 10 visits or no less then four to six months, depending on the frequency of therapy. At the progress evaluation, reassess the visual system and determine if further therapy is needed. If not, schedule a follow-up in three to four months to make certain that the patient is still developing in a timely fashion, and to assess any further need for either the glasses or vision therapy. If the child continues to progress, schedule another follow-up in six months, and then annually.

At the follow-up evaluations educate the parent on what to look for in the coming months as the visual system continues to develop. Suggest that if regression occurs or a problem arises, to push up the appointment, because the earlier an issue is addressed, the better. Often just a change in the glasses prescription or a session or two of "booster therapy" will get a child back on track.

Case Studies

Remember the female patient with very difficult behaviors who Dr. Schulman cited above? When the child put on 10Δ yoked right and left prisms, her behavior changed markedly. Schulman recommends using yoked bases right and left prisms in varying powers, even as low as 1Δ for kids who are big "side-lookers" and "head turners." The child even exclaimed, "No more side-looking!" in her high pitched voice after wearing the new yoked prisms. Her side-looking so diminished that at her last session she was able to sit still long enough to complete every fine motor task wearing the glasses. She also attempted the walking rail, and drew horizontal lines from one side of the paper to the other to connect matching shapes; if they intersected, however, she got stuck.

Kaplan reports a case of a five-year-old boy who had never spoken but interacted using facilitated communication. Upon donning corrective lenses for the first time, he verbalized, "What a bright, sunny day!" When his mother asked, "What color is my dress?" He verbally responded, "Your dress is blue![15] Dramatic breakthroughs such as this serve to emphasize the importance of the visual system in language and behavior.

Eric Another one of Kaplan's patients was Eric, a non-verbal, hyperactive four-year-old diagnosed with PDD. Eric responded extremely well to a variety of yoked prism lenses. Therapy focused initially on Eric's difficulties with spatial orientation. Kaplan believed that the constraints in orientation limited the time and energy Eric had to attend to visual cues, causing him to constrict his peripheral vision and forcing him to make excessive eye movements.

Kaplan's conjecture was that Eric's hyperactivity was a survival mechanism. Eric and others with autism, attempt to establish the limits of "self" by locking onto objects in space with such intensity that they lose awareness of self when standing. The treatment plan starts with anti-gravity procedures to create postural awareness, then movement awareness, next, hearing and moving, and finally, hearing, seeing and moving. Kaplan used activities such as walking on a balance board, marching (progressing from using only single limbs, to same side limbs to opposite side limbs) and angels-in-the-snow with base-left prisms. He integrates auditory and visual system by adding music or a metronome. These activities all served to ground Eric and free up the visual system for a relaxed exploration of the environment.

Eric took two months to establish a body schema and another two months to connect the visual to the vestibular system and finally to audition. Five months after beginning treatment, Eric, previously non-verbal, was producing three and four-word phrases. He was markedly more aware of his surroundings, with far fewer symptoms.

Lydia, an adult patient with autistic behaviors who consulted with Dr. Torgerson, described her world when using base-up and base-down prisms: "With the thick bit at the bottom I felt very aware, but easily lost self control, especially in relation to getting excited in shops, etc. The sound was normal (in my sense of the word) with both, and the periphery more in the middle with both; that is the things that normally would be on the edge were more in front, but more so with the thick bit at the bottom. The thick section at top definitely makes the faces of people more meaningfully complete, and makes for more separation in the foreground."

"Both prisms really make me feel a bit nauseous, which is what I would expect, and, unlikely though it may seem, the thick part at bottom also makes me really silly, in the sense that I have those 'happy' feelings that one associates with being played with. That is why I was finger flicking… being 'happy' in that sense is not 'happy' in the normal sense."[16]

BG One of Dr. Nancy Torgerson's favorite teachers about autism is BG, a 29-year-old adult with autism, referred to her by an auditory integration therapist. BG had little expressive language, although she comprehended quite well. Dr. Torgerson followed her for 10 years, even though she lived 200 miles from her office.

BG did not read but could pick out some letters; she was uncomfortable in a crowded area with a lot of movement, such as a shopping mall; eye/hand coordination sports were very difficult; she was hesitant with stairs; she placed a keyboard off to the right when using facilitated communication; and she had possible visual field problems.

BG only did optometric vision therapy every other week in office due to the distance. She did 30 minutes of home activity four days each week. During the course of her ten years of therapy she became productive at work, learned to follow words using her finger as a pointer, became more verbal. She is active in sports and has been accepted in a new group home.

BG's phenomenal gains made her mother comment that "vision therapy gave her the daughter she had never had." BG was even able to be a bridesmaid in her brother's wedding! Before vision therapy, no one would have ever even have thought that possible. BG's success also changed Dr. Torgerson's view of those with autistic behaviors. She gained hope that vision would be a part of the puzzle in other patients and that lenses, prisms and/or vision therapy could help others reach their potential. For more details on this case see "A Behavioral Approach to Vision and Autism" by Marcy Rose, OD, and Nancy Torgerson, OD.[18]

Summary

Dr. Melvin Kaplan states that "no treatment program for autism, developmental delays or learning disabilities can be complete unless it addresses and corrects the visual dysfunction that underlies so many learning and behavioral problems." By correcting "visual deficits, optometrists facilitate all future learning, and powerfully enhance the ability of patients to maintain and generalize the skills they acquire."[3 (p. 45)]

Whether used in spectacles for part or full time wear, and/or during vision therapy activities, yoked prisms can be very powerful tools for increasing visual awareness and redirecting and extending the range of vision in a person at either end of the spectrum. Using them is an awesome responsibility that can be life-changing for both the patient and the optometrist.

Torgerson believes that her journey learning about those with autistic behaviors, watching them change with yoked prisms, and the rewards of working with them reoriented her thinking and truly changed her perspective for all patients. Schulman recognizes that children with autism spectrum disorders have unique and adaptive visual patterns that may or may not work for them. Vision therapy and appropriate lens and prism application can make all the difference for them in their relationships to others, the environment and to future potential.

Authors agree that vision therapy must be part of an overall treatment plan that includes biomedical intervention and other sensory therapies. Each child is unique and the therapies for an individual must be appropriate for his/her developmental age and history. "To understand autism, or any other human condition you must observe the individual, not just the stereotypes. Our most talented teachers agree when they say, to reach a child with autism, you must first learn to see the world through the student's eye.[17]

References

1. *Personal communication with Dr. Nancy Torgerson, approximately 1994.*

2. *Rowley EV. Integrating Mind, Brain and Body: A Vision Aerobics Program. Woodinville, WA, 1988. (Available through OEP).*

3. *Kaplan M. Seeing Through New Eyes: Changing the Lives of Children with Autism, Asperger Syndrome and other Developmental Disabilities through Vision Therapy. Philadelphia, PA: Jessica Kingley Publishers, 2006:34, 81.*

4. *Kaplan M., Edelson SM, Seip JA. Behavioral changes in autistic individuals as a result of wearing ambient transitional prism lenses. Child Psychiatr Hum Dev 1998;9:65-76.*

5. *Kaplan M, Flach F. The magic of yoked prisms. OEP Curriculum 1985;7:15-9.*

6. *Flach FF, Kaplan M. Visual perceptual dysfunction in psychiatric patients. Comp Psychiatry 1983;24:304-11.*

7. *Van Orden Star. Mast Development Co. Keystone View Division, 2212 E. 12th St., Davenport, IA 52803, or Circle Publishing Co., PO Box 13073, St. Louis, MO 63110.*

8. *Press LJ. Topical review: strabismus. J Optom Vis Dev; 1991;22:5-20.*

9. *Baker JD, De Young-Smith M. Accommodative esotropia following surgical correction of congenital esotropia, frequency and characteristics. Graefe's Arch Clin Exp Ophthalmol 1988;226:175-7.*

10. *Scheiman M, Ciner E, Gallaway M. Surgical success rates in infantile esotropia. J Am Optom Assoc 1989;60:22-31.*

11. *Von Noorden GK. A reassessment of infantile esotropia: XLIV Edward Jackson Memorial Lecure. Am J Ophthalmol 1988;105:1-10.*

12. *Maples WC. Early correction of esotropia: A literature review. Mid-American Vision Conference 1987, Camas, WA·C&R Croisant, 1988:27-36.*

13. *Montecalvo BH. Infant and toddler strabismus and amblyopia. Behavioural Aspects of Vision Care 2000;41:16-20.*

14. *Kavner RM. Strabismus and amblyopia. New Developments 2002-2003 Winter;8:2,5.*

15. *Kaplan M, Edelson SM, Gaydos AM. Postural orientation modifications in autism in response to ambient lenses. Child Psychiatr Hum Dev 1996;27:81-91.*

16. *Personal communication, Dr. Nancy Torgerson.*

17. *Hart C. A Parents Guide to Autism. New York, Simon and Schuster, 1993:1.*

18. *Rose M, Torgerson N. A behavioral approach to vision and autism. J Optom Vis Dev 1994;25:269-75.*

Chapter 10
Sound-Based Therapies for Those
on the Autism Spectrum
Primary author: Dorinne Davis, MA, CCC-A, F-AAA
Contributor: Stephen M. Edelson, PhD

Introduction

Sound-based therapies include interventions that address auditory, listening, and vestibular issues. Some call sound-based therapies "listening therapies" or "auditory retraining therapies." However, they are much more than "listening" to music or "retraining" the ear. The term "sound-based therapies" embraces all components of the other terms as well as includes other therapies that use sound and vibration on the body.

Most individuals with an autism spectrum diagnosis have issues in one or more of the above areas. While the etiology of these difficulties is unclear, they could very well be related to the repeated inner ear infections many experienced as babies and the treatments used to ameliorate them (See Chapter 3).

Sound processing difficulties manifest themselves as the impaired ability to perceive, process and/or respond to sound appropriately. While the term "auditory processing," meaning what the brain does with what it hears, is typically connected to language and communication, the term "sound processing" is more inclusive, encompassing the whole body's responses at a cellular level. Likewise, the symptoms of sound sensitivities and sound processing disorders extend far beyond the perception of sound for speech, language and listening. Table 10-1 lists these symptoms for children and adults.

Table 10-1 Symptoms of Sound Processing Disorders

Children

Language issues – poor memory; auditory discrimination, sequencing rhythm and timing; difficulty learning a foreign language; stuttering; dysfluency

Vestibular problems – poor balance, coordination, muscle tone, posture

Sensory processing disorder – Hyper- or hypo-reactivity to touch, taste, smell, sound or sight; seeking out deep pressure, such as clinginess or burrowing under pillows

Oral motor problems – impaired chewing, articulation, swallowing; lip and tongue mobility, teeth grinding; picky eating

Attention and focusing issues

Social/emotional problems – excessive crying, inability to make and keep friends, using inappropriate words

Academic issues – Poor phonemic awareness, decoding, reading comprehension; spelling, writing, and/or math

Poor athletic skills

Adults

Poor self-confidence, organizational, public speaking, singing skills

Below average ability to stay focused, follow conversations, tune out background noise

Low energy, depression, weak visual motor skills

Many individuals with autism also demonstrate problems with sound sensitivities and/or processing.[1] Both under- and over-sensitivities to sound are common. Those who are hypo-responsive may appear deaf or unresponsive to sound, and "tune out." Others can be bothered by the humming of a fluorescent bulb, experiencing certain sounds as intolerable or even painful. Birthday parties, shopping malls, restaurants, sporting events and other gatherings can be particularly troublesome for them, because of the unpredictability of sound. Symptoms of hyper-sensitivity include crying, covering the ears, running from the sound source, and temper tantrums. Inconsistencies in hearing the various frequencies of sound or lack of synchronicity of the two ears, can result in behavior that is distractible, avoidant, hyperactive, inattentive or bizarre.[2]

Just as distorted visual messages sent to the brain can impair the ability to focus on and give meaning to what is seen, distorted processing of auditory signals impairs the brain's ability to focus on and give meaning to that which is heard. Furthermore, just as those on the spectrum have difficulty with visual discrimination, visual closure, visual sequential, short- and long-term visual memory, they also have difficulty with auditory discrimination, auditory closure, auditory sequential, short- and long-term auditory memory. Obviously, auditory processing problems also impede the acquisition, interpretation and use of language.

In the past 15 years, an increasing number of professionals from a variety of disciplines, including audiology, occupational therapy, psychology and speech-language pathology, are recommending, and have incorporated, sound-based therapies to improve the auditory, listening, and vestibular skills of children with autism spectrum disorders. While some programs are designed to take place in a therapist's office, others can be used at home, under a therapist's supervision.

Utilizing sound to facilitate bodily change is not new. For centuries, almost every culture on earth has developed methods using sound and song to heal. Unfortunately, many of these tools are associated with superstition and mysticism. Today's sophisticated computerized technology allows us to document and record what is happening in the body and brain, thus removing the mystery.

This chapter draws upon the work of top experts in the field of sound-based therapy. Audiologist, Dorinne S. Davis, President and Founder of The Davis Center in New Jersey, <www.thedaviscenter.com>, and author of *Sound Bodies through Sound Therapy*[3] coined the term "sound-based therapy," and is the primary author. The editor consulted with Stephen M. Edelson, PhD, former President of Society for Auditory Intervention Techniques (SAIT), and Director of the Autism Research Institute. She also added the section on music therapy at the end of the chapter.

What is Sound?

A well-used copy of *The American College Dictionary* defines sound as "the sensation produced in the organs of hearing when the surrounding air vibrates."[4] Sound is vibrational energy that impacts the entire body, sometimes without a person's awareness. Vibration produces frequency, and frequency is synonymous with sound. People "hear" or "feel" sound vibrations through their bone structure, sense of touch, and through the interconnected network of cells all through the body.[3 (p.20)]

The Anatomy of the Ear

A short review of the ear and its physiology is important for understanding how sound-based therapies work. The ear is the only fully functioning sensory system in utero, and the last sense to go before death. By its very nature and development, the ear and its response to sound are instrumental in overall development and functioning in everyday life. Assuring the adequate development of the processing and utilization of sound stimulation by the bodies of those with autism spectrum disorders is foundational to their overall growth and development.

Sound travels to the inner ear through both air and bone conduction. First, vibrations move by air conduction through the outer ear, down the ear canal to the eardrum transmitting through the middle ear cavity, along the three tiniest bones in the body. Then, vibrational signals go to the inner ear via bone conduction, where both the vestibular system and the cochlea are located. Fluids in both sense the body's movement, and stimulate both the hearing receptors in the cochlea, and the body movement and positioning receptors in the semi-circular canals and vestibule.

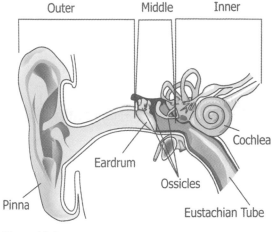

Figure 10-1

Figure 10-1 shows the ear and its parts.

Sound moves faster by bone conduction than by air conduction. The ear's response to sound moving by bone conduction is key to improving the listening process. Some sound-based therapies have mechanisms that allow a practitioner to manipulate the time delay between air and bone conduction. The vibrations then reach the brain more quickly, allowing for a more rapid response.

The last step is for the ear to send responses to the brain along the eighth cranial nerve to the cortex, stimulating both the auditory and vestibular centers, which are the primary integrators of the nervous system. The purpose of these two systems extends far beyond hearing; they synchronize to detect and analyze movement. At the ear level, the vestibular system detects and discriminates the larger movements of the body, while audition's role is to register and regulate the finer movements of sound waves in the air. The brain then interprets this information and sends the needed messages to the rest of the body. Because both centers are located in the ear, audiologists and occupational therapists are two of the professionals most interested in sound therapies.

Sound stimulation affects many sensory, motor and bodily functions: hearing, listening, balance, coordination, vestibular function, movement, rhythm, posture, proprioception, receptive language, expressive language, social/emotional skills, oral motor skills, articulation, speech fluency, taste, touch, smell, and yes…vision. Digestion, blood pressure, hormone secretion, muscle tone and other autonomic nervous system functions also respond to vibration. Sound vibrations impact and are impacted upon by each of the cranial nerves. These vibrations search out those areas in greatest need, and support changes through branches of the cranial nerves that connect to and/or pass through the ear.

Two muscles, the tensor tympani and stapedius, are important in the transmission of sound in the middle ear. The stapedius, also known as the "acoustic reflex" muscle, helps protect the ear from loud sounds. It can over- or under-react, resulting in hyper- or hypo-sensitivity to sound. Both the tensor tympani and stapedius muscles must be working correctly in order to suppress background noise and emphasize high frequencies, a missing outcome in many of those with autism spectrum disorders.

Dr. Stephen Porges, a psychologist at the University of Maryland, found that these two muscles were also important for controlling vocalization, facial expression, heart rate and breathing, as well as developing and maintaining oral motor skills. In the ears of many individuals with autism their lack of efficiency results in the inability to sort out high frequency sounds, such as in human speech, from low- frequency sounds, because these individuals are in a state of high anxiety. Those with autism are thus hyper-vigilant, attending to all sounds in the environment, thus over-exposing their brains to sound.[5] If the cochlea, semi-circular canals, and vestibule in the inner ear over- or under- respond to sound, the vibrations they receive may not be sufficient to process information correctly. Insufficient or excessive vibration can affect the development of language, gross and fine motor skills, oral motor skills, body movement and rhythm, balance, timing, attention, proprioception, and other sensory integration skills.

The pathway to the brain is complex, and problems can occur at any of many cross-over relay stations, due to lack of stimulation or weak responsivity. Each station is responsible for a specific function, such as listening with the two ears together, localizing sound, response time, attention, etc. The thalamus controls the rhythmical brain waves, spreading them throughout the brain and the body. Brain waves help regulate the nervous system, which plays a very important role in the sensation of sound stimulation.

Hearing Versus Listening

Hearing is to listening as eyesight is to vision. Just as the eye is more than an apparatus for sight, the ear is far more than a hearing mechanism. Hearing is the passive reception of sound: the involuntary physical act of sound transmitting to the ear and then to the brain. Listening is an active, dynamic process involving far more than the ear's ability to elicit a response at just a hearing or auditory level. Listening is a mental process that requires the intention and desire to communicate, and the ability to tune in to sounds at both a conscious and an unconscious or cellular level for discrimination and interpretation.[6] Efficient listening, like good vision, requires that the various components of both organs work together. The coordination of sounds allows the ear to send messages to the brain to be interpreted and stored.

The Founders of Sound-Based Therapies

Tomatis Dr. Alfred Tomatis is considered the father of all sound-based therapies. He was the first to define the difference between hearing and listening, the first to recognize the close relationship between the auditory and vestibular systems, the first to recognize the importance of high frequency audition, and the first to identify a connection between the voice, the ear, and the brain. In the 1950s he developed the first technique to "re-educate the ear."

Tomatis stated that while hearing is fully functional at four-and-one-half months in utero, listening, like vision, must be learned. Hearing remains constant as development takes place; listening skills, on the other hand, change over time. Tomatis connected listening to the development of receptive and expressive language, learning, motor control and motivation. He viewed the ear as the source of vibrational energy for the brain, charging it with electrical impulses, and organizing the perceptions for the whole body.

Tomatis, a French ear-nose-and-throat specialist, was the son of an opera singer. Tomatis' research in the mid-1900s focused on the interaction between the ear and the voice to achieve changes in the voices of opera singers. He believed that changes to either organ influenced the other. He found that singers' voice quality improved when he stimulated their ears with their own voice. Tomatis called this the audio-vocal loop, later named the Tomatis Effect, which demonstrates that the ear and the voice are part of the same neurological loop. Tomatis viewed the audio-vocal loop as key in developing the desire to listen. His pioneering work on the voice-ear-brain connection led to the introduction of sound as a treatment modality.

The Tomatis Effect states that:

- "The voice only contains the harmonics that the ear can hear.
- If you give the possibility to the ear to correctly hear the distorted frequencies of sound that are not well heard, these are immediately and unconsciously restored into the voice.
- The imposed audition sufficiently maintained over time, results in permanently modifying the audition and phonation."[7]
- Bottom line: The voice can produce only what the ear hears.[8]

Davis has further validated The Tomatis Effect with "The Davis Addendum to the Tomatis Effect,"[9] which additionally supports the voice as the body's stabilizer. The voice is the mechanism through which one can evaluate and support a person's wellness. Davis' unique combination of training in audiology, the Tomatis Method and BioAcoustics laid the foundation for the discovery of "The Davis Addendum to the Tomatis Effect." Davis' redefinition of the Voice-Ear-Brain connection is the foundation for her "Tree of Sound Enhancement Therapy®," which follows.

The Tomatis Effect has strong implications for autism, attention deficit disorder, dyslexia, and other autism spectrum disorders. The Tomatis Method of therapy evolved from the Tomatis Effect. This approach, and how it ameliorates the many sound- based problems of those on the spectrum, is described in detail later in this chapter.

Madaule   When Tomatis died in 2001, his protégé, Canadian psychologist, Dr. Paul Madaule became the disciple for his work. Dyslexic and clumsy as a child, Madaule studied in France with Tomatis, and, after he conquered his reading disability, vowed to use the Tomatis Method to help others. He views the Tomatis Method as a concrete, efficient, holistic and humanistic "therapy of the future."[6 (p.15)]

Madaule, has opened many Tomatis Centers in North America, including The Listening Centre in Toronto, Ontario, Canada, <www.listeningcentre.com>, which he founded in 1978, and still directs. There, he evaluates and helps many individuals with autism spectrum diagnoses.

Madaule uses a music metaphor to describe what goes wrong in autism: "If the senses are musical instruments, in autism, they lack a conductor. They are not able to play together… In the Tomatis view, the ear is the conductor. When I speak of the ear, I mean the sensory organ and all its connections to the nervous system and the whole body."[10]

Madaule has written about his experiences and his life's work practicing and adapting the Tomatis method in his book, *When Listening Comes Alive: A Guide to Effective Learning and Communication*.[6] It is also available in Spanish as *Terapia de Eschcha*.[11] Madaule's adaptation of the Tomatis Method is called Listening Fitness Training or LiFT™. (See Section on Modified Tomatis "Spin-Offs" later in this chapter.)

Berard Dr. Guy Berard, another French physician who studied with Dr. Tomatis, believed that most of Tomatis' protocol was unnecessary. Based on irregularities in the audiograms of more than 8000 patients, he concluded that some people hear some sound frequencies more clearly than others, and that their combination of hypo- and hyper-sensitivity to sounds negatively impacts their development of phonological awareness and language. The end product is delayed or decreased comprehension, poor articulation, and/or decreased or inappropriate expression.

Berard postulated that the quality of the perception of sound that one hears is equal to the behavior of the individual. He formulated his own theory that "human behavior is greatly conditioned by the way one hears." Berard's theory evolved further as he watched the audiograms of children with disabilities change along with their behavior.

Berard developed his own "hearing retraining device" and treated patients with auditory problems that were more subtle than hearing loss. His method is described in his book, *Hearing Equals Behavior*.[12] Berard described his method as one of hearing re-education. His system, originally called "Auditory Training" was later renamed "Auditory Integration Training" or AIT. The word "integration" was added at the recommendation of Dr. Bernard Rimland of the Autism Research Institute, in order to distinguish this method from another used to rehabilitate the deaf and hard-of-hearing. Annabel Stehli introduced AIT for those with autism in the early 1990's with her daughter Georgiana's remarkable improvement.[2]

Davis and other researchers have evaluated the efficacy of AIT by testing the acoustic reflex muscle, the second muscle in the middle ear, pre- and post- completion of the AIT program. Consistently, this muscle demonstrates a positive 'retrained' functioning after Auditory Integration Training.[3] (pp. 167-171) Whereas Dr. Berard reported the behavioral changes, this retraining of the muscle helps explain the phenomenon from a physiological perspective.

Kemp and Edwards In 1978 audiologist David Kemp began conducting research on otoacoustic emissions. This phenomenon, identified in the late 1940s, states that the ear not only takes in and sends sound to the brain, but also emits a sound, most likely from the cochlea.[13]

About the same time, Sharry Edwards, a college student, was searching for an explanation for why she heard sounds emanating from the people around her. She claimed to be able to identify people by their sound, and believed that each person resonates at a unique frequency. Three different sound laboratories conducted independent testing of Edward's voice; all confirmed that she could produce a pure tone sine wave with her voice.

Edwards postulated that if key frequencies are out-of-balance in the ear, then they are also out-of-balance in the voice. For over 30 years Edwards has increased her unique knowledge of the voice-ear connection and concluded that the voice is a hologram of the body's emotional, physical and spiritual components. Eventually her knowledge led to the development of the science of BioAcoustics™.[14]

BioAcoustics™ uses a "voiceprint" to evaluate a person's state of health by analyzing the frequencies of all cellular structures in the body, and their relationship to each other. After evaluating the voiceprint, and identifying imbalances, a qualified sound health practitioner suggests a combination of specific frequencies that are programmed into a portable tone box designed to support an individual's overall well-being. BioAcoustics is an emerging science with unlimited potential for many wellness fields. It is a useful tool for those practicing integrative medicine, as well as for professionals in nutrition, sports medicine, occupational and physical therapy, and, of course, optometry.

A Review of the Literature on Using Sound-Based Therapies with Autism
Stephen M. Edelson, PhD, and Bernard Rimland, PhD, of the Autism Research Institute (ARI) have reviewed 28 published studies investigating the effectiveness of sound therapies in autism spectrum disorders.[15] Most of the studies showed AIT to be effective. While Drs. Edelson and Rimland found "none of the research of Nobel Prize quality," they believe that, because positive studies are far more credible than those with negative results, that AIT clearly confers improvement in a number of symptoms for a significant proportion of those with disorders on the autism spectrum.

Of the 28 research studies that evaluated physiological, behavioral, and cognitive changes in the subjects, the authors of 23 (82%) studies concluded that their data supported the efficacy of AIT, three (11%) claimed to have found no evidence of efficacy, and two (7%) report ambiguous, contradictory results. None of the studies failed to show discernible benefits.

Table 10-2 summarizes research results.

Table 10-2 Review of Findings in Studies Using AIT in Those with Autism Spectrum Disorders (Number of Studies)				
Disorders	Positive Findings	Ambiguous, Controversial, &/ or Contradictory	Results Unclear/ Questionable	No Effects
Autism	13	2	1	0
AD(H)D	4	0	0	0
Several Populations	2	0	1	0
Animals (chicks)	2	0	0	0

The study probably of most interest to optometrists is co-authored by Dr. Janice Scharre of the Illinois College of Optometry and psychologists Margaret P. Creedon and Stephen M. Edelson. They found significant improvements in horizontal and vertical tracking immediately following and three months post -AIT.[16]

A variety of other changes were noted in other studies, including, but not limited to: reductions in hyperactivity, social withdrawal, restlessness, and anxiety,[17,18,21,24] reduction in sound sensitivity,[19-22] increased attention span,[20,23-24] increase in language output,[20,21] improved speech perception,[26] and biochemical changes, specifically, an increase in norepinephrine, and decrease in serotonin levels.[27]

To read abstracts of all studies, go to <www.beardaitwebsite.com/sait/>.

Anecdotal evidence from therapists and parents reporting significant benefit from sound-based therapies abounds. In general, parents report the same benefits noted in the research: reduction in temper tantrums, sound and tactile sensitivity, hyperactivity, impulsivity and distractibility. Increased eye contact, calmness, coordination, balance, more vocalizations, improved language, oral motor skills, better ability to focus, follow directions, pay attention, remember, speak, socialize, move, draw, and play independently are also reported. Significant changes seen in dyslexia include improvement in all aspects of reading and writing. Occasionally sleep disturbances occur or behavior can become agitated. These side effects are usually temporary, and a return to normality is usually seen in a short time, however.[28]

To read some detailed success stories about the use of Tomatis listening therapy in autism, consult Chapter 10 in *The Natural Medicine Guide to Autism* by Stephanie Marohn.[10] For AIT success stories read *Dancing in the Rain: Stories of Exceptional Progress by Parents of Children with Special Needs* by Annabel Stehli.[29] For those interested in how a combination of sound-based therapies can produce even greater positive changes for 16 individuals with mild to severe autism, read *Every Day A Miracle: Success Stories with Sound Therapy* by Dorinne Davis.[30] This new resource explains how to use of the Diagnostic Evaluation for Therapy Protocol (DETP®) as a tool for choosing appropriate therapies.

Several parents have written complete books, or chapters in books, documenting the role of sound therapies in their children's recovery from autism. Those interested in their stories should read *The Sound of a Miracle: A Child's Triumph over Autism*,[2] by Annabel Stehli, whose daughter Georgiana, now an adult, improved dramatically using AIT, and

Awakening Ashley: Mozart Knocks Autism on its Ear[31] by Sharon Ruben, whose daughter recovered using the Tomatis Method. Finally, *Recovering Autistic Children*,[32] published by the Autism Research Institute (ARI), is a compendium of parent stories detailing the combination of methods they used in recovering their children. Many cite sound-based therapies as instrumental in their positive outcomes.

The Tree of Sound Enhancement Therapy®

Dorinne Davis developed "The Tree of Sound Enhancement Therapy" analogy as a tool to assist in understanding the differences among the many methods using sound as their basis for change.[3 (pp.255-277)] (See Figure 10-2.) Davis includes each of the sound-based therapies described in the next section on a part of The Tree of Sound Enhancement Therapy. Those in brackets offer less support than the others, because they do not exactly duplicate the original method or equipment, and/or, alone, may not achieve all of the desired effects.

Working from the bottom up on The Tree, the **Root system** is comprised of therapies that address the specific physiological function of hearing, i.e. retrains the ear to hear;

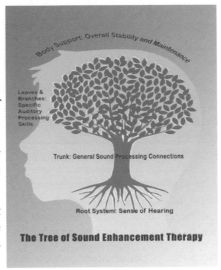

Figure 10-2 The Tree of Sound Enhancement Therapy©Davis, 2004

- Berard Auditory Integration Training - (AIT)
- [The Clark Method - (BGC)]
- [Digital Auditory Aerobics™ - (DAA)]

Trunk includes all the therapies that address how sound energy and processing impacts on bodily functions—all of the vibrational responses that the ear is capable of. This section incorporates the basic connections of the voice-ear-brain foundation.

- The Tomatis Method
- [Dynamic Listening System™ (DLS)]
- [MX Pro]
- [EnListen™]

Leaves and Branches incorporate therapies that address specific auditory processing skills and higher ordered learning skills;

* Upper Trunk/Lower, Leaves and Branches

- Listening Fitness Training (LiFT)
- The Listening Program®
- Samonas®
- [Sound Therapy for the Walkman®]
- [EASe CD's]
- [JoEE®]

*Lower Leaves and Branches

- Fast ForWord
- Interactive Metronome
- Earobics ®

Body Maintenance, surrounds The Tree, and maintains its overall wellness. These supporting therapies are diagnostic and offer therapeutic sound solutions affecting the overall health of the individual. An individual can only reach maximum potential when the whole Tree works together.

- BioAcoustics™

Davis uses her Tree in conjunction with her assessment battery, The Diagnostic Evaluation for Therapy Protocol or DETP,® (patent pending for future distribution), to determine when, if, and in what order, any sound-based therapy is appropriate for an individual. Periodic re-testing assures that an individual is deriving maximum benefit from the therapies.

Types of Sound-Based Therapies

Sound-based therapies all utilize vibration to facilitate change. First the professional runs special tests to determine whether a person has any problems that could benefit from sound-based therapy. If so, then the therapist suggests one or more of the many therapies available.

All sound-based therapies require the use of special equipment that electronically alters music or sound, and/or offers specific tones or beats.[35] All therapies' purpose is to balance the way individuals with autism process sound. The instruments enable a trained professional to approach the auditory/vestibular system directly, thus impacting the whole body vibrationally.

Each sound-based therapy program differs slightly. Some are clinic-based, some home-based. Some inherently contain an active component, while others provide only passive input, unless used in conjunction with a movement therapy, such as occupational therapy. All interventions require specialized training or certification beyond practitioners' professional licensing.

The Tomatis Method, Berard AIT and BioAcoustics are the three foundational types of sound-based therapies. The next section covers these therapies in detail.

The Tomatis® Method

Approach The Tomatis Method takes a psychological approach based on the premise that the ear integrates auditory information at every level of the nervous system. The Tomatis Method emphasizes listening. The five phases of the Tomatis Method establish the audio-vocal loop by taking the listener through the various levels of listening development. The first two stages prepare the individual for relating to the external world, thus establishing a foundation for listening. The third stage is a transition between listening and using the voice.

The last two stages emphasize the voice. When appropriate, programming includes the use of a microphone so that the person hears his/her own voice in order to monitor his/her "listening posture." The voice work is the stabilizing portion of the program and is key to its success.

The Tomatis Method is based on three main principles:

- An acoustical education is necessary to develop true listening;
- The will to communicate must be awakened;
- Re-awakening vibrational memories, experienced in utero through the amniotic fluid, vitalizes the will to communicate.

The goal of a Tomatis listening program is to establish good functional use of the auditory/vestibular system by improving listening and communication skills directly. Because of the vibration and stimulation of sound throughout the entire body, this method brings over-all balance to the listener.

Who Can Benefit The Tomatis Method can help people with listening disorders from infancy through senior citizens. Those at both the mild and severe ends of the autism spectrum, as well as those with a variety of other diagnoses, including, but not limited to general developmental delays, Down syndrome, William syndrome, receptive/expressive language disorder, apraxia, dyspraxia, dyslexia, dysgraphia, and sensory integration dysfunction, can benefit if they have documented listening disorders.

Testing Before starting therapy, a Tomatis Consultant identifies the need for therapy by conducting special testing. The Tomatis Method uses proprietary tests, The Listening Test and The Laterality Test, to determine one's 'listening posture.' The results of these tests guide the consultant in setting up a client's program. The Listening Test is continually used throughout the course of the Tomatis Method. After the initial test, it is administered around the eighth and fifteenth days of the first fifteen days of listening and again at the beginning and end of each session thereafter. The test helps to determine progress.

The Listening Test is different from a hearing test. A hearing test, shown graphically as an audiogram, measures when a person hears a sound 50% of the time, a concept known as a "threshold of hearing." A listening test, is a different type of graph, and measures an individual's motivation to attend to, focus on and organize what he/she hears. The test results also provide information about vestibular functioning, as well as receptive and expressive language skills.

Equipment Tomatis listening therapy utilizes of a device called the Electronic Ear (EE). The EE plays three different types of selections to effect change:

• Mozart, for its special sound energy qualities,
• Gregorian Chants for its slow, rhythmic, relaxing effect,
• the mother's voice, if available, for its ability to trigger primal sound memories.

The EE has two principal channels with a connection between them, which acts as a gate. The first channel allows the listener to hear as he/she normally does; in the second channel the listener hears sounds enhanced with high frequencies. The gate between the channels opens and shuts, switching the sounds one is listening to between channels, thereby exercising the tensor tympani and stapedius muscles and training them to work together.

The capability of filtering out sounds of certain frequencies is a unique feature of the EE. It progressively blocks the lower sound frequencies (below 9000 Hertz) in the music and the mother's voice, to correspond to what the fetus heard in the womb. Tomatis also developed a mechanism on the EE that can change the movement of vibrations from air conduction to bone conduction. This feature, when used in conjunction with filtering and gating permits the practitioner to individualize a listening program for each individual's profile.

To listen, a person dons a headset with earphones attached to a long cord, which is plugged into the EE. The long tether allows participation in a wide variety of developmental activities while listening. Therapists encourage playing with toys, puzzles, or looking at books; gross motor activities like jumping, swinging, rocking; fine motor activities like coloring, legos, peg designs; relaxing activities like lying down; stimulating activities around a particular theme, like oral motor exercises; and more.

Dr. Tomatis discovered that those with a right ear dominance had an advantage over those whose left ear dominates, because a right ear lead offers the shortest physiological connection to the language center, usually located in the left hemisphere of the brain. He postulated that a left-ear lead took longer, used more energy, and was thus less effective. Another goal of the EE is thus to gradually establish a right ear lead.

Frequency and Duration The basic Tomatis Method program is clinic-based, and consists of two sets of 15 days of listening for two hours per day. Some practitioners use a program of 15 days, followed by two eight day programs instead. Some listeners, typically those on the autism spectrum, need more than the basic program and may receive five or eight day continuation programs, spread out over the next few months or years, depending on the severity of the presenting issues. Successful Tomatis programs can take as long as 100 hours. It is extremely important to finish the program so that the body can integrate the desired changes.

Davis believes that during Tomatis therapy, the body finds its own weak spots and self-corrects. She thus does not recommend over-emphasizing a specific area, such as vestibular functioning, but rather guiding the listener towards developing those weak spots in combination with other skills during sessions. When the program emphasizes a person's total development, changes are more well-rounded. Tomatis Consultants often suggest home exercises following the completion of Tomatis sessions, in order to maintain progress.

Resources Over 200 practitioners are trained to deliver Tomatis therapy around the world. For a list, go to <www.tomatis.com> or <www.iarctc.org>.

Auditory Integration Training (AIT)

Approach AIT is a physiological approach in-clinic program based on Dr. Guy Berard's belief that hypersensitivity, distortions and delays in the auditory signal contribute to inefficient learning. The method retrains the ear to process sound without distortions or delays, which, in turn, enhances a person's ability to be alert and to concentrate. AIT works by increasing the intensity levels of music, challenging the acoustic reflex muscle to repattern itself.

Patients are not permitted to use any of their other senses when retraining their sensory modality of hearing, in order to derive maximum benefit from the program. They should not eat, drink, chew or do anything else while listening, because these activities could negate the effect of the therapy by activating the same muscle that AIT retrains. The goal of AIT is to reduce hypersensitivity to sound and equalize the perception of all frequencies.

Who Can Benefit Auditory Integration Training can help people with hearing- related issues, such as hyper- or hypo- responses to sound, age three through adult. Symptoms that may indicate such sensitivities include:

- covering the ears to certain pitches or intensities
- tuning out or ignoring sound
- being uncomfortable in noisy settings or ones in which listening is difficult
- difficulty distinguishing pitch sound differences that impact upon comprehension, articulation, or singing skills
- difficulty localizing sound and/or maintaining auditory attention
- vestibular and balance issues
- gross, fine and oral motor weaknesses

Research has shown AIT to be effective for those with autism and attention deficits, as well as for reading issues, handwriting problems and depression.

Dr. Bernard Rimland suggested that anyone considering AIT also pursue biological interventions (See Chapters 5 and 6), preferably, for some time prior to initiating AIT. First, a well-nourished body, free of toxins, is likely to respond better. Furthermore, sound sensitivity could be the result of magnesium deficiency, mercury toxicity or excitotoxins, such as aspartame. If so, the biological intervention alone could correct the hearing difficulties.

Because some treatments, such as detoxification can take months to years, some children may need to proceed with AIT concurrent with biological interventions, especially if their language is significantly delayed or their hearing hyper-sensitive. In those cases, an AIT "tune up" could stabilize the system at the completion of biomedical intervention.

Davis' "Body Maintenance" of The Tree suggests a similar concept – that maximum wellness supports maximum learning.[3 (pp.273-274)] The Diagnostic Evaluation for Therapy Protocol (DETP) can identify when the bio-chemistry of the body is the best place to start. AIT (or Tomatis) are best begun in conjunction with or after stabilizing the body.

Testing After checking the ears for wax build-up, an audiologist conducts a special Hearing Sensitivity Audiogram (not a typical audiological assessment audiogram) to determine whether an individual is a candidate for AIT. Ear wax can interfere with AIT's effectiveness. AIT uses an audiogram for testing because this method changes hearing.

The audiologist tests each client pre-, mid-, and post- 10 days of listening. Pre-testing identifies specific hearing parameters, establishes a hearing baseline, and suggests the initial individualized programming. The mid-testing helps modify programming and final testing identifies hearing changes. Davis believes that the audiologist should also administer diagnostic acoustic reflex testing.

Equipment Dr. Berard originally developed a device called the Ears Education and Retraining System (EERS), which was later updated and called the AudioKinetron. However, for part of the 1990s, the FDA prohibited distribution of the AudioKinetron in the United States. Currently AIT is considered to be an educational, not a medical application, and both the AudioKinetron and another AIT device called the Earducator, which is manufactured in South Africa, can be used. These two units are the only "Berard approved" devices for AIT.

The AudioKinetron plays music chosen from selected discs at a moderately loud, but not uncomfortable level. The AIT sound amplifier attenuates low and high frequencies randomly, and sends this modified music through headphones to the listener's ears, a technique termed "modulation." AIT also involves using narrow bands to filter out specific frequencies that a person hears too well.

The processed music, which may also be filtered to meet a client's specific profile, is thought to stimulate the auditory and vestibular systems, which in turn, activates the language centers of the brain, eye movements, and the digestive system. Thus, AIT influences far more than hearing. The machine randomly allows sound to bounce back and forth between the ears, requiring the middle ear muscles to unlearn habitual responses and allowing new responses to develop.

Berard specified that AIT use music that has

- a strong tempo/beat
- a large variation in frequency within short intervals
- a strong unpredictability component

Frequency and Duration An AIT program consists of 20 sessions of listening for one half hour in the morning and one half hour in the afternoon, separated by at least three hours in between for 10 days straight. Dr. Stephen M. Edelson of SAIT recommends that AIT is most successful when done as a part of a multi-disciplinary team approach. He suggests that the team should include, but not be limited to specialists in audiology, optometry, psychology, special education and speech/language.

No research supports any home-based follow-up programs at this time. However, AIT practitioners consult with parents during the training to apprise them of possible changes that may occur during and after therapy.

Resources To find an AIT practitioner in your area, go to <www.drguyberard.com>, <www.berardaitwebsite.com> or to <www.georgianainstitute.org>.

BioAcoustics™

Approach BioAcoustics™ is the study of the frequencies all living systems produce. It uses voice spectral analysis, a scientific method for identifying and interpreting the complex frequency interactions constantly occurring in the body. BioAcoustics™ is based on the principle that the body requires a full range of harmonious frequencies, working cooperatively, in order to be healthy.

Everything in an individual's body is impacted by sound: every single cell in the body continuously emits and absorbs sound vibrations that affect the entire body.[35] Every element, pathogen, bacteria, hormone and nutritional factor also manifests a unique vibration, defined by BioAcoustics as its Frequency Equivalent™. Every person's body vibrates with its own unique combination of frequencies. Combined, they produce a distinctive and unique sound blueprint or "voiceprint," representing the totality of those frequencies at that moment in time.

A BioAcoustics Research Associate (BARA) analyzes the voiceprint and identifies frequencies to help a person's body makes changes that support and maintain its overall balance and harmony. BioAcoustics depends upon both individual Frequency Equivalents™, and the relationships among them, to identify imbalances and restore an individual's balance and health.

Frequency Equivalents interact with each other. For example, when you combine the Frequency Equivalents of calcium and magnesium, the result is the Frequency Equivalent of phosphorus, an element that is necessary for calcium and magnesium metabolism. BioAcoustics explores the potential that the body is a mathematical matrix of predictable frequency relationships.[3 (p. 246)]

When a person listens to combinations of specific sound frequencies, programmed into a tone box, his/her brain supports the body to self-correct frequencies that are "out of balance" by sending information back to the brain via the nervous, circulatory, soft tissue, and cellular network.

Who Can Benefit BioAcoustics is particularly useful in diagnosing and helping symptoms related to a variety of seemingly diverse conditions, including autism spectrum disorders, in people of all ages. To date, BioAcoustics has improved many conditions, including heavy metal and chemical toxicity, low muscle tone, and nutritional imbalances. Individuals with arthritis, back injuries, chronic fatigue syndrome, chronic pain, fibromyalgia, gout, hearing loss, high blood pressure, HIV, menopause, multiple sclerosis, nutritional and hormonal imbalances, over-medication, Parkinson's disease, quadriplegia and Tourette syndrome have also benefited. Although not related to autism but of interest to optometrists, is that Bioacoustics has been shown to stabilize and reverse macular degeneration.[3(pp 248-251)]

Testing and Equipment BioAcoustics uses a computerized voice analyzer to capture a 44-second sample of the frequencies of a subject's voice in a "voiceprint" known as his/her Signature Sound™. Because the voice produces what the ear hears, a BioAcoustics' voiceprint also reflects the voice-ear-brain connection.

The BARA prints a graphic representation of the results and reviews it. Computer analysis identifies vibrational discordance: frequencies that are out-of-balance, or "in stress," as well as those that are not supporting the body sufficiently. For instance, a particular vitamin, mineral, or hormone level may show up as too low or high.

After evaluating the voiceprint, and identifying imbalances, the next step is for the BARA to establish a protocol of frequency combinations chosen specifically for that individual. The BARA tests this protocol with the individual connected to biofeedback equipment that monitors his/her body responses. These formulated frequencies are then programmed into a portable tone box that the person listens to at home. Instruments show that BioAcoustics individualized binaural beat frequencies entrain the brain, thus facilitating positive change.

The Bioacoustics voiceprint and tone box are extraordinary tools. The voiceprint can be:

- *Diagnostic* - pinpointing long standing health issues, such as nutritional deficiencies and toxicity. The voiceprint can also identify invaders, like toxins or pathogens, as well as system problems, such as muscle weaknesses. The voiceprint of a three-year-old with autism, who wasn't progressing, showed high levels of fluoride. After taking a history, the practitioner discovered that the family drank only fluoridated water, and that the child liked to eat his fluoride-containing toothpaste.
- *Predictive* - identifying imbalances even when a person has no symptoms, because stress in the body manifests itself at an acoustical level before showing up physically. Some parents and health care professionals are using the BioAcoustics' PreVac® program to predict whether a child is at risk for having a vaccine reaction. This program determines if a child's stressed Frequency Equivalents are related to vaccination factors such as mercury toxicity.

The tone box is

- *Supportive* - resolving a person's innate weaknesses, and even facilitating better absorption of ingested substances, by using the tone box to re-pattern the brain. The end-product is wellness. For example, after listening to a sound Frequency Equivalent of Vitamin C, one child who refused and spit out vitamin C pills and liquid drops, ingested them without difficulty.

Voiceprints are not intended to be used as medical information. However, patients can share the results with their physicians for additional interpretation or to make an informed decision about a child's vaccination schedule, if they so desire.

Frequency and Duration Children with autism make changes both physiologically and psychologically by listening at home daily to the tone box containing their unique protocols. The length of individual protocols varies, as does the frequency. Most programs are under an hour, and are utilized from one to three times a day, depending on the severity of the condition. Patients should repeat their BioAcoustics voiceprints about every three months to measure changes. The practitioner then reformulates the frequency combinations to address the current needs.

Resources BioAcoustics facilities are located throughout the United States and in six other countries. About 3000 people are trained in this technique, but only about 40% use it in a medical practice. Approximately a third learned BioAcoustics to take care of ill family members. To locate a practitioner in your area, go to <www.soundhealthinc.com>.

Other Sound-Based Therapies
During the past 15 years, many contemporary researchers have modified or adapted the Tomatis Method, Berard AIT and BioAcoustics™. They have developed other innovative

sound-based therapies to help people with the auditory/vestibular symptoms of autism, AD(H)D, learning disabilities, developmental delays, and more. The presenting symptoms associated with the diagnosis, rather than the diagnosis itself, is what is important when considering these methods.

Other innovators (and their sound-based therapies) are: Advanced Brain Technologies (The Listening Program™), James Cassily (Interactive Metronome), Chris Faddick (MX Pro and JoEE), Patricia Joudry (Sound Therapy for the Walkman), Paul Madaule (Listening Fitness Training-LiFT®), Kevin McBurnie (Digital Auditory Aerobics™ or DAA), Ronald Minson (Dynamic Listening System™ or DLS), Robert Monroe (Hemi-Sync), Bill Mueller (EASe), Drs. Paula Tallal and Michael Merzenich (Fast ForWord), Drs. Billie and Kirk Thompson (EnListen™) and Jan Wasowicz (Earobics). The next section briefly discusses these sound-based interventions and the benefits of each in three categories:

- Modified Tomatis and Berard spin-offs
- Therapies that develop specific auditory processing skills
- Others.

Modified Tomatis "Spin-offs"

The Tomatis Method has several variations which are also included in the Trunk of The Tree. These therapies, like the Tomatis Method, should include both air and bone conduction vibration, filtered and gated music, as well as active voice work in order to fully establish the necessary connections to learn, grow, and develop one's listening skills. They are considered modified because all do not include these features. All of the following therapies should be administered only under the direct supervision of a qualified practitioner.

Sound Therapy for the Walkman® After experiencing the positive benefits of the Tomatis Method, Patricia Joudry wanted a way to maintain the changes she had made, and to share the method with others. She taped the high frequency music recorded through the Tomatis Electronic Ear, mass-produced the tapes, and offered them for sale. Joudry found that listening to this music throughout the day kept her calm, and thus recommended that others listen to the tapes a minimum of three hours per day, with the volume fairly low.[36] Unfortunately, the sound quality of this method is not good, and because it offers only the filtered and gated music part of the Tomatis Method, some individuals may need as many as 200 hours of listening before they notice any results. To learn more go to <www.toolsforwellness.com>.

Samonas™ Sound Therapy (SST) Samonas was developed by Ingo Steinbach, a German acoustical physicist with a background in music, physics and electronics.[6 (p. 1-4)] Steinbach combined the principles of The Tomatis Method with modern technology to design a special new listening device that filtered sound while enhancing high frequencies. He called this electronic envelope-shaped modulator a System of Optimal Natural Structure or SONAS. While SONAS showed excellent results, it was long and tedious.

From SONAS, Steinbach created a second listening system. Using a series of recordings played on natural instruments, which produced tones rich in harmonics, it includes classical chamber music, Mozart, and nature sounds. This system became known as Spectrally Activated Music of Optimum Natural Structure or SAMONAS. Samonas incorporates high frequency filtered and gated music similar to that used by the Tomatis Method, except that it is not individualized.[37]

SAMONAS CDs have been used in Europe since the mid 1980s; today many therapists use them as both a home listening program and during occupational therapy sessions for those on the autism spectrum. (See section on Therapeutic Listening™ in Chapter 7.) Results include increased vitality, reduction in stress, improved concentration, renewed creativity, and improvement with reading and writing skills. For more information about Samonas, go to <www.samonas.com>.

Listening Fitness Training - LiFT™ Paul Madaule's LiFT™ program is quite similar to the Tomatis Method in that it uses filtered and gated music, and emphasizes a right-ear dominance along with active voice work. Madaule's basic model does not include bone conduction, and programming is not as individualized as the Tomatis Method.

While appropriate for office-based therapy, LiFT is often also used as a home program, under the supervision of a trained practitioner, following the Tomatis Method. The LiFT device is closely related to Tomatis' Electronic Ear. LiFT™ has two phases: auditory processing for receptive listening, and an audio-vocal phase for expressive listening. In the second phase, individuals gain better control over their voices and bodies through humming, singing and reading into a microphone. The LiFT™ program includes about 50-60 hours of listening for one to two hours per day with a short break between two phases. For more information on LiFT, go to <www.listeningfitness.com >.

The Listening Program™ The Listening Program is another generic filtered and gated music and sound stimulation method with a full spectrum of sound frequencies, based on the concepts of the Tomatis Method.[38] It is designed solely as a home listening program. Developed by Advanced Brain Technologies Inc., an outgrowth of the Utah-based National Association for Child Development (NACD), The Listening Program incorporates classical music and nature sounds to balance the workings of the middle ear muscles.

The original program consists of eight CDs that an individual listens to for one half hour per day over an eight-week period. Listeners on the more severe end of the autism spectrum may need extended and modified programs. Changes are subtle, with gains reported in communication and learning skills, attention, behavior, energy levels, coordination, relaxation and sensory integration. For more information go to <www.advancedbrain.com>.

Dynamic Listening System™ (DLS) Ronald Minson, MD, a physician board-certified in Psychiatry and Neurology, developed Dynamic Listening System™ or DLS in 2001. Dr. Minson studied a variety of auditory programs, including Auditory Integration Training, the Tomatis Method and Samonas, and was a co-developer of The Listening Program™.

Minson further altered Dr. Tomatis' equipment using state-of-the-art technology to bring listening to a higher level of quality and clarity. His program varies slightly from Dr. Tomatis' in length and time of listening. Clients listen for 15 days, take a month off, and listen for eight days more. Each session lasts 1.3 hours. DLS training is said to improve tonal abilities, which, in turn, supports auditory sequential and language processing skills. This program is an alternative to the Tomatis Method in geographical areas where trained practitioners do not exist.

Dr. Minson recently partnered with Lucy Miller, OT, PhD, to found The STAR Center in Colorado. In 2006, they plan to embark upon research examining the efficacy of DLS, alone, and DLS combined with occupational therapy. To learn more go to <www.dynamiclistening.com>.

MX Pro® and JoEE® Chris Faddick, an engineer/technician/clinician with about 15 years experience in Tomatis, Berard, Samonas, and other sound therapies, developed two models of portable and affordable listening units with digital signal processing. One has voice capability and the other does not. The JoEE® is a small, compact unit that uses air and bone conduction sound stimulation, and fits neatly into a waistband carrying case. The MX

Pro® is a table top unit that incorporates air and bone conduction sound stimulation, and incorporates active voice work. All recordings are uncompressed and stored on hard drives; thus no CDs or CD players are required. The MX Pro® is designed for professionals, and can accommodate multiple listeners, while the JoEE® is for single listeners. These units are ideal for home usage. For more information, go to <www.bigbangsoundworks.com>.

EnListen™ Drs. Billie and Kirk Thompson, long-time followers of Tomatis, developed a software program called EnListen™ that works on a computer with Windows XP or Windows 2000. EnListen™ incorporates air and bone conduction, voice work, as well as other components found in the Tomatis Method. Its advantage is that by playing on an ordinary computer it can easily be used at home, school, or for in-office therapy. For more information go to <www.soundlistening.com>.

The Mozart Effect Don Campbell, one of the world's foremost authorities on the connection between music and healing, has also taken the music of Mozart and used it to affect the body, mind and spirit not only of individuals on the autism spectrum, but of infants, children, and typically functioning persons, as well.[39] The Mozart Effect is an extension of the Tomatis Method, although it is not considered true sound-based therapy.

In her book on reflexes, Sally Goddard relates a story about a high school science teacher who used Mozart as background music during her class. She observed that the noise level dropped, and students' concentration and behavior improved. She documented that the blood pressure of students who had listened to Mozart was consistently lower after class than those who had not.[40]

In his book, *The Mozart Effect for Children*,[41] Campbell presents a wealth of dynamic, inventive ways for parents and teachers to use music, sounds and songs to improve language, behavior and learning. Mozart Effect tapes and CDs, as well as more information on the Mozart Effect, are available through the Mozart Effect Resource Center at <www.mozarteffect.com>.

Modified Berard Spin-offs
The Clark Method – BGC In 1989 Dr. Bernard Rimland phoned Bill Clark about an early version of the AudioKinetron he had received from Dr. Guy Berard in France, which had been damaged in transit. Dr. Rimland, who knew Clark was both an electronics engineer and the father of an autistic child, asked if he could repair it. He explained that Berard's machine had produced very notable improvement in a number of autistic children. Rimland wanted to use the machine to try to reproduce Dr. Berard's results, and was concerned, since Dr. Berard was about to retire, and the machine was the only one in the United States.

Upon dismantling the device, Clark saw that its design and construction were out-dated. He rebuilt it as a much simpler, more reliable and adaptable device, using state-of-the-art integrated circuits and called it the BGC machine.[42] It works similarly to the AudioKinetron, but programming is slightly different.

EASe CDs Bill Mueller of the Institutes for the Achievement of Human Potential, near Philadelphia, created an affordable, portable listening program based upon Berard AIT. He recorded music with short random bursts of high frequency energy encoded into it through the AudioKinetron, but did not use Berard approved music. He called his recordings Electronic Auditory Stimulation effect CDs or EASe. Benefits of the EASe CDs are a result of the high frequency bursts rather than the muscle retraining of AIT. EASe CDs can be used either in a therapy session or at home, and as an integral part of an occupational therapy session. To learn more, go to <www.vision-audio.com >.

Digital Auditory Aerobics™ (DAA) After the FDA banned the use of the AudioKinetron, Americans searched for other ways to do AIT. A company called EARliest Adventures in Sound, headed by Kevin McBurnie developed a machine called an EQattenuater (for regulating volume to each ear and for filtering specific frequencies). This device was exempt from FDA approval because it was sold as an educational tool and not medical equipment.

DAA applies Dr. Berard's concept of filtering and regulating the volume of the music. It uses a CD player, a set of 20 CDs of selected music and headphones, along with the EQattenuater. Each CD is exactly 30 minutes long, and the music is an exact replication of the auditory output of the AudioKinetron. To learn more go to <www.aitinstitute.com>.

Sound-Based Therapies that Develop Specific Auditory Processing Skills

Fast ForWord® Fast ForWord®, formerly called HAILO, is a family of interactive computer-based training programs, based on 20 years of brain research. Developed by Paula Tallal, PhD, of Rutgers University in New Jersey, and Michael Merzenich, PhD, of the University of California at San Francisco, it is designed to improve language, reading and learning skills in children and adults. Some practitioners recommend that students undergo intensive auditory training prior to starting Fast ForWord®.

Fast ForWord® includes different levels for early language development through advanced language and reading skills; programs build upon each other. While listening through headphones, an individual plays a series of computer games that automatically adjust to his/her improving competence level. Progress is charted daily. The different programs are:

Fast ForWord Language® - For children age five through 12. This original program trains temporal sequencing, sound discrimination, phonological awareness, sustained focus, attention and listening comprehension using an intensive series of adaptive, interactive exercises of acoustically modified speech and speech sounds. A student must complete five of seven 20-minute sessions per day, five days a week. The whole program takes six to eight weeks; children with autism typically need longer.

Fast ForWord Language to Reading® - For children up to age 16. This program targets sound-letter recognition, decoding, vocabulary, grammar, syntax, listening comprehension and beginning word recognition. Training consists of five 18-minute exercises per day for six to eight weeks.

Fast ForWord Reading® Series - For older students. This program helps students master reading through a series of sequentially appropriate reading skills.

Fast ForWord Middle & High School® - For teenagers and adults up to age 21. The program hones advanced language and reading skills leading to improved communication. Participants progress at their own rate working on skills such as organization, participating in group discussions, and sustained attention.

Scientific Learning also has other programs for younger children. Research on a group of children with pervasive developmental disorders and autism, ages five to 13, showed significant gains in both receptive and expressive language following a Fast ForWord® program.[43] To find a Fast ForWord® practitioner, and for more information, go to <www.scilearn.com >.

Earobics® Earobics®, created by Jan Wasowicz, PhD, a speech/language pathologist, consists of multi-media computer games using acoustic enhancement of speech signals and adaptive training. It is aimed at developing many specific auditory processing and phonological skills including auditory attention, discrimination, figure ground, identification, memory, and vigilance. Games also work on phonemic sequencing and synthesis, sound segmentation, sound blending, word closure, pattern recognition, auditory sound-symbol correspondence, rhyming, and phonological awareness.

Earobics® has multi-level programs for ages four to adult.

- *Earobics® Step 1* trains phonological awareness, auditory processing, and beginning phonics skills. It also addresses attention and memory skills.
- *Earobics® Step 2* continues with skills at Step 1 at a more advanced level, along with language processing.
- *Earobics® Step 1 for Adolescents and Adults* is similar to Step 1 with materials that appeal to older students.

The format of Earobics® programs allows students to progress at their own pace. Individuals can use Earobics® games at home or in a clinic at least once a week. Length of sessions depends on the level. The more extended the program, the greater the benefit. In a research study, students with learning disabilities and/or attention deficits, who worked with Earobics® software for eight weeks, showed measurable improvement on measures of auditory processing and exhibited positive changes to speech stimuli in quiet and in noise.[44]

Earobics® is now in use in over 8,000 schools and in more than 50 countries. To learn more and to find a practitioner, go to <www.earobics.com> .

Other Sound-Based Therapies

Hemi-sync® Hemi-Sync® is an audio technology guided approach to listening that subtly leads the brain to various states of awareness. Hemispheric synchronization, or "Hemi-sync" for short, is based on the research of Robert Monroe, who founded the non-profit Monroe Institute in Virginia.

Hemi-sync® works by sending different sounds (tones) to each ear through stereo headphones. The two hemispheres of the brain then act in unison to "hear" a third signal – the difference between the two tones. The third signal is not an actual sound, but rather an electrical signal that can only be perceived within the brain when both brain hemispheres are working together.

The goal of Hemi-Sync® is to induce and improve states of consciousness. EEG-based research documents actual changes in brain waves. Positive behavioral results include increased attention, focus and relaxation, reduction in depression and stress, improved sleep, and enhanced learning and memory skills. In a study with children with developmental disabilities, 18 of 20 had positive responses.[45] The versatility of Hemi-Sync® gives the basic technology an almost limitless range of applications for mental, physical, and emotional well-being. For more information on Hemi-Sync®, go to <www.monroeinstitute.org>.

Interactive Metronome® The Interactive Metronome® (IM) is a structured, goal-oriented training process that is a PC-version of the traditional musical metronome. Created by James Cassily, a former record producer and sound engineer, Interactive Metronome is based on the premise that improving one's ability to plan and sequence motor actions enhances cognitive, learning and social skills.

Behavioral optometrists and occupational therapists have long understood that motor planning and sequencing are key facets in the development of foundational skills for learning. Many already use metronomes in their therapy practices to improve response time and sequencing.

Stanley Greenspan, MD, an internationally renowned psychiatrist, and creator of the Developmental-Individual Difference-Relationship Based (DIR) model and FloorTime (See Chapter 11) has also endorsed IM to improve social interactions in children with autism spectrum disorders. He believes that the skills trained by the IM are essential for adaptive motor and language development, as well as for complex social behavior involving sequential steps, such as sharing toys, complex greeting patterns, or simply playing with others.[46]

A subject wears a special headset that emits signals. The IM computerized program challenges the participant to precisely match the computer's rhythm by tapping hand and/or foot sensors. A different set of tones gives the person feedback as to whether his/her response is too early, too late, or just right. The computer immediately analyzes the difference in milliseconds between the actual beat and the person's motor response, and then averages his/her ability to maintain focus over an extended period of time. During a full training, a person could respond over 35,000 times.

The IM program is for those age seven up. It lasts for 15 days, listening one hour per day over three to five weeks. Some people need up to as many as ten additional sessions. A double-blind, placebo-controlled study of nine to twelve-year-old boys diagnosed with AD(H)D found that those undergoing IM treatment showed significant improvement in attention, coordination, control of aggression/impulsivity, reading and language processing.[47] Interactive Metronome is now in use in more than 1700 clinics in North America. To find a practitioner and to learn more, go to <www.interactivemetronome.com >.

Table 10-3 shows various sound-based therapies and compares the characteristics of each. As is apparent from this chart, each therapy has its advantages.

Music as Therapy
Music therapy, although very different from sound therapy, also has efficacy for those on the autism spectrum. Sally Goddard calls music "one of life's earliest teachers." Pre-natally, the fetus reacts to music with movement; infants respond to music and can imitate simple rhythms, like paddy-cake, before they develop speech. Music supplies the architecture for many aspects of learning.[40(p108-9)]

Music as Communication and Socialization Music is a universal language. Rhythm is basic for speaking, reading, writing and socializing. Singing, dancing and rhythmic movement are natural ways to communicate with those on the spectrum and for them to communicate with and relate to others. Musical activities have many desirable characteristics: they require no verbal interaction, have inherent structure, can be playful, and they facilitate the desired outcomes of increased language, socialization and appropriate behaviors.[48]

Dr. Stanley Greenspan, who recommends using the Interactive Metronome to enhance language and relatedness, is not the only mental health professional integrating music into therapy. Suzi Tortora, a dance therapist with a doctorate in counseling makes music an inherent part of her "dancing dialogue" with children on the autism spectrum. She sees music and its props as tools that foster individual expression and relating. In her work, she uses variations in beat, style, rhythm and volume to connect with both verbal and nonverbal children.[49]

Dr. Stephen Porges, who was credited earlier in this chapter for determining the functions of the muscles of the inner ear, has also developed an intervention, that allows a child to sort sound frequencies, reduce anxiety, and thus be more available socially and emotionally. See Chapter 11 for more on how programs from these and other talented mental health professionals are helping those with autism spectrum disorders.

Table 10-3 Sound-based Therapies Related to Stimulation Type

	Filtered/ Gated Music	Ener-gizing Music	Classical Music	Bone Conduc-tion	Active Voice Work	AP Skills	Sound Frequen-cies	Binaural Beats
AIT	X	X						
Tomatis®	X		X	X	X			
DLS®	X		X	X	X			
MX Pro™	X		X	X	X			
EnListen™	X		X	X	X			
LiFT™	X		X	*	X			
TLP®	X		X	*				
Samonas™	X		X	*				
ST Walkman	X		X					
EASe CD's	X	X						
JoEE™	X		X					
Fast ForWord ®						X		
IM®						X		
Earobics®						X		
Bio Acoustics™							X	X
Hemi-Sync®								X
*Has bone conduction add-on program								
								© Davis 2005

Music and Academics In the 1890s Swiss music teacher, Emile Jacques Dalcroze discovered that students who could not hear music inside their heads could not write the chords on paper. Dalcroze theorized that these students had not had sufficient physical experience with the chords. Providing the students with rhythmic physical exercises, put to music, developed their ability to use the body as an instrument. By harnessing a child's natural movements in walking, running, hopping, skipping, bending and stretching, Dalcroze improved their written language skills.

The Dalcroze Method, known as Eurhythmics, is now taught in many music schools and practiced by a multitude of music teachers. Dalcroze Eurhythmics is also being applied outside the mainstream of general music education, such as in palliative care for terminally ill adults and for emotionally or developmentally handicapped children.[50]

Music is not just related to the language arts, but to numbers, as well. In medieval times, "the science of number was fundamental to all learning. Music was the expression of number in time, giving pitch, duration, rhythm, stress and accent to words. Language regulated by number was song. Number structuring space was geometry."[51]

Musical Giftedness Many individuals with autism are intrinsically attracted to music. Some like David Helfgott, featured in the movie "Shine," and Stephen Shore, a very accomplished adult with Asperger syndrome, are musically gifted. Shore who teaches music to those with autism, writes eloquently about the role music played in his childhood in his autobiography, *Beyond the Wall*. He explains how, when he could not learn the Hebrew necessary for his Bar Mitzvah, he perfectly mimicked an audiotape of a cantor singing the prayers, which he accompanied with the necessary, ceremonial, rhythmic rocking called davening.[52]

What Music Therapy Offers Certified music therapists use a variety of instruments; many like Tortora have training in the behavioral sciences. According to the American Music Therapy Association, "for individuals with diagnoses on the autism spectrum, music therapy provides a unique variety of music experiences in an intentional and developmentally appropriate manner to effect changes in behavior and facilitate development of skills."[53]

Music therapy provides individuals with autism:

- an opportunity to express themselves and their emotions
- concrete, auditory, visual, tactile, proprioceptive and vestibular stimulation in both hemispheres of the brain. This multi-sensory experience is very organizing, enhancing cognitive function, language comprehension and usage, perceptual-, gross- and fine motor skills, and can assist in the remediation of other important areas
- a sense of security and familiarity, encouraging individuals to attempt new tasks within a predictable and malleable framework
- successful experiences

Several types of music therapy are showing success with individuals on the autism spectrum. Two are:

Nordoff-Robbins Method The late Dr. Paul Nordoff, an American composer and music professor, and Dr. Clive Robbins, a British special educator developed this method. The Nordoff-Robbins Music Therapy Clinics in England, Germany and Australia use improvisational music therapy to improve communication in children with autism. Therapists treat patients once a week, both one-on-one and in small groups, at their clinics. Techniques are based on the belief that every human being has the capacity to respond to music. For more information on Nordoff-Robbins, go to <www.nordoff-robbins.org.uk>.

Rhythmic Entrainment Some music therapists practice rhythmic entrainment, which uses drum rhythms that are said to improve brain functioning by altering the body's processing of the beats. For more information about this therapy, contact the REI Institute at <www.reiinstitute.com>.

To find music therapists in your area, go to <www.musictherapy.org>.

Summary

Given the vast volume of information now available on sound interventions, parents have a formidable task in choosing programs most suitable for a child's specific needs. This chapter reviews the many sound-based, and music therapies presently showing efficacy for those on the autism spectrum.

All sound-based therapies are connected through the voice-ear-brain connection. The random application of sound-based therapies without full understanding of the function, purpose, target population, and effect of each one, is inappropriate. The Tree of Sound Enhancement Therapy is a very useful tool designed to help optometrists, other professionals and parents understand the components of each type.

Davis has also designed a Therapy Indicator Form for optometrists and other professionals to use in determining if a sound-based therapy is appropriate for their patients. To obtain a copy of this form, contact info@thedaviscenter.com.

Sound therapies must be utilized from a foundational and developmentally appropriate sequence. Sound is present all around us and impacts our very being. To alter the impact randomly can create change, but not necessarily positive change. As Joshua Leeds states, in his book *The Power of Sound*, "Sound is an ally; it always has been. The question is whether we are ready to embrace it as such."[54]

Without a doubt, maximizing the hearing function to enhance listening abilities is analogous to maximizing vision…both with the goal of maximizing potential and maintaining the wellness of the whole body. Specific auditory processing and academic skills can develop only when all the foundational pieces are in place.

Choosing the potentially most effective sound-based therapy program for a child requires knowledge and input from an experienced clinician. Each of the various sound interventions has advantages. Guidance from a clinician trained in several different forms of sound interventions might be the most helpful.

Sound stimulation, like visual intervention, can make a marked difference when used appropriately for individuals with autism, AD/HD, learning challenges, sensory processing disorders and other developmental delays. The use of sound-based therapies for those on both ends of the autism spectrum is both promising and challenging. Scientists around the world are developing new and improved therapies every year which can make powerful changes in the lives of children and adults with disabilities everywhere.

References

1. Sollier P. *Listening for Wellness: An Introduction to the Tomatis Method.* Walnut Creek, CA: The Mozart Center Press, 2005:129-130.

2. Stehli A. *The Sound of a Miracle: A Child's Triumph over Autism.* New York: Doubleday, 1991.

3. Davis DS. *Sound Bodies through Sound Therapy.* Landing, NJ: Kalco Publishing, LLC, 2004.

4. Barnhart CL. *The American College Dictionary.* New York: Random House, 1960:1153.

5. Edelson S. *Dr. Stephen Porges' research may support Dr. Berard's and Tomatis' theory on middle ear muscle dysfunction. The Sound Connection* 2003;9(4):1- 2.

6. Frick SM, Hacker C. *Listening with the Whole Body.* Madison, WI: Vital Links, 2001:1.

7. www.iarctc.org. Accessed January 11, 2008.

8. Madaule P. *When Listening Comes Alive.* Norval, Ontario Canada: Moulin Publishing,1994.

9. Davis-Kalugin DS. *The Davis Addendum to the Tomatis Effect.* Acoustical Society of America Annual Conference, San Diego, CA., November 2004.

10. Marohn S. *The Natural Medicine Guide to Autism.* Charlottesville, VA: Hampton Roads Publishing Co., 2002:194.

11. Madaule P. *Terapia de Escucha.* Mexico: Editorialis Trillas, 2005.

12. Berard G. *Hearing Equals Behavior.* Georgiana Foundation. Pre-publication issue, 1992:1.

13. Martin FN. *Introduction to Audiology.* Englewood Cliffs, NJ: Prentice-Hall, 1986:278.

14. Edwards S. *Subtle Energy Medicine: Bridging the Gap Between Psychic and Science.* Albany, OH: Sound Health, Inc., 1992:1-7.

15. www.berardwebsite.com/sait/. (Accessed January 30, 2008)

16. Creedon MP, Edelson SM, Scharre J. *Ocular Movements Among Individuals with Autism Pre- and Post-Auditory Integration Training.* Paper presented at the Annual Conference of the Association for the Advancement of Behavioral Therapy, New York, 1993.

17. Veale TK. *Two Studies of the Effects of Auditory Integration Training in Autism.* Paper Presented at the International ASA Conference on Autism, Toronto, Canada, 1993.

18. Edelson SM, et al. *Auditory integration training: a double-blind study of behavioral, electro-physiological, and audiometric effects in autistic subjects. Focus on Autism and Other Developmental Disabilities* 1999;14:73-81.

19. Rimland B, Edelson SM. *The effects of auditory integration training in autism. Am J Speech-Language Path* 1994;5:16-24.

20. Woodward D. *Changes in unilateral and bilateral sound sensitivity as a result of AIT. The Sound Connection* 1994;2:4.

21. Monville D, Nelson N. *Parental Perceptions of Change Following AIT for Autism. Paper presented at the American Speech-Language-Hearing Conference, New Orleans, 1994.*

22. Madell JR, Rose DE. *Auditory integration training. Am J Audiology* 1994 Mar:14-18.

23. Bettison S. *The long-term effects of auditory training on children with autism. J Autism Dev Dis* 1996;26:361-74.

24. Gillberg C, Johansson M, Steffenberg S, Berlin, O. *Auditory integration training in children with autism: brief report of an open pilot study. Autism* 1997;1:97-100.

25. Kirby WJ. *The effects of auditory integration training on children diagnosed with attention deficit/hyperactivity disorder: a pilot study. The Sound Connection* 2000;7:4-5.

26. Madell JR. *Auditory integration training: one clinician's view. Language, Speech, and Hearing Services in Schools* 1999;30:371-7.

27. Panksepp J, Rossi J, Narayanan TK. *Biochemical Changes As a result of AIT-type modulated and unmodulated music. Lost & Found: Perspectives on Brain, Emotion, and Culture* 1996/7;Vol. 2:1,4.

28. Rimland B. *Auditory integration training update: scientific clues, FDA obstruction. Autism Res Rev*;9:4,2.

29. Stehli A. *Dancing in the Rain: Stories of Exceptional Progress by Parents of Children with Special Needs. Roxbury, Ct: Georgiana Institute, 1998.*

30. Davis D. *Every Day a Miracle: Success stories with sound therapy. Landing, NJ: Kalco Publishing, 2006.*

31. Ruben S. *Awakening Ashley: Mozart Knocks Autism on its ear. Lincoln, NE: iUniverse, 2004.*

32. Edelson SM, Rimland B. *Recovering Austic Children. San Diego: Autism Research Institute, 2006.*

33. Davis DS. *How sound-based therapy can help the Isodicentric 15 Individuals. Presentation at Isodicentric 15 and other Chromosomal Imbalances Conference Schaumberg, IL, June 24, 2005.*

34. Edelson SM. *What's before AIT, what's after AIT. The Sound Connection* 2002;9:3.

35. Wheeler M. *Signal discovery? Smithsonian Magazine* 2004 Mar.

36. Joudry P. *Sound Therapy for the Walkman. Saskatchewan, Canada: Steele and Steele Dalmeny: March, 1994.*

37. Steinbach I. *Samonas Sound Therapy: The Way to Health through Sound. Kellinghusen, Germany: Techau Verlag, 1997.*

38. Advanced Brain Technologies. *The Listening Program: Guidebook and Manual. Ogden, UT: Advanced Brain Technologies, LLC, 1999.*

39. Campbell D. *The Mozart Effect. New York: Avon Books, 1997.*

40. Goddard S. *Reflexes, Learning and Behavior. Eugene, OR: Fern Ridge Press, 2005:110.*

41. Campbell D. *The Mozart Effect for Children. New York: Harper Collins, 2000.*

42. Clark W. *A Letter from Bill Clark. The Sound Connection* 1994;2:1.

43. Merzenich MM, Saunders G, Jenkins W, Miller S, et al. In: Broman SH, Fletcher JM, eds. *The Changing Nervous System: Neurobehavioral Consequences of Early Brain Disorders. New York: Oxford University Press, 1999.*

44. Hayes EA, Warrier CM, Nicol TG, Zecker SG, Kraus N. *Neural plasticity following auditory training in children with learning problems Clin Neurophysiol* 2003;114.

45. Morris SE. *Music and Hemi-Sync® in the treatment of children with developmental disabilities. Open Ear* 1996;2:14-7.

46. www.interactivemetronome.com. *(Accessed January 2, 2008)*

47. Shaffer RJ, Jocokes LE, Cassily JF, et al. *Effect of interactive metronome rhythmicity Training on Children with Attention Deficit Hyperactivity Disorder.. Am J Occup Ther* 2001 Mar/Apr;55(2):155-62.

48. Gerlach E. *Autism Treatment Guide-Third edition. Arlington, TX: Future Horizons, 2003: 117-8.*

49. Tortora S. *The Dancing Dialogue: Using the Communicative Power of Movement with Young Children. Baltimore, MD: Brookes Publishing Co., 2005.*

50. www.dalcrozeusa.org. *(Accessed January 3, 2008)*

51. Goddard Blythe S. *The Well-Balanced Child. Gloucestershire, UK: Hawthorn Press, 2004:88.*

52. Shore S. *Beyond the Wall. Shawnee Mission, KS: Autism Asperger Publishing Co., 2003:68-83.*

53. www.musictherapy.org. *(Accessed January 2, 2008)*

54. Leeds J. *The Power of Sound. Healing Arts Press: Rochester, VT, 2001:219.*

Chapter 11
Therapies that Address Communication and Social-Emotional Issues Through Play
Patricia S. Lemer, MEd, NCC

Poor, unusual and absent communication skills and inter-personal relationships are the hallmarks of autism spectrum disorders. To review information presented in Chapter 1, symptoms of autism include:

1. *Impairment in social interaction*

   - Inappropriate eye contact or facial expression
   - Failure to develop peer relationships
   - Lack of spontaneous sharing of enjoyment or interests
   - Lack of social or emotional reciprocity

2. *Impairment in communication*

   - Delayed or non-existent language development
   - Poor conversational abilities, if language is present
   - Stereotypic, repetitive language or idiosyncratic language
   - Lack of make-believe or social imitative play

3. *Repetitive and stereotyped behavior, interests and activities*

   - Abnormally intense preoccupation with one or more interests
   - Seemingly inflexible adherence to routines or rituals
   - Mannerisms such as hand or finger flapping or twisting or whole body movements
   - Preoccupations with object parts

How Children Play

According to Rebecca Klaw, MS, MEd, an autism specialist in Pittsburgh, Pennsylvania, play begins "small and simple" for typically developing children. With input from parents, teachers, siblings and friends, simple play gradually expands over time, becoming rich and very complex. The elaboration of play is fueled by social interaction, and serves as the basis for early learning. The child at play is not idle or aimless, boring or bored, or wasting time. The child is, in fact, engaged in complex activity that develops skills and builds, bit by bit, concepts as complicated as physics and essential as empathy.[1]

Children with autistic spectrum disorders, on the other hand, have difficulty learning from others how to expand their play. They tend to play alone in unusual and repetitive ways. They often miss the social component to play because interaction can be so hard for them. They might be good at manipulating objects and figuring out how they work. They might be great at creating sounds, sights and motions for their own pleasure. What they are not good at, however, is playing with someone else. Children with autistic spectrum disorders tend to get stuck in their play, and they need to learn, through patient and skilled adults, how to play.

General Guidelines for Playing with those with Autism Spectrum Disorders

How do you play with a child who wants to be left alone? Insist that they play with you, using persistence, intelligence, flexibility and humor. Children with autism spectrum disorders need to be guided in memorable ways to explore all aspects of their world, not just how to manipulate objects, but how to share, build, pretend, elaborate, invent, describe and create. Klaw offers strategies that utilize the guidelines from some of the methods

Figure 11-1
Ways to Engage
Children with Autism in Play

- Heighten interest
- Be persistent
- Include repetition
- Establish routines
- Add sensory stimulation
- Minimize language
- Have fun

elaborated upon in this chapter in Figure 11-1. Go to <www.rebeccaklaw.com> to purchase her DVDs on relationship-based intervention and to see her schedule of trainings nationwide.

Laying the Foundations for Play

Many therapists understand that the sensory and biomedical treatments discussed in the previous chapters prepare the body and the brain for communication and interaction by addressing underlying deficits. Biomedical treatments remove stressers from the body by normalizing digestion, detoxification and other bodily functions, thus releasing energies for sensory processing. Visual, auditory and occupational therapies then can be most effective and produce secondary benefits in communication and social emotional interaction.

How *does* a person develop all the skills necessary to talk, engage, relate, converse, imagine and play? That outcome occurs only through the process of sensory integration, with vision emerging as the dominant sense. Efficient sensory integration is imperative for receptive and expressive language development, as well as for appropriate social interactions. Everyone involved with children on the autism spectrum must take the same type of developmental approach to social skills as they do to motor, language, vision and academic skills. Children must crawl before they walk, babble before they talk, and feel good about themselves before they can consider others. As their sensory processing systems mature, so will their social interactions.

In order for a child to *really* own his behavior, he must initiate social interactions from the inside out. Modeling, therapy and social skills training combined with the programs described in this chapter can all help. If we train social skills from the outside in, rather than let children develop them from the inside out, however, we teach them to distrust their own sensory processing. How much better to allow social skills to develop in tandem with good sensory integration.

Three systems are primarily responsible for good social-emotional development: touch, balance and vision. In *The Out-of Sync Child*[2] Carol Kranowitz emphasizes the role of a well-regulated tactile system for getting along well with others. Lacking good regulation, "the child with tactile defensiveness sends out signals that he is unfriendly and prefers to be left alone." Kranowitz believes that he may just be employing a healthy protective mechanism that keeps people from violating his oversensitive touch system. A child who does not return a greeting, such as "hi" may fear that an adult might take the greeting further with a handshake, hug or kiss, which he could find intolerable.

Balance also plays a role. An efficient balance system allows a child to feel grounded and know where his body is in space. When one is gravitationally insecure, feeling emotionally secure is difficult, if not impossible. Cautious interactions could indicate vestibular dysfunction. Because the vestibular system is physiologically connected to the language center of the brain, children with balance issues often have trouble expressing themselves.

Vision is another key to social interaction. Children must not only see another person, but also be able to give appropriate meaning to subtle facial expressions and gestures. They must be able to focus *on* the person's face, not in front of her or over her shoulder. They must be able to judge appropriate "social distance" for conversation.

Some therapists and parents do not realize that focusing and depth perception are a result of two eyes working well together, and that lack of good eye contact could be a sign of binocular dysfunction, not social inhibition. Some children with autism contend with periodic double vision. *Not* looking may be easier than simultaneously unscrambling the competing visual images and interpreting the words of a parent or teacher.

Relationship-Based Therapies

Recognizing the role of efficient sensory processing in language and social-emotional development, a few practitioners in the mental health and language fields have thus developed some highly sophisticated trans-disciplinary programs for relationship building and communication. This chapter covers in depth four long-standing, highly respected programs for which professionals in many fields have received extensive training. They are:

- The **D**evelopmental, **I**ndividual Difference, **R**elationship-based Approach (DIR) and Floortime
- **R**elational **D**evelopment **I**ntervention (RDI)
- The Son Rise Program®
- Social Stories™

This chapter also includes some less well-known programs, including The Dancing Dialogue, The Miller Method, SCERTS, and the Polyvagal Theory.

DIR/Floortime

The **D**evelopmental, **I**ndividual Differences, **R**elationship-based Approach (DIR) is a comprehensive, interdisciplinary approach developed by child psychiatrist, Stanley Greenspan, MD, and psychologist, Serena Wieder, PhD. Greenspan is a Clinical Professor of Psychiatry, Behavioral Sciences and Pediatrics at the George Washington University Medical School, and supervising child psychoanalyst at the Washington Psychoanalytic Institute in Washington DC. Wieder is a clinical psychologist in private practice in the Washington, DC area and the Associate Editor of the *Journal of Developmental Processes*. She is on the faculty of the Washington, DC School of Psychiatry and is Associate Chair of the Interdisciplinary Council on Developmental and Learning Disorders (ICDLD). Greenspan and Wieder are the co-authors of *The Child With Special Needs*[3] and *Engaging Autism*[4], from which the author has drawn much of the information in this section. The interested reader should also go to <www.stanleygreenspan.com>, <www.icdl.com> and <www.floortime.org> for extensive research support of and explanations relating to the DIR model and Floortime approach.

The DIR model offers a framework to assist parents and professionals in creating a comprehensive, intensive therapeutic program. DIR addresses relationships, behaviors, ideas and processing, without dictating any specific interventions. It is fully compatible with, and incorporates many of the therapeutic programs described in previous chapters, especially biomedical intervention, occupational therapy, sound-based therapies and, of course, vision therapy. While the DIR model tailors intervention to the individual needs of each child, it also focuses on the entire family, thus often resolving family issues that may be interfering with a child's growth and development.

Components of DIR

Developmental DIR takes into account six sequential stages of development that denote how well a child engages with others, initiates interaction and uses gestures to communicate. First, a child masters the early non-verbal developmental stages of communication, and learns to maintain a continuous flow of interaction and engagement. Early on, DIR focuses on getting the child to play symbolically. At the second stage, a child moves to understanding the full range of feelings and develops interpersonal problem solving.

The latter stages focus on helping children to develop abstract thinking through making comparisons and judgments based on their own emotional experiences.

The six stages are:

1. *Shared attention* – Utilize all the senses and motor abilities, stretching the child's capabilities for interaction.

2. *Engagement* – Follow the child's lead, building upon pleasurable interactions. Match the child's rhythm, deepen the warmth, add physical closeness.

3. *Two-way purposeful interaction with gestures* – Exaggerate emotion, become animated, support initiative, facilitate goal achievement.

4. *Two-way purposeful problem solving interaction* – Add extra steps to play, such as acting dumb, playing obstructively and creating barriers, forcing the child to solve problems.

5. *Emotional ideas* – Encourage imaginary play, combining words with ideas and affect with action.

6. *Emotional thinking* – Build bridges between ideas and development of abstract reasoning. Challenge with "wh" questions. This high level of development is the ultimate goal for all children.

Individual Differences Each child brings individual differences that affect learning and behavior. Individual differences occur in:

- auditory processing
- gestural non-verbal communication
- ability to understand and use language
- visual-spatial processing
- motor planning and sequencing
- sensory reactivity and modulation

Relationship-based A child's unique individual differences and developmental challenges combine to affect how he/she relates to others. Understanding each child's unique set is crucial in planning emotionally based interactions, which are at the heart of intervention. The DIR approach assists caregivers in developing adult/child relationships, which then allow a child to develop meaningful relationships with peers and siblings.

Sensory and Affective Experiences Take Place Simultaneously

According to Greenspan and Wieder, all individuals categorize experiences by their sensory and affective qualities simultaneously. Sensory perception focuses on physical properties (bright, loud, big, smooth, etc.) and emotional qualities may be perceived as soothing, jarring, happy, tense, etc. Affective categories essentially function as sense organs. As experiences accumulate, sensory impressions become increasingly tied to feelings. Making sense of an experience is an immediate emotional reaction, which probably precedes any cognition. Intelligence is the connection between a feeling (or a desire) and an action (or a symbol).

Whereas a majority of mental health professionals consider emotional reactions secondary to cognitive perceptions, Greenspan believes that in many instances they are primary. Dual coding of experiences is the key to understanding how emotions organize intellectual capacity and create a sense of self, because it allows children to "cross-reference" each memory or experience in a mental catalogue of phenomena and feelings, and to reconstruct it when needed. This process theoretically also provides the basis for generalization, abstraction, logic and reasoning.

DIR Theory and Autism

In the Greenspan model of autism, aberrant sensory perceptions, including vision, are processed by a brain that has not mastered the ability to attach emotions to relevant experiences. When sensory processing is disrupted, the emotional organization of experiences can be compromised. Compare this to typical development, where each sensation registered by a child, including visual perception, gives rise to an affect or emotion, which organizes experience and behavior.

Because the development of symbol formation, language and intelligence is based on a series of critical emotional interactions early in life, when a child does not master these emotional interactions, essential learning abilities and behavior suffer. Greenspan, Wieder and Stuart Shanker, DPhil, have observed and written extensively on how children diagnosed with autism spectrum disorders consistently have not mastered early critical emotional interactions.[5,6,7]

DIR focuses on the child's ability to interact with others. DIR holds that children must be emotionally attached to the people in their world and have the ability to interact with them in order to develop cognitively and emotionally. Learning is an inherent part of emotional development.

In the DIR approach, the first goal is to help the child work around sensory processing difficulties to reestablish a meaningful relationship with parents. For a child who is in his own world and not relating to others, the first emphasis is on enticing him into the world by giving him a greater degree of pleasure in relating.

DIR takes into account the child's feelings, relationships with caregivers, developmental level and individual differences in his ability to process and respond to sensory information. It focuses on the child's skills in all developmental areas, including social-emotional functioning, communication, thinking and learning, motor skills, body awareness, and attention. It is less focused on specific skills, such as reading and writing, recognizing that those skills will develop more readily when the child has a solid foundation from which to learn.

The DIR Approach

The primary goal of a DIR-based intervention program is to enable children to form a sense of themselves as intentional, interactive individuals, and thus to develop cognitive, language and social capacities. At the foundation of the intervention are protective, stable, developmentally supportive relationships from family and others. This foundation includes both physical protection and security, as well as ongoing, nurturing and consistent interactions, adapted to the child's developmental level and individual differences. Caregivers can easily misperceive children's attempts to cope with the world as rejecting of their love, and may need guidance in supporting, relating and interacting to children with autism or related disorders. DIR offers such support.

Floortime

The heart of the DIR approach for infants and children with a variety of developmental challenges, including autism spectrum disorders is Floortime. The guidelines for Floortime allow the child to develop spontaneous interactive behaviors that are purposeful and intentional. The basic principles of Floortime are to

1. *Follow a child's lead.* The child is the leader; do what the child does. The role of the adult is to facilitate communication and problem solving, and to keep the play interactive, not to direct the child's play. If a child spins, take his hand and dance with him,

singing, "Ring around the Rosy." If he runs back and forth, play tag or "London Bridge" and "lock him up." When he lies down, dim the lights, provide a blanket, and sing a lullaby; when he arises, exclaim, "Good morning!" Every child will recognize these gestures that open the door to symbolic meanings. As interaction increases, respond to real desires with pretend actions and props. If she wants to leave, offer the keys. Ask her to turn off the lights and help open the door. If she seems to search for food, offer pretend cookies. Use every opportunity to encourage the imitation of symbolic actions, even in the bathtub, where she is a captive audience in a familiar and supportive sensory environment. As he becomes more symbolic or more able to sequence actions, new meanings will emerge.

2. *Join in at a child's developmental level and build on his natural interests*. Treat whatever the child is doing as intentional and purposeful. A child may not know hot to initiate purposeful behaviors. Use affect and action to woo the child into interacting. Express pleasure for every move the child makes. By giving every move the utmost attention, interest and energy, adults convey that actions are meaningful, and can elicit a response.

3. *Open and close circles of communication.* Build upon the child's natural interests, always focusing on maintaining a continuous flow of interaction. When a child avoids or rejects adult interaction, treat it as an error. Say, "Oh, you don't want this! Sorry! Here, try this toy." If at first, adult involvement triggers anger, avoidance, whining or tantrums, continue anyway. Anger is an acceptable response and often precedes the ability to express pleasure. Persistence pays off as the child realizes you will not stop pursuing her and treating what she does as intentional. Be indirect without imposing upon or overwhelming a child while opening and closing circles of communication.

4. *Help the child do what he wants to do*. Motor planning difficulties, low muscle tone, and poor "self-other differentiation" may cause a child to take an adult's hand to do something. Guide by putting hand over hand. Work face-to-face, or at a mirror so the child can see adult expressions. When a child is purposeful, hand him another object.

5. *Create a play environment.* Use rattles, balls, dolls, action figures, cars, trucks… anything that peaks a child's natural interests, motivation and curiosity. Initially, a child may reject a toy that he finds interesting later. Focus on creative interaction; avoid structured games.

6. *Extend the circles of communication.* Interact in such ways that help a child reach individual goals such as obtaining a toy. Interact playfully, sometimes playing dumb, or obstructing avoidance behavior, such as moving between a child and a desired toy to encourage interaction. When a child communicates the desire for something (taking your hand, looking, vocalizing, pointing), respond quickly, but not necessarily accurately, to stretch the desire into as many interactions as possible.

7. *Broaden the child's range of interactive experience.* Extend the child's desire to expand upon emotional, sensory and motor responses. Help a passive child become more outgoing, even aggressive, or an impulsive child to move in slow motion.

8. *Tailor interactions to a child's unique sensory processing differences.* Informally assess a child's auditory, visual, sequential processing and sensory modulation. Add sound, touch, vision and movement to the play with sensory, wind-up, and simple cause-and-effect toys to entice a passive child's interest and attention. Use sensory toys such as whistles, bubbles, textured blocks and beanbags to capitalize upon strengths and to remediate weaknesses.

9. ***Mobilize the six developmental stages simultaneously.*** Share attention, engage the child with gestures and pre-verbal problem-solving to encourage two-way purposeful interaction, emotions, ideas and thinking. Build bridges between ideas and the development of abstract reasoning, with the ultimate objective of maintaining mutual attention and engagement.

Floortime enables the child and the adult to feel connected and to communicate with each other. Floortime helps the child see the value of non-verbal communication through facial expressions, gestures, and other cues, and encourages the child to use these tools to communicate with others.

The Home Program

Unlike many "in office" therapy programs, most DIR sessions take place as an intensive home program. Parents, caregivers and therapists typically interact with children in Floortime activities for at least 20 minutes eight or more times a day. For children attending school, the program can be integrated into the classroom, which allows interactions with typically developing children, when the child is ready.

The role of parents in DIR is crucial. Both mother and father often need to make significant changes in the way they interact with their child throughout the day. DIR teaches them to respond to every utterance or gesture, in an effort to spark a response, giving endless choices to close one more circle, or engaging in endless debates and negotiations to help a child develop the ability to reason. DIR becomes a way of life, one that is both demanding and exhilarating, as families watch their children climb the developmental ladder, one rung at a time. In order to achieve success, it is essential that parents, caregivers and extended family all make a commitment to spend a considerable amount of time on the floor, playing and becoming part of the child's world, even if activities are limited.

Once a child begins to be interactive, peer play becomes an important part of the program. Children on the autism spectrum need to learn how to communicate with peers, who may be less forgiving than adults. Normally developing children provide good role models for language and social-emotional development. "Play dates" are opportunities for the skills developed with adults to generalize to other kids. At first, adults must be available to orchestrate children's interactions. As peer interaction improves, less adult intervention is necessary.

A well-balanced DIR program includes both spontaneous and semi-structured activities designed to facilitate mastery of specific processing abilities and emotional, cognitive, language and motor skills. The recipe for balance depends upon a child's developmental profile. DIR includes structured activities at least three times a day to address the following areas:

- ***Motor and sensory skills*** – activities include running, jumping on a trampoline, spinning, navigating obstacle courses,
- ***Balance, coordination and left-right integration*** – exercises include walking on a beam, standing on one leg with eyes open and closed, throwing, catching, and kicking balls with each and both hands, drawing standing and sitting with hands alone and together.
- ***Rhythm*** – games such as patty-cake, dancing to music, clapping and playing percussion instruments.
- ***Modulation*** – sessions that require the child to move at different rates of speed. Use of a drum or special music can facilitate these games.
- ***Visual-spatial skills*** – search and other visual-spatial games, such as a treasure hunt. Harry Wachs, OD, has worked closely with Greenspan and Wieder in developing a visual-spatial curriculum to include in Floortime, which is based on *Thinking Goes to School*.[8]

The Affect-Based Language Curriculum

Dr. Greenspan has collaborated with speech-language pathologist Diane Lewis, MA, CCC/SLP to develop the Affect-based Language Curriculum (ABLC), which is based on the premise that emotion is critical for many elements of language acquisition and use. Without affect and engagement, a child will encounter difficulty developing purposeful and meaningful language. The ABLC is designed to be implemented at home.

The ABLC includes a series of structured and semi-structured activities undertaken with high affect and motivation so that they generalize quickly. In implementing the ABLC caretakers first create a supportive environment in which a child is engaged in a pleasurable activity. While adhering to the DIR principles of attention, engagement and closing circles, the adult introduces activities to enhance such specific skills as oral motor capacities, imitation, receptive, expressive and pragmatic language.

The ABLC moves through five developmental levels from Level A (0-9 months) to Level D2 (36-48 months). Sequential skills and activities comprise the program. Caregivers use comprehensive checklists to chart progress and plan an individual child's program.

The ABLC focuses on traditional elements of language, such as phonology, syntax, grammar and semantics, while also addressing reflective and abstract thinking. Those interested in learning more about the ABLC should refer to *The Affect-Based Language Curriculum (ABLC): An Intensive Program for Families, Therapists and Teachers*.[9]

Who are Candidates for DIR/Floortime?

The DIR/Floortime model is useful in working with children at all levels of severity on the autistic spectrum. Greenspan and Wieder found that the degree of autism does not necessarily determine prognosis with DIR. In a review of 200 children who received DIR treatment, Greenspan and Wieder, found that 58% achieved excellent or good outcomes. These children showed warmth, and related to their environment with joy and pleasure. They were able to use ideas creatively, engage in spontaneous back & forth conversation, and answer questions (including "why" questions). They showed less self-absorption and repetitive behaviors.[5]

Those supporting the DIR approach believe that it is most effective when all therapists providing a child's therapies are knowledgeable about DIR principles, and that a child's program be coordinated by a DIR-trained clinician. Those interested in ongoing training institutes should go to <www.icdl.com> for a schedule.

Vision Therapy Using Floortime Techniques

Mehrnaz Green, OD, and her therapists at the Vision and Conceptual Development Center, in Washington, DC, have created some vision therapy techniques incorporating Floortime principles. The therapists sited with each procedure conceptualized the activity applying Floortime theory learned by attending DIR conferences. Harry Wachs, OD, is the founder of the DC Center and is also on the Board of the Interdisciplinary Council on Developmental and Learning Disorders (ICDLD), co-founded by Drs. Greenspan and Wieder.

Many vision therapy activities can be adapted according to DIR principles. The optometrist can modify the demands and complexity of VT activities by skill level, building upon each other in a hierarchical manner. Dr. Green believes that adding Floortime to vision therapy can be extremely helpful in encouraging, motivating, and engaging the more resistant patients on the autism spectrum in thinking, conversation, and play. The therapist creates an inviting atmosphere for a child by using exaggerated body language, vocal inflection, and facial expressions, thus establishing a connection.

Guided Directions Activities for Receptive/Expressive Language – by Mollie Straff Vision therapy focusing on remediating the receptive and expressive communication difficulties seen in children on the autism spectrum naturally lend themselves to a Floortime approach. A therapist uses circles outlined on transparency paper or hula hoops, to define spaces, placing them in a pattern. Depending upon a child's developmental level, the circles can form a single row, a three by three matrix, or any other pattern. For less mature patients, directions concentrate on top/bottom and right/left concepts; at higher levels, work focuses on understanding complex directions from another person's perspective.

The circles and a child's favorite story or movie can provide the setting for receiving and giving directions, with each person taking on the role of a character. Having an imagination helps, although that level of abstract thought is not necessary for the activity to be successful. Using an imaginary scenario for receptive-expressive circles allows participants to get involved in the game and enjoy it, while at the same time incorporating expression and interpretation of directions accurately.

Directions are titled "challenges," which move a player to a "goal" circle in a specified number of steps. For example, using a Harry Potter theme say, "Harry, your next challenge is to go two steps from your bottom and one step to your right." A child receives a point for each challenge completed correctly on the first try. After six rounds, the child and therapist exchange roles, with the child giving directions. The child then moves through the challenge to prove he has mastered it.

This activity can also be done as a peer interaction where the therapist or clinician may take a less active role and simply mediate the game. Allowing children to influence the setting and details of the game's realm opens the lines of communication and increases their involvement in the activity. Increased involvement provides them with a greater sense of ownership and responsibility, thus encouraging them to attend fully put in their best effort.

Island and Lily Pads – by Lauren Gonzales This is a visuo-spatial logic activity that also offers the opportunity to use receptive and expressive communication. The therapist can do it one-to-one or with peers to encourage group problem solving.

Explain an imaginary situation in which both therapist and child are frogs stranded on an island, (inside a hula hoop) without food. Another island across the room, (a second hula hoop) has food. The therapist presents five hula hoops as lily pads to help the frog get to the other island, without explaining how this can be done.

Ground rules are as follows. The frogs can throw or drop the lily pads wherever they like, but cannot step outside a lily pad to retrieve another. When a lily pad is placed on the floor, the frog can step inside the hoop and it will stay afloat. The Lily pad cannot be moved while a frog is standing on it.

At first, the child will have enough hoops to line them up like a bridge and walk to the other island. Once accomplished, the therapist removes one of the hula hoops and asks the child to return to the other island. This step will require the child to plan the spacing of the remaining hoops. Some children evenly space the hoops while others chose to repeat what they've done but jump the remaining distance. Once successful with four lily pads, remove another.

Throughout the activity, the therapist should ask the child about his plan of action. Eventually, the child should be left with only two hoops, and the goal is for the child to realize he can pick the hoop up from behind him and place it in front of him. Often, children will try to place the remaining two hoops evenly apart, taking large jumps from one to the other. If this is the case, the therapist could congratulate this achievement and then prohibit jumping as a more difficult challenge, by saying something such as, "Now pretend that you are an old frog and you cannot jump that high."

Negative Space   Understanding negative space as a visual, mental construct or concept developmentally follows using the sense of sight meaningfully, reasoning visually, mathematically and logically, and being able to manipulate objects using the fingers.

Draw a 4" x 4" square on the piece of paper, and create a story describing the space. It could be a "parking lot" for racecars, a "garden" for flowers, or a classroom for desks. Have a pile of one inch cubes. Ask the child to estimate how many cubes would be necessary to completely fill the space. If necessary, hand the child a block and encourage using it to estimate.

After a guess is recorded, ask the child to place blocks in the square, and count them, all along, observing the child's thought processes. For example, does the child place cubes adjacent to each, thus fully covering the space or are there gaps between cubes? Does the child extend blocks outside the border? Does the child lack visually guided movement or lack attention to detail? Does the child not see the line as a limit or barrier? As the child continues to place the cubes, ask for a revised estimate until he is sure of the exact number of cubes that will fill the area. Determine whether the child is using addition or multiplication to figure out the answer.

Next, adhere some of the cubes to the board, using tape, and quickly remove the remaining cubes. Put the board with the adhered cubes on the table, and ask the child how many cubes are missing. Observe what the child does: count the open spaces; counting the number of visible cubes; guess? After the child has given the correct number, return the cubes and have the child place them in the empty spaces to cross check.

Mental Mapping – John Balsley   Activities using large exercise balls of varying sizes can stimulate a child's curiosity and encourage Floortime-based discovery of gross motor function, logic, and mental map of the body. First, use any size ball to engage the patient. Apply pressure by rolling or bouncing on the ball, thus opening a circle of communication. Once the child is engaged, switch to a large 50" diameter ball and a small ball, such as a Marsden ball, suspended by a string from the ceiling.

Use the large ball to bounce the Marsden ball as many times as possible without letting the Marsden ball strike the player. The game can be set up so that the child is a super hero protecting the city and the ball is his/her shield from the bullets/fireballs/etc. from the villains. This procedure promotes ocular tracking, bilateral coordination, and mental map of the body (ducking and dodging the approaching Marsden ball).

The Dancing Dialogue

Suzi Tortora, EdD, a dance psychotherapist with practices in New York City and in Cold Spring, New York combines her training with Greenspan's DIR techniques to use the communicative power of movement with young children on the autism spectrum. She calls her program "The Dancing Dialogue." Tortora became fascinated with the connection between mind and body by observing children's non-verbal cues to uncover critical information about their physical, social-emotional, cognitive and communication skills. She holds that all nonverbal acts have the potential to be communicative.

Tortora believes that the body and its sensations are the reference point from which nonverbal children decode experiences. Body awareness, posture, and movement style are all reflections of emotional expression. By paying attention to rhythm, tempo, muscular tension, effort and use of space, she gains insight into how children with autism spectrum disorders organize and experience their world. Dance is the communication between the self and the other. Simply by moving with a child, she creates a dancing dialogue between child and adult, as well as between the child and the environment. As a result, the child becomes more self-aware, conscious of the environment and of the relationship between the two. Eye contact increases, and verbal interactions become more appropriate.

Assessing Individual Communication and Emotional Bonds

Tortora first evaluates a child's feelings and the messages behind them. She informally assesses a child's developmental levels and preferred style of relating by looking at visual, auditory, olfactory, gustatory, proprioceptive and vestibular sensitivities, noting which senses are hyper-reactive and which are hypo-reactive.

Next, she chooses therapeutic techniques and activities that enhance relating and make interactions fun. Her goal is to expand all aspects of abilities by engaging a child in movement, dance, play and music by regulating his/her senses through body and spatial awareness. Initially, she matches a child's actions; then she modifies them. For example, running transforms into leaping, then into fast marching, and lastly, into slow marching, with a strong, focused beat. Verbally narrating actions during the interaction provides the child with symbolic verbal cues that label and follow the experience.

When following a child's lead, she watches for fragmentation, disorganization and chaotic behavior. If the dancing dialogue does not include mutual, sharing movements, affective reactions, and expressivity, then she looks for new avenues with which to connect to a child.

Group Sessions

Groups help develop a sense of self and others by increasing body awareness and control. The improvisational nature of group sessions supports free expression, while, at the same time, encouraging greater social relatedness. Tortora includes the following elements to encourage social interactions. All can be adapted to vision, speech-language or occupational therapy sessions.

- *Start and end each session with relaxation activities.* Intersperse periodic moments of relaxation, stretching and breath awareness.
- *Shift between free individual movement explorations and structured group movement explorations.* Alternate activities with individuals, dyads, small and large groups.
- *Include movements requiring gradually more complex body control.* As children gain better body awareness and control, they are ready for challenges.
- *Identify a child's "signature" action for the day.* Individual non-verbal expressive movements may vary each session or may be similar for a period of time.
- *Ask each child to lead.* Visualizing and carrying out a specific movement requires a great deal of organization. Mimicking the movements of a peer incorporates both attention and motor planning.
- *Focus children on a specific movement activity.* Simultaneously be ready to change focus, if necessary, to keep children engaged and interacting.
- *Keep the group moving together, whenever possible.* Relating to others builds group cohesion. Allow for spontaneous breaks from relating, that individual children may need.
- *Use music and/or props.* Relating to something outside of self helps foster individual expression.
- *Use variations in music beat, style, rhythm and volume to redirect and/or reconnect children.* A strong, clear rhythm with a moderate tempo enhances internal organization and creates full body-body part coordination.
- *Create a theme.* Animals, space, the beach or a holiday, will all do fine.

Dancing as therapy draws from the principles of sensory integration theory, vision training and speech-language therapy, put to music. Children of all ages have fun as they learn where they and their peers are in space. For more on this exciting intervention, go to <www.suzitortora.org> and read Tortora's *The Dancing Dialogue: Using the Communicative Power of Movement with Young Children*.[10]

Solving the Relationship Puzzle: Relational Development Intervention (RDI) ©

"I knew each child with autism could not make the same progress or reach the same goals. But, regardless of his or her abilities and limits, I wanted to give each of them something." So began the journey of psychologist Steven E. Gutstein, PhD, the innovator of Relational Development Intervention or RDI©, which helps those with autism learn the social skills that come easily to others. It is based upon the ways in which typical children become socially competent, steers children on the autism spectrum down a path of self discovery and social awareness to a world of meaningful friendships, shared emotions and heartfelt connection with people in their lives.

Dr. Gutstein is a nationally renowned developer of innovative clinical programs for children with high-risk conditions. In 1995, he co-founded The Connections Center in Houston, Texas, which began as a multi-disciplinary private outpatient practice serving local children and families. In recent years, The Connections Center has evolved into the home of the RDI Program©, and now serves as an international consultation and training center for professionals and families. Currently, over 3000 families world-wide participate in an RDI Program©, and over 100 professionals in child development are certified as RDI Program© Consultants.

Gutstein describes RDI© in his book, *Autism Asperger's: Solving the Relationship Puzzle*.[11] This synopsis of RDI is taken from that book and from Gutstein's website, <www.rdiconnect.com>.

Experience Sharing

Experience sharing is the innate pleasure derived from a variety of social encounters. For typically developing children, Gutstein believes that *experience sharing* takes place in levels, each with four distinct stages, starting at birth. He has systematically analyzed and labeled many levels of *experience sharing*, starting with "emotional attunement" and "social referencing," among others, at the early months, to "fluid transitions" in the second year of life, "unique selves" in the fifth year, and "enduring friendships" by age 11 or 12. While this model is clearly a gross oversimplification of the millions of situations children experience, it provides a useful framework for understanding emotional development.

Autism: Life without Experiencing Sharing

According to Gutstein's model, individuals with autism have deficits in the understanding and appreciation of *experience sharing*. Gutstein believes that sometime during the first year of life, children with autism go down a developmental road that does not include the endless hours a typical child spends with social referencing, or "you-me" thinking and emotional attunement. By the end of the first year of life, when objects begin to compete with people for a child's attention, the typical child enters the object world looking for enhancement, while at this stage, the child with autism chooses objects over the people, and departs from the world of experience sharing. Typical children already know that adults are good reference points for safety, meaning, excitement and resolving, while those with autism have not made that connection.

What is the Relational Development Intervention® Program?

RDI® shares many features with other treatment approaches. Gutstein has adapted other programs described in this chapter. Like DIR, RDI educates and coaches adults to interact and work with children with autism. Its goal is the remediation of specific deficits that define autism spectrum disorders by creating numerous daily opportunities for the child to respond in flexible, thoughtful ways. In addition, it helps children capture and stockpile critical memories that build a repository of competence, in gradually more complex environments. RDI® is not wedded to any series of techniques, but rather to developing effective methods to remediate those specific deficits which impede people on the autism spectrum from productive employment, independent living, marriage and intimate social relationships.

The RDI® Program Protocol consists of nine essential elements. All nine must be in place for the intervention to be classified as an RDI® Program:

1. *Diagnostic evaluation* The first step is for the child to undergo comprehensive language, cognitive, neurological, perceptual, motor and medical evaluations. A Relationship Development Assessment™ (RDA), numerous questionnaires, rating scales, a video segment of the home, a consultation session with parents, and a few other procedures are also required.

2. *Parent education* Prior to beginning a program, all parents must attend a series of workshops, or if impossible, view a comprehensive DVD about how to incorporate RDI® into their daily lives.

3. *RDI® program planning* A certified RDI® consultant reviews the results of the RDA™, and provides a written intervention plan with lengthy recommendations. RDA™ results are used for intervention planning, formulating objectives and developing *customized* modifications for environments and activity frameworks, based upon a child's unique needs. Parents collect data daily, and summarize it weekly. Videotapes of a child's program are made and reviewed at least every two weeks. Objectives are updated regularly, with RDA™ reassessments conducted at a minimum of six month intervals.

4. *Consultation* Intervention is guided by a certified RDI® Program consultant, or by someone who is currently receiving supervision from staff or designees of the Connections Center. The consultant must be highly familiar with the child and family and consult with parents on a regular basis.

5. *Parents use RDI as a lifestyle and function as facilitators* Parents are encouraged to spend three to six hours per week interacting with the child using RDI methods. These include the utilization of declarative communication, rather than questioning, directing or demanding, and creating frequent periods of "productive uncertainty" that emphasize a child's present objectives.

6. ***Children work individually with adults, and then in therapeutic peer dyads or groups when developmentally ready*** The consultant monitors the stage at which a child is functioning. Eventually, children are matched by stage to work together.

7. *Episodic Memory* Intervention plans include specific methods designed to strengthen Episodic Memories (EM). This includes regular addition to and review of Memory Journals that are constructed to be developmentally appropriate for the child.

8. ***Emphasis on Self Development*** Self and social development objectives are clearly balanced and sufficient time is spent to work on objectives in both areas. Primary emphasis is given to development of relative thinking and executive functioning skills.

9. ***The RDI® Program is a Primary Intervention*** The RDI® Program is carried out as a primary (but not necessarily the only) intervention. The RDI® Program is not treated or considered adjunctive or secondary to any other intervention. Most participants in RDI® Programs receive other interventions such as dietary modification, occupational therapy, vision therapy, and/or speech and language intervention.

The Three Cardinal Principles of RDI

RDI recognizes that learning to be proficient in even the simplest forms of experience sharing requires many different abilities, and it is thus far more complex than most social skills programs. RDI provides a special therapeutic setting which amplifies critical information, minimizes distractions, and slows down the pace of interaction. Continued change and unpredictability, rather than scripted or discrete learning are inherent aspects of *experience sharing* encounters.

Gutstein has classified the three major principles that lay the foundation for RDI as "social referencing," "functions precede means" and "co-regulation."

- ***Social Referencing*** The desire and capacity for social referencing is the foundation of experience sharing. Gutstein defines "social referencing" as a highly specialized form of perception and information processing that allows a person to evaluate the state of a relationship. In the process, a child is constantly reading the degree of similarity between something he is doing, feeling, perceiving or thinking and to interpret the relationship with social partners.

  For example, individuals with good social referencing skills are simultaneously noting facial expressions, bodily movements, focus of attention, etc. prior to and following any interaction. They make rapid comparisons between themselves and others, rather than watching for specific cues. Referencing takes place subliminally, while social partners and their environments are constantly moving and changing. Life, unlike football, offers no instant replays; interactions keep moving without time outs for regrouping.

  RDI helps children with autism understand how to operate in a fluid system, where important information occurs in an ongoing feedback loop. The ability to socially reference with ease opens up a whole new world and changes the entire nature of social interaction from being dependent upon a series of rote responses that may or may not be applicable to the situation, to independently making choices. For instance, the therapist may deliberately lag behind a child when taking a walk, forcing the child to notice and process what it means, and say something like, "Hurry up!"

- ***Functions Precede Means*** At each developmental level of *experience sharing* RDI introduces the child to new aspects of experiences to be shared, thus establishing greater emotional connections. Eventually, children with autism, like their typical peers, develop a desire for deeper emotional experiences, leading them to pursue and spend many hours mastering new skills. They then learn to interact for the sole purpose of sharing their world with others, and become eager to apply newly learned skills both in and out of treatment settings.

- ***Co-Regulation*** Once children have mastered "social referencing," and "functions precede means," RDI introduces "co-regulation," the ability to understand how one partner's actions impact upon the actions of another, in order to maintain the relationship. Co-regulation requires constant referencing of a partner. Give-and-take interaction produces curiosity about the other person. As co-regulation becomes more and more proficient, it provides the foundation for moving into exploring another person's mind. What will he do next? What is he thinking? How is he feeling?

Adults often take responsibility for maintaining coordination of interactions with children. In RDI, children learn to take responsibility for their part of keeping an interaction intact; they become co-regulators. Most importantly, they learn how to self-regulate, or to take actions that alter their own behavior so that it coordinates with that of their partner.

The most crucial part of co-regulation for children with autism is learning how to observe when coordination has been lost, or is in jeopardy. In early work on co-regulation, RDI, like DIR, recommends exaggerating non-coordination. For example, adults should deliberately and playfully impede a child's desired goal.

In all three areas, RDI, introduces new skills only after determining that a child is developmentally ready for them. Prior to working on any new skill, the adult should always make sure the child understands its functions and value. As in typical development, each step is built upon a prior stage of accomplishment. RDI introduces improvisational activities only after a child has learned many ways of coordinating his actions with others, and has sufficient reasons to take specific actions.

Trained RDI counselors are integral to the process to carefully and gradually introduce the child to social referencing and gradually allow him to take on more responsibility for co-regulation. Activities focus the child on the enjoyment of *experience sharing*, as well as provide opportunities for the child to successfully practice communication and self-regulation for coordination in slow and gradual ways.

The Goals of RDI
RDI's goals are for those with autism to
- Understand and appreciate the many levels of experience sharing
- Become an equal partner in co-regulating experience sharing interactions
- Value the uniqueness of others' perspectives, ideas and feelings
- Work to maintain enduring relationships
- Become adaptable and flexible in both social and non-social problem solving
- Recognize that their own unique identity can continue to grow and develop

The Relationship Curriculum
In developing his intervention program, Gutstein has painstakingly analyzed how each stage of experience sharing develops at six different levels, and applies this knowledge to facilitating the child with autism to grow emotionally. The RDI "curriculum" is composed of hundreds of step-by-step treatment objectives and customized activities developed after a child undergoes the Relationship Development Assessment (RDA). Activities and objectives at each of the six levels represents a dramatic developmental shift in the central focus of relationships. As a reference, Gutstein has labeled the six levels in the curriculum as: Novice; Apprentice; Challenger; Voyager; Explorer; and Partner.

- *Novice* This foundational level establishes parents as the emotional and reference center of the child's world. Components are emotional attunements, social referencing, excitement sharing and simple games. As rapidly as possible, parents frame the importance of their faces and voices in every activity. This goal cues the child to reference the parent's face to anticipate what will happen next.

- *Apprentice* At level two, children gradually learn to enjoy synchronized activities. They also coordinate their movements with those of their parents, and share in co-regulation. Components include taking, reversing and changing roles, participating as a partner in regulating activities and moving together, such as in running or falling down simultaneously.
- *Challenger* At the third level, children share novelty, make fluid transitions, modify rules and regulations, create new games and improvise, all while working together as partners. For instance, together the child and an adult may decide to build a fort, then one person changes his/her mind, and suggests that the structure be a store. At this level, children experience the strength of working together.
- *Voyager* Level four marks a dramatic change from referencing outward facial expressions, gestures and movements to looking inward to the private world of ideas, feeling and thoughts. At this step a child learns to ask questions such as "What are you looking at?" and begins to realize that others' emotions are as interesting as his own. He attempts to take another's perspective and, as work progresses to use language efficiently for experience sharing.
- *Explorer* At the fifth level, the child makes the shift from objects to people by sharing ideas, opinions and feelings. This level is often not reached until the teenage years, even for typically developing individuals. Competence at this stage spawns the ability to have a real conversation where inner thoughts, feelings and ideas can be shared, and differences appreciated.
- **Partner** A the final level of emotional development, life becomes truly worthwhile. Many people never reach this stage, which allows the integration of a life with others in a variety of ways. This level sets the stage for enduring friendships, belonging and marriage. This is an especially important step for those at the high functioning end of the autism spectrum. Gutstein believes that it is important for those with autism to confront their disability, speak openly about it, and reflect upon the progress they have made.

The End Product of RDI

RDI provides a structured path for people on the autism spectrum to learn friendship, empathy and a love of sharing their world with others. The program begins at an individual's level of capability, and carefully, systematically teaches them the skills they need for competence and fulfillment in a complex world. Eventually, they learn not only to tolerate, but to enjoy change, transition and going with the flow.

The Son-Rise Program®

Like other professionals and psychologists in this book, Barry Neil Kaufman and Samahria Lyte Kaufman refused to listen in the 1970s, when, at 18 months old, their son, Raun, was diagnosed as severely and incurably autistic. Experts advised the Kaufmans to institutionalize Raun because of his "hopeless, lifelong condition." Instead, they designed an innovative, unique home-based, child-centered program to reach their son. It transformed Raun from a mute, withdrawn child with a very low IQ into a highly verbal, socially interactive youngster with a near-genius IQ. Bearing no traces of his former condition, Raun graduated from an Ivy League college.

Responding to the demand to teach others their program, The Kaufman family established The Option Institute and the Autism Treatment Center of America™, where they have been offering The Son-Rise Program® since 1983. Raun now teaches families and individuals there, and following the publication of his story, "Son-Rise®," now updated to *Son-Rise®: The Miracle Continues,*[12] and the award-winning NBC-TV movie *Son-Rise®: A Miracle of Love*, lectures internationally.

What Are the Principles of the Son-Rise Program®?

The Son-Rise Program® is based on the idea that adults must enter the world of autism instead of asking the child with autism to enter the "real" world. By mirroring repetitive and ritualistic behaviors, and interacting with the child through play, accompanied by an optimistic, trusting, respectful and non-judgmental attitude of love and enthusiasm, adults can gradually lead a child toward a more normal life.

Son-Rise® encourages parents to follow the child's lead or actions, while simultaneously directing him or her into an expanded world. The unique feature of this program is the commitment to happiness. Parents are encouraged to explore their own belief systems and to question judgments that limit them.

The guiding principles of the Son-Rise Program® are
- *Autism is a relational, not a behavioral disorder.* Son-Rise® views autism as an inter-actional disorder in which children have difficulty relating and connecting to those around them. Most of the so-called "behavioral challenges" stem from this relational deficit. That's why dynamic, enthusiastic, play-oriented methods focus so extensively on socialization and rapport building. The goal is for parents to enjoy their child, and for the child to enjoy interacting with adults.
- *Motivation, not repetition, holds the key to all learning.* Son-Rise® strives to uncover each child's unique motivations, and use these to teach children the skills they need to learn. While many traditional modalities endeavor to teach through endless repetition, the Son-Rise Program® does not provide the child with information, or teach the child predetermined skills. Instead, it views the child's current level of performance as being the best that the child can do. The child thus participates willingly, demonstrating an increasing long attention span, better retention and the generalization of skills. The Son-Rise Program® emphasizes total acceptance of the child, and encourages the child to become a more motivated and participating individual.
- *"Stimming" behaviors have important meaning and value.* Son-Rise® accepts and respects children's behaviors. The program thus encourages joining, rather than stop-ping, a child's repetitive, ritualistic behaviors. Doing so builds rapport and connection, the platform for all future education and development. Participating with a child in repetitive behaviors facilitates eye contact, social development and inclusion of others in play.
- *Parents are a child's best resource.* Nothing equals the power of parents. No one else can match the unparalleled love, deep dedication, long-term commitment and day in, day out experiences with their children that parents possess. Son-Rise® empowers parents to be confident directors and teachers by listening to them, and providing them with skills training.
- *Parents and professionals are most effective when they feel comfortable with a child, optimistic about a child's capabilities and hopeful about a child's future.* Caring professionals often do not have the resources, guidance or support they need to help the children they are working with. Son-Rise® offers a unique attitudinal perspec-tive that re-energizes adults and arms them with excellent tools to help their students.
- *All children can progress in the right environment.* Most children on the autism spec-trum are over stimulated by a plethora of distractions that others do not even notice. Son-Rise® eliminates environmental distractions, thus creating an optimal work/play-room that facilitates positive interactions and reduces control battles.
- *A child's potential is limitless.* Experts sometimes give parents frightening and nega-tive diagnoses and prognoses. Son-Rise® believes that no one has the right to predict what a child can and cannot achieve. Son-Rise® focuses parents on their own attitudes, striving to help them reclaim their optimism and hopefulness, and see the potential in

their children. While Son-Rise® does not give parents "false" hopes, they refuse to predict what level of competence any given child can achieve. From this perspective all things are possible.

Son-Rise® can be combined effectively with other therapies including biomedical interventions, sensory integration therapy, a gluten- and casein-free or other diets, auditory therapy, and of course, vision therapy. When complimentary therapies are included, and applied using The Son-Rise Program® principles, the intervention is even more effective than when used individually. However, some approaches, which contain principles and techniques which are contradictory to the Son-Rise® approach, can undermine the effectiveness of the program and confuse the child.[13]

The Son-Rise Program® is customized to each child's needs. Families come to and stay at the Option Institute for a week or more at a time, and are trained to use skills that allow them to accept their child and become his/her teacher. Son-Rise® begins with a five-day start-up program, a group seminar that outlines the basic components of the home-based program. Next is an intensive one week seminar, which provides 40 hours of one-on-one work with a trained facilitator and the child. The advanced training seminar is a follow up program after the implementation of a home-based program.

Son-Rise® is an intensive program requiring an enormous commitment of time and money. While I am aware of no studies of the Son-Rise Program's® effectiveness, many families who use it, swear by it, and like the Kaufmans, report recovery from autism.

Social Stories™

Carol Gray, a former consultant to students with autism spectrum disorders in Jenison, MI, and Director of The Gray Center for Social Learning and Understanding in Grand Rapids, MI, became interested in the difficulty autistic individuals have assuming the perspective of another person. In 1991 she devised a technique to help them learn how to understand others' behaviors called "Social Stories™."

What are Social Stories™?

Social Stories™ help individuals with autism learn to "read" and understand social situations by answering questions "who," "what," "when," "where," and "why" questions to a variety of situations presented in the form of a stories. Each story describes a scenario, skill, or concept in terms of relevant social cues, perspectives, and common responses in a specifically defined style and format.

The goal of a Social Story™ is to impart accurate social information in a patient and reassuring manner, not to change an individual's behavior. However, heightened understanding of social events and expectations often leads to more mature behavior. Social Stories™ can be individualized to the needs of the person with autism to teach routines, instructions for a specific activity, how to ask for assistance, and socially appropriate emotional responses to feelings such as anger and frustration.

Social Stories use four types of sentences: descriptive, directive, perspective, and control.

- *Descriptive sentences* express what people do in particular social situations. They are used to explain a social setting, step-by-step directions for completing an activity, etc. *Example:* "When the bell rings, the children come in from recess and go to their classrooms, where the teacher reads a story."
- *Directive sentences* move a person toward a desired appropriate social response. They state in positive terms what the behavior is. *Example:* "When the bell rings, I stop playing and line up to come in from recess."

Descriptive and directive sentences often occur together, in what Gray calls the Social Story™ ratio. She suggests that for every directive sentence, a story should have two to five descriptive sentences. This proportion minimally limits an individual's choices. The greater the number of descriptive statements, the greater the opportunity for the individual to supply his/her own responses to the social situation. The greater the number of directive statements, the more specific the cues for how the individual should respond.

> *Example of combination:* "I am playing during recess. The bell rings. I stop playing and line up to come in. I follow the other children and quietly go to the classroom. When we get to the classroom, I sit down at my desk and listen as my teacher reads a story."

- ***Perspective sentences*** present others' reactions to a situation so that the individual can learn how others' perceive various events. *Examples:* "The teacher is happy to see all the children line up quietly and walk to their classroom." "Many children are excited that they get to hear a story."

Perspective sentences are combined with descriptive sentences in the same ratio as directive sentences.

> *Example of perspective sentences in combination*: "When the bell rings for recess to end, the teacher is happy to see all the children line up quietly and walk to their classroom. Many children are excited that they are going to hear a story. The teacher likes it when children sit quietly and listen."

- The final type of sentence is the ***Control sentence***. This sentence identifies strategies the person can use to facilitate memory and comprehension of the social story. Thus, these sentences are added by the individual after reviewing the social story. *Example:* "I remember that the bell means it's time for recess to end by thinking of a teapot. I know that when it whistles, the water is done. The bell is like the whistle; when it rings, recess is done. "

Directive or control sentences may be omitted entirely as the functioning level of the person with autism increases.

Who are candidates for Social Stories™?

Although Gray developed Social Stories™ for use with children with autism spectrum disorders, her approach has also been successful with adolescents, and adults, as well as with others who have social and communication delays. Social stories are applicable for both readers and non-readers.

How are Social Stories Implemented?

For a person who can read, the author introduces the story by reading it aloud twice. The person with autism then reads it once a day independently. For a person who cannot read, the author records the story on a tape or CD with a verbal cue or bell indicating when to turn the page. The person listens to the story and follows along daily.

Once an individual with autism successfully enacts the skills, or appropriately responds in a particular type of social situation, use of the number of times a story is read a week can be reduced, or the story can be reviewed once a month or as necessary. Fading can also be accomplished by rewriting the story, and gradually removing directive sentences.

Carol Gray and her associates have written two books with collections of Social Stories™ Topics in *My Social Stories Book*[14] include:
- *Taking Care of Myself* Using the toilet, washing hands, brushing teeth, taking medicine, blowing your nose, wearing new clothes, dressing for the weather, taking a nap,

getting a haircut, clipping fingernails and toenails, taking a bath, washing your hair, bedtime and sleeping.

- *Home* Dealing with unexpected noises such as the telephone, doorbell, dogs barking, the vacuum cleaner, etc, managing time, appropriate behavior with playdates and baby-sitters and even divorce.
- *Going Places* Why do adults forget and what helps them remember, running errands, checking out in line, visiting places like the zoo, beach and movie theatre, eating out in a restaurant, going to school and to the doctor.

The New Social Story Book[15] covers topics such as learning to chew gum, giving a gift, how to give a hug, how to use the telephone, sharing, when to say, "Thank you" and "Excuse me," pets, personal care, cooking, helping around the house, picking flowers, school issues such as fire drills, recess and homework, escalators, seat belts, going to church, getting a haircut, going shopping, new shoes, understanding the weather, holidays, vacations, and others. Gray also teaches the reader how to construct a Social Story™.

The Gray Center offers workshops, support groups, DVDs and other educational materials. Carol Gray travels extensively to teach her method. Studies are currently assessing the effectiveness of Social Stories. They appear to be a promising method for improving the social behaviors of autistic individuals. For additional information about Social Stories, go to <www.thegraycenter.org>.

The Miller Method

Arnold Miller, PhD, a Boston psychologist, and his late wife, Eileen Eller-Miller, MA, CCC, a speech and language pathologist, developed the Miller Method at their Language and Cognitive Development Center (LCDC) in the 1960's. They describe this approach as a cognitive-developmental approach for children with body organization, social and communication issues.

Cognitive-developmental theory assumes that typical development depends on children's ability to form systems, or organized chunks of behavior. Initially, these systems are repetitive and circular, triggered only by the environment. As children develop, and become increasingly aware of the distinction between themselves and their immediate surroundings, their systems expand and become more complex. They then gradually learn to take control of their environment, and combine their systems in new ways. Early gesture language, problem solving, social exchanges and complex communication all emerge as a child directs body action toward or with objects and events.

The Miller Method Philosophy

Miller maintains that every child, no matter how withdrawn or disorganized, is trying to find ways to cope with the world. The ability to assess and respond to the outside world is essential for survival.

The Miller Method is based on a belief that optometrists would most certainly agree with: that children learn most effectively when their whole bodies are physically and repetitively involved in the learning process. While the reader may argue that this therapy should right-fully be included along with those that integrate sensory processing, its place in this chapter is due to the fact that the founders are a psychologist and speech-language therapist who emphasize the end-product skills of social interaction and communication. While visual processing is not a primary component of the therapy, the approach certainly depends upon and builds visual skills in many areas.

The Miller Method and Autism

Miller theorizes that children with autism become stalled at early stages of development, and progress to more advanced stages in an incomplete or distorted fashion. Their spotty development leads to impairments in the ability to react to and influence the world. Lacking a sense of where they are in space, external stimuli drive them into scattered or stereotypic behavior from which, unassisted, they cannot extricate themselves. This results in aberrant systems involving people and/or objects, as well as a "hardening" of transitory formations seen in typical development, such as hand inspection, twiddling or intense object preoccupation.[16]

The Miller Method Procedures

Miller has developed special assessments to evaluate the unique way in which a child with autism reacts to various situations. He then prescribes a program that addresses that child's specific body organization, social interaction, communication, and representation issues in both clinical and classroom settings.

The Miller Method gradually transforms a child's limited reality systems by expanding his/her repertoire of activities. As a child with autism gradually tolerates and accepts new reality systems through repetitive activity, and can makes transitions from event to event without distress, the ability to cope with different life situations improves dramatically.

Miller has developed specialized training systems and instructional equipment to help children maximize their capacity to learn. The Miller Method uses two major strategies to restore typical developmental progressions. The first extinguishes children's aberrant systems, such as lining up blocks, and transforms them into functional behaviors, such as putting blocks into cups. The other introduces developmentally appropriate activities involving objects and people to fill in gaps in development.

All activities take place with children elevated two and one-half feet off the ground on a special structure. Elevation enhances body awareness, focus, motor-planning and social-emotional contact, thus increasing the ability to cope with obstacles and demands. Children with autism transition from one object or event to another, and from object involvement to representational play when placed on elevated boards.

Miller's therapists facilitate the systematic and repetitive process by teaching particular functions in a specified sequence, all the while narrating a child's actions. They thus build in the ability to generalize. For example, if they are teaching a child to put cups on cup hooks, the worker might first help put the cup on the hook by working hand-over-hand until the child can do it without support. Then, the worker moves a foot or two away, so that the child must turn toward the adult to get the cup and then turn toward the cup hooks to hang the cup. Ultimately, the child learns to perform the cup-on-hook task while accepting cups of varied shapes and colors presented from different points in space and by different people.

Because a disorganized child affects all around him, the Miller Method, like many of the other therapies in this chapter, works closely with parents and families. At least one parent interacts with the child during the above process, thus allowing new capacities to cope that have begun to flourish at the Center to generalize to the home and elsewhere. Parents also play an integral role in the program by creating a supportive and sufficiently demanding home life.

Miller views tantrums and other negative behaviors as a failure in the child's ability to cope with people or things in his or her surroundings. The Miller Method always looks for the meaning underlying the behavior, which varies from child to child. Some children cannot cope with the shift from one situation to the next; others may a feel a loss when a teacher turns to another child. Once the need is identified, Miller uses repetitive and reassuring rituals to help a child reorganize. As a last resort, the therapist holds and talks calmly to the child, explaining what is happening and what will happen next.

The Sign and Spoken Language ™ Program

The ability to understand others and to express oneself is fundamental. Miller has thus developed some unique methods for teaching communication through videotapes of signed and spoken language. He uses "narratives" accompanied by manual signs and words that guide children's actions. His little patients thus quickly learn to communicate as signs, spoken words, and related objects are presented simultaneously.

Miller's experience is that children who cannot follow directions on the ground can often do so on elevated boards. When obstacles are placed in the their paths, and a therapist "narrates" what a child is doing as he/she moves over, in, through and across obstacles, the child develops a repertoire of meaning which can readily be transferred to the ground. Eventually, children begin to respond to spoken words and express themselves without signing or object accompaniment, for the first time.

Training films teach receptive and expressive communication of four clusters of concepts using manual signs adapted from the American Sign Language (ASL) for the deaf. Signs and their objects are associated with spoken words designed to establish certain linguistic functions:

- *Signs, Sounds and their Actions* of 18 action meanings: come, go, stop, up, down, get up, sit down, open, close, pick up, drop, walk, run, jump, fall, push, pull and break.
- *Food Situations* teaches 17 signs and word meanings that permit those with autism to function more appropriately in eating situations: knife, fork, spoon, plate, glass, table, chair, eat, pour, drink, bread, salt, ketchup, roll, cookie, egg and pie.
- *Familiar Objects and Events* extends understanding and use to include familiar objects and events in their immediate surroundings: comb, toothbrush, sleep, wash, awake, hot, sweep, house, cat, tree, car, boat, ball, man and boy.
- *Two-Sign/Two-Word Combinations* helps children achieve basic syntactical constructions involving two sign/two word combinations such as verb/noun (eat cookie), noun/verb (man sleeps), adjective/noun (little chair), noun/adverb (table up/down), adverb + noun (more pie), possessive pronoun/noun (my chair), and noun/ preposition (cat in). Miller demonstrates situations that relate directly to each grammatical construction, such as showing a cat going into a paper bag.

Symbol Accentuation ™ Reading Program

Once children can speak or sign two and three word sentences, Miller uses his *Symbol Accentuation™ Reading Program* to teach them the symbolic function of printed words by living the meaning of a group of familiar words. A teacher facilitates interplay between a child and animated sequences presented on a CD ROM, with flashcards and workbook materials to help a child compose sentences. First children develop a sight vocabulary; they then learn to sound out unfamiliar words using phonetics. Finally they combine the two methods for reading and writing.

The Miller Method was first described in the book *From Ritual to Repertoire*[17]. A new book on The Miller Method ®[18] by Dr. Miller with Kristina Chretien, a long time LCDC staff member, is due out in 2008. Chapters outline the underlying principles of the Miller Method® and its practical application to developing communication skills and social play. The book also addresses such behavioral issues as temper tantrums, aggression, and toilet training. A chapter on research outcomes demonstrates the efficacy of the method in practice.

This information and more is available at <www.millermethod.org>.

The SCERTS® Model

SCERTS® is a comprehensive, multidisciplinary, integrative team approach that offers a framework for enhancing communication and social emotional abilities. It is derived from approaches and techniques in the fields of communication disorders, special education, occupational therapy, and developmental/behavioral psychology. SCERTS® is an acronym for Social Communication (SC), Emotional Regulation (ER) and Transactional Support (TS), developed by speech-language pathologist Barry Prizant, PhD, CCC-SLP.

SCERTS® is a product of Prizant's 25 years experience as a clinical scholar, researcher and consultant to families of young children with autism spectrum disorders. He is currently the Director of Childhood Communication Services and Adjunct Professor in the Center for the Study of Human Development, Brown University, and a Fellow of the American Speech-Language-Hearing Association.

SCERTS® promotes social communication and emotional competence by building meaning into daily experiences from the preverbal to conversational level. Carol Gray believes that the strength of this program is in its ability recognize individual differences and to focus on the family, capitalizing on its ability to form a solid foundation of mutual respect, meaning, logic and predictability for the individual with autism.

All activities and strategies are designed to enhance the development of emotional self- and mutual regulatory capacities, and to modify attentional, arousal and emotional states. SCERTS® borrows from other sensory, motor, vision and language models, always looking at an individual child's strengths and needs. Prizant may thus recommend that one child jump on a trampoline for arousal, and that another listen to soothing music for calming.

SCERTS® provides support to assure that behaviors generalize across settings, thus fostering successful interpersonal interactions, relationships, and productive learning experiences at school, in the community and elsewhere.[19] The SCERTS® model encourages professionals from different disciplines to collaborate with each other, and is thus totally compatible with other treatment approaches in this book. Families measure progress by noting the number of functional activities a child with autism can do with a variety of partners.

For a complete overview of SCERTS®, watch the three video or DVD set, *The SCERTS™ Model: A Comprehensive Educational Approach for Children with Autism Spectrum Disorders*[20], or read *Autism Spectrum Disorders: A Transactional Developmental Perspective*.[21] Prizant has developed workshops and seminars of various lengths in many cities. Go to <www.barryprizant.com> for a complete schedule of presentations and to order materials.

Porges' Theory of Socio-Emotional and Communications Disorders

Stephen W. Porges, PhD, Director of the Center for Developmental Psychobiology at the University of Illinois at Chicago, developed an intervention model for socio-emotional and communication disorders while at the University of Maryland. His Polyvagal Theory is derived from neuroanatomical, neurophysiological, and behavioral research on brainstem abnormalities. Dr. Porges' research, discussed briefly in Chapter 10, focuses on the two muscles in the middle ear - the tensor tympani and the stapedius. Porges has found that the same nerves that control these two muscles also control vocalization, facial expression, heart rate and breathing.[22]

According to Dr. Porges, many children with developmental disabilities are in a constant state of high anxiety, in which they attend to all sounds in their environment, not only to the higher frequency sounds that are human speech. His intervention, similar to the Tomatis method, provides acoustic stimulation to children during a quiet, free-play session. The child dons headphones and listens to specific sounds or music within a narrow frequency range, similar to that of human speech. Gradually, the therapist widens the frequency range, thus vigorously exercising the two muscles in the middle ear.

In preliminary data collected on 40 children fitting the criteria of autism, 75-80% of the children showed positive changes using this approach. While intervention varied markedly, many children had dramatic changes in facial affect, spontaneity, listening, communication, and behavioral state. Parents reported that the effects persisted at least three months after intervention, in most children who experienced changes. Although the initial study was conducted with children diagnosed as autistic, Porges believes that the intervention has a much broader application for both children and adults at the mild end of the spectrum, as well[23].

Dr. Porges concludes that improvement in communication and social-emotional interaction is a result of an improvement in middle ear function. Gains in social and communication skills will in turn, make the child more available to other forms of treatment. Since the middle ear muscles share the same neural connection with facial expression and vocalization, stimulating the middle ear allows a child to sort sound frequencies, regulate listening, reduce anxiety, and be more available socially and emotionally.[24]

Conclusion

The emergence of appropriate interpersonal interaction is typically the final step on the path to resolving autism spectrum disorders. While it is tempting to address deficient communication and interpersonal skills aggressively at a young age, these skills must wait until a child's immune system works efficiently, and motor and vision skills develop. Unfortunately, consulting with an optometrist, occupational therapist, Defeat Autism Now! doctor or audiologist may not make as much sense to parents as making an appointment with a speech-language pathologist or mental health professional.

For adults, especially parents, trying to interact with a young child who doesn't look at, laugh with, talk to or imitate you, can be very frustrating. Observing a child "in his own world" can be heart-breaking. Watching a child botch an interaction can be most embarrassing. Acknowledging that a child has few friends can be extremely painful. Imagining how a teenager's social awkwardness might affect personal relationships and job performance in the future is downright frightening.

This chapter summarizes some extremely innovative programs based on a solid understanding of sensory processing. Most importantly, they respect a child's inefficient sensory systems, and view "aberrant" behaviors as attempts at coping with a confusing world. Joining a child in what appears to be purposeless play following DIR, RDI, the Son Rise Program® or Miller Method guidelines, often yields remarkable results. While intensive, demanding, and costly, these models can initially be the core of the therapy for an unresponsive child, and then adjuncts to a transdisiplinary program. Parents are the key to their success. Social Stories™ can be utilized by educators or parents, while principles of The Dancing Dialogue, SCERTS, and the Polyvagal Theory combine well with almost any communication-based model.

According to Daniel Goleman, author of *Emotional Intelligence*,[25] social intelligence is a better predictor of success than SAT scores. Most people with disabilities lose jobs because of social-emotional, rather than skill deficits. Applying some of the brilliant methodologies described in this chapter empowers children on the autism spectrum to develop those skills necessary to join others, interact in socially acceptable ways, have friends, and eventually marry, and hold a good job. Best of all they can realize whatever potential they have to become confident, happy, productive individuals in a demanding society.

References

1. Klaw R. *Playing with young children with autism spectrum disorders. New Developments Newsletter. 2002;8:1,4.*

2. Kranowitz CS. *The Out-of-Sync Child. New York, NY: Perigee, 1998.*

3. Greenspan SI, Wieder S. *The Child with Special Needs: Encouraging Intellectual and Emotional Growth. Cambridge, MA: Perseus Books, 1998.*

4. Greenspan SI, Wieder S. *Engaging Autism: Using The Floortime Approach to Help Children Relate, Communicate and Think. Cambridge, MA: Perseus Books, 2006.*

5. Greenspan SI. *The affect diathesis hypothesis: The role of emotions in the core deficit in autism and the development of intelligence and social skills. J Dev Learn Dis 2001;5:1-45.*

6. Greenspan SI, Shanker, SG. *The First Idea: How Symbols, Language and Intelligence Evolved from our Primate Ancestors to Modern Humans. Cambridge, MA: Perseus Books, 2004.*

7. Greenspan SI, Wieder S. *Developmental patterns and outcomes in infants and children with disorders relating to communicating: A chart review of 200 cases of children with autistic spectrum diagnoses. J Dev Learn Dis 1997;1:87-141.*

8. Furth H, Wachs H. *Thinking Goes to School: Piaget's Theory in Practice. New York, NY: Oxford University Press, 1974.*

9. Greenspan SI, Lewis D. *The affect-based language curriculum (ABLC): An intensive program for families, therapists and teachers. Bethesda, MD: Interdisciplinary Council on Developmental and Learning Disorders (ICDL), 2005.*

10. Tortora S. *The Dancing Dialogue: Using the Communicative Power of Movement with Young Children. Baltimore, MD: Brookes Publishing, 2006.*

11. Gutstein S. *Autism Asperger's: Solving the Relationship Puzzle. Arlington, TX: Future Horizons, 2000.*

12. Kaufman BN, Kaufman R. *Son-Rise: The Miracle Continues. Tiburon, CA: HJ Kramer, Inc., 1994.*

13. *<www.theautismtreatmentcenter.org> Accessed December 27, 2006.*

14. Gray C, White AL. *My Social Stories Book. New York, NY: Jessica Kingsley Publishers, 2002.*

15. Gray C. *The New Social Story Book. Arlington TX: Future Horizons, 2000.*

16. *<www.millermethod.org> Accessed January 8, 2007..*

17. Miller A, Eller-Miller E.. *From Ritual to Repertoire. Boston, MA: John Wiley & Sons, 1989.*

18. Miller A. Chretien K. *The Miller Method ®. Developing the Capacities of Children on the Autism Spectrum. New York., NY: Jessica Kingsley, 2007.*

19. Gray C. *The Scerts® Model. Jenison Autism Journal, Winter 2002:1-19.*

20. Prizant BM, Wetherby AM, Rubin E, Laurent AC, et al. *The SCERTS™ Model: A Comprehensive Educational Approach For Children With Autism Spectrum Disorders. Baltimore, MD: Brookes Publishing, 2005.*

21. Prizant BM, Wetherby AM. *Autism Spectrum Disorders: A Transactional Developmental Perspective. Baltimore, MD: Brookes Publishing, 2000.*

22. Porges SW. *Orienting in a defensive world: mammalian modifications of our evolutionary heritage. A polyvagal theory. Psychophysiol 1995;32:301-18.*

23. Porges, SW, Bazhenova OV. *Evolution and the autonomic nervous system: A neurobiological model of socio-emotional and communication disorders. <http://www.icdl.com/porges.html>. Accessed February 13, 2007.*

24. Edelson, S. *Dr. Stephen Porges' research may support Berard's and Tomatis' Theory on middle ear muscle dysfunction. The Sound Connection 2003;9(4):1-2.*

25. Goleman D. *Emotional Intelligence. New York: Bantam, 2005.*

Chapter 12
Homeopathy:
A Tool to Help Children Heal Naturally

Principal author: Patricia Lemer, MEd, NCC
Contributing authors:
Barbara Brewitt, PhD
Judyth Reichenberg-Ullman, ND, DHANP, LCSW
Robert Ullman, ND, DHANP

Homeopathy is a 250-year-old tool used by a small number of medical and osteopathic doctors, by many naturopathic physicians, and by a growing number of lay professionals without medical licenses. Several recent books have informed the public about this extremely efficacious treatment for people on the autism spectrum. *The Impossible Cure,* by Amy Lansky,[1] a mother of a child with autism who educated herself about this therapy, offers hope to others. Her story follows. *The Natural Medicine Guide to Autism*[2] includes an extensive section on homeopathy, parts of which are referenced here. The co-authors of *A Drug-Free Approach to Asperger's and Autism: Homeopathic Medicine for Exceptional Kids*[3] contributed greatly to this chapter, including several case studies.

Dr. Paul Herscu, the co-founder of the New England School of Homeopathy, is convinced that all patients on the autism spectrum should receive homeopathic treatment as a part of their therapy protocol. He feels strongly that other therapies, such as dietary modification, nutritional supplementation, and sensory integration therapy work much better after homeopathic treatment.[4] A video of Dr. Herscu's approach to autism is available at <www.nesh.com>.

The History of Homeopathy

Homeopathy is a 250-year-old systematic approach to healing developed by Dr. Samuel Hahnemann, a German physician searching for a safe, effective alternative to conventional medicine. The word "homeopathy" comes from the Greek words "homoio," meaning "similar" and "pathos," meaning "suffering or disease." Homeopathy is a complete system of healing targeted at achieving homeostasis and balance, resulting in the optimal healthy functioning of the entire body.

Perhaps one of the best known principles of homeopathy is the Law of Similars, also known as the "similarity principle."[5] The principle that "like shall be cured by like" is the basis for Hahnemann's homeopathic doctrine. Loosely translated, the Law of Similars states that a substance that produces symptoms of illness in a well person when administered in large doses will cure the illness in a sick person when administered in minute quantities.

Double-blind, placebo controlled clinical research studies during the past decade prove homeopathy's safety and effectiveness.[6,7] The latest one, conducted in Switzerland on 62 children with ADD and ADHD found that those treated homeopathically showed measurable improvement on a behavioral rating scale, while children taking a placebo showed none.[8]

The father of American homeopathy is Constantine Hering, a German who immigrated to the United States in the mid 1800's. Hering observed that as his patients became sick, physical problems, which were least severe, appeared first, followed by cognitive problems and "emotional" illness, which appeared later. Applying this concept to autism spectrum disorders, constipation, diarrhea, bronchitis and asthma often precede children's language delays, which likewise appear before hyperactivity, autistic-like behaviors and cognitive problems. Hering also found that "dis-ease" manifested itself first on the outside, and then moved inward to increasingly more vital internal organs. Again, looking at autism from a homeopathic point of view, practitioners believe that when a baby's diaper rash or eczema clears up externally, a problem may exist later in the digestive or respiratory tract, as sickness deepens.

Three general principles of the homeopathic healing process became known as Hering's Laws of Cure:

- Recovery progresses in the opposite sequence as illness, from the inside outward, from the most important organ to the least. The deepest "sickness" in the mental and emotional parts of the organism (the brain) clear first; the external parts, such as the skin and the extremities return to health last;
- As healing progresses, symptoms reappear in reverse order to that of onset;
- Healing progresses from the upper to the lower parts of the body.[9]

While Hering's law has long been a guiding principle for homeopaths, it is not true 100% of the time in autism spectrum disorders. Most children on the autism spectrum follow the expected sequence, and show clearing of cognitive and behavioral symptoms before the physical ones, and with skin issues being the last to subside.[10] As healing occurs, however, some kids show improvement in digestion first, while others begin speaking or put words together for the first time shortly after homeopathic treatment. Some of the cases in this chapter demonstrate this concept clearly.

Most homeopathic practitioners are open-minded about combining their treatments with other therapies, especially nutritional supplementation and dietary modification. They probably would also collaborate with behavioral optometrists if they knew of their interest.

Classical Homeopathy

Many health care professionals practice "classical homeopathy" which focuses on determining the correct homeopathic medicine, or remedy for a patient. (*Editor's note:* Some homeopathic practitioners use the term "remedy." The contributors to this chapter prefer the terms "homeopathic medicines" and "homeopathic drugs." These three terms are used synonymously in this chapter.) Remedies are made from plant, mineral, metabolic or animal substances that stimulate a person's "vital force," enhancing the body's ability to heal itself. Remedies produce symptoms of a specific disease in a healthy person.

Almost anything can be a homeopathic medicine if it has known "homeopathic provings" and/or known effects which mimic the symptoms, syndromes or conditions which it is administered to treat. Remedies come in pellets, tablets, creams, ointments, salves, or liquids, in different potencies. They are prepared through a process of dilution and potentization. The higher the number of dilutions, the greater the potency, and the more powerful the remedy.

Homeopathic medicines strive to reinforce the body's own healing capacity by providing minute doses of a drug that enhance benefits, without stimulating any adverse, toxic side effects. In contrast, many allopathic medicines have well-documented toxicities which often outweigh the benefits.

Homeopathy, like other treatments in this book, appreciates, assesses and treats the whole person, not individual parts, symptoms, or the diagnosis. Two children with autism may be given different remedies, depending on what symptoms cluster together. The child's unique symptoms and history, as well as the practitioner's interview with the child, provide the most important information. Homeopathic medicine affects the physical, mental and emotional body. Thus, the classical homeopath evaluates all of these areas before prescribing.[11]

How Homeopathy Helps Those with Autism Spectrum Disorders

Two eminent classical homeopaths, Judyth Reichenberg-Ullman, ND, DHANP, LCSW and her husband Robert Ullman, ND, DHANP believe that homeopathy can help children from the mild to severe end of the autism spectrum make marked improvements academically, behaviorally, and socially.[3] Whether they exhibit delays in reading, math, spelling, or writing, have dyslexia, difficulty with comprehension and retention of material, are simply slow learners, or have Asperger syndrome, or other autism spectrum disorders, a homeopathic remedy can make an important difference in the lives of these children.

Homeopathy is especially effective for healing the physical and behavioral problems of children on the severe end of the spectrum. One can expect a significant decrease in seizures, bowel and behavioral problems, along with improvement in language and social interaction. Some children in the mid-range of the spectrum, including those with Asperger syndrome, can manifest the most dramatic changes in all of these areas. Experience shows that kids with learning disabilities and attention deficits often begin to enjoy reading, develop heightened confidence and self-assuredness, along with more legible handwriting, and an overall more rapid social maturation after correct homeopathic treatment.[12]

Changes usually appear within one to four weeks after the administration of the correct homeopathic medicine. Improvement continues and builds over time. Many children who were in special education settings can be happy and successful in mainstream classrooms, and establish and maintain friendships for the first time, as a result of homeopathic treatment. Benefits such as an improved desire to engage in age-appropriate activities, increased communication skills, decreased obsessiveness and diminished quirky habits, enable some of these kids to blend with their peers. Parents are overjoyed to have their children back with such minor and non-toxic intervention.

How far can a child on the autism spectrum progress under the care of a homeopath? It depends upon three criteria: 1) where the child initially falls on the spectrum; 2) how clear an understanding the homeopath has of the child; and 3) how well the homeopathic remedy fits the child.

The next section includes key points by the Ullmans. Both are licensed naturopathic physicians, board certified in homeopathy, and co-authors of a number of books on using homeopathy with children who have attention issues and autism.[3,7] Readers interested in a more in-depth look at using homeopathy for those on the autism spectrum are encouraged to read their book, *A Drug-Free Approach to Asperger's and Autism: Homeopathic Medicine for Exceptional Kids*, co-authored with Ian Luepker, ND, DHANP.[3]

Matching a Child's Unique Symptoms with a Homeopathic Drug

One of the first things a classical homeopath treating a child with autism looks for are "exceptional features" that make an autistic child unique. Classic autistic behaviors such as perseveration, lack of flexibility, fascination with fans, flapping, lack of eye contact and incessant movements are only of mild interest. Rather unusual behaviors, such as attachments to a particular object, odd routines, rituals, use of language, as well as positive and endearing qualities, interest homeopaths the most. Homeopaths love people who are "out of the box" - whose symptoms are quirky. The timing between the onset of autism and vaccines is an important concern for the homeopath. Those children who were perfectly healthy prior to the measles/mumps /rubella (MMR) vaccine, and then appeared autistic immediately afterwards, are of particular interest. Once a homeopath determines a child's unique combination of interests, expressions, and behaviors he/she matches this picture with a homeopathic drug.

The right homeopathic drug can address language delays, learning challenges and impaired social functioning along with physical problems such as headaches, allergies, heightened sensitivities or chronic constipation. The beauty of homeopathy is that a single homeopathic medicine, when properly identified, addresses all of these concerns at the same time.

A homeopath speaks with the parent(s) and the child, if possible, to get as clear a picture as possible about the child's problems, health, academic performance, behavior, social interactions, habits, and nature. Often youngsters have the ability to express their feelings in a fresh, spontaneous, and honest way, providing images and glimpses into their inner worlds. The more expressive and open the child, the greater the possibility of finding an exact remedy match based on the child's specific symptoms, sensations, hobbies, fascinations, fantasies, images, and dreams. Once the child starts talking, regardless of the subject matter, he/she reveals him- or herself and starts giving clues about which remedy he/she needs. Explaining the intricacies of a favorite video game or describing in detail how it feels to be unable to get the words out, both offer clues to matching the child with a remedy.

Children who are unable to communicate verbally are more challenging. The homeopath then must depend solely upon the parents' understanding and descriptions of their child's developmental history, symptoms, experiences, behaviors, and reactions. Sometimes the combination of observations and descriptions are so unique that the correct remedy is obvious even without a child's direct input.

Examples of Homeopathic Remedies

The following three remedies provide instances of matches between a homeopathic medicine and symptoms.

Baryta carbonica

Medicines from the barium family, of which the best known is Baryta carbonica (Barium carbonate), can often make a tremendous difference in a child's learning. Youngsters for whom this is the right remedy are typically:

- shy about raising their hands in class for fear of giving the wrong answer and making a fool of themselves
- self-conscious about their intelligence, as well as their social skills
- physically awkward, resulting in ostracism by other children
- delayed in walking, talking, speaking, and other developmental milestones
- less mature than their peers
- challenged with grade-level materials
- slow-paced
- sweet kids who usually do not have behavioral problems

Calcarea carbonica and Calcarea phosphorica

The Calcium group of remedies, including Calcarea carbonica (Calcium carbonate) and Calcarea phosphorica (Calcium phosphate), are excellent for older children with learning disabilities.

Children who may benefit from Calcarea carbonica are typically:

- slow-paced - the last to finish tests, homework or to leave the house
- cautious about trying physically adventurous activities
- kind and caring, with the most challenging temperamental features being obstinacy and dawdling
- well-intentioned and sincere about learning, even though they just can't keep up the pace
- couch potatoes who would rather not push themselves into vigorous physical challenges

- afraid of heights, dogs, bugs, and ghosts
- cheese lovers!

Children who may benefit from Calcarea phosphorica share some features with those using Calcarea carbonica. However, there are some clearly distinguishing characteristics.

Calcarea phosphorica children tend to:

- be much more athletic and often excel in a number of sports
- get fractures
- complain of growing pains
- have knee pain due to Osgood-Schlatter's disease
- use the word "frustrated" in describing their ability to perform in school
- get headaches and stomachaches in school
- have a particular fondness for smoked meat such as bacon or pepperoni pizza!

Three Children Who Improved

In order to better understand homeopathy, three cases of children with autism who were treated successfully with homeopathy by the Ullmans follow:

Alan

Alan, age seven, had been formally diagnosed with Asperger Syndrome. He had suffered an intractable nine-month bout of hives following an MMR immunization.

Exceptional Features Alan exhibited both a number of common characteristics of those with Asperger syndrome and some that were unique:

- difficulty with social cues and interactions
- fixation on computers, Nintendo and technology
- lack of eye contact
- self-absorption
- a lack of interest in sports

Choosing a Homeopathic Medicine for Alan Alan had symptoms of two common homeopathic medicines, Baryta carbonica (barium carbonate) and Sulphur (sulfur). The symptoms of those who need Baryta carbonica are listed in the previous section on choosing a homeopathic treatment.

When a patient exhibits characteristics of two different homeopathic medicines made from minerals, the doctor chooses a mineral salt containing both components. In this case, the medicine was Baryta sulphuricum (barium sulfate). Alan took three doses of the Baryta sulphuricum over the course of a year. His response to the first two doses of Baryta sulphuricum was promising and he became more aware and less "in his own world."

Over the next four months, Alan continued to improve academically, behaviorally, and socially. He excelled in math, science and spelling, though writing was still challenging. He began socializing with his peers. Alan improved further with a once or twice a year dose of Baryta sulphuricum. He was successful in a mainstream classroom; his parents, and teachers were all pleased with his development.

Drew

Drew was diagnosed with autism at the age of four, when he was not yet speaking. His diagnosis was later changed to ADHD, and shortly before his homeopathic evaluation, to Asperger syndrome (ASD). Drew's problems had eluded his parents because he blended in so well. He did however enter a kindergarten class for children with developmental delays.

Exceptional Features Drew was remarkably bright, articulate, and imaginative, exhibiting the typical Asperger profile of pedantic, professorial tendencies. He often put himself right in the faces of his peers, grimacing, gesturing, and making odd noises. Drew could devour the encyclopedia for hours at a time. In addition, he had recurrent, vivid, violent dreams which were so intense that he was afraid to fall asleep.

Choosing Homeopathic Medicines for Drew The first medicine prescribed was Stramonium (thorn apple), one of the most common homeopathic medicines for intense, fearful, violent children. The fears of a child needing this medicine often include wild animals, the dark and water.

Within an hour of taking Stramonium, Drew's speech was noticeably different. That evening his eye contact improved. Drew blushed for the first time in his life. His behavior and conversation were more appropriate; his tendency to fixate dramatically lessened. His childish jokes were replaced with much more mature conversation. Drew told his mother that he was very happy she had taken him for homeopathic treatment.

The improvement with Stramonium lasted a little over a month. Drew's mother reported that he was a different kid. After taking the medicine, he was more aggressive for a day or two, followed by a wonderful month. His report card showed improvement in 20 different areas. He started hanging out with the other kids at church and school.

Then he regressed. He started saying repetitive, goofy things again and crawling around on the floor, howling. His disconnectedness with others reappeared, and his speech became more babyish and choppy.

While Drew showed a definite benefit from the Stramonium, his improvement was not yet complete. He still had good and bad days at school. The original dramatic positive changes lasted only temporarily. Three other medicines were tried before settling on a final one, which helped Drew the most.

Homeopathic Panther was next. Two aspects of Drew's features caught our attention. He reported feelings of being chased and had a habit of stealing food. Drew explained that he didn't like using up all of his muscles and fuel. It felt to him as if he was wearing a little, magnetic tracking device that allowed others to get him.

Within two months of the original dose, Drew was getting along much better with his peers: no fighting, kicking, or shoving. He was noticeably more flexible when things didn't go according to his plan. The chasing theme in his dreams had been replaced by the occasional UFO or spaceship. Nine months later, Drew continued to respond dramatically.

Another dose of Panther accelerated this course. Drew became much more able to assess relationships and sort out friendships. Happier, more interactive, and just plain fun to be around, Drew lost the goofy, alienating behaviors he once displayed. He became more interested in being with people: just "one of the guys." He actually asked to accompany his mother on errands. Drew was much more willing to experiment with different foods, and learned to keep his mouth closed when eating. His eye contact was still fleeting and his speech was still not linear. In all, however, Drew made tremendous strides with homeopathic treatment.

Sam

Sam, age five, could calculate cube roots in his head and was interested in prime numbers, often counting series of numbers to himself in the back seat of the car. He could multiply numbers in the millions, while most children hhis age were not even adding or subtracting. Sam's intense interest in numbers was not the only unusual thing about him.

Exceptional Features
- Sam was obviously intelligent, eccentric, especially focused on math.
- He was rigid, fearful, aggressive and distraught and only came alive when you spoke about his specific interests.
- He had poor emotional stability.

Sam's history included a severe reaction to Amoxicillin and, later, a high fever induced by the MMR vaccine. The antibiotic or vaccine might have played a role in either creating or worsening Sam's autism.

Choosing a Homeopathic Medicine for Sam
Silica was prescribed for Sam. He became calmer, cried, and banged his head less often. His play was more creative. Sam's language greatly improved. He began asking questions using "why" and "because" and describing his own and other people's actions. He also expressed reasons for actions, and he became more reasonable in general.

Sam showed more interest in other people, and enjoyed playing with other children, who accepted him more easily. He was interactive 75% of the time. The other 25% he spoke only about what interested him. Surprisingly, Sam gave up his obsession with mathematics, without losing his mathematical ability. Silica helped Sam with language, behavior and social-emotional skills, and enhanced his thinking, as well.

Judyth Reichenberg-Ullman and Robert Ullman's Recommendations
Optometrists who wish to collaborate with a health care practitioner trained in homeopathy should:

- Find a homeopath with experience treating kids with autism spectrum disorders. Children with learning disabilities, attention deficits and autism require homeopathic care from an experienced practitioner.
- Work with a practitioner for at least a full year. It may take the homeopath time to find the right remedy.
- Inform the homeopath when adding other therapies to homeopathy, especially at the beginning of treatment while your homeopath is trying to find the best remedy.
- If a child becomes ill during the course of homeopathic treatment, consult with the homeopath before administering conventional medications, except in emergency situations.
- Become an astute, impartial observer who reports symptoms and changes objectively. Note how vision development differs before and after homeopathic treatment.
- Encourage families to maintain balance and harmony. Raising a child with autism, especially one with siblings, can be high-maintenance. While the demands of a youngster with autism may seem pressing and urgent, make sure that the needs all members of the family are met.
- Remind parents to breathe deeply, and take one step at a time. Everyone is doing the best they can!

The Impossible Cure
Probably the most well-known use of homeopathy with autism is Max, the son of Amy Lanksy, PhD, the author of *The Impossible Cure*.[1] With a doctorate in computer science, Amy had an unusual background to become a homeopath. When her son, Max was still not talking at age two and one-half, she knew something was wrong. Max had many of the risk factors for autism, including an MMR shot at 18 months as he was recovering from roseola, a relative of the measles. He also had an addiction to milk, some days consuming a half gallon. Removing cow's milk from his diet helped, and so did some early speech/language therapy.

Max's unique features included his strong craving for milk, which also upset his digestion. He had a love of dancing and music, night sweats, an odd sleeping position, a strong restlessness and intensity, a family history of cancer, schizophrenia and diabetes, all in the presence of a stubborn, yet sweet, personality.

Max's characteristics are associated with the remedy Carcinosin. Two days after his first dose, Max began using some new phrases and was more socially aware. Five days post-remedy, Max was able to follow a two-step command. Each day brought new improvements. After a few months, changes were undeniable. Six months after starting Carcinosin, Max's language and social awareness were far better. He still was restless and socially distanced, however. Osteopathic treatments helped calm him. Nine months after treatment began, Max no longer qualified for special education, testing at or near age level.

At his five year check-up, the pediatrician did not argue with Amy's request to skip the MMR and DPT boosters. However, he insisted that Max receive the tuberculosis test required for kindergarten entrance in California. This injection set Max back, with persistent crying, withdrawn and fearful behavior. A single dose of Carcinsosin put him back on track. Auditory processing problems in second grade resolved. Today at age 14, Max exhibits no behaviors associated with autism. He is a "typical teenager" who is a sociable, excellent student who takes piano lessons and plays sports.

Amy has become well known in her new-found field of homeopathy. Her book holds the "promise of homeopathy" for everyone working with those on the autism spectrum.

Nosodes- A Specialty Subclass of Homeopathy

The therapeutic administration of homeopathic nosodes is another way to practice homeopathy. While homeopathic medicines are derivatives of substances that occur in nature, nosodes are derived from the pathogens which cause a disease. Neither nosodes nor homeopathic medicines contain any biochemical trace of the substance from which they are derived, but are rather energetic imprints of those substances. Homeopathy falls into the category of energy medicine, as it works on an energetic level.[2]

Homeopathic nosodes have two applications in autism: as prophylactic alternatives to vaccines, and as a possible way to mitigate adverse vaccine reactions. Amy Lansky reports that in the early 1900s Variolinum, made from a smallpox pustule was used successfully to prevent smallpox, Diptherinum was used to prevent diphtheria, Pertussinum to prevent pertussis (whooping cough), and Morbillinum was used to prevent measles.[1]

Only a very small number of physicians use homeopathic nosodes in lieu of vaccines.[2] Few of those physicians practice in the United States, primarily because they cannot get nosodes here.

A Dutch physician, Tinus Smits, MD, has treated post-vaccination problems of all kinds with homeopathic nosodes for more than 20 years. He uses the term "post-vaccination syndrome" to describe the relationship between vaccination and behavioral problems in children on the autism spectrum. His website <www.tinussmits.com> contains 30 short case histories of those with mild to severe problems. His experience has convinced him that "homeopathy, through the use of homeopathic dilutions of the relevant vaccines, is a perfect tool to cure post-vaccination damage, and by doing so, can deliver proof of a relationship between complaints and a given vaccination." Three of his cases follow.

1. Wiebe received an MMR shot at 14 months, and was diagnosed with autism at age two and one-half. He was non-verbal and severely retarded both physically and mentally. Behaviors included head banging, shrieking and hand flapping. He was in his own inaccessible world.

Wiebe's problems started after the fourth DPT/HIB at age 11 months. He had a high fever for three days after the first injection.

A first course of potentized MMR elicited no change. However, the potentized DPT/HIB brought an enormous transformation. Wiebe began to react clearly to external stimuli, his muscular tension improved, and he began walking, despite the pediatrician's prediction that he would never walk. His head banging stopped completely, his eye contact improved and he said three words.

2. Jeroen was diagnosed with ADHD at age nine, following MMR and DPT injections. Before, he was a calm boy, without any problems in school. After this double injection he didn't want to go to school, complained of headaches and abdominal pains, became aggressive, awkward and uncertain in contact with other children. He was tired, had no day-night rhythm, shut himself in his bedroom, and refused to do what he was told. He was very restless and had difficulties falling asleep. Often he was absent-minded, inaccessible and easily irritated. Jeroen was on Ritalin, which made his behavior in school more acceptable.

After treatment with potentized DPT and MMR, Jeroen became much calmer. He was able to stop Ritalin, had better concentration, was no longer aggressive, and became a perfectly normal adolescent.

3. Rik was diagnosed autistic at four and one-half years of age. He was developmentally normal until the MMR injection at 16 months. The following week he declined rapidly both physically and psychologically. He became aggressive, threw toys, made shrill sounds, and withdrew in front of strangers. His speech disappeared completely and his physical development deteriorated. He slept poorly, no longer made eye contact, and his pupils no longer reacted to light. He had soft stools and frequent nosebleeds.

After five courses of potentized MMR, the pupils of Rik's eyes began reacting to light and his eye contact returned. He began talking in two and three word phrases. He cuddled with his parents. His nosebleeds stopped, his stools were more normal and he was sleeping soundly.

Smits states that "vaccination damage can take months to express itself, starting very insidiously, almost imperceptibly." He believes that "the sacrosanct conviction among the medical profession that vaccinations are completely safe and cannot have serious side-effects is causing much suffering and much unnecessary and costly medical investigation that could be avoided if the diagnosis 'post-vaccination syndrome' would figure in the top ten of possible causes of childhood illnesses."[13]

Sarcodes – Another Subclass of Homeopathy

A sarcode is a metabolic factor from healthy cells or tissues, made into a homeopathic medicine. Barbara Brewitt, Ph.D. is using homeopathic growth factors, classified as homeopathic sarcodes that yield significant benefits for children with autism spectrum disorders. Dr. Brewitt has nine International and US patents to her name. Her peer-reviewed published work is translated into seven languages. Dr. Brewitt's innovative discoveries and applications of homeopathic principles which arose from her work as a scientist, visionary, minister, and socially responsible activist, are unique. Dr. Brewitt's work is diversified, ranging from autism to HIV, diabetes, PMS and healthy aging. She is the founder and CEO of Biomed Comm, Inc., a Seattle-based biotechnology company in the natural products industry, whose homeopathic products strengthen the body's immune, nervous and hormonal systems.

A Sarcode Approach to Autism Spectrum Disorders
By Barbara Brewitt, PhD

Some homeopaths apply the Law of Similars to cell-to-cell communication, or "cell signaling," the natural way cells talk to each other. Cell signaling utilizes over 150 small information-carrying proteins called growth factors, sometimes known as cytokines, and neuro-peptides. For simplicity, in this discussion, the continuous sending and receiving of feedback to adjust and maintain healthy homeostasis is called "cell signaling" and all growth factors will be called "cell signalers."

Cell signalers regulate information flow into cells, and monitor all cell activities, including nutrient in-take. This continuous feedback pinpoints and repairs any dis-harmony in the body's nervous, immune and endocrine systems, thus adjusting for and maintaining healthy homeostasis in the body. Cell signaling is like balancing on a teeter-totter; one cell talks to the cell on the other side of the teeter-totter with the shared goal of balance. Too much rocking up and down of the teeter-totter can cause dis-harmony, which the body does not like.

Cell signaling modulates DNA expression and continuously changes cell behavior in the context of its neighboring cells. Cell signalers never need to enter the cell to have their effects. Highly specific cell surface receptors wait for unique instruction from cell signalers about the cell's ultimate fate. Each cell signaler carries a specific message. Once a cell receives a signal it carries the message down to the nucleus through a cascade of secondary messengers until the message reaches the regulatory sites on the DNA, instructing the DNA what segments to read and express.

Cell signalers have multiple functions throughout the body, some of which are to initiate processes related to enzyme activation, utilization of vitamins, minerals, natural supplements, drugs and expression of RNA or DNA and their repair. Without cell signaling, metabolic activities do not occur. Normally, growth factors are potent within the body and throughout the brain at extremely low concentrations in the homeopathic range.

How Does Cell Signaling Work?

Cells' ability to process a broad array of diverse cell signals into an appropriate small array of intracellular responses depends upon a unique cascade of events in the signaling pathway.

1. First, the cell signaler (growth factor) communicates a message.

2. Then, unique cell surface receptors for each signaler located on the bi-lipid cell surface membrane are activated by each cell signal, and in response, change their shape.

3. Almost simultaneously, G-proteins located within the bi-lipid cell surface membrane mobilize and bind to the activated cell receptor as it changes its shape.

4. Finally, G-protein signaling activates a cascade of many secondary messenger molecules which further carry the cell signaler's information through the cell's interior to the DNA. When the DNA receives the information, the cell's behavior changes. This instruction must take place before cell nutrition, cell growth, cell repair, cell division, cell differentiation and cell death can occur.

Cell signaling underlies all mental and physical activities;[14] it's ultimate goal is balance, allowing cells to remain harmonious with each other.

What Does Cell Signaling Have to Do with Autism Spectrum Disorders?

Cell-to-cell interactions are known to be severely compromised in autism. Mary Megson, M.D., first reported,[15] and other experts on autism now agree, that damage to G-proteins plays a significant role in the impaired cell-to-cell communications in autism.[16,17] Boyd

Haley, PhD, at the University of Kentucky demonstrated by video in 2002[18] the damage that rapidly occurs to neuronal axons and microfilaments, key components of G-proteins, by low concentration mercury exposure. Damage to the microfilament disrupts the signal transduction pathway of G-proteins. Autism can occur very shortly after an environmental shock such as mercury exposure or damage to the cell membrane by viruses or other pathogens. Such damage is known to be associated also with numerous other human diseases involving vision, immune function, and olfaction.

Homeopathic Fibroblast Growth Factor-2 (FGF2) and Vision in Autism

Research shows that growth factors are critical to the maintenance of vision and cell-to-cell communication.[19] Many visual problems involve an imbalance and over-production of cell signaling growth factors.

One of the most significant growth factors related to ocular health is fibroblast growth factor-2, FGF2 for short. FGF2 is found in the posterior vitreous humor, as well as in the kidneys, adrenals, cartilage, muscles, ovaries and prostate. An excessive amount of FGF2 has been identified as a contributor to retinal vascular pathology.[20]

FGF2 provides multiple positive functions throughout the body, all relevant to children with autism.[21] In addition to regulating G-proteins, FGF2 is key to cell activities related to new vascular and neuronal sprouting, epithelial and endothelial cell healing, cell repair, survival and differentiation, increased serotonin uptake, intestinal, fibroblast and epithelial cell healing. FGF2 also participates in thyroid, thymus and pituitary gland development, and targets communication networking throughout the limbic system.

Creating a homeostasis of cell signaling by using homeopathic FGF2 may be an efficacious treatment for visual and other problems in children with autism for several reasons. Growth factor cell signaling:

- assists in visual acuity and visual repair
- regulates general nervous, immune and organ functions
- contributes significantly to the orientation of cells, since it directs cell-to-cell interactions and cell positioning inside a tissue
- modulates cellular processes directed at homeostasis
- optimizes the body's ability to achieve homeostasis without toxic or adverse side effects

A Pilot Study Shows Promising Results

In 2000 Brewitt conducted a pilot study using a homeopathic FGF2 with 12 children diagnosed with mild to severe autism, ages four to 19 years old. Each received the homeopathic FGF2 liquid drops three times daily. Parents used a standardized scoring sheet every two weeks to rate any changes in severity of symptoms.

Findings showed a 20% increase in positive observations versus a 5% increase predicted if observations were by random occurrence. Subjects showed the following improvements within two weeks and up to four months. Initial improvements occurred very quickly, with continual positive trends thereafter:

- Doubling of external awareness, reciprocal sharing and social interactions with continued increases up to three fold by the end of the study, six weeks to six months later
- Quadrupling of understanding, including abstract ideas
- Increase in communication by greater than 1.5 fold
- Two-fold decrease in frustration and acting out behaviors
- Decrease in fixations by 1.5 fold

Improvements in the broad array of social interactions during this study suggest that homeopathic FGF2 impacts the limbic system, a complex part of the brain responsible for controlling emotions. The research of Dr. Margaret Bauman and Dr. Thomas Kemper confirm that the amygdala, called the social part of the brain, and a part of the limbic system, acts abnormally in those with autism.[22] Social interactions and facial expressions require activation of the limbic system. Improvements in social interactions during this study suggest that homeopathic FGF2, administered orally, impact upon the limbic system, especially the amygdala.

This pilot study demonstrates the broad spectrum applications possible when using a sarcode approach to treating autism. Homeopathic cell signaling integrates three areas: molecular biology's detailed structure, functional cell membrane electrophysiology, and the discipline of homeopathy. Further research into this innovative approach to neurobiology and immunology is warranted in effectively, safely treating children with autism.

Homotoxicology

Homotoxicology is a "bridge" between allopathic and homeopathic medicine. When Samuel Hahnemann founded homeopathy, he knew very little science, including biology or chemistry. He thus placed more emphasis on the mental and emotional issues of a patient than on physical symptoms. From the late 1930s to the early 1970s Dr. Hans-Heinrich Reckeweg of Germany combined modern knowledge of the basic medical sciences with the principals of homeopathy.

Based on the principles of homeopathy, homotoxicology has similarities to classical homeopathy as well as some major differences. Consistent with classical homeopathy, Reckeweg prescribed homeopathic remedies designed to restore a patient's vital energy and to balance the body's systems. Unlike Hahnemann's classical homeopathy, homotoxicology emphasizes the physical manifestations of disease. Reckeweg believed that until the vital force or the body's defense systems are restored, single homeopathic remedies may be limited in their effectiveness.

Following the classical homeopathic model, Reckeweg observed that many patients required more than one remedy to get well. He also concluded that many of the conditions he treated were caused or exacerbated by an exposure to toxins. He thus named his form of homeopathy, homotoxicology: or the study of toxins in humans.[23]

Since it is becoming clearer that in autism spectrum disorders, toxins have disrupted intracellular regulatory and metabolic function, today's medical practitioners are embracing this approach. It is a very common treatment in Europe, and is slowly gaining recognition in the United States.

Reckeweg developed over 1,000 combination remedies derived from, among other things, the body's own enzymes, allopathic medicines and nosodes, as well as traditional homeopathic remedies. When a single remedy fails, prescribing a combination of remedies, all with the potential of producing the same outcome, allows the body to choose which one it wants.[24] Low-potency combination formulas increase metabolic function and circulation. Drainage remedies, which are organ-specific detoxifiers, are often integrated into the program to assist in the removal of toxic build-up.

Those using combination remedies believe that these formulas trigger the self-healing process while addressing a broad range of functions, thus allowing the body to put more of its energy into learning, socializing and focusing. Single homeopathic medicines, nutritional supplements and other detoxification substances can then do their work more efficiently.

Research validates the efficacy of this approach A review of 105 published studies on cellular detoxification concluded that 80% of the outcomes were positive.[25] Even when physical symptoms are absent, a combination of nosodes, sarcodes, and other remedies may help clear acute metal toxicity.

Reckeweg also developed the concept of the Hommaccord: combining multiple potencies of the same substance, allowing the patient's system to choose not only which remedy it wants, but which potency of the remedy it needs.[26] Reckeweg's formulas are produced by Heel, the company he founded in Germany. His products were introduced to the United States about 25 years ago.

Some professionals believe that homotoxicology is one of the safest ways to assist the body in removing heavy metals.[27] Many use laboratory tests that measure blood and urine levels of toxins to evaluate a person's detoxification pathways. Levels of heavy metals can actually rise temporarily as toxins are released from the cells and eliminated from the body. Testing the presence and levels of heavy metals, especially mercury, gauges the outcome of homeopathic detoxification.[28]

Over the past 10 years a number of children on both ends of the autism spectrum have recovered from autism through the use of homotoxicology.

David, almost four, was diagnosed at age 19 months with PDD/autism by three different experts, one of whom recommended institutionalization. He had many of the early warning signs, including an allergy to cow's milk, eczema, and an unexplained high fever. According to his mother, her son "fell off a cliff" a month after receiving five vaccines, losing all words and affect.

After starting a GF/CF diet, David regained waving, pointing and clapping. Further dietary modification and nutritional supplementation resulted in improved sleeping and expressive language. Intensive behavioral and sensory therapies brought him back further. However, anti-fungals were still necessary to control yeast overgrowth, and his speech was stilted with many pronoun reversals.

David started a slow regime of homotoxicology soon after his third birthday. After treatment with homeopathic bacteria, viruses, parasites, yeast and fungus, he was free of anti-fungal medication for the first time. Miraculously, his speech became error free almost overnight without pronoun errors. By age three and one-half, a world-renowned autism specialist declared him "recovered" with only minor subtle motor and sensory issues, for which he still receives occupational and physical therapy. Most remarkably, David's play skills have expanded, he is flexibile, funny and social. He continues with the homotoxicology program showing daily subtle improvements in learning and behavior.

Michael, age 14, is a very bright ninth grade boy with subtle learning disabilities and social awkwardness. As a young child, he began waving his hands in front of his face and danced around in space when frustrated. Although he learned to read and write on time, he worked extremely slowly.

In fifth grade, Michael completed several rounds of Tomatis auditory therapy, which helped his information processing skills. In the sixth grade, he completed 80 hours of vision therapy for a binocular dysfunction. There is still a huge discrepancy between the eyesight in his two eyes, and even though he wears one contact lens for distance, his eyes still do not work well together. Although organized, Michael still finds it difficult to work quickly.

Michael began homeopathic detoxification in the eighth grade. By then, most of his academic kinks had been worked out. Socially, he was still a bit reticent and lacked confidence, however. The remedies were given in 14-21 day mini-segments. At first he appeared tired and acted grumpy. He also experienced some physical symptoms, such as unexplained rashes, pimples, and a runny nose. Following each segment, he took a break for a couple of weeks. Each time, he returned to a higher level of energy and was more "present." Over the summer, Michael's hand waving and dancing completely disappeared. When Michael returned to school in the fall, he was more positive and confident in his ability to do the work.

Sequential Therapy

Three other books which describe complex approaches to homeopathy not covered in this chapter, are worth mentioning for those who wish to delve deep into this topic. They are *Autism: Body-Brain Connection: How Stress Plays a Role in the Development of Autism and What You Can Do About It* by Gregory Ellis,[29] *Autism: The Journey Back* by Rudi and Patty Verspoor,[30] and *Rediscovering Real Medicine: The New Horizons of Homeopathy*, by Dr. Jean Elmiger.[31] Ellis is a nutritionist who has embraced homeopathy. The Verspoors, who practice in Canada, describe Heilkunst, a little known system combining homeopathy with other aspects of healing.

Elminger coined the term "sequential therapy" to describe the process of undoing the damage from the most recent exposure or toxin first and "peeling the onion" down to the genetic influences. Individual remedies are given to address each "event," in reverse order. A patient is given a remedy to treat one vaccine, then a month later another remedy to treat the previous vaccine, etc.

These interesting books all focus on identifying underlying causes of disease, or miasms. Hahnemann identified miasms as "noxious influences," the energy of which is thought to be passed down from generation to generation. Heilkunst looks also at traumas to the body from mental, physical and emotional shocks, including vaccinations, heavy metal toxicity and stressors possibly inherited energetically from previous generations. Contemporary homeopaths are having great success applying these principles to children on the autism spectrum, especially those whose parents believe that their difficulties are a result of heavy metal toxicity.

Conclusions

The 250-year-old practice of homeopathy has a great deal to offer those with autism spectrum disorders. Classical homeopathy pinpoints a single medicine based upon an individual's physical, mental and emotional uniqueness. Nosodes, sarcodes, homeopathic cell signaling growth factors, and homotoxicology focus on pieces of the autism puzzle. Homeopathy is based on the principle that illness is a manifestation of lack of harmony in the vital flow of the body's energy. When the harmony breaks, illness follows; when harmonious flow is restored, health is established. Homeopaths identify the disturbing elements and neutralize them using packets of energy called "remedies" or homeopathic medicines.[26]

To learn more about homeopathy, read the books cited in this chapter, and contact the practitioners who have contributed. Visit the websites of Dr. Judyth Reichenberg-Ullman and Dr. Robert Ullman at: <www.healthyhomeopathy.com> and <www.drugfreeasperger.com>, and Amy Lansky at <www.impossiblecure.com>. Both also have monthly radio shows on Autism One Radio. Amy's is on the third Friday of each month, 2-2:30pm EST, and the Ullman's is on the first Wednesday, 9-9:30pm EST. Shows are both archived for later listening. Tune in at <www.autismone.org/radio>.

To find a classical homeopath in your area, go to The National Center for Homeopathy at <www.homeopathic.org>. For more on Dr. Brewitt's approach go to <www.biomedcomm.com> or write to her at drbrewitt@biomedcomm.com.

Those interested in learning more about homotoxicology should go to <www.heelbhi.com> and contact Mary Coyle, a homeopathic practitioner using this method, by e-mail at: wellnessny@aol.com or phone at 917-733-8473. You can also listen to her on Autism One Radio on the third Thursday of the month at 1:00 pm by going to <www.autismone.org/radio>. To find a practitioner in your area who practices homotoxicology, contact Marco Pharma International at <www.marcopharma.net>, (800-999-3001) or Energetix at <www.goenergetix.com>, (800-990-7085).

References

1. Lansky A. The Impossible Cure: The Promise of Homeopathy. Portola Valley, CA: R.L. Ranch Press, 2003.

2. Marohn S. The Natural Medicine Guide to Autism. Charlottesville, VA:Hampton Roads, 2002:137.

3. Reichenberg-Ullman J, Ullman R, Luepker I. A Drug-Free Approach to Asperger's and Autism: Homeopathic Medicine for Exceptional Kids. Edmonds, WA: Picnic Point Press, 2005.

4. Herscu P. Homeopathy and autism. Homeopathy Today. 2001 Nov;21(10).

5. Hahnemann S. Organon of Medicine. Philadelphia: Boericke and Tafel, 1901:65.

6. Jonas WB, Ernst E. The safety of homeopathy. In: Jonas WB, Levin JS, eds. Essentials of Complementary and Alternative Medicine. Philadelphia: Lippincott Williams & Wilkins; 1999:167-71.

7. Lamont J. Homeopathic treatment of attention deficit hyperactivity disorder. British Homeopathic J 1997 Oct;86:196-200.

8. Frei H, Everts, R, von Ammon, K., Kaufmann, F., et al. Homeopathic treatment of children with attention deficit hyperactivity disorder: a randomized, double blind, placebo controlled crossover trial. Online version EuroJ Pediatr July 27, 2005. www.springerlink.com. Accessed, August 4, 2005.

9. Bianchi I. Principles of Homotoxicology. Baden-Baden, West Germany: Aurelia-Verlag GmbH D-7570, 1988:10-12.

10. Ullman J, Ullman R. Ritalin-free kids: safe and effective homeopathic medicine for ADD and other behavioral and learning problems. Rocklin, CA: Prima Publishing,1996.

11. Zand J, Walton R, Rountree, B. Smart medicine for a healthier child. Garden City, NY: Avery Publishing Group, 1994:33.

12. Reichenberg-Ullman J, An epidemic of autism: how homeopathy can help. Homepathy Today 2003 Apr;23:12-14.

13. www.tinussmits.com. (Accessed January 30, 2008)

14. Kuznetsov AV, Janakiraman M, Margreiter R, Troppmair J. Regulating cell survival by controlling cellular energy production: novel functions for ancient signaling pathways? FEBS Lett 2004;577:1-4.

15. Megson M. Is autism a G-alpha protein defect reversible with natural vitamin A? Med Hypotheses. 2000 Jun;54:979-83.

16. Rutter M. Autism: neural basis and treatment possibilities. Novartis Foundation Symposium 251;2003.

17. Brasic JR, Wong D, Eroglu A PET Scanning in Autism Spectrum Disorders 2005. Www.emedicine.com/neuro/topic440.htm. Accessed 6/24/05.

18. Haley B. The biochemistry of mercury toxicity and removal. Defeat Autism Now Conference. San Diego CA, 2002.

19. Regulation of tight junctions and loss of barrier function in pathophysiology. Int J Biochem Cell Biol 2004 36:1206-37.

20. Song E, Yu D, Han LH, Sui DM, et al. Diabetic retinopathy: VEGF, bFGF and retinal vascular pathology. Chin Med J (Engl) 2004;117:247-51.

21. Pimentel E. Handbook of Growth Factors: Volume II: Peptide Growth Factors. Ann Arbor MI: CRC Press, 1994:187-216.

22. Edelson SM. Autism and the Limbic System. www.autism.org/limbic.HTML. Accessed 6/24/05.

23. Reckeweg HH. Illness and Healing through Antihomotoxic Therapy. Albuquerque, NM: Menaco Publishing Co, Inc. 1980.

24. Reckeweg HH. Materia Medica Homoeopathia Antihomotoxica. Vol II, A Selective Pharmacology. Baden-Baden, West Germany: Aurelia-Verlag GmbH D-7570, 1983. (1st English edition 1991.)

25. Linde K, Jonas WB, Melchart D, Worku F, et al. Critical review and meta-analysis of serial agitated dilutions in experimental toxicology. Human Experimental Toxicolo 1994;13:481-92.

26. Shelton BH. Homeopathy. Explore 2002;11(4).

27. Coyle, M. Personal communication.

28. Kratz AM. Clearing & Cellular Detoxification. In Health, newsletter of the International Academy of Nutrition and Preventive Medicine 1995 Feb;XVI(1).

29. Ellis GS. Autism Body Brain Connection. Mountainview, CA: Targeted Body Systems Publishing, 2003.

30. Verspoor R, Verspoor P. Autism: The Journey Back-Recovering the Self through Heilkunst. www.heilkunst. com. (Accessed January 30, 2008)

31. Elmiger J. Rediscovering Real Medicine. Boston: Element Books, 1998.

Chapter 13
Educational Kinesiology
Mary Rentschler, MEd

Introduction
The common ground shared by behavioral optometry and educational kinesiology (Edu-K) is extensive. Aspects of their clinical practice, their underlying philosophy and sometimes even their patients are similar. This chapter presents a brief history, the basic philosophy, and the components of Edu-K as it relates to working with those who have autism spectrum disorders.

Edu-K is the fruit of 20 years of study and experimentation with learners of all abilities by educator, Paul Dennison, PhD. Dennison first became interested in the role of movement in learning through his own personal struggles, and later through his observations of the children at the Valley Remedial Group Learning Center in southern California, which he directed in the 60s and 70s. Dennison observed direct connections between his students' learning difficulties and the subtle dysfunctional movement patterns they displayed.

Since Dennison and his wife Gail founded the Educational Kinesiology Foundation (now Brain Gym® International) in 1987, their belief in the interdependence of movement development, language acquisition and academic achievement has fueled the worldwide growth of interest in their ideas and techniques.[1(p.113)] According to their website, "Today...Brain Gym is used in more than 80 countries and is taught in thousands of public and private schools worldwide as well as in corporate, performing arts, and athletic training programs."[2]

Some Definitions
Kinesiology is the study of movement, the mechanics of how muscles and bones interact to enable us to move.

Educational Kinesiology (Edu-K) is both the study of movement as it relates to brain integration and the application of movement to the learning process[3(p.15)] as well as to intellectual and athletic skills, communication, interpersonal relations and creativity. The Edu-K umbrella also covers Brain Gym, Vision Gym and numerous advanced techniques for enhancing learning and performance.

Brain Gym®, a registered trademark of the Educational Kinesiology Foundation, refers to the introductory level of Edu-K and the 26 activities/movements taught in the Brain Gym 101 workshop.[2]

The Role of Stress
Central to the conceptual grounding of Educational Kinesiology is the relationship between dysfunctional behavior and stress. Most of us know the experience of feeling muddled and less efficient when we are tense. No other population knows this as well as those with ADD, ADHD, LD, PDD and autism. The way they experience the world every day is what we know only during extreme stress, when unconscious survival centers of the brain take over and our ability to act intentionally and skillfully disappears.

Low gear and high gear: Dennison found that underachievers in his school were frequently in just such a survival mode. He uses the term "low gear" to describe the state of imbalance that results when the higher brain switches off. This imbalance has many causes. One common activity that leads to switching off in children is "excessive involvement in two-dimensional activities (those that involve a flat surface, like TV, video games, reading)."

Stress results, as the reader will recognize, because the human visual system is designed primarily for three-dimensional, not two-dimensional, vision.

Sometimes schools and parents introduce two dimensional activities prematurely, before their children have learned to alternate between foveal focus and distance vision. The trance induced by TV and video games can be so compelling that children abandon other forms of play that require depth perception. The chronic stress that results pushes the child into a compensatory switched-off pattern which, once learned, is difficult to break.[4(p.44a)] Behavioral optometrists are all too familiar with this syndrome.

Muscle checking: The stress or blockage that individuals on the autism spectrum experience in every day activities and academic tasks is often all too obvious. Other times require sensitive exploration to tease out precisely what aspect of a task may be too challenging. To facilitate this detective work Brain Gym practitioners sometimes use a tool from applied kinesiology called muscle checking. Dr. George Goodheart, the father of applied kinesiology, developed this technique in the 60s. Muscle checking is now widely used by chiropractors, allergy specialists, kinesiologists and other professionals. Some optometrists depend on this practice to determine the precise gradient for a lens prescription.

Brain Gym practitioners usually use the anterior deltoid muscle; that is, the client holds an arm out to the front at a thirty degree angle to the body, and resists against light downward pressure, causing the muscle to contract to hold its position. In the absence of stress, the muscle locks and the arm stays in place easily, because the nervous system is efficiently communicating its intention to the muscle fibers. This state is called "high gear." In the presence of stress the muscle is weak, and the arm wobbles or gives way under pressure: a "low gear" state.

The same principle operates when someone is told to sit down before receiving bad news. In response to severe stress, muscles give way and a person might fall over and get hurt. In response to a subtle stress, there is a subtle response at the level of the muscles. If an otherwise strong muscle gives way after 10 or 20 seconds of horizontal tracking, for example, an optometrist recognizes that the effort of using both eyes to follow a moving object is stressful. Such a response would indicate a "low gear" state for tracking.[5(p.155-8)]

A "low gear" state is appropriate for activities not yet mastered. Beginning third graders, for instance, might be "high gear" for addition and subtraction and "low gear" for multiplication until they have practiced it enough to acquire mastery. The Brain Gym practitioner's goal is for clients to gain easy access to a "high gear" state for all the physical, postural and gross and fine motor components of the tasks they are asked to perform. Making eye contact, "low gear" for many children with autism, is an example of a visual skill that depends on more basic capabilities such as proprioception and balance. Edu-K addresses the integrity of these underlying physical/mechanical systems.

Alleviating stress: The Dennisons believe, as many behavioral optometrists do, that students can master what they need to learn in school only when the body mechanics are in place. They have adapted many familiar vision training activities and added them to their own innovative techniques. In the early 80s Paul Dennison began teaching 26 Brain Gym movements designed to counter the stress response by moving attention and energy away from the survival centers of the brain. He found that more energy was then available to activate the cortex and promote integrated visual, auditory and kinesthetic functioning. All attentional, perceptual and cognitive skills have a muscular component related to the body's ability to maintain itself in an appropriate posture and to engage appropriate musculature. Brain Gym enhances this muscular component, which must be in place for efficient learning.[2]

In practice then, Edu-K is a whole brain integration program that utilizes simple body movements, postures and stimulation of acupuncture points to integrate the functions of the brain. Optometrists and practitioners from many other disciplines have found in Brain Gym activities an engaging and powerful addition to their own techniques of intervention.

The Edu-K Dimensions

Edu-K recognizes three primary dimensions of brain function: focus (front/back), centering (top/bottom), and laterality (left/right).

Focus Dimension: Focus involves the integration of the front and back of the body and the front (frontal lobes) and back (brain stem) of the brain. Practically, focus dimension relates to participation and comprehension, to the ability to act on the details of a situation, while at the same time understanding new information in the context of previous experience.[2] Reading comprehension is the quintessential focus dimension task.

When children develop normally, their bodies' proprioceptors give them reliable information about position in and movement through space, resulting in integrated postural and spatial awareness. For learning to take place, one must be supported at this most basic level of neurological function. Children with integrated postural and spatial awareness, unlike many on the autism spectrum, feel safe within their bodies. They process sensory information efficiently, easily find appropriate muscular support for their activities, and have a clear sense of physical boundaries. All of these conditions are necessary foundations for attention, concentration and retrieval of information stored in the back brain.

At the less severe end of the spectrum, children who lack integration in the focus dimension may be responding to some form of internal or external stimulation that makes them feel unsafe. Some squirm interminably because their energy is all gathered in their long muscles; part of the fight-or-flight survival response. Some constantly scan their surroundings, over attentive to peripheral visual stimulation in order to detect any potential danger. Others jump up and run to the window at the sound of a car or a lawn mower because their auditory systems are constantly scanning for any sound that might signal a threat in the environment. No amount of asking these children to sit still and pay attention will work, because their bodies are maintaining them in a state of constant arousal oriented toward survival. At the more severe end of the spectrum bright lights, loud noises, strong odors and certain tastes and textures can seem threatening to a poorly calibrated sensory system. A student with Asperger syndrome once described tactile hyper sensitivity as living with a constant feeling that "my clothing is attacking me."

A child who has difficulty with transitions or perseverates, making the same mistake again and again, is unbalanced in the direction of over-focus rather than under-focus. In children who are either unable to keep perspective or unable to attend, the Dennisons would see a lack of integration in the focus dimension. Such children are sometimes labeled ADD, ADHD or OCD (obsessive/compulsive disorder). An optometrist might describe their behavior in terms of vergence and figure/ground difficulties.[6(p.28)]

Centering Dimension: Centering refers to integration of the top and bottom halves of the body, and the rational top (cortex) and emotional bottom (limbic system) of the brain. This integration arises from the interrelationships among proprioception, balance and vision.[7(p.21)] These systems work together to provide a sense of the center of one's body as a point of reference for the directions up, down, back, front, left, right, in and out. Individuals with problems in centering often lack coordination between emotional content and abstract thought.[8(p.35)] Like some children with autism, those who are either cut off from their emotions or too easily flooded with feelings are unbalanced in this dimension. Handwriting in which words and letters float chaotically out of alignment on the page mirrors an uncentered internal state. In the Edu-K model one would expect uncentered, poorly grounded patients to have difficulty with accommodation, vertical tracking and binocularity.[7(p.23)]

Laterality Dimension: Laterality, familiar to most readers, is concerned with the coordination of the right and left sides of the body and the right and left hemispheres of the cortex. Joined by the corpus callosum, the right hemisphere controls the left side of the body, and the left hemisphere controls the right side. Integration of the two hemispheres is essential for the development of all bilateral skills, including binocular vision and binaural hearing. Binocularity and lateral integration become the foundations for reading, writing, and communicating. Lateral integration is also essential for fluid gross motor activity and for moving and thinking at the same time. A student with deficient bilateral skills may have difficulty crossing the midline and be labeled learning disabled or dyslexic.[9(p.5)]

Some students write with their heads tipped down to one side almost on the table and their papers turned so that the line of script goes straight out from their noses. These students are processing information with only one eye and one hemisphere. Their compensatory posture helps them to suppress confusing information from the unfocused eye, but it also keeps them from activating and using the resources of the other hemisphere. An optometric exam would probably show poor binocularity for horizontal tracking across the midline for these cases. In the Brain Gym model, fluent oral reading with poor comprehension, hesitant error-filled oral reading with relatively good comprehension, and reversed letters also signal a lack of hemispheric balance: of poor integration in the laterality dimension.

Brain Gym

The ideal "high gear" state for learning, playing and interacting is one of whole brain integration with access to all resources. Dennison found that certain ways of moving could bring students with dysfunctional learning patterns into balance and enable them to experience that integration. Then ease in learning and performance is natural, because the body is relaxed and good physical and mental posture supports access to all parts of the brain. According to the Dennisons, Brain Gym activities promote such a state.

PACE

Four Brain Gym activities are used frequently as a warm-up. Called PACE for Positive, Active, Clear, Energetic, this sequence is a quick, easy, efficient way to achieve readiness for any activities from eating and dressing to athletics and academics. Brain Gym instructors recommend performing them in the order indicated below:

Energetic-Water: Drink a sip of water. (Best done throughout the day.)
Optimal hydration enhances the brain's ability to process information efficiently. Water ionizes salts, providing the electrolyte environment needed for electrochemical conduction of nerve impulses. It increases the polarity of membranes, resulting in more effective nerve firing (a higher signal-to-noise ratio). Water also increases the affinity of hemoglobin for oxygen, improving oxygenation of the blood and brain tissues.

Clear-Brain Buttons: While holding navel with one hand, rub thumb and finger of other hand in hollow area on either side of the sternum just below the collar bone for 30 - 60 seconds.
Massaging the Brain Buttons, which lie above the carotid arteries, increases the flow of freshly oxygenated blood to the brain. These indentations, the kidney-27 acupressure points, connect with clusters of glial cells which send electrical messages to the pituitary, the body's master gland. The navel, with nerve connections to the vestibular (balance) and

reticular activating (wake-up) systems, tells the brain where the body's center of equilibrium is located.

Active-Cross Crawl: Touch hand to opposite knee, alternately moving one arm and opposite leg. Even better: touch elbow to knee. Continue for 1 minute.
Done standing, the movement is more like marching in place than crawling. The alternating right and left hand touching the opposite knee activates the left and right sides of the brain and body simultaneously, and connects the upper and lower halves of the body. The combination of movement and touch stimulates both the motor and sensory cortex, and increases hemispheric communication across the corpus colossum. Movement also promotes myelination of neurons by glial cells.

Positive-Hook-ups: Part 1: Cross ankles, hold arms out with hands back to back, cross one arm over the other so that palms touch, clasp hands and bring them to the chest. Touch the roof of your mouth with your tongue. Sit this way for one half to one minute listening to your breath. Part 2: Uncross legs, place feet squarely on the ground, release arms, and hold finger tips together. Sit this way for another half to one minute.

Hook-ups activates the sensory and motor cortex, stimulating the right and left hemispheres of the neocortex. It connects and balances the body's electrical circuits, allowing calm relaxation. The tongue on the roof of the mouth connects the limbic system (emotional centers) with the neocortex (reasoning centers), allowing rational processing of emotionally charged issues and increased choice of responses and actions.[10]

Anyone, including optometrists' patients, can complete this brain warm-up in less than four minutes. Many Edu-K practitioners and their students use it as a daily practice, or as needed to enhance their performance under stress. Other professionals; educators, occupational therapists, and psychotherapists, find that they accomplish more in a lesson or therapy session when they and their students or patients start out from the internal posture of alertness and calm that the PACE exercises promote.

Although the Dennisons particularly recommend PACE, any of the 26 Brain Gym exercises can be used with those on the autism spectrum to "warm up" before school, before meals, before a doctor's appointment, a social event, or any challenging task. Obvious uses for an optometrist are preparation for the eye exam, regrouping during transitions, and keeping the patient moving through the therapy session.

Some Brain Gym movements seem to be more helpful with particular skills. Eleven "Midline Movements" (among them Cross Crawl) enhance lateral integration through various ways of crossing the body's midline. Nine "Energy Exercises" (among them Water, Brain Buttons and Hook-ups) stimulate acupuncture points to provide grounding, helping one to stay centered and organized. Six "Lengthening Activities" work with muscles to promote integration of primitive reflexes, enabling learners to take the risks necessary for self expression and full participation in the learning process. The Dennisons claim that "Once an individual learns to move correctly, integration becomes an automatic choice, and the learner does not depend upon Brain Gym movements to maintain integration. People find Brain Gym helpful over a short period of time to establish a positive behavior; many use the activities daily."[9(p.5)] Parents, teachers and therapists can return to Brain Gym routines again and again when new stresses or challenges appear in the developmental process.

Modifications of Brain Gym are possible for individuals with special needs and severe challenges. Over a two year period in a public school special education classroom of children who had complex developmental delays, Cecilia Koester (formerly Freeman) used Brain Gym to help her students achieve both higher levels of functioning in the world and greater inner stability and peace. Among the eleven children, five were diagnosed with cerebral palsy, two with autism, and one each with spina bifida, Angelman's syndrome, brain damage, and mental retardation with impairment of hearing and vision. Several of them were confined to wheelchairs. Koester's work, documented in her inspirational book, *I am the Child*, demonstrates the adaptability and effectiveness of Edu-K in the hands of a talented and creative practitioner.[11]

Vision Gym and Visioncircles

Vision Gym™, taught in the Visioncircles workshop, adds 31 complementary exercises for drawing out natural integrated visual function. Like Brain Gym, they use eye and body movements, stimulation of acupuncture points and breathing.[2]

The 31 Vision Gym exercises are designed to develop all the perceptual skills that comprise and support efficient vision. They promote relaxation and flexibility in the vision system, integration of vision with movement and the other senses, binocularity, near focus skills, peripheral vision, perception of color and depth, and visualization.[12(p.4)] Many Vision Gym exercises are very different from what is usually seen in vision therapy; others would be familiar to most optometrists.

The Visioncircles Workshop is open to graduates of the introductory Brain Gym 101 course. In addition to learning Vision Gym, participants in the workshop focus on eight aspects of perceptual intelligence that contribute to vision.

Figure 13-1 Visioncircles

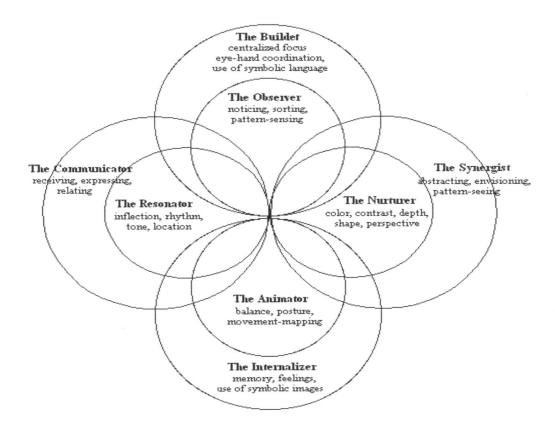

"The first three circles are aimed at letting go of visual dependence and control, balancing these through more efficient kinesthetic and auditory processing. Circles four to six focus on...big picture, vision of details, and internalizing vision through memory and imagination. Circles seven and eight integrate...perceptions in the context of one to one relationships and self-expression within our community and world."[13(p.4)]

Table 13-1 presents the name, skill and summary for each circle. Figure 13-1 represents this concept graphically.

Table 13-1 The Visioncircles[14]

Circle	Skill	Summary
1. The Observer	To notice	All learning begins with discovery.
2. The Animator	To move	Proprioceptive and vestibular awareness are kinesthetic "vision."
3. The Resonantor	To listen	The soft focus of hearing, sensing, and feeling is another kind of vision.
4. The Nurturer	To grow	Memory and peripheral awareness provide background and perspective to support and enrich vision.
5. The Builder	To create	When sensory experience is integrated with abstract thought we can manifest a vision.
6. The Internalizer	To feel	Memory and imagination combine to create inner vision.
7. The Communicator	To relate	Expressive & receptive eye contact, visual gesture, body language, listening & speech bring shared vision.
8. The Synergist	To see	Vision results when all the skills work in concert.

The concept of a Venn diagram representing interactive modules is not new to behavioral optometrists; they will recall Skeffington's Circles (See Chapter 2) where the interactions result in the emergent, vision.[15]

The Dennisons relate Skeffington's Circles to Visioncircles as follows:

- Antigravity corresponds to the Edu-K concept of bilateral development explored in Visioncircles #2 and #5.
- Centering corresponds to the Edu-K concept of centering, emphasizing interpretations of spatial information through kinesthesia and is explored in circles #2, #3, #4 and #8.
- Identification skills are developed through the fine motor and noticing processes in Circles #1, #5 and #6.
- Speech-Auditory symbolizes the development of language. In Visioncircles, these audition processes are explored in Circles #1 and #7.[12(p.56)]

The Balance Process
Another way to use Edu-K is through the five step balance process. Unlike warm-ups for general learning readiness, a "balance" aims the exercises or other activities at particular energy blocks relative to success in areas of every day behavior, performance and socialization. A goal for

the balance should be the child's, not the therapist's or parents' choice. These interventions would be appropriate for those on the high end of the autism spectrum. Simply articulating a goal provides stimulation to areas of the brain that support focus, engagement and productivity. When a child mobilizes all his/her resources of energy, motivation and intention, then the work has deep relevance and personal meaning.

After deciding on a goal, the child performs a number of pre-activities designed to elicit the physical disarray she usually experiences in the context of that goal. Often she can identify discomfort or tightness in a particular part of her body. Other times the facilitator uses the kinesiological response, or muscle checking, to make inferences about the presence or absence of stress. This part of the "balance" provides an opportunity for education and insight about dysfunctional patterns of behavior that arise under stress.

The child then chooses corrective interventions from a "learning menu" including Brain Gym, Vision Gym, Repatterning (see below) and various other activities. The menu procedures redirect energy to the parts of the mind/body system that tend to shut down during the goal activity. Afterwards the child revisits the pre-activities, experiencing a new ease in functioning and, through either noticing or muscle checking, a clear indication of reduced stress. "Homeplay" activities (from Brain Gym or Vision Gym) to perform daily for a week or two help to maintain the new level of integration. Balances can be done with individuals or groups.

Case Report: A Balance for Handwriting

Kristen, age 8, presented with issues of organization and extremely illegible handwriting similar to what might appear in a child with learning disabilities. A "Vision Report" from her optometrist cited visual fixation skills definitely below expected. At her balance session her goal was to "write cursive easily and legibly." Muscle checking pre-activities identified a "low gear" response for holding a pen in her hand and for writing a short sentence. Kristen noticed that she was gripping the pen with tense muscles. In a further test for proprioception, pouring water from one glass to another, Kristen's movement was clumsy. She seemed not to be getting precise enough feedback about the changing weight of the two glasses and she poured too quickly, spilling a few drops of water.

From the "menu" of corrective activities, Kristen chose two Brain Gym activities: The Thinking Cap and Positive Points, followed by drawing for fun. The Thinking Cap involves massage all around the outside of the ear, stimulating over 400 acupuncture points in the ears and giving the entire brain/body system an energetic tune-up. Positive Points calls for gentle holding of stomach meridian points on the forehead. In Applied Kinesiology these points alleviate emotional stress by redirecting blood flow from the brain stem to the rational centers in the frontal lobes and reducing the fight-or-flight response. After calming and balancing her energy in the centering dimension with these Brain Gym Energy Exercises, Kristen enjoyed some drawing for fun. She noticed how comfortable her grip on the pen was and the ease with which she manipulated it. We talked about transferring that comfort and ease to "writing cursive."

When she had completed the menu, Kristen revisited the pre-activities, noticing improved integration and a "high gear" state for pouring water from one glass to another and for writing, as well as improved fluency and neatness in her writing. The corrective activities Kristen chose related to vision only insofar as her visual system would be affected by anything that promoted overall relaxation. To the extent that she had developed a pattern of "low gear" over-focus for handwriting, this overall relaxation would be beneficial.

Brain Gym practitioners generally find that it is easy to elicit noticeable improvement during a balance session and that reinforcement is often essential for that change to become lasting. For "homeplay" Kristen agreed to perform the two Brain Gym activities every day for two weeks before doing homework. Kristen's mother reported remarkable improvement a few weeks later and sent stunning before and after handwriting samples.

Before　　　　　　　　　　　　　　　　**After**

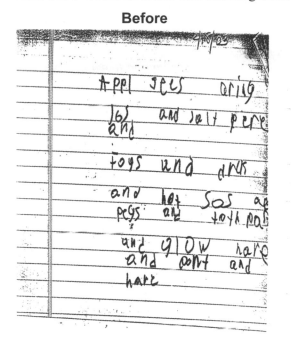

A "balance" such as the above is facilitated by someone who has taken at least Brain Gym 101, the 24-hour introductory course offered through Brain Gym International. However, many licensed Brain Gym consultants and instructors have hundreds of hours of training in Educational Kinesiology and related fields. Their clients benefit from an array of skills and techniques well beyond the 26 Brain Gym movements.

Repatterning

Another key element in Edu-K is Dennison Laterality Repatterning, a process designed to enhance or awaken cross-lateral movement and eye teaming skills that may not have developed in infancy and early childhood. Dennison Laterality Repatterning "stimulates key stages of laterality from infancy through walking, and helps to free compensatory visual or postural habits."[3](p.15) In her book on the neurophysiology of movement, Carla Hannaford, Ph.D., describes repatterning: [1](pp.129-130)

Infant crawling has long been known to be crucial for activating full sensory functioning and learning. Crawling involves movements that cross the body's midline and use both sides of the brain in concert. Our cross-lateral movements help us to build the capacities that allow full sensory access (auditory, visual, proprioceptive) from both sides of the body. (Later on, walking incorporates all of our early stages of development from infancy to toddling.)

Dr. Dennison discovered that some people he worked with were unable to Cross Crawl but were proficient at homolateral movement (arm and leg on the same side of the body moving together). These people generally accessed brain hemispheres in a one-sided way, and suffered stress from lack of full sensory-motor functioning.

Dennison also discovered a high correlation between the inability to Cross Crawl and the tendency toward learning difficulty.

Drs. Doman and Delacato coined the term "patterning" to describe the process of repeating a natural movement again and again in order to imprint it in the body's physiology, even years after the developmentally appropriate time has passed. In 1981, Dr. Dennison coined the term "repatterning," meaning a return to the natural, integrated pattern imprinted within the nervous system during normal development. For many people, stress disrupts cross-lateral patterning. They must compensate for this disruption with less efficient patterns of movement, sensing and learning.

Dennison Laterality Repatterning is a specific series of activities that reestablish efficient, integrated patterns among cross-lateral movements, vision, and hearing. The Laterality Repatterning activities (some of which are homolateral, i.e., on one side only) are performed with the help of a trained instructor. This experience enables the learner to recognize the inefficiency of homolateral movement and homolateral sensory processing, which contrasts strikingly with the more efficient, integrated state as learning becomes easier.

Reflexes
Edu-K workshops offer not only Dennison Laterality Repatterning, but also four related processes, 3D Repatterning, Core Muscle Repatterning, 42 Muscle Repatterning and Homolateral Reflex Repatterning. In the advanced Total Core Repatterning and Creative Vision workshops, Dr. Dennison teaches the use of these techniques for integrating the tonic neck and other reflexes. Optometrists may be familiar with the relationship among vision, learning problems and childhood reflexes through the work of Sam Berne, Al Sutton, Carol Marusich or Sally Goddard and her husband Peter Blythe.[16] (See Chapter 8 on reflexes)

Svetlana Masgutova, Ph.D., Director of The International Dr. Svetlana Masgutova Institute of Movement Development and Reflex Integration (Poland), and The Svetlana Masgutova Educational Institute of Neuro-Sensory-Motor and Reflex Integration (USA), and Edu-K International faculty member, teaches other advanced workshops on the integration of dynamic and postural reflexes into the whole body movement system. In her research from 1994 to 1999 at Ascension Institute in Moscow, Dr. Masgutova identified correlations between Dennison's Three Dimensions and seventeen different infant reflexes, eleven specific muscles, and the twenty-six Brain Gym activities. In her population of 522 (240 kindergartners, 42 elementary school children, and 240 youths and adults) for example, she found that 87% of the 362 who lacked integration in the Centering Dimension also demonstrated patterns of an unintegrated Bauer crawling reflex and had a "switched off" pectoralis major clavicular muscle.[17(p.12-7)]

Dennison's Repatterning or Dr. Musgutova's reflex integration work by a Brain Gym consultant could be an adjunct to vision therapy for ODs who do not include reflex integration in their practices. Some ODs report that vision therapy proceeds faster and more efficiently once key reflexes have been integrated.[18]

Brain Gym and Sensory Integration
Chapter 7 explains the role of sensory integration (SI) in autism spectrum disorders. Rita Edwards, Dip. OT, D.T.S.E., Brain Gym Consultant, and Edu-K International Faculty member, developed a workshop, "In Synch: Integrating The Senses Through Movement" which combines SI with Brain Gym. Rita was a founding member of the South African Institute for Sensory Integration. The work of Paul and Gail Dennison, Carla Hannaford, Jean Ayres, and Carol Kranowitz provides conceptual and practical support for her method.

Rita has developed "balances" for integration of the cranial-sacral, vestibular, proprioceptive, visual, auditory, tactile, olfactory and gustatory systems.[19]

A Balance for Vestibular Integration

Suppose that a seven-year-old with low muscle tone wants to ride her bike around corners and stop easily. First the practitioner makes sure that her goal is appropriate and realistic and that she is in PACE. Muscle checking might lead to vestibular integration as a priority. Next, the child identifies aspects of bike riding that cause stress in her system. Simply walking the bike or sitting on it might produce a weak muscle check (MC). She would also perform various pre-activities that stimulate the vestibular system, each time noticing or muscle checking to establish awareness of stress and provide a base line for measuring progress.

Pre-activities

- Hold left, then right mastoid, bringing attention to the semicircular canals - part of the vestibular system - just beneath this bone. (MC)
- Prone extension posture. (how many seconds?)
- Standing balance, eyes open and closed. (how many seconds?)
- Spinning with eyes closed. (MC or notice loss of balance)
- Leaning forward. (MC)
- Resist being pushed.

Intervention

The child could choose, or muscle checks could lead to a choice, among activities that would foster integration by providing physical, environmental, emotional and/or energetic support:

- **Physical**: Brain Gym (Midline Movements and Lengthening Activities) or other movement stimulation (bouncing, rolling, spinning, jumping)
- **Environmental**: Vestibular stimulation in daily home, playground and classroom routines. Drinking more water.
- **Emotional**: Brain Gym (Positive Points and Hook-ups), integrating music, free movement, dance, resonation.
- **Energetic**: Brain Gym (Energy Exercises)[19] (p. 1-4)

Post-activities

After her menu of chosen activities, the last step would be to revisit the pre-activities, noticing the absence of stress, changes in duration and MCs, and new overall ease with the goal activity. She could then practice bike riding and choose Brain Gym or other home activities to reinforce her new skills.

Case Report: A Balance for Auditory Integration

Danny (name changed), also age seven, experienced dramatic progress in reading through a similar process. He read haltingly, nearly breathless with effort. Pre-checks showed ease for vision, but significant stress for auditory integration, particularly for the right ear, which feeds primarily into the brain's language hemisphere.

An important element in the Brain Gym SI balance format is attention to emotional elements that may influence a child's performance. Danny was able to identify his feelings when he read as "confused" and "frustrated." To see if this might be an echo of past stress, the practitioner explored, through muscle checking. Using guided visualization, she helped him to imagine himself at each age, birth through seven years. When his arm checked weak at ages three and four, his mother said, "Oh, that's the year I was sick." She had, in fact, been critically ill, in and out of the hospital, so ill that a little boy could very well have wanted to block his ears against the voices of worried adults in his house.

To integrate his hearing, Danny needed "Temporal Tapping," firm tapping on the skull all around the outline of his ears as he revisited that time in his imagination. Afterwards he picked up his book again and began reading with obvious pleasure, never stopping until it was time to leave. He could now "hear" the story. At home Danny greeted his father saying, "Dad! I used to hate to read! Now I love to read."

Though this may sound too good to be true, many Brain Gym practitioners have experienced similar nearly magical responses in their clients. Because integration is a natural state, and because Danny's current situation was no longer generating the stress that originally caused his ears to "switch off," a minimal intervention easily brought his auditory system back to a healthy level of relaxation and receptivity.

SI Balances for Other Goals

Goals involving vision would require checks for tracking, looking in all directions, and far/near pursuits. Physical interventions could be Brain Gym, Vision Gym, or other eye exercises. Nurturing the eyes with more time outside, less TV, and improved diet could address environmental issues. For the tactile system pre/post-checks might include wearing a sweater, standing close to someone, hugging, stroking or brushing. Balances for other senses would have different goals, pre/post-checks, interventions, and reinforcement. The approach is infinitely adaptable.[19(p49-62)]

Creative Vision

In further application of their work to visual issues, the Dennisons developed the advanced Edu-K course, Creative Vision. According to its manual, the Creative Vision workshop "explores the use of Edu-Kinesthetics to improve visual information processing by unveiling hidden perceptual gifts blocked by the survival mechanism. The Creative Vision material draws deeply from Dr. Dennison's experience working with behavioral optometrists. This course also offers more in-depth applications of movement to specific learning, drawn from the theories of Doman and Delacato, Jean Ayres, Maria Montessori, and other pioneers in the field of sensory/motor development."[7(p.1)]

A practitioner offering a Creative Vision balance would relate visual skills to the three Edu-K dimensions in the following ways:

Dimension	Skills
Focus	Expressive Abilities: Total Attention, Analysis, Projection
	Receptive Abilities: Perspective, Exploration, Assimilation
Centering	Visual recovery, Visual unity
Laterality	Crossing the midline, Figure/Ground, Visualization, Sensory involvement

An original contribution from the Dennisons to the field of vision improvement is their combined use of color, eye movement, and stimulation of specific points on the head, face and upper body. Called "Edu-K Eye Points," they are related to alertness, balance, grounding, sensory integration and stress reduction. Most of the points are located on acupuncture meridians.

In a Creative Vision balance for example, a practitioner might check a student's muscle resistance while stimulating cones in the fovea of the eye with the color red, followed by another check with blue to stimulate the rods in the retina's periphery. If one color results in a "low gear" response, then the student would do pursuits with that color, while at the same time firmly holding or rubbing the "Edu-K Eye Points" that reverse the low gear response. The result should be new ease and comfort in using the eyes for either near or distance vision.[6(p.45)] The Dennisons claim that "Creative Vision work has proven its value as a tool for release of visual/postural compensations and reestablishment of whole brain visual processing."[7(Preface)]

Edu-Kinesthetics In-Depth: The Seven Dimensions of Intelligence

The In-Depth Balance adds four other dimensions of brain/body intelligence to Laterality, Centering and Focus, as well as a much expanded menu. The result is a process of remarkable scope, depth and flexibility. Because it requires a deeper level of engagement and some capacity for insight, this balance is more appropriate for those at the high functioning end of the autism spectrum.

Four New Dimensions

Motivation Lack of integration relative to motivation, in the Edu-K sense, in no way implies laziness or a need to "just buckle down and get on with it." Instead, it is about unconscious emotional and physical responses operating without input from the rational centers of the brain; something most of us experience on a regular basis. Usually we get over it quickly, but when such patterns arise over and over again, they can become reflexes that sabotage our best intentions.

Cranial Movement Cerebral-spinal fluid moves through membranes of the cranial-sacral system in a constant rhythm, expanding and contracting our cranial bones and nourishing and maintaining balance in our central nervous system. When stress related blockages restrict or inhibit this cranial-sacral rhythm a corresponding disruption in activity level, vision, allergic sensitivity, sleep patterns, repetitive behaviors, and self expression can occur. Traumatic injury, stress (physical or emotional), toxins in the body (environmental pollutants, drugs, etc.), prenatal problems, or a difficult birth can all cause restrictions. Frequently, children with the diagnosis of autism or autistic tendencies have been found to have high tension in the meninges of the head.

Breathing Efficient breathing is key to smooth functioning of all our mind/body intelligences. Relaxed deep breathing supplies oxygen to our blood and gives us energy and strength. When we habitually hold our breath or breathe in a shallow way due to stress, we are more likely to experience exhaustion. We literally lack inspiration. Interventions in the Breathing Dimension aim to reset our internal alarm button so that relaxed and more efficient breathing patterns can become automatic.

Body Regulators The Body Regulator dimension addresses the chemical aspect of brain/body intelligence relating to the balance between intake of nutrients and release of waste. This system is sensitive to excess of all kinds; worry, eye strain, self criticism, as well as poor nutrition and environmental toxins. Physical, emotional and mental activity is reflected in the autonomic nervous system, the endocrine system, and the immune system. Many people on the autism spectrum experience a lack of integration in body regulation and function consistently with a state of body chemistry more appropriate for conditions of extreme danger than for ordinary daily life.

The In-Depth Menu

In addition to the 26 Brain Gym activities plus versions of Repatterning, the In-Depth menu is expanded to include expressive activities that an individual performs on his own and receptive interventions facilitated by a practitioner in four different realms (described below). As in other balances, the menu supports the achievement of a behavioral, academic, athletic or interpersonal goal.

Structure/Movement Realm The aim of the Structure/Movement Realm is to develop physical awareness of muscles working in synergy with the whole brain/body system in service of the goal. Brain Gym movements and Repatterning fit into the expressive part of this realm along with 12 Integrated Movements, each related to a different acupuncture meridian. Processes experienced receptively involve "Movement Re-education," a type of body work in which the facilitator helps the student to reset one or more of twenty different muscles to increase range of motion or to promote relaxation where chronic contraction may exist. Aspects of Creative Vision also can figure in the In-Depth Structure/Movement realm.

Personal Ecology Realm Like other living systems, humans experience a rhythm of fluctuation between periods of stability and change. Change can mean either breaking down or reorganizing at a higher level of complexity. This realm looks at how individuals choose to relate to their external and internal ecosystems and how those choices support or undermine them. The external influence of diet, environmental toxins, ergonomics, amount of time spent in various activities (too much TV? not enough time in nature?), and attitudes inherent in habitual self talk may be important. Internally, allergies, phobias, emotional or chemical residue from past trauma or illness, and recurring family patterns may need attention. Pre- and post-activities and an expanded menu provide the student with both insight and a felt experience of integration.

Emotional Realm The emotional realm receptive process is a ritual-like procedure which allows an uncoupling of the goal issue from the stress response. A combination of supportive touch, holding of neurovascular points on the head, affirmations, memories, projection into the future, eye movements, guided visualization and integrative music enable the student to regulate her internal posture relative to the goal in a way that is free from the domination of the survival brain. The expressive process uses creative resources in the form of drawing, writing, free form movement/dance, integrated movements, resonation, or role play to evoke an internal shift and movement toward a higher level of integration.

Acu Realm Being stuck often indicates a lack or excess of energy somewhere in the acupuncture meridian system itself. Brain Gym energy exercises and/or holding, tapping or massaging various points along certain meridians can help to open blocked circuits in this system. Sometimes the subtle stimulation of an Acu Realm procedure is enough to both soothe and enliven the internal electrical system in a way that can support new goal-oriented behavior.[8(p33-124)]

A single balance is not likely to involve all seven dimensions and all four realms, since it would only address areas where there is a lack of integration relevant to the goal. Because of the way prioritizing is built into the process, the exploratory educational part of the balance moves through the dimensions very quickly to uncover the most salient issues. Similarly the choice of menu activities from four different realms leads economically to the least invasive and most effective interventions. One client described the experience of an In-Depth balance as "an amazing tour around my brain."

Conclusion

Educational Kinesiology is intimately allied with behavioral optometry and a fantastic adjunct to other therapies for those on the autism spectrum. The Dennisons credit the work of over 70 years of research by pioneers in behavioral optometry, including G.N. Getman, Darrell Boyd Harmon, and Moses Albalas. They were also strongly influenced by other important thinkers including John Ott, Arnold Gesell, William Bates, Janet Goodrich, and Noel Kephart. In Edu-K, the Dennisons have created an elegant and powerful synthesis of ideas and techniques from the fields of child development, chiropractic, brain research, applied kinesiology, yoga and acupuncture as well as developmental optometry.

Brain Gym and Vision Gym exercises are easy to learn, easy to teach, noninvasive and non-aerobic. They consume very little time and require no equipment. For the most part children find them enjoyable and quickly learn which ones are most effective for their own particular needs. They are easy to incorporate into the daily home, office or classroom routine. Promoters of Edu-K claim that simply using the four PACE exercises can bring individuals of all ages and abilities into a state of learning readiness. Balances with a trained facilitator can address sensory integration, integration of primitive reflexes, or a specific academic goal. An In-Depth balance goes even deeper. Considerable anecdotal evidence and a growing body of serious research is available at <www.braingym.org> to support these claims.

When patients are not yet ready for or able to benefit from vision training, referral to a Brain Gym practitioner is an option to consider. For those on the autism spectrum, Educational Kinesiology can have a remarkable impact on overall performance in the clinic, at home and at school. Visit <www.braingym.org> for more information and a directory of practitioners around the world.

Brain Gym® and Vision Gym™ are registered trademarks of Brain Gym® International/ Educational Kinesiology Foundation.

References

1. Hannaford C. Smart Moves: Why Learning Is Not All in Your Head. Arlington, VA: Great Ocean Publishers, 1995:113.

2. Frequently asked questions Educational Kinesiology Foundation website: http://www.braingym.org/faq. html. Accessed 3/15/04.

3. Unattributed. A reference List of Edu-K Terms.Brain Gym® J 2004; XVII(3):15.

4. Dennison PE, Dennison GE. Brain Gym Handbook, 2nd ed. Ventura CA: Edu-Kinesthetics, Inc., 1997:44a.

5. Hannaford C. The Dominance Factor. Marshall, NC: Great River Books (formerly Great Ocean Publishers), 1997.

6. Cobb, S. Visions of educational kinesiology. In: Barber A, ed. Vision Therapist Hot Topics. Santa Ana, CA: Optometric Extension Program, 1993:28.

7. Dennison PE, Dennison GE. Creative Vision. Ventura, CA: Edu-Kinesthetics, Inc., 1993.

8. Dennison Pe, Dennison Ge. Edu-kinesthetics In-depth: The Seven Dimensions of Intelligence. Ventura, CA: Edu-Kinesthetics, Inc., 1990:35.

9. Carroll DHL, Erickson CA. Brain Gym for Educators Student Manual. Ventura, CA: Educational Kinesiology Foundation, 1992:5.

10. Miekka S. Workshop Handout. Brain Gym 101. Gaithersburg, MD, 1985.

11. Freeman C. I Am the Child. Ventura, CA:Edu-Kinesthetics, Inc., 1998.

12. Dennison PE, Dennison, GE. The Visioncircles Handbook. Ventura, CA: Edu-Kinesthetics, Inc., 1993:4.

13. Dennison, PE and Dennison, GE. The Visioncircles Teacher Manual. Ventura, CA. Edu-Kinesthetics, Inc. 1993:4.

14. McGee W. Handout at Visioncircles workshop, Alexandria, VA., May 1998.

15. Skeffington AM. Introduction to Clinical Optometry. Santa Ana, CA: Optometric Extension Program Continuing Education Courses. Curriculum II 1964; 54 Series 1, Number 2.

16. Goddard S. A Teacher's Window into the Child's Mind. Eugene, OR. Fern Ridge Press, 1996.

17. Musgutova S. A study on the influence of brain gym movements on muscles and on dynamic and postural reflexes. Brain Gym J July 2001;XV(1 & 2).

18. Personal communication with Harry Wachs, O.D., 12/16/04.

19. Edwards R. In-synch 1: integrating the senses through movement. Spectrum Whole Person Training. Hout Bay. South Africa: Spectrum Whole Person training, 2003.

Chapter 14
Therapies Based on Operant Conditioning: EEG Neurofeedback and Applied Behavioral Analysis (ABA)

Patricia S. Lemer, MEd, NCC

Introduction

Conditioning is the use of consequences to modify behavior. Remember Pavlov's dogs that salivated at the sound of a bell? Researchers trained them by ringing the bell as they moved toward food. Eventually, the food was no longer necessary to make the dogs salivate. This technique is called classical conditioning, and works for behavior over which one has no voluntary control. Operant conditioning uses reinforcement to promote behaviors under voluntary control.

The person probably best known for the application of the principles of operant conditioning to humans is twentieth century Harvard psychologist, B.F. Skinner. Using his operant conditioning chamber, or "Skinner Box," this brilliant man even used his offspring as research subjects.

EEG neurofeedback and ABA are forms of operant conditioning, because both reward behavior that approximates a behavioral goal. In EEG neurofeedback, the brain is the active agent; in ABA the child is the agent. If a child's brain is producing too many low frequency waves, a therapist rewards him with points or a desirable tone each time the brain makes some high frequency waves. If a teacher wishes a child to ask for a treat, initially she may give it to him if he grunts. Gradually, he must make the sound more intelligible to receive a reward. Finally, he must say an approximation of "please" to be rewarded.

Operant conditioning is a common teaching method, so it is no surprise that applying it to children with autism spectrum disorders has become very popular. What is surprising, however, is that so many parents and practitioners are using the following methods in isolation, when they are so compatible with the other therapies described in this book. For most people with autism and attention deficits, these therapies should be considered complementary, not primary. Complementary also does not mean optional, as functional improvements may be available more quickly with EEG operant conditioning than with other methods.

EEG Neurofeedback

Patricia S. Lemer, , MEd, NCC
Contributors: Siegfried Othmer, PhD, Judy Chiswell, EdD, OTR

What if it was possible for individuals diagnosed with AD(H)D, learning disabilities and autism to learn how to control their brainwaves to sustain attention, increase concentration, improve sleep and decrease anxiety? Due to the advent of super fast computers, which are capable of handling real time data from the brain, it is!

Scientists have now developed biofeedback technology utilizing a device called an electro-encephalogram (EEG), which records and feeds back information about the brain's electrical activity. Neurofeedback is a highly sophisticated version of biofeedback that allows the brain to "eavesdrop on itself,"[1] and learn how to alter its own timing and the frequency of its brainwave activity. Improved coordination of cerebral communication causes changes in behavior, motor coordination, language and other cognitive skills.

Neurofeedback has recently emerged as a powerful therapy for teaching the brains of those on the autism spectrum to function more efficiently. Individuals from a number of disciplines have embraced it because it complements many of the biomedical and sensory methods and approaches described in earlier chapters of this book, including vision therapy.

What is Biofeedback?

Biofeedback is a method by which electronic or mechanical instruments relay information to an individual about some aspect of physiological activity, such as heart rate, temperature changes, sweat gland activity, muscle tone, or electrical action in the brain. Biofeedback provides the brain with direct access to its own physiological activity.

Biofeedback training is an educational process developed in the 1970s, during which individuals acquire specialized mind/body skills, by learning to recognize physiological responses and alter them. It is a painless and non-invasive procedure. When the sensors are placed on the scalp to derive information about brainwave activity, it is referred to as EEG biofeedback or neurofeedback.

The client receives immediate visual and auditory feedback on both a video monitor and through headphones. As activity in a desirable frequency band increases, the display moves faster, or the patient receives a reward of some type. As activity in an adverse band increases, no reward materializes. Gradually, the brain learns to respond to the sensory cues, and new brain wave patterns emerge. Through practice, individuals become familiar with their bodies' unique patterns and responses, and learn to alter them to improve function.

Brainwaves and their Frequencies

The EEG is an instrument similar to a car's tachometer; both show how fast the machinery is working. The car's engine revs slowly when idling, and more quickly when one begins driving. The revolutions increase the faster the car goes. Likewise, the EEG shows the brain, an extraordinarily complex communication system, at work. When the body is sleeping, brainwaves are slow; when a person is actively alert, they are faster.

Brainwave frequencies are measured in cycles per second, or Hertz. Thus one Hertz equals one cycle per second. EEG signals are composed of many different frequencies, which are organized in frequency bands. These all occur simultaneously; under certain circumstances some are dominant. Figure 14-1 shows these bands and the mental state associated with each band. The boundaries of bands may differ slightly from practitioner to practitioner.

Figure 14-1: **Brainwave Bands and their Mental States**

Frequency Name	Cycles per second (Hertz)	Mental State
Delta	< 4	Sleep
Theta	4 – 7	Drowsy
Alpha	8 – 11	Inattentive
SMR (Sensori-motor rhythm)	12 – 15	Calm
Beta	16 – 20	Focused
High Beta	> 20	Excited

Brainwave patterns and behavioral issues differ at the different parts of the autism spectrum. Figure 14-2 shows typical brainwave patterns at the mild, moderate and severe ends and areas of deficit that neurofeedback training addresses.

Figure14- 2 **Brainwave Differences in Autism Spectrum Disorders**

Diagnosis	Neurofeedback Patterns	Goals
ADD & ADHD LD & Asperger's	Too much Theta; Too little Beta Too much Theta; Too little Alpha	Improve focus Visual retention Mathematics skills Spatial reasoning Language processing
PDD/Autism		Decrease over-arousal

The brains of those with attention deficits demonstrate a dominance of low-frequency theta waves, which produce a drowsy mental state, resulting in symptoms such as lethargy, poor focus and compromised memory.[2] While an abundance of theta waves are appropriate before sleep, they are inappropriate for the classroom. It may seem paradoxical that kids with AD(H)D are in a state of under-arousal; however, their hyperactive behavior may be compensatory, functioning to keep their brains awake.

Too many theta waves can also disturb sleep. In order to sleep the brain must slow down and produce delta waves. Too much theta can cause trouble falling asleep, staying asleep, and restless sleep, symptoms that are very familiar to parents of AD(H)D children.

A study comparing brainwaves in 18 adults with autism to 18 typical controls found that the autism group exhibited a significantly greater number of brainwaves in the three to six Hz and 13-17 Hz ranges, and significantly fewer between nine and 12 Hz. Some typical children share these features. The conclusion was that those with autism experience both over- and under-connectivity.[3]

EEG Neurofeedback
Neurofeedback training, utilizing today's high speed computers, has increased the range and complexity of biofeedback options for the clinician. Neurofeedback takes the form of a visual display with auditory signals, and occasionally tactile feedback. The visual display serves the dual purpose of entertaining the subject and training the brain. The dual nature of this process makes it possible for the training to proceed even with non-verbal individuals with autism. The brain continuously does its best, primarily at an unconscious level, to adjust to the demands of its environment, regardless of the cognitive level of the patient.

Individuals on the autism spectrum often appear calmer after just the first few minutes of training. As sessions continue, many demonstrate the ability to focus and concentrate for longer periods of time, exhibit less or no self-stimulatory behaviors, and respond with appropriate reactions, even in interpersonal relationships.

Other Types of Neurofeedback
Three new forms of neurofeedback which are showing promise for those with autism are hemoencephalography (blood-brain-image) or HEG, the Low Energy Neurofeedback System (LENS), and passive infrared thermal training (pIR). HEG uses a headband with infrared heat sensors that can detect blood flow within the brain. In HEG biofeedback sessions the goal of treatment is to increase either blood perfusion or oxygenation at specific sites, such as the frontal cortex. Infrared photos confirm that effects last for days and are cumulative.

HEG training for increased brain metabolism can lead to improved neural function, which, in turn, leads to more appropriate behavior and higher levels of achievement. This form of neurofeedback allegedly also affects frustration tolerance, habits, sleep, cognitive, social-emotional, behavioral and mental functioning.[4] For more information on HEG, go to <http://www.biocompresearch.org/>.

The LENS system, the invention of Len Ochs, Ph.D., uses very low power electromagnetic fields, no larger than those that surround digital watches, to carry feedback to the subject. Although the feedback signal is weak, it produces measurable changes in brainwave frequencies without conscious effort from the subject. The result of exposure to very low power EMFs is a changed brainwave state, and much greater ability for the brain to regulate itself.

The high frequencies of the LENS system have information about the EEG frequencies impressed upon them. The high-frequency information travels from the computer system back to the scalp via the same electrode leads that conduct the EEG signal from the scalp to the computer. The software determines just how the trainee's brain is to be challenged. [5] For more information on LENS, go to <www.ochslabs.com>.

Autism Deficits from a Neurofeedback Perspective

Any professional who has referred a patient for neurological testing knows from experience that the EEGs, CAT scans, and MRIs of individuals on the autism spectrum rarely show prominent "abnormalities." This finding is corroborated by research.[6]

Optometrists are familiar with, and can understand this phenomenon, as frequently they see patients who have been told by ophthalmologists that their "vision" is fine, even though it is obvious to parents and teachers that something is wrong. The reason that little or nothing shows up is that medicine has taken a structural point of view. New imaging techniques, such as a functional MRI, are changing this, and revealing more features relevant to behavior.

Neurofeedback, like behavioral optometry, treats underlying causes, dysfunction in a patient's brain, its central processing mechanism, and views patients and their bodies functionally, not structurally. If balance, memory, or emotional status is dysfunctional, the reason(s) could be that the system as a whole, not an individual part, is malfunctioning. For example, the high arousal levels seen in individuals with autism have no localized representation within the brain.

Breakdown in the left hemisphere causes deficits in the development of laterality, sequencing skills, and language acquisition. Right hemisphere problems include sensory over-arousal, communication deficits, lack of emotional connectedness, sleep dysregulation and a poor sense of body in space.

Neurotherapists and optometrists have both studied brain physiology, and know whether a patient's issues are right or left brain problems. Just like the optometrist knows which lenses and prisms to use for testing and remediation, so does the neurotherapist know where to place the electrodes on the scalp. Specific frequencies and locations on the scalp, just like certain lenses and prisms, are more effective than others when training those with autism. While therapists direct most neurofeedback for the autistic patient at the right hemisphere, and at increasing relatively low EEG frequencies, treatment varies from individual to individual.

The History of Biofeedback and Neurofeedback

Researchers have been trying to unlock the mysteries of the brain since ancient times. Anthropologists have discovered century old skulls with carefully drilled holes, in Egypt, France and Peru, suggesting that curious scientists have been looking into the relationship between brains and behavior in ancient cultures for many years.[7]

The first notion that the brain was electrical in nature came in 1791 when Luigi Galvani, an Italian researcher, proposed that an inherent energy exists in all living organisms. While not conclusive, his theory was validated in the 1850s by a German physiologist, Emil Du Bois Reymond. The ability to measure electrical nerve impulses then took off, and in the early twentieth century, scientists were able to show signals from an intact skull for the first time. Furthermore, they could demonstrate differences in brainwave frequencies depending upon the emotional state of an individual.[1 (p. 16-20)]

Eventually, scientists began mapping the brain, and learned that specific centers of the brain controlled specific functions. By stimulating or disabling various parts of the cortex, they were able to increase and decrease abilities in motor, language, sensory and emotional abilities.[1 (p. 17-23)]

It was not until the 1950s that researchers got the idea to use the power of the brain's own electricity to treat undesirable behaviors. When doctors stimulated specific centers in the brains of schizophrenics, the patients reported general feelings of well-being and a reduction in symptoms, such as anxiety, palpitations and rage.

Barry Sterman, PhD, is considered the father of modern neurofeedback training. Like many discoveries, his was scientific serendipity when experimenting with cats. In the late 1960s he identified some unique qualities of the brainwave frequency band of 12 to 15 cycles per second. He labeled this band "sensorimotor rhythm" or SMR, because the location runs across the top of the head, on the area of the brain that controls sensory and motor activity.

Sterman found that he could reduce and eliminate seizures in those with epilepsy by stimulating the SMR band. Applying this finding to humans, he was again successful in reducing, and sometimes eliminating, the need for medications by giving adults feedback on their brain rhythms using biofeedback techniques on the SMR region.[8]

Dr. Sterman's work laid the foundation for using biofeedback techniques to remediate what was then called "minimal brain dysfunction," the predecessor to attention deficit hyperactivity disorder. The slow brainwaves of patients with ADD resembled those of patients with epilepsy. In the 1970s, Joel Lubar, PhD, and his associates[9] and others[10] successfully applied this technique to those with AD(H)D, with the SMR band the target of therapy.

The new EEG neurofeedback is showing positive outcomes with those diagnosed with not only with attention deficits, but also with learning disabilities,[11] Asperger syndrome[12] and autism.[13,14] In 1995, Rossiter and La Vaque compared matched samples of children receiving medication with another doing neurofeedback found both treatments to yield positive changes.[15] Rossiter replicated this study ten years later with a larger sample, and the same results.[16]

Neurofeedback, unlike Ritalin, has long-lasting gains, without any negative side effects. Even though research is still scant and samples small, practitioners are optimistic about neurofeedback being an efficacious treatment for those on the whole continuum of autism spectrum disorders.

The Mind Body Connection

Neurofeedback therapy is based on the basic underlying premise of this book: a mind-body connection to disease and disability. The body is like a city: an interdependent information communication system. When a single system breaks down in a city or human body, other systems dysfunction.

The brain is centrally involved in regulating all bodily functions: it thus determines and reflects the body's health. A healthy brain is flexible, and has the ability to change its arousal and attention in response to the demands of the environment. An unhealthy, dysregulated (and autistic) brain is inflexible and "out-of-sync" with itself. Its inability to process information at the right speed produces a discontinuity in communication, and inappropriate responses to its surroundings.[1 (p. 75,76)]

Brain dysregulation produces systemic mind/body effects, clearly demonstrated in patients on the autism spectrum who show symptoms in virtually every system. Almost no one would argue today about dysregulation in the gut. Dysregulated gut function ultimately degrades brain function in autism, and the reverse can be true, as well.

Dr. Othmer believes that one way the dysregulated brain can dysregulate the gut is by shifting the balance between the sympathetic and parasympathetic nervous system. As neurofeedback gradually decreases arousal levels, and restores a healthier balance between the two parts of the autonomic nervous system, gut dysbiosis alleviates. Neurofeedback training can potentially affect every bodily system by regulating the central rhythmic activity of the brain.

The next section explains the use of neurofeedback techniques for training the brain of those on the autism spectrum. The contributors shared their work and knowledge through conversations, lectures, writings and websites. In addition, the editor gleaned additional information from two articles about and by Dr. Othmer, appearing in *Latitudes*, the publication of the Association for Comprehensive Neurotherapy (ACN).[17,18] *Latitudes* editor Sheila Rogers is a wealth of information, and has worked tirelessly for many years in support of non-drug alternatives for autism spectrum disorders and Tourette syndrome. Her website is <www.latitudes.org>.

Neurofeedback Training for Autistic Spectrum Disorders
Neurofeedback practitioners have a choice of using standard training protocols that address different common brain wave patterns, or formulating individualized training programs specifically designed to treat a patient's unique needs. One way they can develop a program is by using a new EEG called a quantitative electro-encephalograph, or qEEG, which aids in the diagnostic process, and guides the neurofeedback treatment program. Some clinicians use a qEEG as a pre-test prior to a session; others use it only as a aide for patients making slow progress.[1(p.280,281)]

Neurofeedback itself is simple and painless. First the patient sits in a comfortable chair, like a recliner, in a small, dimly lit, well-isolated room. The neurofeedback equipment, consists of two computer monitors on a desktop, one for the patient to watch the visual display, and the other to show brainwave activity to the therapist.

The therapist applies conductive paste to the sensors, which are wired to an amplifier and then to the computer. The number of sensors attached to areas of the scalp is dependent on the individual needs of the patient and the therapist's therapeutic plan. As the patient relaxes, the sensors act like tiny receivers conducting electricity produced by the brain through the wires. The EEG shows the therapist within seconds how a patient's brain is communicating. At the same time the information about the EEG goes back to the trainee, whose brain recognizes itself as an active agent in the process.

The purpose of each session is to train the brain to communicate more efficiently by regulating specific brain regions. Many patients on the autism spectrum need to train their brains to calm down; others need to make their brains more active. This is not a contradiction. Appropriate activation allows the brain to do its job: regulate its state to match the needs of the moment. Training always starts with the parts of the brain that are the most troublesome, as a "trickle-down effect" can favorably affect less problematic issues.

The following generalized benefits are often seen with neurofeedback training:

- Progression toward calming
- Normalization of sleep patterns
- Increased flexibility, resilience and emotional well being
- Improvement in ability to interact with others
- Reduction in self-stimulating behaviors
- Improvement in attention

Sessions for those on the autism spectrum last from 30-50 minutes, depending upon the functioning level of the subject. Allow at least 20 sessions to achieve noteworthy results. The cost of diagnostic testing and treatment sessions are about the same as for academic tutoring. Many insurance companies are now covering neurofeedback for certain conditions like anxiety disorders and chronic pain, and only a few recognize neurotherapy as an acceptable treatment for autism. However, patients are finding ways around this problem, in the same way they are finding ways to pay for vision therapy, using methods such as a medical savings account.

Who are Candidates for Neurofeedback?

While nearly everyone, with or without a disability, is capable of responding positively to neurofeedback, among the disabled, high functioning individuals at the less severe end of the spectrum, who enjoy computer tasks, are the best candidates. Some practitioners are using neurofeedback for non-verbal individuals with autism, however. Those who have higher potential than is evident superficially, and those who are facile with and attracted to computers and other gadgets, are often excellent responders.

Children adopted from orphanages in foreign countries and other severely impacted children are also a particularly interesting and very promising group. Progress with this population is often striking and unexpected. Neurofeedback awakens dormant messages in their brains and shows success in eliciting sociability and language processing because of better brain organization.

Impediments to Success with Neurofeedback

The following are the most common reasons for failure of neurofeedback training with those on the autism spectrum:

- **Sensory defensiveness** – Individuals with autism may dislike various aspects of the sensors – how they feel on the scalp or the smell of the paste, or even the sound made by the machine. However, just like the optometrist can gradually overcome sensory issues to allow the use of lenses, so does the neurotherapist who is intent upon working with autistic patients.
- **Poor sustained attention** – This hallmark symptom of autism can easily interfere with neurofeedback therapy. Being able to pay attention to a screen for lengthy periods of time is a function of progressive training. A graded program to improve attention by increasing time in training enables many autistic children to gain skill and improve flexibility without frustrating them.
- **Medications** interfere only infrequently because an autistic patient's poor response to drugs or a preference for a holistic approach may be what brought him/her to neurofeedback in the first place. Some individuals however, are on medications that interfere with their ability to sustain attention as described above. A few neurofeedback practitioners, like many optometrists, refuse to work with patients on medications because

of their side effects. Other professionals inform patients that as the brain learns how to control itself more efficiently that medication dosages may be able to be lowered, or that they may no longer be necessary. Collaboration with the patient's physician is key to this process.

- **Attitude** – People who question whether neurofeedback has efficacy or is worth their money, especially if it is not covered by insurance, can sabotage training. Their belief system simply interferes psychologically with the brain's willingness to accept the challenges that neurofeedback training presents.

Collaboration with Optometry

Professional collaboration between neurofeedback practitioners and developmental optometrists can be an extremely successful two-way street when both professionals recognize the potential of the others' services. Clues of potential vision issues can present themselves both in the initial intake interview and during neurofeedback training. The neurofeedback practitioner can observe obvious functional behaviors, such as a head tilt, squinting or postural issues. Fast moving images, changes in figure-ground, or difficulties with peripheral vision during neurofeedback training could cause rapid visual fatigue, eye watering and headaches. Writing or drawing tasks may demonstrate visual-motor and visual-spatial problems.

Case Studies

- *Case 1:* S.T. is an eight-year-old boy, diagnosed with autism. Upon initial intake he demonstrated little eye contact, and waved his hands and feet, while sitting in the chair. His mother agreed to position him on her lap for the first session of neurofeedback. She was encouraged when he allowed the therapist to apply the sensors to his scalp and ears, and even more surprised when he became very calm after several intervals of training.

After only two training sessions, S.T. came hurrying into the office to get started, and was able to sit by himself. By the end of 40 sessions S.T. was able to sit calmly for the training period. Eye contact had improved, he conversed easily with his therapists, showed improved attention, focus and concentrated for longer periods of time. Self-stimulatory behaviors decreased markedly. As behavioral issues decreased, specific vision issues became obvious, and the therapist referred him to a local behavioral optometrist for an evaluation.

The following three cases come from Donna Troisi, LCSW/C, a neurofeedback specialist in Maryland.

- *Case 2:* A.C. is a 13-year-old boy with autism who is non-verbal. At first he was extremely impulsive, and the slightest emotional distress over-activated his autonomic nervous system, causing him to vomit. He also had very sweaty palms, and could not close his eyes voluntarily. A.C. worked for over a year with Donna, one to two times a week, using specialized equipment. After approximately 20 sessions, A.C.'s parents were able to put a rug in his room for the first time, because he no longer threw up frequently. He gradually became more expressive and interactive, and demonstrated increased awareness of his environment. Interestingly, he was also able to close his eyes independently.

- *Case 3:* P.T. is a sixth grade boy diagnosed with Asperger syndrome, who never became dizzy, even when spinning on equipment, and who also demonstrated a low frustration tolerance. After 40 sessions of neurofeedback, he tolerated longer and longer sessions, and now gets dizzy when spinning. These new symptoms are attributed to a more integrated vestibular system as a result of neurofeedback training.

- *Case 4:* Serena is a bright fourth grade girl, diagnosed with ADHD. Parents and teachers were disturbed that she was mouthing objects and clothing. After several months of neurofeedback therapy, this behavior disappeared.

Cases demonstrate the power of neurofeedback in challenging the brain to organize itself for better functionality. The largest gains occur when neurofeedback is combined with biomedical and other therapies, such as behavioral optometry. Changes because of the normalization of the communication pathways of the neuronal networks, with respect to the domains of timing and frequency, impact favorably not only on cortical function directly, but also on autonomic, endocrine, and immune system regulation as well.

Summary and Conclusions

Neurofeedback is an emerging new treatment modality for those on the autism spectrum. It is a brain-training technique that complements both behavioral methods and biomedical approaches. Brain training enhances a child's regulatory function broadly, with resulting favorable outcomes across the board. This broad impact is traceable to the central role of the brain in the expression of autistic features.

By working with the EEG, the therapist observes the brain in its role of organizing its own internal state, managing other bodily functions, and directing overt behavior. By shaping brain behavior toward more normal patterns through neurofeedback, we can alter the brain's capacity to communicate both internally and externally, thus bringing about better functional integration.

The response to brain training can be both profound and relatively quick. Devotees of EEG neurofeedback believe it to be one of the best pathways toward an improved quality of life for an autistic child and the family. It also has the potential to render other therapies more effective. Any child on the autistic spectrum is a candidate for an early trial of neurofeedback. The challenge to future researchers will be to determine the longevity of neurofeedback training. Does this intervention hold over time, or are occasional "booster shots" necessary?

Several books extol the virtues of neurofeedback for those searching out alternatives to prescription medications for attention deficits and autism. The first of these is *A Symphony in the Brain* by Jim Robbins,[7] published in 1999, with a second edition due out in 2008. Two newer books, focusing on ADD are *The ADD Book* by Sears and Thompson,[19] and *Getting Rid of Ritalin* by Hill and Castro.[1]

Websites with current research, professional training courses, certification, and directories of neurofeedback therapists all over the world include the following: <www.bcia.org>, <www.eeginfo.com>, <www.eeginstitute.com>, <www.eegdirectory.com>, <www.isnr.org>, <www.eegspectrum.com>, <www.aapb.org>, <www.brianothmerfoundation.org>.

All are excellent references for anyone desiring more complete information about this treatment.

Applied Behavior Analysis

Editor's note: This overview of ABA is a compilation from many sources, including the Lovaas Institute <www.lovaas.com> and the Center for Autism and Related Disorders <www.centerforautism.com>. Susan Varsames, M.A. Ed., of the Holistic Learning Center in Eastchester, NY <www.hlcinfo.com> is a contributor.

Behavior Analysis is the systematic study of variables that influence the behavior of an organism.[20] *Applied Behavior Analysis* (ABA) is the process of systematically applying what scientists have learned in the laboratory to significant behaviors in real life situations, such as home, school and work.[21] ABA, like neurofeedback, traces its roots back to the principles of operant conditioning (see introduction to this chapter).

The umbrella term "ABA" includes many interventions based on direct observations of behavior which comprise a "functional behavioral assessment," or a "functional analysis of behavior." All ABA programs utilize the manipulation of antecedents and consequences of behavior to

- reduce inappropriate, self-injurious and stereotypical behaviors
- modify conditions under which interfering behaviors occur
- teach new skills
- transfer and generalize behavior from one situation to another

ABA is a therapy that is appropriate from an early age, and is proving effective even for older individuals on the autism spectrum.

A Historical Overview of ABA and Autism

Clinical psychologist Ivar Lovaas, PhD, is considered the father of Applied Behavior Analysis therapy for autism. Today the term "Lovaas therapy," or simply "Lovaas," is often used synonymously with "Applied Behavior Analysis." Lovaas therapy is only one type of ABA, however, as psychologists and educators have modified the original therapy, resulting in many hybrids.

In 1987, when a Professor of Psychology at the University of California at Los Angeles (UCLA), Lovaas demonstrated scientifically what no one believed possible: that the behavior of autistic children could be modified through teaching. Working intensively with 19 seven-year-old children with autism and 19 controls, 90% of the children in his study substantially improved, compared to the control group. In this study, 40 hours of therapy per week for three years, with the original Lovaas method of behavioral analysis, was necessary for close to one half (47%) to attain normal IQs and test within the normal range on adaptive and social skills.[22]

A follow-up study on these same children four years later, at an average age of 11.5, showed that eight of nine were indistinguishable from average children on tests of intelligence and adaptive behavior.[23] A later study with 28 children receiving intensive ABA therapy for four years found the same results, with 48% being able to succeed in regular classroom settings.[24]

An independent author completed the most recent replication study of the Lovaas Model in 2006. Children in behavioral treatment scored significantly higher in IQ and adaptive behavior scores than the comparison group. Further, 29% (6 of 21) children were fully included in regular education without assistance and another 52% (11 of 21) were included with support. This compares to only 5% (1 of 21) children in the control group who were placed in regular education.[25]

Research shows that when ABA is compared in effectiveness to a combination of other treatments for pre-schoolers, it also is more effective. In 2005, researchers at California State University, Stanislaus found that intensive ABA for 14 months was a substantially more effective treatment for a group of 61 preschool children with autism than "eclectic treatments." The children not receiving ABA were administered a combination of Picture Exchange Communication System (PECS), sensory integration therapy, speech and language therapy, discrete trial training, play therapy, and techniques drawn from the Teaching and Education of Autism and related Communication handicapped Children (TEACCH). [26]

Over the past 40 years, several thousand published research studies have documented the effectiveness of ABA for treating autism across a wide range of

- *behaviors*, that are self-injurious,[27] stereotypical,[28] communicative,[29] social, academic, leisure and functional
- *populations*, including children and adults with a variety of behavioral, learning and developmental disorders, as well as attention deficit hyperactivity disorder[30]
- *therapists and educators*, including parents, teachers and remedial specialists
- *settings*, including schools,[31] homes, institutions, residential placements, hospitals,[32] and businesses.[33]

Doreen Granpeesheh, PhD, Founder and Director of the Center for Autism and Related Disorders (CARD) divides the copious research on ABA for autism into two categories:

- *Large-scale outcome studies* with over 10 subjects, intensive therapy for over a year, and a comprehensive treatment program
- *Small-scale treatment studies* with one to three subjects, for one to two months only, and with treatment focused on only one or two skills.

In every large-scale study published, subjects showed substantial progress. However, intensity matters; at least 30 hours of treatment for more than a year are necessary for positive outcomes. Small-scale studies showed that almost any child can show improvement in some area of skill acquisition by using ABA principles, even for a short time.

A meta-analysis summarizing about 250 articles on long- and short-term ABA therapy starting in 1980,[34] and a review of almost 1000 articles through the present are available at <http://www.nationalautismcenter.org> for anyone interested in reviewing ABA research in depth.

ABA therapy became the therapy of choice in the 1990s. In 1999, the late Bernard Rimland, PhD, Founder and Director of the Autism Research Institute (ARI) wrote a passionate letter in his newsletter that he entitled "The ABA Controversy." He urged therapists, schools and others recommending ABA as the *only* scientifically based therapy for autism to consider biomedical treatments as well. By that point in time, much research on the benefits of B6, magnesium and DMG had been published. (See Chapter 6 for those studies.) Rimland's letter is reprinted here in its entirety, with permission from ARI.

I am a long-time and ardent supporter of what is now called the "ABA" (Applied Behavior Analysis) method of teaching autistic children.

I remember very clearly the day in October 1964 (35 years ago), when I first visited Ivar Lovaas in his clinic at UCLA. I met the autistic children Billie, Rickie, and Pam, who resided there. Their speech was sparse and stilted, but the children were miles ahead of where they had been when they were filmed (this was before videotape) at intake. I spent the day with Ivar, and came away impressed. I returned home and started using "operant conditioning" with my then eight-year-old son Mark. He, too, began to improve.

A year later, in November 1965, I spoke to a group of parents in Teaneck, New Jersey, a suburb of New York City, and proposed that we start a national organization, the National Society for Autistic Children (now the Autism Society of America) dedicated to helping, not just baby-sitting, our children. The talk I gave was titled "Operant conditioning: breakthrough in the treatment of mentally ill children." (I said "mentally ill" because few were aware of the term "autism" then.) I traveled to city after city, giving the "Breakthrough" talk and starting a new chapter of the society in each city. My "Breakthrough" talk was translated into many languages in the '60s and '70s, and helped educate parents and educators around the world.

In 1987, when Lovaas' landmark study of ABA was published, we featured it in the Autism Research Review International (ARRI). I wrote dozens of letters of support for parents who wished to obtain ABA for their children, and in ARRI Vol. 8, No. 3, in 1994, I published a generic letter of support which was helpful, I'm told, to innumerable families fighting to get ABA for their children.

As a long-time advocate and supporter of ABA, I take a back seat to no one. Having said that, I must tell you that I am dismayed and appalled at the ludicrous position taken by many other supporters of ABA, who claim that ABA is the only scientifically validated treatment for autism. Not so! That position is not only false, it is absurd. Believe it or not, the Early Intervention Program of the New York State Department of Health has published a series of Clinical Practice Guidelines which makes that claim.

Considering the weight of scientific evidence, there are several treatment approaches which clearly meet the criterion of scientific validation, and of these, at least two surpass ABA in terms of scientific supportability. I will confine my comments here to the treatment modalities which most clearly exceed ABA in terms of level of scientific support (not necessarily in terms of percentage of children helped, nor in terms of the degree to which they are helped, but only in terms of weight of scientifically valid evidence that the treatment effect is real).

The New York State Guidelines, which recommend ABA as the only effective treatment, explicitly reject vitamin therapy, gluten- and casein-free diets, anti-fungal treatment, auditory integration training, sensory integration, and many other interventions.

The Lovaas 1987 study, the centerpiece of the ABA early intervention movement, attracted a great deal of attention because it employed a control group of more-or-less equally impaired children who were given less intensive (fewer hours per week) treatment. This represented an important advance in methodology over no control group at all (the usual approach), but the study did not employ double-blind procedures. Those involved in the study knew how intensive the treatment was for each child. I am aware that it would have been exceedingly difficult, if not impossible, to develop a double-blind evaluation of intensive ABA treatment, but that does not change the fact that a double blind was not used. The results were thus to some extent contaminated by participant bias and expectancy.

Further, all of the methods of measuring the effect of the treatments were to some degree subjective-and a source of error. No study of the effectiveness of ABA has used double-blind procedures or scientific laboratory analytical equipment.

In contrast, of the 18 studies showing vitamin B6 and magnesium to be effective, 11 employed the double-blind procedure. Further, in addition to using soft behavioral and observational criteria such as were employed in the ABA evaluation studies, 10 of the studies of B6 and magnesium measured the presence of abnormal substances in the blood and urine of autistic children, and found the B6/magnesium to have improved the children's metabolism. Five studies of B6/magnesium in autism have shown normalization of brainwave activity in the autistic children. These are hard, objective, measurable, scientifically replicable findings. Show me the equivalent of such solid scientific evidence in the ABA literature. It is absent.

The situation is similar with regard to the efficacy of the casein- and gluten-free diet. Study after study has documented the presence of abnormal substances in the urine of autistic children, with improvement in the children's urine and in the children's behavior when the special diets are implemented. There are over 40 such studies, yet the New York State report claims the diets are ineffective. Very strange.

Recently an organization has been formed with the title Association for Science in Autism Treatment (ASAT). Their literature espouses the same nonsensical, counterfactual position as the aforementioned New York State report: ABA is the only scientifically valid intervention for autism. Their position is indefensible: it requires a distorted view of what science is all about, as well as a willingness to ignore all relevant evidence.

The "ABA is the only way" folks are wrong, not only because of their lack of information about research on the validity of other interventions, but because of their failure to recognize that parents have a right and an obligation to consider all possible forms of intervention, including those which may not yet have won the stamp of approval of whatever person or committee feels qualified to pass judgment on candidate interventions.

A case in point: ABA itself. I can't help but wonder how the ABA-only folks would view my efforts to have ABA accepted between 1964 and 1987. Though there were no control group studies, and certainly no double-blind studies to point to, the evidence was clear enough to compel me to fight for ABA. Should I have abandoned my efforts for more than two decades while waiting for a control group study to appear? I'm glad I didn't.

It is a major mistake to think of ABA as being competitive with, rather than complementary to, many other interventions, particularly such biologically based interventions as vitamin B6 and magnesium therapy. For years, our publications have urged parents who are about to undertake megavitamin therapy to refrain from mentioning the new intervention to teachers, therapists, grandparents, sitters, etc., so they would be able to obtain objective input from these "blind" observers. Each such case is a mini double-blind single-subject experiment. We have heard from hundreds of parents who have reported, "Our therapist, who did not know about the B6 we started last week, said our child has made more progress in one week than in the prior three months.

If you really want to be scientific, do a mini double-blind trial on your child." [35]

Today the CARD program at Thoughtful House in Austin, TX, headed by Drs. Andrew Wakefield and Doreen Granpeesheh combines ABA and the Defeat Autism Now! approach. (See section on CARD.) Centers where patients with autism could receive a biomedical approach combined with ABA was one of Dr. Rimland's dying wishes. The newest multidisciplinary center, open in September, 2007, is The Rimland Center in Lynchburg, VA, named in his honor.

The Language of ABA

Learning, as defined by behaviorists, is a change of behavior as a result of experience. Target behaviors are anything which is observable and measurable, and can include receptive and expressive communication, adaptive living skills (toileting and grooming), learning academics, and social skills, such as sharing and taking turns. Examples of target behaviors are: "When given the direction 'Touch your nose,' the child will do so independently." "When asked to count out one, two, or three items, the child will do so with accuracy." "Karen will count the family members present for dinner, and set the table with the correct number of place settings."

Behaviors have definable and measurable frequency rates, durations and intensities, and consist of specific actions that can be maintained, increased or decreased. Behavioral descriptors, such as moody, angry, sad, etc. are not used in ABA, as they cannot be accurately measured by any of the above criteria.

ABA is not a specific program, but rather many programs that follow a set of principles and guidelines,[36] and use some very specific terms to describe actions therapists take with their clients.

- *Task analysis* – Breaking skills down into small attainable parts.
- *Reinforcement* – A consequence that increases the probability of a desired response.
- *Positive reinforcement* – Getting a reward of something viewed as pleasurable as a consequence of doing something new or in a different way. Example: Getting to swing for matching a block to a picture of the same color.
- *Negative reinforcement* – Getting a reward of something viewed as pleasurable for *not* doing something the adult wants to diminish. Example: getting a piece of candy for not flapping arms when excited.
- *Punishment* – A consequence that decreases the probability of a desired response.
- *Errorless learning* – A process that presents information in a way that reduces trial and error and avoids mistakes.
- *Prompting* – A technique used to help the child get a correct response to insure errorless learning. Therapists use several types of prompts: physical (touching), verbal (providing the answer for the student to repeat), gestural (pointing with exaggerated facial expressions) or modeling (showing how to do something), are just a few.
- *Fading a prompt* – Or getting a child to give the correct response with less assistance or without a prompt is the goal.
- *Redirection* – A non-intrusive method of interrupting self-stimulatory or repetitive behaviors, and diverting attention toward an acceptable behavior. Example: When a child exhibits self-stimulatory behavior, put something interesting in his hand to redirect the behavior.
- *Shaping* – A way of adding a new behavior to a person's repertoire by reinforcing a successful approximation of the target behavior. Shaping is like playing "hot and cold." The closer the person comes to the behavior, the closer he is to the reward.
- *Chaining* – The combining of simple, sequenced component behaviors into a more complex, composite behavior. Example: putting on pants, shirt, socks, and shoes to the request, "get dressed."
- *Expansion Activities* – Generalizing and combining skill sets to new materials and a variety of conditions. Example: if a child masters "turn taking" and "matching colors," teach a game such as *Candyland* to maintain both skills with a functional application. Or, if a child learns to independently complete a jigsaw puzzle at a table, provide opportunities to learn how to do a floor puzzle, a puzzle with a peer, or a different type of puzzle.

The delivery of ABA techniques includes errorless learning, prompting, chaining behaviors, using task analysis, and reinforcing desired behaviors. While treatment is always based on the principles of Applied Behavior Analysis, its implementation varies based on a child's unique needs. Educators have the responsibility to deliver experiences that are appropriate for individual learners. The "magic" of ABA comes from a "good fit" between the teacher's methodology and the student's learning style.

Educators utilizing ABA teaching procedures often fade and reintroduce techniques according to a student's progress. As students demonstrate reliability and consistency with skills, less structured techniques are necessary to maintain behavior. Teachers can also use more flexible instructions and different settings to assure that students are able to demonstrate their skills in a variety of environmental conditions. As new skills are added, a therapist may need to reintroduce specific ABA techniques in order to assist students in adding new information into their repertoire of skills that they can functionally apply on demand.

Consider this example: A teenager must learn to walk on city streets back and forth between his home and school. An ABA therapist analyzing this task might break it down into the following measurable target behaviors: responding to walk/don't walk signals, not talking to strangers, not crossing if an emergency vehicle with a siren is present, etc. The teacher prompts each target behavior sequentially, gradually fading them out until the student memorizes the route, the signs, and masters the task completely, and can do it independently. One day, the city tears up the street on the corner that the student has learned to manage, and barricades the area with a detour, requiring pedestrians to walk on planks to get to the opposite corner. The student freezes and is unable to employ flexible thinking to manage the new route with the detour. A new target behavior in ABA now needs to be taught that states, "When walking to a learned destination on a learned route, and a detour is present, the student will independently follow the detour and get back to learned route." As skills require new demands or when there are exceptions to a learned procedure, it is necessary to reintroduce the necessary trials to teach the new skill.

The Components of an ABA Program
The essential elements of a good ABA program are
- Selection of a specific interfering behavior or a behavioral skill deficit that has some social significance
- Establishment of a baseline of present levels of targeted behaviors or skills
- Identification of behavioral goals and objectives
- Design and implementation of interventions that reduce interfering behaviors and/or teach new skills
- Measurement of levels of target behaviors to determine the effectiveness of the intervention
- Evaluation of the effectiveness of the intervention, with modifications, made as necessary, to maintain and/or increase both the effectiveness and the efficiency of the intervention
- Generalization of behaviors or skills in a variety of environments and across related or similar behaviors or skills[37]

ABA and Autism
Programs grounded in ABA are now extremely popular assessment and therapeutic/educational interventions for children, teens and adults with autism. The popularity of ABA is a result of the scientific evidence that it is effective. Just like vision therapy for those with autism can take place in-office, at home, include motor or computer-based activities, lenses and/or prisms, a child who is receiving ABA could be involved in one of many types of interventions that follow the ABA guidelines.

Individuals, clinics, and even entire school systems are using an ABA approach to the assessment and evaluation of an autistic child's behavior, and to the application of interventions that alter behavior. ABA focuses on the reduction of maladaptive behaviors and on the development of adaptive, socially significant behaviors.

ABA, like many other therapies, is most effective with children diagnosed with autism at a young age. However, it usually begins between the ages of two and eight, continuing through elementary school, up until about age twelve.

For *children younger than three*, therapists use an interactive play-based approach. Goals include developing skills such as imitating, pointing, verbalizing, requesting, playing, interacting, relating, and regulating sensory input. Treatment typically begins with 10-15 hours per week and gradually increases to 35-40 hours per week, by the age of three. Instructors use any opportunity to take advantage of situations occurring in the natural environment, to teach new behaviors. This is called "incidental teaching." For example, when a child demonstrates interest in a toy, the instructor prompts the child to request the toy using an appropriate form of communication.

In the beginning, instructors use "pairing techniques" to build rapport with a child. These provide a high rate of reinforcement for behaviors, and follow a child's lead as much as possible, building upon a child's initiations, both non-verbal and verbal, no matter how small or subtle. At this age, adults often rely on redirection. Once a learning environment has become positive for both the child and instructor, and the child enjoys being with the instructor because of positive experiences, the adult increases the amount of structured time, emphasizing effective reinforcers and motivating activities.

For children ages three to five, therapy increases in length and intensity, and interactions become more elaborate. Language advances from one-word responses to simple questions, to speaking in complete sentences. Children learn turn taking, how to learn in groups and how to make and keep friends.

At this age, therapists use ABA methodology to teach a pre-school curriculum, including every imaginable skill. Areas include
- *color, number and letter identification*
- *vocabulary development* for items such as animals, clothing, food, people, etc.
- *gross motor development with essential safety awareness skills* for behaviors such as riding a tricycle (and stopping at the end of the driveway), throwing a ball, (but not at windows!) and independently getting on and off a swing (without walking in front of a peer on a moving swing)
- *fine motor development* such as manipulation of beads and puzzle pieces, using crayons and markers, snipping and cutting with scissors, (but not cutting Grandma's lace table cloth or giving the dog a haircut!)
- *language and organization* such as listening to stories, predicting outcomes, following directions and the routine of a pre-school class and even toilet training

Therapy takes place in sessions of two to four hours, including many play breaks. ABA specialists recommend an integrated approach of five to eight hours per day, approximately 35-40 hours per week, including breaks. An individualized schedule fits the needs of a child, and may, for instance, include an afternoon nap.

Typically, a child and instructor work on a specific task for two to five minutes and then take a one to two minute break. Different settings, including a small table, the floor, different rooms in the house or school, and the out-of-doors, provide variety. Lengthier play breaks of 10-20 minutes occur every hour or so, during which a child and instructor might swing, play a game, or eat a snack. Breaks offer opportunities for a child to generalize new-found skills.

Behavioral therapy, while originally used only with children under five, is also an effective intervention for *older children,*[38] with some modifications. With pre-teens, high school students and adults, collaboration with educators and other professionals at school and in the community increases. Those with autism are no longer isolated and working one-on-one. Rather, inclusion in a classroom or job setting, for at least a part of the day, in family life, in the community, and with peers, are all goals for older children. In these settings, they improve their self- help skills, learn to use leisure time independently, and increase functional communication. In order to accomplish these outcomes, a "shadow" or trained 1:1 aide, may be necessary.

ABA is certainly compatible with other therapies. Integrating it with biomedical interventions, for which the CARD program is the model, is extremely effective.[39]

However, some practitioners have reservations about using it with "inside-out" therapies, such as sensory integration based occupational therapy, sound therapy and some vision therapy, Critics believe that ALL behaviors are meaningful, and that the ABA approach to extinguishing socially unacceptable behaviors is disrespectful of the body's attempts to self-regulate.

Incorporating Sensory Integration into ABA

ABA therapists and other professionals are finding ways of accommodating a child with sensory issues by incorporating sensory integration (SI) theory into ABA.[40] Many of these are similar to the environmental changes optometrists make during vision therapy.

- *Modify environmental stimuli.* Be aware of sounds and sights which may distract a child. Use a quiet voice for the hypersensitive child. Organize or limit the use of visual materials that are too exciting or distracting. Use light or heavy touch depending on the child's level of sensitivity.
- *Encourage proper posture during seated activities to enhance attention.* Stabilize a child's feet on the ground for maximum sensory feedback and support. Use a Move N' Sit™ cushion or wedge to help the child with low muscle tone or inadequate postural stability, and to keep the pelvis in a position that will facilitate muscular activation and arousal.
- *Provide opportunities for individualized sensory input.* Children need different sensory inputs at different moments throughout the day, depending upon their physiological state. Sometimes touch will help a child focus, while at other times movement is more helpful. Each child has a unique sensory profile and requires an individualized sensory diet. (See Chapter 7.)
- *Allow a child to choose, rather than prescribe input in a standardized manner.* This small step can greatly enhance regulation. Some children with motor planning difficulties may be unable to initiate or sequence the steps, however. It may be necessary to prompt them to obtain the input their bodies need to be calm and attentive.
- *Use imitation and pair actions with objects.* Imitation is a stage of communicative interaction that increases social interest and eye contact, and becomes increasingly intentional and referential throughout early childhood. If a child has difficulty imitating, play patty-cake and peek-a-boo. Next, have the child imitate the therapist putting glasses or silly hats on and off, or giving and receiving objects paired with exaggerated affect cues. Form dyads of children, using two identical objects in the context of object manipulation/imitation to enhance social reciprocity as well as imitation.
- *Use reciprocal social praise.* Wait both for a child to give a response, and to give praise, to enhance purposeful communication. Ample wait time gives a child with autism the

natural experience of conversation. Once he/she provides an affect cue by gaze, gesture, or vocalization, "rhythmic praise" is effective because it does not overwhelm. This type of interaction enhances self-regulation, attention, and social responsivity.

Case Study Combining ABA, SI and Vision Therapy

The Holistic Learning Center in Eastchester, New York uses a multi-disciplinary model which successfully combines ABA with both sensory integration techniques and vision therapy. The following case demonstrates the role of behavioral optometry in the successful implementation of ABA.

TJ is a six-year-old boy diagnosed with PDD-NOS at age three. He had a history of mild pre-eclampsia during pregnancy, a normal delivery, multiple ear infections from infancy through the toddler years, general good health, and significant developmental delays. TJ had received 30 hours of ABA in a home program for two years as a preschooler, and out-patient occupational and speech-language therapy. He began kindergarten in a self-contained classroom in his school district where teachers used ABA methodology for 10 hours weekly, as well as the TEACCH approach for independent demonstration of skills. They also used behavioral strategies for compliance with wearing his prescribed glasses. TJ practiced his vision goals daily with his teachers, parents, and occupational therapist. However, TJ's hypersensitive auditory system over-reacted to the sounds of the heat coming through the air vents, the buzz of the fluorescent lights, and the birds chirping outside.

Special educators increased levels of reinforcement in an attempt to elicit even a few seconds of on-task behavior, but without success. Visually, TJ could no longer maintain eye contact, or focus on tasks. TJ's ABA record book showed that, despite program modifications, increases in his reinforcement schedules, and the use of 1:1 teaching, he was unable to learn at the same rate as during home schooling.

The special education team agreed with parents and teachers to home school TJ for the remainder for the school year. During that period, he received listening therapy and significantly reduced his auditory sensitivities. In the fall, TJ returned to school in a self-contained first grade using an ABA model.

Although auditory skills had improved, visual self stimulatory behaviors were still present, and poor visual attending skills still prevented TJ from fully exploring toys or cutting on a line. Staff from The Holistic Learning Center referred TJ to Randy Schulman, MS, OD, FCOVD of Vision Works in Norwalk, Connecticut for a functional vision evaluation.

Dr. Schulman's initial evaluation findings are as follows:

Presenting issues squinting his eyes, light sensitivity, poor focus, difficulty making eye contact, and visually stimulatory behaviors.

Initial Optometric findings
- *Acuity* at distance was not possible to assess; acuity at near was 20/40 in both eyes. TJ exhibited very mild nearsightedness in both eyes, although refraction was difficult to assess.
- *Accommodative skills* were very poor. TJ had great difficulty getting objects clear at near such as written words on Bell retinoscopy; the reflex was a dull with motion.
- *Oculomotor skills* were inadequate. TJ was able to track an object with both eyes in all positions but ability to sustain tracking was very limited. Saccadic eye movements were jumpy and he exhibited poor fixation and limited eye contact.
- *Binocular testing* revealed significant difficulty converging as measured on the near point of convergence test. He exhibited a left exotropia or eye turn out on Hirschberg testing and could not hold fixation for with base in and base out measures at distance

and near using a prism bar. He also exhibited very limited stereoscopic depth perception. He did not respond to gross stereopsis as measured on the Stereo Butterfly, saw only one out of three animals and none of nine Wirt circles.

- *Visual motor integration and visual perceptual skills* such as *spatial organization* appeared delayed as well. On the Copy Forms Test TJ was only able to scribble on the paper. Observation of peg play revealed that he had great difficulty attempting the task; it was hard for him to get started. He was able to identify colors and shapes but had difficulty placing pegs accurately. During ball-on-string play, he demonstrated very limited tracking, limited attention and poor awareness of where the ball was in space, being unable to catch the ball with his hands.
- *Lens and prism probing* revealed improved visual skills while wearing glasses. Observations with lens and prism glasses revealed improved eye contact, better visual attention and better visual awareness.

Overall, at the initial visual evaluation TJ had good receptive language and limited use of expressive language. He toe walked, was very distractible and made many stimulatory behaviors with his hands. He made very limited eye contact and his left eye turned out often.

Conclusions TJ was experiencing significant difficulties with the following visual skills: fixation, saccadic and pursuit eye movements, accommodation or focusing skills, stereoscopic depth perception, and binocular or eye teaming skills. He also had inadequate visual motor and visual perceptual skills.

Recommendations An individualized in-office monthly vision therapy program was recommended with daily home-based support. A list of activities were given at each monthly visit and lens and prism glasses in loaner form were also prescribed for home and school for all concentrated visual tasks.

Follow Up After nine months TJ showed many improvements in many areas of his visual skills.

- *Acuity* at distance was 20/25 both eyes and acuity at near was 20/20 both eyes. He did not avoid cover of either eye.
- *Accommodative skills* were improved as observed on Bell retinoscopy. He exhibited a bright, albeit brief reflex at 14 inches.
- *Oculomotor skills* were also improved as TJ was able to track an object smoothly with both eyes in all positions, exhibit appropriate saccadic eye movements and sustained eye contact. He continued to have limited ability to sustain his pursuit eye movements.
- *Binocular testing* revealed that TJ still exhibited an intermittent left exotropia or eye turn out and had difficulty with convergence but eye teaming skills were significantly improved and he was able to get and keep the two eyes working together as a team some of the time as observed on testable prism bar findings. He exhibited base out and base in at distance of 10/4 and 12/4, respectively and base out and base in at near of 6/4 and 6/-, respectively. He responded to gross stereopsis as measured on the Stereo Butterfly, saw all three animals and five of nine Wirt circles.
- *Visual motor integration and spatial organization* were also slightly improved. TJ still was only able to scribble on the paper with a whole hand grasp high up on the pencil. On ball on string play he had limited tracking and still could not catch the ball; however, his attention and awareness were good. He also tended to look while catching better while wearing his lens and prism glasses.

TJ's expressive language skills have improved, although articulation is poor; receptive language is better. He continues to toe walk, albeit less. In therapy, he is quite focused on tasks, is rarely distracted, and makes very limited stimulatory behaviors with his hands.

His eye contact and visual attention are excellent, and he exhibits good compliance with therapeutic glasses.

As the report indicates, TJ's development over time is impressive. His skills in school have improved in several domains of development: cognitive, visual motor, gross and fine motor, and receptive and expressive vocabulary. In school, the use of reinforcement was used to increase TJ's compliance to wearing his lens and prism glasses, and his school tasks were modified to assist with visual attention, awareness of depth and distance, and to stimulate eye teaming skills. His occupational therapist modified tasks as well and designed specific activities to "drill" the necessary skills outline in Dr. Schulman's report. Collaboration between the various practitioners involved in TJ's care was crucial to a successful outcome in a relatively short period of time.

Lovaas and Discrete Trial Training

Lovaas Therapy or Discrete Trial Training (DTT) is a specific one-on-one intensive behavioral ABA teaching strategy that breaks down a complex skill set of behaviors into small, manageable tasks, according to a child's level of ability, and teaches these components sequentially. A discrete trial consists of an instruction or question to the child, the child's response, reinforcement, consequences, and prompting, followed by fading prompts, as necessary. [41]

DTT is a comprehensive, integrated program in which skills complement and build upon each other. The intervention progresses systematically through developmental stages, and is customized to meet the needs of each child and his/her family. If, for instance, a parent wishes a child to make a request, such as "I want to play," she first may teach the individual sounds of each word of the request, or label activities that fall into the category of "play." The goal is that the learner is gradually able to complete all subcomponent skills independently, and then link them together to enable mastery of the targeted complex and functional skill.

With discrete trial teaching, repetition of the target behavior provides multiple opportunities to "get it right" and associate the language of the direction with the expected appropriate behavior. This approach teaches young children how to learn because it requires attending, imitating and being socially responsive to an instructor. These pre-requisite behaviors become the foundation for future learning.

Recent Innovations in ABA Therapy

Initially, ABA programs for children with autism included any and all forms of "behavioral therapy." Some consider only Discrete Trial Teaching (DTT), where the curriculum focuses on a child learning basic communication, play, motor, and daily living skills, as true ABA.

While discrete trials are an essential element of ABA-based interventions, they are not the whole program. In recent years, the strict DTT approach has given way to more flexible treatments that are still based on the science of ABA. These programs alleviate some of the issues that caused criticism of DTT: that target skills are limited, DTT is primarily adult, not child initiated, and that edible reinforcers often contain colors, dyes, sugars, gluten or casein, to which many autistic children react negatively.

Good programs utilize many teaching approaches, all based on the principles of Applied Behavior Analysis. Programs continue to evolve as children progress and develop more complex social skills. Many of the newer ones place greater emphasis on the generalization and spontaneity of skills. Sometimes, therapists set up a specific environment in the clinic, so that learning in a given situation can generalize. They may also take therapy out of a clinical setting to more familiar environments, such as the playground, where a child is already interacting. Most importantly, GF/CF treats, playtime with a favorite toy or watching a video have replaced M+Ms, Cheerios and gummy worms as reinforcers.

Each of the following ABA methodologies identifies and focuses upon different behaviors, and applies a unique system of instruction.

- ***The Center for Autism and Related Disorders, Inc. (C.A.R.D.)*** is one of the largest organizations in the world providing treatment to children with Autism, PDD and Asperger's Syndrome. Doreen Granpeesheh, Ph.D., who studied with Dr. Lovaas at UCLA, is the Founder and Executive Director. She has dedicated over 25 years to the study and treatment of Autism Spectrum Disorders using ABA techniques.

CARD employs over 350 therapists worldwide, and has provided services to tens of thousands of children since opening its doors in 1990. At CARD, therapists develop unique and individualized behavioral programs based on each child's particular strengths and weaknesses. The goal is to teach all children the functional skills necessary to replace previously learned maladaptive behaviors, enabling them to live independent and productive lives.

CARD provides a variety of services:
- o ***Supervision and consultation*** for families approximately every three months
- o ***Direct 1:1 therapy*** in the home and school settings, providing individual behavior therapy and school shadowing
- o ***Workshops*** to serve families not living near a CARD location
- o ***Assessments*** for families suspecting that their child is showing symptoms of autism
- o ***Referrals*** to medical doctors for patients interested in pursuing biomedical treatment
- o ***District training and consultation*** to school district employees and Departments of Health and Education throughout the United States and abroad, re ABA theory and implementation
- o ***Parent training*** in behavior management
- o ***External collaboration*** with service providers, such as medical doctors or educators

CARD recommends one-on-one behavioral therapy initially in the home setting, and then generalized to other settings such as school. Instruction covers the following skills: speech and language, gross and fine motor, academic, self-care, and most importantly, socialization. Basic skills are taught in the first years and advanced social and language skills are taught in the final years.

CARD treatment starts between 20-59 months old, and is intensive: 20-40 hours per week, and continues for at least two years. A typical schedule, allowing variance depending on each child's particular symptoms and rapidity of learning is as follows:

	Services	Skills Taught
YEAR ONE	40 hours of 1:1 in-home behavioral intervention.	Simple compliance, self-help, motor imitation, receptive and expressive object and action labeling, simple requests, and basic toy manipulation.
YEAR TWO	5-10 hours of preschool with a CARD shadow targeting social skills, and 30-35 hours of 1:1 in-home intervention.	Complex skills including imaginary play, describing and complex language, emotion recognition, and basic cause and effect, with an emphasis on generalization.
YEAR THREE	15 hours of general education Kindergarten with a CARD shadow, and 20 hours of 1:1 in-home behavioral intervention.	Abstract skills such as reasoning and observational learning. Other areas include attention, behavior and social development.
YEAR FOUR	30 hours of attendance in general education First Grade, and 10-15 hours of in-home therapy.	The final treatment year focuses entirely on social skills and academic achievement in first grade. Typically, theory of mind and executive functioning skills, understanding cause and effect relationships, and comprehending social cues are the primary focus. Parent and teacher training to maintain gains after therapy is terminated.

Unique Characteristics of CARD

CARD is fully focused on the flexible, individualized treatment of each child, and inclusion of parents as an integral part of the treatment team. Regular monitoring and supervision is an essential component of each patient's program. The patient, parents and entire therapy team meet two to four times per month to discuss progress, modify the program, conduct parent training, and provide skill reinforcement to CARD therapy staff.

CARD insists upon frequent parent contact, collaboration with teachers and district representatives and regular meetings with adjunct therapy providers including occupational therapists, speech pathologists, dieticians, and physicians. CARD aggressively troubleshoots for those patients not progressing in the program. Each child's program is constantly monitored and adjusted in order to assure the best possible outcome.

CARD utilizes a comprehensive alternative communication program to ensure that nonvocal children have effective means of communication. This program incorporates the Picture Exchange Communication System (PECS) and an advanced reading/literacy program. CARD Supervisors are certified by Scientific Learning Corporation to provide and monitor the FastForWord program. (See Chapter 10.)

CARD is one of the most comprehensive ABA programs in the world. It is probably also the only one that is respectful of children's sensory needs. Most importantly, CARD strongly recommends that children in their programs work with health care professionals to ameliorate biomedical issues that interfere with function. For more information, go to <www.centerforautism.com> .

- **Pivotal Response Treatment (PRT)** is a variation of ABA that is the product of 20 years of research from Robert and Lynn Koegel PhD, co-founders of the Koegel Autism Research Center at the School of Education, University of California, Santa Barbara. PRT emerged to address the acquisition of complex skills that go beyond the basics.

PRT stresses functional communication over rote learning, by working with each child's natural motivations in natural learning opportunities. It targets and modifies communication/language, behavior, and social skills by capitalizing upon an individual child's idiosyncratic interests and obsessions.

PRT rewards children by creating less structured, playful opportunities to do more of what they already enjoy. For instance, in one study, therapists played a game of tag on a huge map. Because the child was a geography expert, he was motivated to move in the game from place to place. Increased social interactions he learned during the game of tag continued after the game ended.[42] In another study, children used more appropriate conversation following PRT training than with DTT.[43]

For more information on PRT read *Pivotal Response Treatments for Autism* by the Koegels[44] and go to <http://www.education.ucsb.edu/autism/index.html>.

- **TEACCH** is a result of the work of the late Eric Schopler, Ph.D., Psychology Professor at the University of North Carolina, Chapel Hill. The acronym stands for **T**reatment and **E**ducation of **A**utistic and Related **C**ommunication Handicapped **Ch**ildren. Schopler's heir and Director of UNC's Division TEACCH today is Gary Mesibov, Ph.D.

A less intensive form of ABA, the TEACCH philosophy embraces and accommodates, rather than remediates the "culture of autism," which it denotes as

- ***Relative strengths in and preferences for processing visual information*** (compared to difficulties with auditory processing, particularly of language)

- ***Strong attention to details*** with difficulty understanding the meaning of how those details fit together
- ***Difficulty combining and organizing ideas***, materials, and activities
- ***Difficulties with maintaining and shifting attention***
- ***Problems with pragmatic language***
- ***Difficulty with concepts of time***
- ***Routine driven*** with the result that disruptions in routines are upsetting
- ***Strong and rigid interests*** in favored activities
- ***Marked sensory preferences and dislikes***[45]

With TEACCH, children sit at workstations, and therapists reward them for completing activities such as matching tasks. The TEACCH program relies on small laminated squares with picture symbols on them depicting everything from locations in the classroom to curriculum materials and self-help skills. These "prompts" guide students through their days. The long-term goals of the TEACCH approach are both skill development and fulfillment of fundamental human needs such as dignity, engagement in productive and personally meaningful activities, and feelings of security, self-efficacy, and self-confidence.

Because those on the autism spectrum do well with these visual materials, the TEACCH conclusion is that vision is a strength. However, optometrists and others recognize that a majority of these "cultural" characteristics of autism relate to deficiencies in visual processing skills. This profound misunderstanding of vision frequently prevents students working in a TEACCH environment from receiving the vital visual intervention they require.

Any optometrists working in TEACCH territory, around Chapel Hill, NC, and in school systems using TEACCH, should consider attempting to educate practitioners how they might work together in the best interest of children with autism.

For more information on TEACCH, read *The TEACCH Approach to Autism Spectrum Disorders*,[46] and go to <www.teacch.com>.

- **Verbal Behavior** is a methodology designed by Vincent Carbone, Ed.D., Director of the Carbone Clinic in suburban New York City. Verbal Behavior places an emphasis on day-to-day activities and learning information in context. In Verbal Behavior, learning is functional. Verbal Behavior uses a systematic, highly structured teaching approach, that moves away from the traditional ABA and DTT by combining behavioral principles with the functionality and generalization of Floortime (see Chapter 11), to emphasize language development.

Like Floortime, Verbal Behavior uses children's own motivations for reinforcement by encouraging therapists to probe a child's skill level and fade prompts as quickly as possible. This technique allows for fast-paced learning and quick success, and permits the child to be more flexible and less rote, because of the variety of topics presented.[47]

The principles of Verbal Behavior are as follows:
1. All learners have the potential to develop skills beyond current levels and should be free of behaviors and activities that cause injury, pain, or limit opportunities for full social interaction and community involvement.

2. Communication and other skills that lead to rewarding personal relationships, well being, vocational productivity, and self-determined daily activities should be targeted.

3. Reliance on the evidenced-based literature of the science of applied behavior analysis and its underlying assumptions lead to the best possible learner outcomes.

4. Functional communication is the foundation that supports the development of skills in all areas. B.F. Skinner's analysis of verbal behavior and the supporting empirical work of Michael, Sundberg and Partington,[48,49,50] among others, lay the foundation for effective treatment strategies and success.

5. Reliable data, gathered and analyzed on a schedule sufficient to make informed decisions, is necessary to achieve the best outcomes for learners.[51]

Verbal Behavior therapists first conduct a Behavioral Language Assessment, then select the most appropriate form of communication for a child (vocal, signing, pointing to or exchanging pictures, or activating an augmentative device), and lastly select the communication responses and supporting skills that should be taught first.

Verbal behavior relies on a fast tempo and is peppered with many questions from both the adult and child. In order to reinforce correct answers and decrease frustration, therapists vary simple and difficult demands by a ratio of 80% easy to 20% hard. This ratio challenges children in areas of weakness, while allowing success. Carbone uses prompting and fading procedures, and his version of discrete trial training in both natural environments and during intensive teaching sessions to increase spontaneous language and to develop conversational skills. Videotaping is a technique upon which he relies heavily.

Dr. Carbone specializes in the assessment of children with language delays and disorders, and the clinical application of procedures for language acquisition. He also lectures worldwide on Verbal Behavior. Visit <www.drcarbone.net> for more information.

Summary
EEG Neurofeedback and Applied Behavior Analysis, two therapies based upon the science of operant conditioning, are very popular for children and adults of all ages, and on both ends of the autism spectrum. Using the brain's ability to process and change its behavior, those with attention deficits, learning difficulties, social skills problems and inappropriate behaviors are fitting in better. When these therapies are adjuncts to reducing total load factors, including toxicity, dietary issues, and sensory problems, including visual dysfunction, "recovery" may be a word that will be appropriate with increased frequency for those on the autism spectrum.

References
1. Hill RW, Castro E. Getting Rid of Ritalin. How Neurofeedback Can Successfully Treat Attention Deficit Disorder without Drugs. Charlottesville, VA: Hampton Roads Pub. Co., 2002:71.

2. Mann CA, Lubar JF, Zimmerman AW, Miller CA, Muenchen RA. Quantitative analysis of EEG in boys with attention-deficit/hyperactivity disorder: controlled study with clinical implications. Pediatr Neurol 1992;8:30-36.

3. Murias M, Webb SJ, Greenson J, Dawson G. Resting state cortical connectivity reflected in EEG coherence in individuals with autism. Biol Psychiatry 2007 Mar;62:270-73.

4. Ames G. Biofeedback and autism. New Visions Magazine 2006 Nov/Dec.

5. Larsen S. The Healing Power of Neurofeedback: The Revolutionary Lens Technique for Restoring Optimal Brain Function. Rochester, VT: Healing Arts Press, 2006.

6. Denckla MB, LeMay M., Chapman A. Few CT scan abnormalities found even in neurologically impaired learning disabled children. J Learn Disabil 1985; 18:132-35.

7. Robbins JA. Symphony in the Brain. New York: Grove Press, 1990:9.

8. Sterman MB, Friar L. Suppression of seizures in an epileptic following sensorimotor EEG feedback training. Electroencephalopgraphy Clin Neurophysiol 1972;33, 89-95.

9. Lubar JF, Shouse MN. EEG and behavioral changes in a hyperactive child concurrent training of the sensorimotor rhythm (SMR), a preliminary report. Biofeedback Self-Regulation 1976;1: 293-306.

10. Tansey MA, Bruner, RL. EMG and EEG biofeedback training in the treatment of a 10-year-old hyperactive boy with a developmental reading disorder. Biofeedback and Self Regulation 1984;2:1-23.

11. Fernandez T, Herrera W, Harmony T, Diaz-Comas L et al. *EEG and behavioral changes following neurofeedback treatment in learning disabled children. Clin Electroencephalogr 2003 Jul;34:145-52.*

12. Scolnick B. *Effects of electroencephalogram biofeedback with Asperger's syndrome. Int J Rehabil Res 2005 Jun;28:159-63.*

13. Jarusiewicz B. *Efficacy of neurofeedback for children in the autistic spectrum: A pilot study. J Neurotherapy 2002;6:39-49.*

14. Sichel AG, Fehmi G. Goldstein DM. *Positive outcome with neurofeedback treatment in a case of mild autism. J Neurotherapy Sum 1995;1:60-4.*

15. Rossiter TR, La Vaque TJ. *A comparison of EEG Biofeedback and psychostimulants in treating attention deficit/hyperactivity disorder. J Neurotherapy 1995;1.*

16. Rossiter TR. *The effectiveness of neurofeedback and stimulant drugs in treating AD/HD: part II. Replication. Appl Psychophysiol Biofeedback 2004;29:233-43.*

17. Spencer J. *EEG Biofeedback, an interview with Siegfried Othmer, Ph.D. Latitudes 1996;2:8-10.*

18. Othmer S. *The emerging frontier of neurofeedback. Latitudes 2003;6:13-16.*

19. Sears W, Thompson L. *The A.D.D. Book: New Understandings, New Approaches to Parenting Your Child. Boston, MA: Little Brown and Co., 1998.*

20. Sulzer-Azaroff B, Mayer R. *Behavior Analysis for Lasting Change. Fort Worth, TX: Holt, Reinhart & Winston, 1991.*

21. Baer D, Wolf M, Risley R. *Some current dimensions of applied behavior analysis. J Applied Behav Analy 1968;1:91-7.*

22. Lovaas OI. *Behavioral treatment and normal educational and intellectual functioning in young autistic children. J Consult Clin Psychol 1987;55:3-9.*

23. McEachin JJ, Smith T Lovaas OI *Long-term outcome for children with autism who received early intensive behavioral treatment. Am J Mental Retardation 1993;97:359-72.*

24. Sallows GO, Graupner TD. *Intensive behavioral treatment for children with autism. Four-year outcome and predictors. Am J Mental Retardation 2005;110:417-28.*

25. Cohen H, Amerine-Dickens M, Smith T. *Early intensive behavioral treatment: replication of the UCLA model in a community setting. J Dev Behav Pediatr 2006;27:145-55.*

26. Howard JS, Sparkman CR, Cohen HG, Green G, Stanislaw H. *A comparison of intensive behavior analytic and eclectic treatments for young children with autism. Res Dev Disabil 2005;26:359-83.*

27. Kahng SW, Iwata BA, Lewin AB. *Behavioral treatment of self-injury, 1964 to 2000. Am J Mental Retardation 2002;107:212 21.*

28. Ahearn WH, Clark KM, DeBar R, Florentino CJ.. *On the role of preference in response competition. Appl Behav Anal 2005;38:247-50.*

29. Hagopian LP, Fisher WW, Sullivan MT, Acquisto J. *Effectiveness of functional communication training with and without extinction and punishment: J Appl Behav Anal 1998;31:211-35.*

30. Hupp SD, Reitman, D, Northup, J, O'Callaghan P, et al. *The effects of delayed rewards, tokens, and stimulant medication on sportsmanlike behavior with ADHD-diagnosed children. Behav Modification, 2002;26:148-62.*

31. Boyajian AE, DuPaul GJ, Handler MW, Eckert TL et al. *The use of classroom-based brief functional analyses with preschoolers at-risk for attention deficit hyperactivity disorder. School Psychol Rev 2001; 30:278-93.*

32. Horner RH, Carr EG, Strain PS, Todd AW et al. *Problem behavior interventions for young children with autism: A research synthesis. J Autism Dev Dis 2002;32:423-46.*

33. www.centerforautism.com (Accessed March 18, 2007).

34. Matson O, Benavidez JL, Compton DA, Paclawskyj LS, et al. *Behavioral treatment of autistic persons: A review of research from 1980 to the present. Res Dev Dis 1996;17:433-65.*

35. Rimland B. *The ABA Controversy. Autism Research Review International, 1999. 13:3.*

36. www.polyxo.com *Teaching Children with Autism: Applied Behavior Analysis. (Accessed July 25,2007)*

37. Wolf M, Risley T, Mees HL. *Application of operant conditioning procedures to the behavior problems of an autistic child. Behav Res Ther 1964;1:305-12.*

38. Eikeseth S, Smith T, Jahr E, Eldevik S. *Intensive behavioral treatment at school for 4-7-year-old children with autism: A 1-year comparison controlled study. Behav Modification 2002;26:49-68.*

39. Granpeesheh D. *Bringing Applied Behavioral Analysis Therapy and Biomedical Treatments Together. Presentation at Autism Vancouver Biennial conference. March 2, 2007. Vancouver, BC, Canada.*

40. Zier A, Hoehne K. *Bridging Sensory Processing Theory and Practice with Discrete Trial Teaching.* New Developments Newsletter 1998;6:4.

41. www.lovaas.com (Accessed July 26, 2007)

42. Baker M, Koegel RL, Koegel LK. *Increasing social behavior of young children with autism using their obsessive behaviors.* Jrl Assoc persons severe handicaps 1998;23:300-8.

43. Koegel RL, Camarta S, Koegel L, Ben-Tall A, et al. *.Increasing speech intelligibility in children with autism.* J Autism Dev Dis 1998;28:241-51.

44. Koegel LK, Koegel RL. *Pivotal Response Treatments For Autism.* Baltimore MD: Brookes Publishing company, 2006.

45. www.teacch.com (Accessed July 28, 2007)

46. Mesibov G, Shea V, Schopler E. *The TEACCH Approach to Autism Spectrum Disorders.* New York NY: Springer, 2004.

47. www.stopthatbehavior.com (Accessed July 31, 2007)

48. Sundberg ML, Michael J. *The benefits of Skinner's analysis of verbal behavior for children with autism.* BehavModification, 2001;25:698-724.

49. Sundberg ML, Michael J, Partington, JW, Sundberg, CA. *The role of automatic reinforcement in early language acquisition. The Analysis of Verbal Behavior* 1996:13:21-38.

50. Sundberg M L, Partington JW. *Teaching Language To Children With Autism Or Other Developmental Disabilities.* Danville, CA: Behavior Analysts, Inc., 1998.

51. www.drcarbone.ne (Accessed July 31, 2007)

Chapter 15
Healing with Animals
Patricia S. Lemer, MEd, NCC

In July, 2007 police arrested a Ventura, CA man on suspicion of stealing and torturing Bob, a 42-pound pet tortoise. Bob is the "special friend" of six-year-old William Sullivan, a boy with autism who is wary of talking to people. William freely chats with 25-year-old Bob who grunts, whistles and croaks in response. Bob is recovering after receiving treatment at an animal rehabilitation center, where they are doing everything in their power to get him back to his owner.[1]

Colorado occupational therapist Lois Hickman, MS, OTR, FAOTA, has a chicken that shies away from people on her farm. A 10-year-old boy with articulation difficulties and Asperger syndrome, whom Hickman treats for sensory processing problems, also has difficulty interacting with others. These two unlikely friends connected when the boy named the chicken after his beloved music therapist, declaring one day at school that, "My chicken's name is Judith." Two goals accomplished: social connectedness and intelligible speech!

"Each of the animals on my farm has taught me a little of what naturalist Loren Eiseley meant when he said that we never truly know ourselves until we find ourselves 'reflected in eyes other than human.'[2] Every animal is special. They aren't simply chickens or ducks or pigs or goats or cats or dogs or rabbits. They are, each of them, both members of the flock and uniquely themselves. And, I think to myself, each of the humans who lives on this farm, and each one who visits, becomes more compassionate through the caring human-animal interactions that happen here."[3]

Research shows that both normally developing children[4] and children with autism[5] exhibit natural interests toward animals. "People and animals are supposed to be together. We spent quite a long time evolving together, and we used to be partners," says Temple Grandin, Ph.D., arguably the most famous living adult with autism. Grandin believes that the bond between animals and those with autism is even stronger than for other people. "Animals are like autistic savants. (They) have special talents normal people don't, the same way autistic people have special talents normal people don't. Autistic people can think the way animals think. Autism is like a kind of way station on the road from animals to human, which puts autistic people like me in a perfect position to translate animal talk into English."[6]

According to Grandin, animals and people with autism share two traits of interest to optometrists: the ability to "think in pictures" and a "hyper-specificity" to visual details. The ability to use pictorial communication is also attributed to dolphins. According to Bobby Matherne, dolphins "spizualize" or "speak-visualize" by "bouncing high frequency sounds off their surroundings, converting the echoed waves into visual information, and using the 3-D images as a real-time map to navigate in dark waters of the sea. Those echoed waves are sounds in the same frequency range that the dolphin can both hear and speak, so by speaking the sounds of something they see (or saw earlier), dolphins can communicate where they are located to someone who is distant from them by many miles or they can equally communicate a situation from some earlier time to those present now. The hearers will be enveloped in the image created by the dolphin speaker as if they were inside of a holographic image, which indeed they would be. Just as humans communicate by speaking the sounds they heard someone else say, dolphins would be able to communicate the images some other dolphin had shared with them."[7]

Making the ability to think in pictures and be acutely aware of visual details into assets, rather than liabilities, has allowed Grandin to apply her talents to her successful career as an animal scientist. Focusing on these gifts on a larger scale has also motivated individuals in a variety of professions to pair individuals with autism with horses, dogs, dolphins and a myriad of other animals, with the result of benefiting both man and beast.

Most of the research in this area involves occupational therapists. One pilot investigation in the Roanoke, VA public schools compared outcomes for 22 children age seven to 13 with autism receiving two forms of occupational therapy (OT): school-based traditional techniques, and OT incorporating animals. Both groups participated in activities targeting proprioceptive, tactile, vestibular and sensory-motor function, as well as those designed to enhance language and social interaction. In addition, those receiving animal therapy interacted in a variety of ways with llamas, dogs and rabbits, in such activities as riding, brushing, feeding, petting and stroking the animals. Results showed that children whose therapy incorporated animals showed significantly greater use of language and social interaction than those receiving standard OT techniques.[8]

This chapter focuses on several therapies resulting from the animal/autism bond.
- **Hippotherapy**, or therapeutic horseback riding;
- **Dolphin Assisted therapy**, or swimming with dolphins, and
- **Service dogs** for autism

Together these therapies address the core deficits for those on the autism spectrum: sensory processing issues, language, social-emotional and behavioral problems, all in a recreational milieu that is neither threatening nor competitive. Children appear to enjoy the activities immensely, and benefits are observable.

Hippotherapy

Therapeutic horseback riding is an intervention that uses the multidimensional movement of a horse to address sensory processing and other issues in those with autism spectrum disorders. Derived from the Greek word "hippos," meaning horse, hippotherapy translates as "therapy with the help of a horse." Classical hippotherapy, based on a medical model, originated in Germany and Switzerland, and emphasized postural alignment and symmetry.

In the United States, hippotherapy may also include vaulting, which combines gymnastics and dance on a moving horse. Hippotherapy is practiced by specially trained physical, occupational and speech therapists who combine classical principles with those of neuro-motor function, sensory integration therapy (see Chapter 7), and with other programs, such as RDI (see Chapter 11) and TEACCH (see Chapter 14).[3]

An Historical Overview Health care practitioners recognized the therapeutic benefits of the horse as early as 460 BC. Little is known about early practices. The use of the horse as therapy quickly spread throughout Europe, the United States and Canada in the 1960's. While therapeutic riding has been used since the early 1950s as a tool for improving the lives of individuals with disabilities, prior to the 1980s, no studies supporting its efficacy are known.[9]

The first published scientific investigation evaluating behavioral changes in children with autism did not take place until 1997. Two children with autism diagnoses participating in therapeutic riding an hour a week for eight weeks showed a decrease in echolalic speech and self-stimulatory behaviors, as well as an increase in appropriate interactions.[10]

A more recent study with 12 participants age four through 10, diagnosed with PDD-NOS and autism, evaluated the impact of combining therapeutic horseback riding with sensory-based activities, such as therapeutic listening, tactile, proprioceptive and vestibular activities on auditory processing skills. Examiners conducted pre- and post-testing using *The Sensory Profile*, a standardized instrument that assesses sensory processing, modulation and behavioral responses based upon parent/caretaker observations, using a Likert scale.[11] After including therapeutic horseback riding once a week for 10 weeks, the experimental group showed more improvement in all areas than the group receiving the sensory interventions alone.[12]

While not conclusive, because it relied on parental/caretaker observations and expectations, the study's results are encouraging. Several participants continued the riding therapy, and one even requested that therapeutic riding be a part of the occupational therapy program in her child's Individualized Education Plan (IEP).

Temple Grandin, who has always had a special connection to animals, reports that her love of horses really helped her get through her special high school boarding school for kids with "emotional" problems. Looking back at her experiences, she notes that many of the horses, like the students, also had serious psychological problems. The school's owner had been able to buy them cheaply because of their bad behavior. Ironically, the "emotionally disturbed" kids were able to connect with horses that no one else could reach.

Grandin believes that horses are especially good for teenagers. A psychiatrist she knows found that if you take two troubled teens with similar issues and the same degree of severity, and one of them rides regularly, the rider will do better psychologically than the non-rider. She thinks this is because the teen looking after and riding a horse is learning about responsibility and relationship building.[6]

What Happens in Hippotherapy? Participants groom, dress, ride, care for and love their horses, but do not control their horses' movements. The horse's walk provides sensory input through movement which is variable, rhythmic and repetitive, moving the rider's body in a manner similar to the movement patterns of human walking.

According to the owner of one stable, "a horse's movement has the potential to mitigate sensory integration issues. A smooth-gaited, consistently paced horse can provide the input needed to help a rider establish rhythm. A rough-gaited horse may provide the stimulation needed to help organize and integrate sensory input. Movement exploration while on the horse can help improve overall body awareness. The variability of the horse's gait enables the therapist to monitor sensory input to elicit appropriate adaptive responses from the client."[13]

Through adapting to the horse's movements, the rider develops better balance and coordination,[14] and then generalizes function to areas such as more independence, leading to improved performance in a wide range of daily activities. Therapists' goals do not focus on specific riding skills, but rather on establishing the neurological foundations for improved function and sensory processing. Activities take place in a controlled environment.

Each facility has its own style. Deborah Kohn, a therapist working at Winslow Therapeutic Riding Unlimited in Warwick, NY, in 1996, adapted the TEACCH approach to work with her students. Children used visual schedules to assist with putting on their helmets, mounting and riding their horses.[15] To see what is happening at Winslow today, go to <www.winslow.org>.

At Hidden Hollow Farms in Milan, NY, Stephanie Fitzpatrick works with an occupational therapist to set therapeutic goals for each child. Some children ride the horses; others groom, walk and control them without ever mounting. Her barn is a training center for the NY Special Olympics. To find out about her programs call 845-758-0619.

Who are Candidates? Specially trained therapists evaluate individuals with almost any disability to determine whether hippotherapy is appropriate. Those with global developmental delays, autism, attention deficits and learning/language disabilities, cerebral palsy and traumatic brain injury can all benefit from therapeutic riding, vaulting, competition and other purposeful, safe and supervised interaction with equines.

What are the outcomes of Hippotherapy? This intervention improves balance, flexibility, posture, muscle strength, mobility and overall physical function by providing proprioceptive, vestibular, tactile, visual, auditory and olfactory stimuli that are beneficial to the rider.[16] Caring for and riding a horse is especially helpful in improving organizational skills in those with autism spectrum disorders.[17] The unique relationship formed with the horse can also increase confidence, patience and self-esteem, and affect other psychological, cognitive, behavioral and communication skills for clients of all ages.

More information Contact the North American Riding for the Handicapped Association (NARHA), founded in 1969 to promote and support therapeutic riding in the United States and Canada. NAHRA has accredited over 600 therapeutic riding centers to ensure high quality and safe instruction. NARHA holds an annual conference and workshops on a variety of topics and advocates to increase awareness of therapeutic riding and other equine facilitated therapy and activities.

Dolphin Assisted Therapy

Most people like dolphins; most dolphins like people. People think of dolphins as loveable, playful animals that appear on television, in movies and in shows at sea parks. Until we can communicate better with these creatures, we don't know how they perceive us. What we do know is that dolphins are among the most intelligent of all creatures, and their bodies are true sensory processing machines.

One of the unique characteristics of dolphins is their exceptional ability to emit and use sound and its echoes (SONAR) to communicate and navigate their environment. Since the use of ultrasound has gained progressive popularity in departments of Physical Medicine and Rehabilitation throughout the United States and Europe since the early 1950s,[18] using dolphins as ultrasound therapy machines is a natural! The variable modulation of the ultrasound frequencies that dolphins emit is thought to contribute to the release of tissue and membrane restrictions in the water, where gravity is not in play.[19]

Laboratory studies confirm that vision, as well as taste and touch are important information sources for the dolphin.[20] Dolphins can attend to and interpret human gestures, follow the direction in which a human is pointing, monitor rapidly occurring visual symbols appearing on a television screen and report the occurrence of certain key symbols, and easily recognize the same objects across the senses of vision and echolocation.[21] Dolphins can see equally well both underwater and in air. Dolphin eyes are laterally placed, providing a wide field of view enabling the dolphin to see forward, sideways, and even behind them. Also, unlike human eyes, the dolphins' eyes work independently, allowing them to have one eye see underwater while the other sees in air.[22]

An Historical Overview Throughout history, humans have been fascinated by dolphins. The ancient Greeks revered them so, that they dedicated their most sacred temple, the oracle at Delphi, to them. In Greek, the root meaning of "dolphin" is "the womb of all."[23]

Dolphins have been reported to save people from drowning, guide ships, take children to school in ancient Greece, fish with fisherman, and most recently, escort a castaway boy on an inner-tube at sea, drifting from Cuba to the United States. No one knows whether these are myths or the truth. Nonetheless, dolphins have an impeccable reputation!

Dolphins as therapists, or dolphin assisted therapy (DAT), began with the founding of the World Dolphin Foundation in the early 1970s. Dr. Hank Truby, a linguist and acoustic phonetician, began working with Dr. John Lilly, a scientist who was attempting to teach English to dolphins. In 1973, these two men took two boys with autism to play with the dolphins at the Miami Seaquarium.

To everyone's astonishment, these children with very limited attention spans immediately established a close rapport with the dolphins. The boys fed the dolphins and played water games with them, cooperating for over an hour. Gradually, others became intrigued by these results, including Dr. Betsy Smith, an educational anthropologist, who noticed the therapeutic effects of dolphins on her disabled brother. [24]

David E. Nathanson, Ph.D is credited with popularizing dolphin assisted therapy. A licensed psychologist, he treated hundreds of individuals with disabilities, including over 450 with autism, at his facility in Key Largo, FL, until hurricanes forced him to close in 2006. He still maintains a website at <www.dolphinhumantherapy.com>.

One of the world's experts on dolphin therapy is Dr. Michael Hyson, Research Director at the Sirius Institute in Hawaii, a human-dolphin habitat where people live closely with the dolphins and they learn from and communicate with each other. There scientists study the nature of the "dolphin effect" on autism, brain trauma, and other conditions.

Hyson has provided much of the information for this section through his website at <www.planetpuna.com>. His involvement with dolphins began when he read John Lilly's works as a child and was privileged to be with dolphins in Texas for a summer when he was 14. Dolphins have been part of his life ever since. Later, at the University of Miami, pursuing degrees in neuroscience, he met and worked with Dr. Truby on the Dolphin Project of the World Dolphin Foundation which Dr. Truby and his team created.

Other DAT programs operate in Florida and elsewhere. At the Upledger Institute's Ruth M. Smith Dolphin-Assisted Therapy intensive programs in Freeport, Grand Bahama Island, select teams of CranioSacral therapists work together in four-day intensive programs designed to address the specific health concerns of individuals with medical and other conditions, including autism.

Participants spend each day in multiple-therapist sessions both in the water where dolphins are present and free to interact with the group, and on land. Working in water limits the effects of gravity. Therapists find that the dolphins' innate ability to scan a person's body allows them to detect and release bodily restrictions, which the CranioSacral therapist can feel. The dolphin and the therapist become a rehabilitation team. At times they defer to a dolphin's decision regarding where and when to approach a client, as the dolphin's scanning ability provides the more accurate image of the tissues than the therapist's palpation skills. For more on CranioSacral therapy, refer back to Chapter 3. For more information on the Upledger program go to <www.upledger.com>.

What Happens in Dolphin Assisted Therapy? Generally an individual swims with dolphins and has on-land lessons. Details vary with the condition being treated. The swims can occur for an hour, a day, over several days to weeks. Consistently, dolphins treat humans with complete and utter respect.

Dr. Nathanson believes that current DAT is too structured, if included as part of behavioral programs that use dolphins as positive reinforcement. This approach limits the time clients have in the water with the dolphins and forces the animals to perform stereotypical behaviors on cue, which, in turn, minimizes the chance the dolphins can interact spontaneously.

His approach is to let humans become friends with the dolphins by allowing as much time as possible in the water with them over as many days as possible.[25]

What Are the Positive Outcomes of DAT? The JF2 Dolphin Therapy Project at Florida's Gulfararium in Fort Walton Beach, is the culmination of many years of research focusing on decreasing response time and increasing expressive communication skills by speech-language pathologist, Dr. Janet Flowers. She has children complete 10 dolphin assisted therapy sessions. Parents and classroom teachers of participating children considered time on task, motivation and communication skills to be the key areas of growth during their child/student's dolphin assisted therapy experience. Children in her studies exhibit

- increases from 25% to 250% in time on task
- significant increases in mean length of utterance as well as in the complexity of expressive skills
- greater long term retention than six months of conventional therapy, and is also more cost effective than conventional therapy.[26]

Flowers believes that having a positive emotional experience during therapy increases a child's motivation and confidence, and also enhances long-term memory. Her experience is that a dolphin's unconditional acceptance of a child with a disability in a safe environment provides exceptional motivation to overcome obstacles and increase confidence.

An objective of the JF2 Dolphin Project is to achieve greater results than traditional therapy in specific behaviors related to: attention span, communication, speech, language, gross or fine motor skills, and academics, as well as other areas. The program motivates and "jump starts" a child, complements and reinforces therapy, and provides a stimulating reward. The achievements a child makes with dolphin therapy also assist other professionals, who may be working with the child. She concludes that human-dolphin therapy is a cost efficient program that achieves long term retention of learned skills by qualified students. For more information on this program, go to <http://www.gulfarium.com/jfdolphin.htm>.

Scientists have conducted few controlled experiments on using dolphin therapy with individuals with autism, so our understanding of this interaction is still quite rudimentary, especially in relation to what aspects of dolphin behavior affects changes in humans. Results such as those above are based on anecdotal evidence. However, most show at least some short term improvement, and lasting specific effects. Some hug their parents for the first time; some say their first words soon after dolphin contact. Learning takes place more quickly.[27] These outcomes show that dolphins are capable of profoundly benefiting those with even severe disabilities.

Who Are Candidates for DAT? Anyone with or without a disability is a candidate for dolphin assisted therapy. Just like a therapeutic massage can be deeply healing, DAT benefits sensory, psychological and cognitive functioning through touch, affection and love. Being with the dolphins can also be a deeply spiritual experience. Many individuals who swim with dolphins have experience profound transformations.

The Future of Dolphin Assisted Therapy Dolphins are complex creatures and our knowledge of them far from complete. Most in the field believe that dolphin therapy is still at an early stage of development; many factors remain to be understood, especially how the sensory rich environment produced by the dolphins contributes to the therapy and human-dolphin interaction. While similar therapy using horses or dogs shows positive results, what part of the results of DAT is unique to dolphins? With increased experience, knowledge, better communication and communion with the dolphins, therapeutic results will-most certainly improve and expand. On-going research is of utmost importance.

Autism Service Dogs

"Man's best friend" can be invaluable in the lives of individuals of all ages and abilities. A dog or other pet can make a huge difference in the quality of life for the elderly.[28] "Seeing-eye" dogs have helped those with limited sight for decades. More recently, well-trained service dogs have become trusted companions and are providing a wide range of services for individuals with disabilities, including hearing impairments, social disabilities, mobility limitations and autism. These dogs can make substantial improvement in the quality of the lives of those they serve.

Service dogs for autism provide the opportunity for those on the spectrum to access a variety of environments safely. Added benefits are an increase in mobility, socialization, independence and autonomy. The dog serves as a positive social link to home, school and the community. In most cases the dog accompanies the child at all times, including to school. The animal's presence calms the child, reduces emotional outbursts, and provides a sense of security to both the child and the family.

Agencies that can Help Finding a good match between a family and an agency, and between a dog and a child, requires time and some research. Agencies work with families to find funds for the service dog, either through fund-raising or other means. Here are a few well-respected resources.

- *4 Paws* was the first agency to begin placing skilled Autism Assistance Dogs and continues to be the largest organization in the United States. Their mission is to enrich the lives of people with a variety of disabilities by training and placing service animals for companionship and to promote independent living. 4 Paws specializes in "hard-to-place individuals who may have been turned away by other agencies." All that is required is that a child's physician approves the home as a safe place for a dog.

4 Paws Families has an online membership group of over 100 families who either have a dog, or are in the process of obtaining a service dog from the agency. For more go to <http://www.4pawsforability.org/autismdogs.htm>.

- *Autism Service Dogs of America (ASDA)* is a non-profit organization based in Oregon. Priscilla Taylor founded it in 2002 and directs it today. This special educator recognized that placement of a dog with a child with autism enables both the child individually and the family as a unit.

ASDA provides uniquely trained Golden retrievers, Labrador retrievers and Golden Lab mixes to children living with autism and their families. Those dogs selected for the ASDA program are specifically trained and nurtured as soon as they enter the program. Service dog training continues while the dogs are in puppy-raising foster care homes. When dogs are approximately 20 months old they are returned to the Autism Service Dog program trainer for advanced service dog training. Upon completion of basic training dogs are matched to a child.

To ensure successful matches ASDA carefully screens applicant families for whether the child will benefit from a service dog. If a placement seems appropriate, ASDA provides a week of intensive training for a parent, followed by a week of training in the home with the parent, child and dog, and the integration of the service dog into the family.

The full cost to breed, raise and train an ASDA assistance dog can range from $15,000 to $20,000; the ASDA service, training and equipment fee is $13,500. To learn more, go to <www.autismservicedogsofamerica.com.>

National Service Dogs is an agency in Canada that has been training Labrador and Golden retrievers to assist children and families living with autism since 1996. They have established the following criteria to obtain the best results in placing dogs:

- *o* The child with autism is between the ages of two and eight at the time of application
- *o* The child has had previous positive exposure to large dogs
- *o* The home has no other family dog and a fenced yard
- *o* The family devotes time to understanding how to add a service dog into their lives
- *o* One or both parents is willing to travel without the child to the training facility for an one day pre-placement seminar, and for five days when receiving the dog
- *o* For pre-school children, one parent, not multiple caregivers, should stay home with the child and dog to promote bonding

Canadian residents should go to <www.nsd.on.ca> to learn about National Service Dogs. This site also has some wonderful stories about how dogs have enriched the lives of children with autism.

This story extrapolated from the "4 Paws" website tells it all. Autism service dogs can make a huge difference in the quality of life for a child with autism.

Noah has autism and is in second grade in a large public school. The school administration was very reluctant to have a dog in school. However, after a meeting with the School Board and Superintendent, they finally agreed upon a trial with Noah's dog, Harry, along with careful data keeping.

At the 30-day-review, Noah's incidents of escaping from staff decreased from 15-20 times per day to zero - except for the day he learned to take Harry's harness off! In August Noah was also averaging over 100 aggressive acts (pinching, hitting or kicking) per day towards staff, and that number fell to 10-20.

Harry was the only intervention during the trial period - so there was no arguing that he was the reason for the drastic turnaround. The IEP team kept saying they couldn't believe how smooth of a transition Harry made into the school day and they were all amazed at how well trained and gentle he is. After the first few weeks the 900+ kids acted like Harry was just another student. The only issue has been with Physical Education, because Harry gets pretty excited when the balls start flying.

The main goal in getting Harry was Noah's safety and behavior. Everyone during the meeting commented on how much calmer Noah was during the school day when he was with Harry. He has also started to interact more with his peers, initiates and returns greetings spontaneously, and is more willing to participate.

Harry has definitely made a huge difference for Noah in a few short weeks. The school has a Hero Award board for staff members and Harry received the sweetest award for his hard work. Everyone who works with Noah just loves Harry and the peace of mind he brings when he's tethered to Noah. They are finally able to focus more on academics and less on behaviors.

Cathy Foust
St. Peters MO

Summary and Conclusions

More and more support for using animals to heal those on the autism spectrum is becoming available each year. Whether therapy is with dogs, horses, dolphins, tortoises, chickens, ducks, rabbits, or other furry creatures, humans of all ages can benefit.

As the present epidemic of individuals with autism inspires a search for ways to maximize function, the strong bond between man and beast makes animal therapies truly a "natural" alternative. Further research will be helpful in better understanding the sensory processing, social-emotional and communication benefits animal therapies have to offer.

References

1. http://www.sciencedaily.com/upi/index.php?feed=Quirks&article=UPI-1-20070720-15052000-bc-us-tortoise.xml (Accessed September 29, 2007)

2. Eiseley LC. The unexpected universe. Orlando, FL: Harcourt Brace, 1969:24.

3. Henry DA, Sava DI. Sensory Tools for Pets: Animals and people helping each other. Goodyear, AZ: Henry Occupational Services, Inc., 2006:19, 25.

4. Melson GF. Child development and the human-companion animal bond. Am Behav Sci 2003;47:31-39.

5. Martin F, Farnum J. Animal-assisted therapy for children with pervasive developmental disorders. Western J Nurs Res 2002;26:657-70.

6. Grandin T. Animals in Translation. New York, NY: Scribner, 2005:6-8.

7. http://www.doyletics.com/arj/starthro.htm. (Accessed October 7, 2007)

8. Sams MJ, Fortney EV, Willenbring S. Occupational therapy incorporating animals for children with autism: a pilot investigation. J Am Occup Ther Assoc2006;60:268-74.

9. DePauw K. Horseback riding for individuals with disabilities: programs, philosophy and research. Adapt Phys Act Qtly 1986;3:217-26.

10. Tolson Pl Therapeutic horseback riding and behavior change in children with autism: a single subject study. In: Engel B, ed. Rehabilitation with the aid of a horse: a collection of studies. Durango, CO: B. Engel Therapy Services, 1997:15-23.

11. Dunn W. The Sensory Profile Users Manual, San Antonio, TX: The Psychological Corporation, 1997.

12. Stoner J. Riding high: a new study shows promise for kids with autism. Advance Occup Ther 2004;20:42.

13. www.highhopestr.org What is therapeutic riding? (Accessed September 29, 2007)

14. Biery, MJ, Kauffman, N. The effects of therapeutic horseback riding on balance. Adapt Phys Act Qtly 1989;6:221-29.

15. Kohn D. Medical considerations for therapeutic riding. NARHA Strides 1996;2:6.

16. Shkedi A. Sensory input through riding. Proceedings for the 7th International Therapeutic Riding Congress, Aarhus, Denmark 1991:129-32.

17. Hubbard S. Sensory integration as a frame of reference for the practice of hippotherapy with pediatric clientele. In: Engel B, ed. Therapeutic riding strategies for instruction. Durango, CO: B. Engel Therapy Services, 1997:273-84.

18. http://www.ob-ultrasound.net/therapy.html. (Accessed October 14, 2007)

19. Bourne RA, Mercurio R. Dolphin-assisted therapy opens new vistas in cranioSacral therapy. Massage & Bodywork Magazine 1997:83-86.

20. Pack AA,.Herman LM. Sensory integration in the bottlenosed dolphin: Immediate recognition of complex shapes across the senses of echolocation and vision. J Acoust Soc Am 1995;98:722-33.

21. Pack AA,.Herman LM. The dolphin's (Tursiops truncatus) understanding of human gaze and pointing: Knowing what and where. J Comp Psychol 2007;121:34-45.

22. www.dophin-institute.org (Accessed October 8, 2007)

23. Hyson M. Dolphins, Therapy and Autism, 2003. http://www.planetpuna.com (Accessed October 7, 2007)

24. http://www.henryspink.org/dolphin_therapy.htm 99Accessed October 7, 2007)

25. www.dolphinhumantherapy.com (Accessed October 7, 2007)

26. Nathanson DE, de Castro D, Friend H, McMahon M. Effectiveness of short-term dolphin assisted therapy for children with severe disabilities. Anthrozoos 1997;10:90-100.

27. Nathanson D.E.. Long term effectiveness of dolphin assisted therapy for children with severe disabilities. Anthrozoos 1998;11:22-32.

28. www.petsfortheelderly.org (Accessed October 7, 2007)

Chapter 16
The Autism Protocol of Dietrich Klinghardt
Contributers: Dietrich Klinghardt, MD, PhD
with Elizabeth Hesse-Sheehan, DC, CCN

Editor's note:

Dietrich Klinghardt MD, PhD is "a kind and gentle spirit who is authentically motivated to provide the most foundational treatments for patients to resolve their illnesses at the deepest level." [1]

Klinghardt is in agreement with the concept of an autism spectrum. In addition to those diagnoses included in this book, he suggests adding allergies, atopic skin diseases, asthma and seizure disorders, to the list of conditions that have similar causes, and are thus responsive to similar treatment strategies.

The Etiology of Autism

Klinghardt believes that autism is a man-made condition, and is therefore preventable. He states unequivocally that autism is not multi-factorial. It has a single cause: mercury toxicity. All problems: nutritional, metabolic, immunological, behavioral, emotional, gastro-intestinal, etc. can be explained by the evils of mercury. The occurrence and severity of autism is directly related to toxic exposure in an individual with inadequate genes that code for detoxification.

The role of mercury toxicity is central in autism.[2] Depending upon an individual's vulnerability, a single molecule is enough to cause significant destruction. NO amount of mercury is safe. At levels as low as less than a nanogram, both ethyl and methyl mercury can cause autism by destroying tubulin, the most abundant protein in the brain.

Mercury interacts with brain tubulin and disassembles microtubules that maintain neuronal structure. Tubulin destruction disconnects the body from higher levels of intelligence. If tubulin isn't working, no systems can function well. Antibodies to tubulin are present and elevated in autism, thus signaling the presence of mercury. Studies in rats have shown that doses of mercury corresponding to those seen in humans can cause a 75% increase in tubulin inhibition.[3]

Klinghardt calls the mercury exposure to those with autism a "triple strike injury." He blames three main sources

1. ***A mother's environment and mercury burden before pregnancy*** From conception, a woman accumulates mercury in her body. Swedish studies show that mothers use their unborn babies as "garbage disposals," dumping an estimated two-thirds of their body burdens of mercury and other toxins into their first children.[4] That could be why many first pregnancies result in miscarriages. Later children have less accumulation of toxins. A classic study done in Texas showed that the incidence of high levels of mercury content in the soil is identical geographically to high incidence of autism.[5] Klinghardt strongly recommends that every woman undergo a metal detoxification program well before becoming pregnant. His paper "Advice to Expectant and New Parents" is available on his website, <www.neuraltherapy.com>.

2. ***Mercury in vaccines and other medical products*** Using thimerosal as a preservative in vaccines was clearly an extremely bad idea. Klinghardt believes that introducing the thimerosal containing Hepatitis B vaccine to the childhood vaccine schedule in the late

1980s, adding mercury to rhogam, and mandating a more aggressive vaccine schedule, have combined to put American children at great risk.

3. ***Mercury in amalgam fillings*** Mothers with multiple "silver" fillings in their mouths also put their unborn babies at risk. These fillings off-gas and the mercury vapor crosses the placental barrier.

Surprisingly, Klinghardt believes that exposure to mercury in fish presents minimal risk because the high essential fatty acids, selenium, amino acids and peptides in fish are protective. He feels that it is better to eat fish with mercury than not to eat fish at all. He cautions, however to eat only fresh, small fish, which are at the lower end of the food chain. Go to <www.mercola.com> for a list of safe fish. Unfortunately, sardines in cans lined with plastic outgas phthylates which are dangerous to the nervous system.

Toxic metals, especially mercury, harm the cells of the body, and create breeding grounds for opportunistic harmful micro-organisms to thrive in their favorite milieu, a heavy metal environment. Klinghardt's research shows that micro-organisms tend to set up their housekeeping in those body compartments that have the highest pollution from toxic metals. Virtually any illness seems to be caused by or exacerbated by a chronic infection.[6]

Micro-organisms multiply and thrive undisturbed in areas where the body's own immune cells are incapacitated. The teeth, jawbone, gut wall, connective tissue, and the autonomic ganglia are common sites of metal storage, and places where micro-organisms thrive. Furthermore, those bodily areas, vaso-constricted and hypo-perfused by blood, lacking in sufficient nutrients and oxygen, provide an ideal environment for the growth of anaerobic germs, fungi and viruses.

Klinghardt suggests simultaneous diagnosis and treatment of the toxic metal residues and the micro-organisms. As long as compartmentalized toxic metals are present in the body, micro-organisms have a fortress that is very difficult to conquer.

Foundations for Klinghardt's Model

Klinghardt's model originates with one of his teachers, Gerhard Koehler, MD, PhD,[7] who believed that doctors choose among three types of healing:

1. **Suppression** – The type practiced by allopathic medicine, which uses *anti*- inflammatories, *anti*biotics, *anti*fungals, and other treatments that work "against life."

2. **Substitution** – The type represented by a biomedical approach, such as Defeat Autism Now!, which uses vitamins, minerals, hormones and other supplements.

3. **Regulation** – The type practiced by truly holistic healers where homeopathy, chiropractic, herbs, neural therapy, acupuncture and other plants and techniques stimulate the body to heal itself. This type of healing is missing in most protocols.

Klinghardt believes that autism spectrum disorders can only be fully healed by restoring the self-regulation of the system and making it fully functional.

The core of this model is Klinghardt's "Five Levels of Healing," shown in Figure 16-1, Autonomic Response Testing (ART), and Applied Psychoneurobiology (APN), all described below. This innovative system of diagnostic and therapeutic tools is applicable to anyone with physical, behavioral or mental issues, regardless of diagnosis. In the early 1990s, Klinghardt became aware of the increasing numbers of children with autism and related disorders, studied the effects of heavy metal toxicity on the brain, and adapted his model to treating these children.

The Vertical Healing System: The Five Levels of Healing

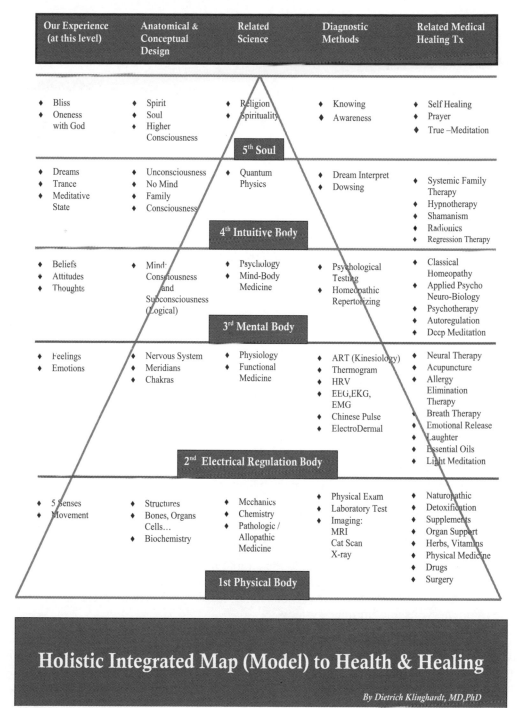

Our Experience (at this level)	Anatomical & Conceptual Design	Related Science	Diagnostic Methods	Related Medical Healing Tx
• Bliss • Oneness with God	• Spirit • Soul • Higher Consciousness	• Religion • Spirituality	• Knowing • Awareness	• Self Healing • Prayer • True –Meditation

5th Soul

| • Dreams
• Trance
• Meditative State | • Unconsciousness
• No Mind
• Family Consciousness | • Quantum Physics | • Dream Interpret
• Dowsing | • Systemic Family Therapy
• Hypnotherapy
• Shamanism
• Radionics
• Regression Therapy |

4th Intuitive Body

| • Beliefs
• Attitudes
• Thoughts | • Mind-Consciousness and Subconsciousness (Logical) | • Psychology
• Mind-Body Medicine | • Psychological Testing
• Homeopathic Repertorizing | • Classical Homeopathy
• Applied Psycho Neuro-Biology
• Psychotherapy
• Autoregulation
• Deep Meditation |

3rd Mental Body

| • Feelings
• Emotions | • Nervous System
• Meridians
• Chakras | • Physiology
• Functional Medicine | • ART (Kinesiology)
• Thermogram
• HRV
• EEG,EKG, EMG
• Chinese Pulse
• ElectroDermal | • Neural Therapy
• Acupuncture
• Allergy Elimination Therapy
• Breath Therapy
• Emotional Release
• Laughter
• Essential Oils
• Light Meditation |

2nd Electrical Regulation Body

| • 5 Senses
• Movement | • Structures
• Bones, Organs Cells…
• Biochemistry | • Mechanics
• Chemistry
• Pathologic / Allopathic Medicine | • Physical Exam
• Laboratory Test
• Imaging: MRI Cat Scan X-ray | • Naturopathic
• Detoxification
• Supplements
• Organ Support
• Herbs, Vitamins
• Physical Medicine
• Drugs
• Surgery |

1st Physical Body

Holistic Integrated Map (Model) to Health & Healing

By Dietrich Klinghardt, MD,PhD

Figure 16-1
Reprinted with permission.

The Five Levels of Healing

- *Physical* The lowest level is the physical body. It is the foundation upon which everything else rests. It is our connection to the earth and the source of our physical energy. The physical body is identical to what we sense: see, feel, hear, smell and taste. It ends at the skin.

The physical level includes the body's structure and functions. This is the level where mercury begins wrecking havoc, and conventional, alternative, and the Defeat Autism Now! approach intervene.

- *Electromagnetic* The second level is the electromagnetic body, or the body's energy field. It is the summation of all electric and magnetic events caused by the neuronal activity of the nervous system. Since most somatic and autonomic nerves in the body travel along the longitudinal axis of the body, and the nerve currents spread as electric fields along these nerves, the magnetic fields created by these forces travel perpendicular to this axis into space. Even though their strength decreases with distance from the body, they extend into space beyond the skin, theoretically into infinity.

Nerves in the physical body fire with an electrical charge, which mercury can both disturb and destroy physically and functionally. Klinghardt believes strongly that electromagnetic fields, such as wall sockets, televisions, computers, cell phones and their towers, and other invisible energy sources interfere with and impede the body's flow of energy, sometimes to the point of illness. Without addressing this level, most patients on the autism spectrum cannot get well.

Klinghardt contends that the electro-magnetic level is the key to answering the question, "If mercury impacts the physical body so strongly, why don't all kids exposed to mercury become autistic?" The bodies of affected individuals have disturbed energetic fields that have a synergistic relationship with factors at the physical level, thus making the ideal "Petri dish" in which autism can develop. In these patients, even with the best nutritional, dietary and other physical interventions, healing does not occur because energetic disturbances are interfering with absorption. See the next section on "Energetic Findings in Autism."

Therapies that address the electromagnetic level are acupuncture, and another one of Klinghardt's major contributions: neural therapy. He injects a form of "liquid electricity" into scars, root canals and ganglia to break up electromagnetic disturbances that gather there. (See section on "neural therapy" later in this chapter.)

- *Mental* The third level is the mental body, the home of thoughts, beliefs, attitudes and childhood memories. Disturbances at this level come from unresolved traumatic experiences, such as a difficult birth, divorce, separation, abuse or witnessing a death.

Laws that govern the third level include the simple natural rules of parent-child relationships: nurture and love a child, keep him/her safe, nourished and warm, and provide opportunities to learn. Each violation has consequences, leading to fairly predictable distortions of the mind, nervous and immune systems.

The brain replays trauma, constantly sending stress signals into the electromagnetic and physical bodies, disrupting the flow of energy, nutrients, blood and other essential components of health. While autism almost never starts at this level, working on mental issues can contribute to a child's complete recovery by the trickle-down effect to lower levels. Food allergies or dysbiosis can be symptoms in cases where mental body disturbances play a significant role.

Therapies that work at this level are homeopathy, psychotherapy, hypnosis, and applied psycho-neurobiology (APN). Klinghardt uses a complicated sequence of muscle testing of organs and their associated emotions to diagnose and treat disturbances at this level.

- *Intuitive* The fourth level is the dream or intuitive body: what Carl Jung called the "collective unconscious."[8] This is the highest level, at which an interaction between physician and client is possible.

The laws that govern the fourth level come from Family Systems Theory conceived by Murray Bowen in the 1970s and 1980s,[9] and expanded by German psychoanalyst, Bert Hellinger in the 1990s.[10] According to this model, a family system is comprised of the genetically linked persons of the last three generations and all of their respective partners. Every member of a family has an equal right to belong. If someone denies this right to one of the members, another member will try to balance the family by self-excluding him/herself.

Ever know a family that seemed "cursed?" Forces that acted upon them, sometimes going back several generations, come from this level. These forces present themselves as an energetic, rather than a genetic legacy. Examples are such injustices as a murder that was never discovered, a stillborn child who was never mourned, a suicide that was never acknowledged, or a secret, shady business deal. Three generations later, a family has a child diagnosed with autism. This child is very often the "sacrifice" for unresolved guilt and grief.

Klinghardt strongly recommends that families of children with autism have a family constellation, a Hellinger invention. Practiced widely in Europe, constellations are slowly becoming tools of many mental health professionals in the United States today.

- *Spiritual* The fifth level is the plane of self-healing. Klinghardt calls this level the "spirit-body." It is a person's relationship with the divine. Not implicated in autism, this level is very personal and not affected by any outside therapies. However, Klinghardt believes that it requires recognition. After resolution of the physical problems, both the physician and the client should do something "good" with the newly gained hope and vitality, and exhibit an attitude of gratefulness. Without this conclusion, a gradual relapse of the condition could occur.

Influences flow in both up and down directions. Each phenomenon in the physical realm seems to occur simultaneously on the other four levels. For instance, removing interference at the electromagnetic level can dissipate problems at the physical level and vice versa. However, some problems in the higher levels, may not be apparent at lower levels. An acupuncturist, for instance may pick up energetic problems before physical symptoms occur. The traditional Chinese medicine doctor was only paid when the patient's physical body remained healthy. He/she had to identify and resolve the disturbance on the second level before it penetrated down to the first.

True healing requires simultaneous work on all five levels. Families should pump as much energy as possible into the lower three levels: eat, sleep and exercise well, and take supplements. Nurture the electric body with massage, acupuncture, neural therapy, sit by a waterfall, listen to good music and do yoga stretches. See a therapist to work through confusion and unresolved conflicts on the mental level. Make sure that the home, work and study area, especially the bedroom, are free of electromagnetic fields.

Klinghardt focuses his autism protocol primarily on the first two levels. For a child to fully recover, mercury poisoning must be treated at both the physical and energetic levels.

The vertical healing system can be a valuable foundation for understanding truly what holistic medicine is, and gives the practitioner a road map to navigate the sometimes chaotic landscape of healing techniques. The lower levels supply energy to the higher levels. Each level has an order, its own laws, and an organizing influence on the lower levels.

Energetic Findings in Autism

In addition to the more commonly recognized physical symptoms of autism reviewed in previous chapters of this book, Klinghardt notes that a majority of those "on the spectrum" have the following unusual energetic characteristics.

- An overly large energy field – The individual with autism has an "energy body" that is displaced from the physical body, and inhibits perceptions and communications from being received and/or downloaded into the physical body. The physical body is thus being driven by toxins to do something different than what the energy body wants it to.
- Blocked mirror neurons in the brain – Mirror neurons are those nerve cells mostly in the frontal cortex or language center of the brain, that allow someone to show a positive emotional response to another person.[11]   One result of tubulin disrupted by mercury toxicity is the inability to return a smile or gaze.
- Enhanced energetic perception and capability for telepathic communication – Kids "know" where things are without using their eyes.
- Greater responsivity to properly used Energy Medicine applications.
- Unusual patterns of regulation.
- Hyperactivity in most meridian systems.
- Autonomic nervous system dysfunction.
- Severe second and sixth charka abnormalities affecting feelings, intimacy, boundaries and mental clarity.
- Recipient of unhealed transgenerational family issues because of their extraordinary energetic sensitivities. This perpetuates the illness.

6 Areas of Stress

Klinghardt categorizes the many "total load" factors described in Chapter 3 into six areas.

1. ***Environmental toxic exposures*** to heavy metals and solvents, pesticides, wood preservatives, off-gassing from plastics, teflon or textiles, molds, etc., which have a synergistic effect with most toxic metals. Metals will often accumulate in body parts that have been chemically injured at a prior time.

2. ***Biochemical and nutritional deficiencies*** – well acknowledged stressors on the body.

3. ***Structural abnormalities in facial development,*** involving the head, neck and jaw, which can cause defective dentition, and problems with the temporal mandibular joint. These cranio-sacral dysfunctions are often responsible for impairment of blood flow and lymphatic drainage in affected areas through low pressure vessels called lymphatics, which are easily compressed.

Elizabeth Sheehan, DC, CCN, one of Dr. Klinghardt's top practitioners, believes that cranio, upper cervical and pelvic misalignments are always present in autism. These stressors on the nervous system, derived from birth and other trauma, can weaken the brain's defenses, making them susceptible to invasion by lead, aluminum and mercury and the micro-organisms that feed on them, as well as set the body up for ear and other infections.

She strongly believes that structure and function work hand in hand. Structure determines function, and function determines structure. When structure is comprised, the body must utilize much of its energy to stay structurally intact, sucking whatever energy it can out of the immune system and elsewhere. The structural organization of the bones of the skull determines the tension of the membranes that suspend the pituitary gland and the hypothalamus, and anchor the brain in place. The ability of the hypothalamus to release and transport its hormones is extremely vulnerable to positional changes of the pituitary.

Dr. Sheehan routinely evaluates the spine globally, including all 12 of the cranial nerves in children with autism spectrum disorders. The inability of any of the cranial nerves to process sensory stimuli efficiently could cause fatigue and stress. Assuring that these nerves have the structural capacity to receive and integrate information, and treating them if they do not, ensures their capacity to handle appropriate therapeutic sensory interventions functionally. She believes that after structural treatment the nerves facilitate quicker and more efficient responses to many sound therapies, as well as to vision and occupational therapy.

Interference from scars and other unhealed focal areas from the umbilical cord, circumcision, tonsil removal, and ganglia can create abnormal electrical signals that often alter the function of the autonomic nervous system. The abnormal impulses cause these areas to become metal and toxic storage sites.

4. *Food intolerances and allergies,* which often cause a low-grade encephalitis and/or joint inflammation, setting up those areas to become targets for toxic deposits.

5. *Geopathic stress and Electromagnetic Fields (EMF)* - Electric and magnetic fields have different effects on the growing nervous systems of young children. A body can resist only about 20 milli-volts of resistance and stay healthy. When measurements are 300-500 milli-volts, people get sick.

Health conscious consumers should check their neighborhoods for placement of overhead powerlines and their transformers, as well as for cell phone towers. Go to <www.antennasearch.com> to find those nearest to you. Sometimes neighbors' radar or security systems encroach upon personal space, as well.

Inside, many homes register thousands, not hundreds of milli-volts of electrical voltage. Sources of household electro-magnetic fields include electrical wiring in the wall, fluorescent lights, large appliances such as computers, TVs and refrigerators, and small appliances, such as hair driers, electric razors and lamps. Klinghardt recommends that children with autism, for whom these machines sound like freight trains, be protected from these invaders, as well as from wireless Internet, alarm systems, cordless phones, and microwave ovens.

One of the most important ingredients to restoring health is a safe sleeping location. The average bedroom nightstand holds many possible EMF sources, including an alarm clock, wristwatch, reading light, CD player, radio and wireless telephone. Everyone is 100 times more vulnerable to EMFs when asleep, because EMFs decrease pineal function, causing it to stop producing melatonin, the most powerful neuro-protective chemical in the Central Nervous System. Klinghardt found that a significant number of his patients were sleeping over underground water lines or too close to electrical equipment, and that their sleep improved markedly when these problems were mitigated.

Geopathic and magnetic stress also open the blood brain barrier, increase leukemia and cancer rates, cause brain fog, and have a negative synergistic effect with other types of radiation. And if that is not enough, they also disturb brain waves, heart rate variability, breathing patterns and bowel movements. Finally, EMFs foster mold growth in homes as microbes crank up their own production of neurotoxins in defense.[12]

To measure EMFs and geopathic stress, have an expert from the International Institute of Building Biology (www.buildingbiology.net) test the home. If this is impossible, ask a patient to close his eyes and picture himself in bed; use autonomic response testing (see next section) to measure the stress.

Unfortunately, another hidden source of EMFs are the new, gas efficient hybrid cars. These put both driver and passengers at risk, as well.

6. ***Unresolved trans-generational trauma in the family system*** – Psychological stressors are by far the most common factor determining where specific metals and infectious agents will take up housekeeping in the body. Klinghardt believes that the impact of this stressor is grossly underestimated. He utilizes some elegant interventions that address this stressor. See below.

In summary:
- The symptom is the reason the patient seeks medical help.
- Underlying or within the symptom is often a chronic infection.
- Underneath the infection is an altered milieu and the presence of mercury and other toxic metals.
- Other than the obvious necessary exposure, the reason why the infection takes hold is inferred from the location of the affected organ, and the type of toxicity present.
- When the body's heavy metal burden exceeds its ability to detoxify, the toxins are drawn to areas where the immune system is weak. Unresolved psycho-emotional conflicts have a role here. Different acupuncture meridians/organ systems are vulnerable to different types of emotional disturbance. Unresolved grief is more likely to affect the lung, for example, and chronic anxiety or fear, the kidney; shame affects the bladder, while pent up anger is associated with the liver. Thus the nature of the emotional issues determines the location of the immune system vulnerability.
- In most cases, mercury toxicity is exponentially strengthened by its synergistic relationship with any other sources of stress.

Autonomic Response Testing
Klinghardt co-developed Autonomic Response Testing (ART), a form of muscle testing or kinesiology, which measures stress responses in the body and nervous system. ART is an extremely accurate, elegant, sophisticated, quick, reliable and comprehensive diagnostic system that is the leading bio-energetic technique in Europe today. ART is the only type of muscle testing that can measure the biophotonic field of a patient, establish a diagnosis and prescribe treatment simultaneously.

Fritz-Albert Popp, a leading European physicist, showed that the bio-photon field surrounding the physical body is the central regulating agency of all metabolic processes.[13] Our cells create a bio-photon field around us, which, in turn, regulates our metabolic enzymes. Any stress at the cellular level creates a disturbance in signals in the autonomic nervous system, which are measurable as distortions in the electromagnetic field around the body. Popp's discovery is the basis for ART.

ART neatly lays out the pieces of the puzzle. Practitioners can then use lab work to confirm and back up findings.

Based on the work of Dr. Yoshiaki Omura's resonance phenomenon between identical substances,[14] ART can determine which of the stressors are blocking the proper functioning of the autonomic nervous system in an individual patient. A practitioner can use Klinghardt's system to prioritize stressors and the order in which to address them.

The Three Laws of ART

ART is based on three laws:

1. ***The Law of Resonance between two identical substances*** – If a substance is held in a person's energy field, and an indicator muscle weakens, the identical substance is in the body. If the substance is only in a particular organ, ganglion or other structure, the test-substance has to be held exactly over this area to get a reaction. With ART the practitioner locates a structure that when held makes the indicator muscle weaken. Then, when a substance is placed anywhere on the patient, the same indicator muscle becomes strong if that substance is also present in the body.

2. ***Variation of the first law*** – If the examiner localizes more then one organ, structure or ganglion during the ART body scan or examination, multiple structures may be affected by the same toxin or infection, or one structure may affect one or more others. The indicator muscle might weaken when one organ is held, and strengthen when held together with another organ that caused it to weaken when held alone. Two negatives make a positive. In that case, there is either a cause/effect relationship between the two, or they are both affected by the same toxin or infection.

3. ***The Law of Resonance between the Examiner and the Patient*** – The examiner's body acts exactly like any other substance held into the energy field of the patient. If the examiner is toxic with the same substance that is either causing the patient's illness, or is stored in one or more of the patient's tissues, the test is invalid. Thus, no two examiners can find the same problems in a given patient, unless both examiners are free of stored toxins, infections, mercury filled teeth, untreated scars, active psycho-emotional conflicts, have not recently consumed foods they are allergic to, etc. This possibility is often overlooked in other schools of kinesiology.

The third law results in a simple postulate: the ART practitioner must continuously strive to stay healthy.

How ART is Done

From an observer's point of view, ART looks like an examiner is pushing on an outstretched arm of a patient, standing, sitting or lying down, with an arm raised at a 90 degree angle to his body. The examiner gives the cue for the patient to "hold" or "resist" about ½ second before pushing on the arm with about two pounds of pressure for about two seconds. The pressure either does or does not engage the muscle group. If the muscle engages, the arm remains straight. If not, the arm weakens. For young children, an adult "surrogate" can act as a circuit between the examiner and the child, by touching the child's body while the examiner tests his or her outstretched arm.

In-depth testing of the stress areas, which allows a practitioner to identify the type and location of stressors, and which antidote to use, is most easily accomplished using a polarized filter with one or more cell signal enhancers. These tools are available from Biopure at <www.biopureus.com>.

A practitioner scans the body, testing all major organs for stress: brain, thyroid, kidneys, adrenals, liver, stomach, spleen, pancreas, small intestine, large intestine and pelvic floor to determine which fields are disorganized, pushing on the individual's arm as each location is held. Simultaneously, the body reveals which areas are stressed, and which agents are beneficial in relieving the stress. In this rapid, non-invasive, inexpensive, yet reliable process, the site and type of toxic metal, micro-organisms, trauma, etc. becomes apparent.

Any of the stress factors, especially heavy metal toxicity, food reactions and psychological factors can block regulation in the patient's pathways. The tester must deal with each one as it comes up before moving to the next level. When regulation is blocked, the examiner looks for an antidote to the problem, from one of the five levels of healing. Antidotes are

- *primary toxic metal removal agents* such as garlic, chlorella, cilantro, EDTA, DMPS or NDF
- *synergistic methods and agents*, such as kidney drainage remedies, blood protective agents, agents that increase fecal absorption and excretion of mobilized Hg
- *treatments for secondary infections*, including viruses, parasites, and bacteria, such as antibiotics, antifungals, antivirals, herbs and homeopathics
- *treatments for psychological trauma*, such as tapping on acupuncture points, repeating affirmations, eye movements with colored glasses and family constellations
- *treatments for geopathic stress and electromagnetic fields,* such as avoidance, relocation or metal shielding

The examiner places each antidote in actual or symbolic form in the patient's field until one product or procedure opens regulation. If more than one is successful, ART has techniques to determine which one works best. Testing then proceeds until the patient is in what is called a "yin state," when regulation is fully open, nothing blocks it, and the body begins to heal itself. *The sum of all the antidotes is the patient's "prescription."*

Klinghardt recommends using ART to fine tune the results of testing, or as a "stand alone" diagnostic tool to further evaluate any of the stressors. Any professional can use ART as an adjunct to standard in-office laboratory and diagnostic testing, as it can be done without any instruments. Some optometrists use simple muscle testing in addition to other visual apparatuses, and without other special tools, to evaluate whether a lens adds to or relieves stress on a patient's body, assuming that the patient's regulation is NOT blocked. Like any technique, skillful autonomic response testing requires study, practice and discipline.

Klinghardt's Five Step Autism Treatment Protocol
According to Klinghardt, a treatment protocol for autism or any other chronic condition must address all risk factors at all five levels of healing focusing on:

1. Symptomatic relief

2. Treatment of all areas of stress

3. Metal detoxification

4. Treatment of infections

5. Restoration of damaged nervous, immune, and gastro-intestinal systems.

1. Symptomatic Relief
Klinghardt adds a new dimension to relieving immediate problems by using every non-invasive method currently available. While treatments at this stage do not reach deep levels of dysfunction, they can cause surprisingly strong positive reactions. In addition, unlike drugs, which often exacerbate symptoms or cause new ones, the following natural treatments can often have a synergistic effect with other interventions.

- *Dietary modification with digestive enzymes and probiotics* – Eat a protein rich diet, corrected for blood type and food sensitivities. Find a diet plan that works; a diet should be gluten- and casein-free at the minimum. Test all foods with ART monthly. Supplement with digestive enzymes and probiotics at the end of every meal. See Chapter 5 for a complete description of dietary, enzyme and probiotic options.

- *Create a biomedical regimen,* such as The Defeat Autism Now! approach to supplement vitamin B6, DMG, zinc and magnesium - Klinghardt recommends magnesium citrate, low dose zinc, along with a little copper. He warns that too much zinc can be harmful, as it has a synergistic toxic effect with mercury. Also, use ART to find the right type of B6 to avoid triggering seizures. See Chapter 6 for the The Defeat Autism Now! approach.
- *Modify the The Defeat Autism Now! approach to other supplements* – Dr. Klinghardt has partnered with College Pharmacy's Center for Advanced Medical Therapeutics (AMT) to ensure the highest quality of supplements in his protocol. Go to their website at <www.amtrx.com> and contact Melanie Gentile, Pharmacist, and mother of a daughter with Rett's syndrome at 866-828-8203.
  - o Vitamin C at 100 mg/kg body weight minimum.
  - o B-complex as high doses of pantothenic acid, niacin and B2 only, or nutritional yeast, if tolerated.
  - o Sublingual Hydroxy-B12 with folic acid in a 5:2 ratio. (AMT can provide this protocol.) Klinghardt believes that the folic acid de-methylates toxic substances, while hydroxy-B12 removes toxic nitric oxide compounds from the brain. He recommends using ART to determine the proper form of folic acid for each patient.
  - o Multi-minerals in high doses.
- *IV Methyl B-12* as recommended by James Neubrander, MD in Chapter 5.
- *Oils* – Klinghardt has strong opinions about fish and other therapeutic oils, since each fish, nut and seed oil has unique qualities. He recommends an oil test kit, kept refrigerated, to use with ART to test pumpkinseed, flaxseed, hemp, primrose, cod liver, Udo's and other oils to see which works best with an individual patient.
- *Other supplements,* including calcium citrate, Vitamins E and A, selenium and low dose Naltrexone (LDN). See Chapters 5 and 6 for more on these supplements.

2. Treating the Areas of Stress

- *Environmental toxic exposures* – Identify and eliminate every possible location in the home of toxins, mold, and chemicals. Klinghardt recommends an indoor air quality inspection by an expert in the field. The inspector should look for insufficient ventilation, polluted crawl spaces, gas leaks, volatile organic compounds from carpets, floors, furniture and building materials, and any other toxins that might have synergistic effects with mercury.

One synergistic toxin, mentioned briefly in Chapter 5, is fluoride, which accumulates in the fat cells, attacking and destroying enzymes. When fluoride enters the body, it hydrolyzes the hydrogen bonds that allow each enzyme to maintain its shape. The body treats these deformed enzymes as foreign invaders, thus triggering an auto-immune response.

Studies have indicted fluoride as a carcinogen, which may also be responsible for symptoms resembling Alzheimer's disease and attention deficit disorder.[15] One researcher found that seven ounces of toothpaste contain enough fluoride to kill a small child.[16] In the early 1990s, the Canadian Dental Association concluded that fluoride supplements were unsafe for children under age three.[17]

Dr. George Waldbott, who warned the public in the 1950s about the dangers of smoking and possible allergic reactions to penicillin, believes that like mercury, even extremely low concentrations of fluoride can do harm. Migraines, stiffness, and gastric distress all diminished in Waldbott's patients when they stopped drinking fluoridated water.[18]
- *Biochemical* (vitamin/mineral) and nutritional deficiencies – these have been discussed in Chapter 5.
- *Structural abnormalities* – Any vertebral and other bony subluxations and defects in facial development or dental occlusion, such as an overbite, can affect bodily systems

profoundly by disrupting lymph flow and adding a huge load factor of stress to the nervous system.

If ART pinpoints any structural abnormalities, Klinghardt strongly recommends a whole body evaluation by a well-trained chiropractor, such as Elizabeth Sheehan, DC, as well as a bite assessment for occlusional problems by a cranial osteopath or a very experienced orthodontist. Dr. Sheehan and others combine many chiropractic procedures to address structural and functional abnormalities simultaneously, Her tools include Koren Specific Technique (KST) and Gonzalez Rehabilitation Technique (GRT) as well as Laser Energetic Detoxification (LED). Using these allows her to obtain optimal results with each patient.

a. *Koren Specific Technique*, developed by chiropractor Ted Koren, enables the practitioner to evaluate and treat the position of every joint in the body, including the spine, extremities, cranial and facial bones, and sutures. Using KST, one of the main subluxations Dr. Sheehan sees in her patients with autism spectrum disorders is a combination of misalignments called the sphenoid pattern, because it includes the sphenoid and occipital bones. This subluxation pattern can occur from subtle of frank birth injury and/or head trauma, as well as from swelling and inflammation in the brain and lymph system from a variety of toxins. Misalignments in this joint complex negatively affect pumping of the cerebrospinal fluid, and can cause impairment of taste, smell, hearing and speech, disturbance of temperature regulation, increased intracranial pressure, and imbalances of neurotransmitters and hormones.

Once Sheehan identifies misalignments or subluxations in the structure, she then uses a very light adjusting instrument, called an ArthroStim™, to gently tap the segment back into place, thus restoring the structure and the function of that area. The ArthroStim™ is an FDA approved instrument that has been continuously refined and perfected over its 22 year history. It provides a fast, accurate, low force and controlled adjustment, and introduces energy/force/information into the body to realign segments and remove nerve pressure at a speed of 12 "taps" per second (12 hertz). The ArthroStim™ gives patients a very specific adjustment by addressing only the segment that is out of position, without any twisting, turning or "cracking" of joints. This technique permits adjusting in many different postures, such as sitting, standing or lying down.

KST is an especially quick and effective way of evaluating and treating cranial bone issues, especially for those autistic children who are unable to tolerate cranial sacral therapy. Dr. Sheehan has observed drastic improvements in children with autism by adjusting them using KST. For more information on this technique, go to <www.teddkorenseminars.com>.

b. *Gonzalez Rehabilitation Technique (GRT)* is a revolutionary "new neurology" system of diagnosis and treatment of the nervous system developed by George Gonzalez, DC. This unique technique closely evaluates and treats the entire nervous system, including the spinal cord, as well as motor, sensory, and cranial nerves. Twenty percent of the nerves in the body are motor nerves that supply muscles for motor control and movement, while the other eighty percent are sensory nerves, which affect the ability to process sensory information.

While some children with autism have motor issues, the vast majority of them have sensory nerve or sensory integration issues with touch, vibration, proprioception and other sensory information. (See Chapter 7.) GRT is crucial in autism because treating the sensory nerves often results in fewer incidences and lessened severity of self-stimulatory behavior.

GRT also evaluates and corrects functional cranial nerve deficits. The 12 cranial nerves originate in the brain and control functions such as sight, smell, eye movements, hearing, balance, motor and sensory control to the face, swallowing, and vocalization. Once a practitioner discovers a functional weakness in a nerve, she uses a powerful infrared device called a GRT light. Treatment with this instrument rapidly up-regulates (strengthens) the nerve and nerve impulses, reduces inflammation, increases intracellular ATP production and effectively retrains the body to better multi task and integrate information. For more information about GRT, go to <www.grtseminars.com>.

c. *Laser Energetic Detoxification (LED)* is a technique originally developed in Germany, and further perfected by W. Lee Cowden, MD. It involves homeopathic preparations of detoxification support in the forms of flower and color remedies, dilutions of toxins and heavy metals, sensitivities, allergens and preparations of healthy glands, hormones, organs and neurotransmitters.

Cowden retrofits a device to hold the homeopathic preparations and laser them into the body in a process called photonphoresis. He "beams" the light through the vial onto targeted acupuncture points on the ears, soles of the feet, and palms of the hands. This procedure facilitates getting the energetic information from the homeopathic remedy into the body, and elicits rapid and deep effects.

A practitioner can use ART or other techniques to determine components of an individual's protocol, including the appropriate toxins, as well as the order and timing in which to treat. The LED speeds up and amplifies the process of frequency-based detoxification because the power of light affects the body's biophoton field, stimulating it to specifically dump a toxin out of the cells and matrix (extra-cellular space) of the body.

Coupling LED with oral chelating agents such as chlorella, charcoal, pectin or other products, binds the toxins and shuttles them out of the body at a much quicker rate than with chelation alone. Rapid removal of metals and other toxins is vital for children with autism spectrum disorders, as it allows the nervous system to repair that much sooner. The beauty of LED is that it is very safe; side effects are greatly minimized because of all the detoxification support built into the protocol.

Dr. Sheehan's approach is to begin with correction of structural issues, followed by LED to strengthen the nervous system. She suggests starting with one chiropractic and one GRT session, and then adding one to two LED sessions a week, so that as the body detoxifies, the nervous system is being stimulated to heal at a quicker rate. Dr. Sheehan has seen very encouraging results with this approach, especially when done as a part of an ART based treatment protocol.

Chiropractic, cranio-sacral therapy, osteopathy or any of a number of gentle structural interventions can all correct misalignments. The guiding principle is always that once function (normal movement) is restored, changes in structure follow. When structure heals, physiology normalizes, with hormones, enzymes, and other fluids flowing freely, allowing detoxification to take place. For a complete overview of structural therapies, refer back to Chapter 3.

• *Scars and other unhealed focal areas* – Klinghardt believes that scars on traumatized body parts create abnormal input into the autonomic nervous system with resultant adverse multi-system effects. Everyone has scars, starting with the place where the umbilical cord was cut. Other scars occur as a result of circumcision, tonsil removal, surgery, infections and accidents.

Neural therapy is a powerful Klinghardt invention that involves the injection of procaine, diluted medications and homeopathics into scars and acupuncture points. Scars and other unhealed focal areas are magnets for heavy metals, which Klinghardt demonstrates eloquently with ART. Injecting scars with healing substances helps the body mobilize the toxins and excrete them. The injections are superficial, safe, easy to learn, and effective for alleviating a wide variety of medical problems associated with toxicity.

Dr. Klinghardt is President of the American Academy of Neural Therapy and the only fully trained teacher of this work in the United States. Tonsils and their scars present a complex problem in a cascade of issues starting with faulty structural organization in the skull, neck and face. Detoxification of the brain occurs through the cribriform plate into the adenoids, and from there, via the tonsils, into the lymphatic vessels accompanying the sterno-cleido-mastoid muscle, and from there into the subclavian vein. When mis-alignment disrupts lymph drainage and neurotoxin transport, tonsils become congested and infected.

Klinghardt believes that chronically infected and degenerated tonsils are a major contributing factor in food allergies, attention issues and autism. Congestion in the tonsils leads to further back-up of lymph flow, and serves as a breeding ground for multiple bacterial and viral colonies that produce potent brain neurotoxins.

The first choices for tonsil treatment are lymph drainage and homeopathic remedies, removing allergic foods (especially dairy products), using an air filter in the bedroom, supplementing vitamins and minerals to boost immunity, and neural therapy. Surgical removal, although out of vogue today, is also an option. However, if congestion does not clear, Klinghardt's choice is regenerative cryotherapy, a procedure available only in Germany. Burning the tonsils allows them to regenerate and start anew doing the filtering job they were meant to do. Go to <www.kryopraxis.de> to learn more. Also see his paper on tonsils at <www.neuraltherapy.com>.

- *Food intolerances and allergies* – Klinghardt believes that the home should be free of any foods that are forbidden for the child with autism, and that food choices will change as the child heals. He recommends a simple food rotation diet that eliminates all gluten and casein containing foods, even if no allergies are apparent. He also recommends metabolic and blood typing (http://www.biotype.net/diets/) as tools for dietary modification. If ART shows no negative reactions, fermented dairy products such as kefir can be added as the child gets well.
- *Geopathic stress and "electrosmog"* – In an earlier section, the authors enumerated the many negative effects that geopathic stress and electromagnetic fields have on the organ systems of the body. Those with autism spectrum disorders are highly sensitive to abnormal electric fields, so the effects on them are even worse. Under geopathic stress, detoxification cannot occur.

Because electromagnetic stress has such profoundly negative effects on sleep, Klinghardt believes that creating a safe, stress-free sleeping location is imperative for healing. First and foremost, families must replace laptop computers with desktops at home, eliminate cordless telephones and wireless Internet, locate and mitigate any stress from nearby cell phone towers, and correct any faulty wiring.

In the bedroom itself,
- o Install a demand switch next to the bed to turn off the current in the walls at night.
- o Use only battery operated clocks and lights; never use night-lights.
- o Remove all cordless telephones, computers, and other electronic equipment.
- o Place the head of the bed on walls without electrical outlets.
- o Buy organic flame-retardant- and metal- free mattresses; add metalicized grounding sheets under natural fiber bedsheets for seriously sensitive children. Surround the

bed with metalicized mosquito netting that prevents microwaves from entering the bedroom.

o Paint walls and floor with graphite paint, and place natural fiber curtains on the windows.

o De-clutter the bedroom.

o Take melatonin before going to sleep. This supplement prevents damage from heavy metals, viruses, bacteria, toxins, outgasing of plastics, etc.[19]

If all else fails, move to a different house.

- *Unresolved trans-generational trauma in the family system* – Traumatic family issues from the past predispose members to childhood diseases, including autism. Often therapy and biomedical intervention do not progress until a healing family constellation is done by an experienced facilitator.

3. Metal Detoxification

Dietrich Klinghardt, MD, PhD is considered one of the leading experts in the world on detoxification. He sees little need to do laboratory testing to determine which metals are in the body. He starts all patients on a gentle detoxification program, using mild agents like chlorella and cilantro first, to jump start lymphatic and organ drainage, and stronger ones like calcium EDTA and TD-DMPS, later.

In Chapter 5, the authors wrote about the use of chlorella in detoxification. This amazing natural substance is one of Klinghardt's favorite detoxification supplements, and a staple for anyone interested in maintaining good health. He believes that some products are better than others, and prefers the BioPure brand, as it is treated with ultrasound and not oxidized.

Each phase of detoxification lasts about three months. Klinghardt then uses hair analysis to monitor which metals the body is excreting. His experience is that toxic mineral levels register low at first, and then begin rising, with lead and nickel showing up before mercury.

During detoxification, Klinghardt makes sure that he

- Removes only one toxic agent at a time. Pulling multiple toxic compounds simultaneously increases the opportunity for a synergistic effect from which a patient may have difficulty recovering.
- Clears the excretory organs first of lead, then mercury, and finally other toxins like pesticides.
- Uses multiple detox agents sequentially to address various forms of mercury in the body, because mercury is bound in the tissues, cells and organs in virtually hundreds of ways, and no single agent can clear all forms of mercury.
- Protects the brain and gut with agents such as electrolyte enhanced drinking water, high doses of essential minerals to compete with toxic metals at the binding site, and to replace the ones that are chelated out, anti-oxidants, especially high doses of vitamin C, as well as turmeric and glutathione.
- Applies techniques such as homeopathy, acupuncture and EMDR at an energetic level, as well as family constellation work to address emotional issues.
- Supports detoxification generally in other ways with Epsom salt baths, ionic footbaths, and far infared saunas. Klilnghardt has found that his footbaths from Switzerland energize the autonomic nervous system and acupuncture meridians in the feet, activating the detox function of the kidneys, liver, gut and skin. The scum in the water after the footbath has no toxic metals in it. However, following a footbath, patients excrete more toxins through their urine and feces. Using cilantro with a footbath brings out lesser known toxic metals such as nickel.

4. Treating the Infections

Detox agents above are successful in treating more than the heavy metals; they also clear out the neurotoxins excreted by the molds, Lyme and other viruses, and bacteria. Molds hold metals in their cell walls. That is why Klinghardt never treats mold without putting a detoxification agent on board.

Once cells wake up, regain their intelligence and use their inborn ability to communicate and clear themselves of toxins, Klinghardt focuses on treating infections. He believes that antibiotics alone cannot break through the toxic metals to treat infections. He thus relies on many other methods and substances, previously not used in the United States. In order to attain healing, Klinghardt believes that microbial agents must come from plants and herbs with a life spirit, not artificial substances. To learn more about the spirit of plants in healing, read *Plant Spirit Medicine: The Healing Power of Plants* by Eliot Cowan.[20]

Some common opportunistic infections in Autism Spectrum Disorders are

* *Lyme Infection from Borrelia burgdorferi (Bb)* – In Chapter 3, the authors stated that Klinghardt believes Lyme disease to be much more common in autism than previously was thought, with seven out of eight of his patients testing positive. He says that a doctor should always suspect Bb infection in a child who is not responding positively to the Defeat Autism Now! protocol or chelation.

After treating many of his families with children exhibiting autism, Klinghardt has concluded the following: if the firstborn is male and has autism, mercury is at fault, as it has a synergistic effect with testosterone. If a mother has a typical child first, however, and one of her other children has autism, mercury is not the sole cause. The culprit is probably Lyme, an infection that adds to the neurotoxin pool in the mother, potentiates mercury, and passes through the placenta to her unborn baby.

Klinghardt has developed a complex Lyme treatment protocol.[21] To reduce the total body burden, he recommends treating Lyme, as well as other infections from viruses and bacteria, with herbs, rather than with antibiotics.

Others are following Klinghardt's lead in treating Lyme disease in autism. The non-profit Lyme-Induced Autism Foundation (L.I.A.) is a clearinghouse for research, and educates the public with periodic conferences and seminars. Go to <www.lymeinducedautism.org>.

* *Measles virus* – Treat with Vitamin A palmitate in a prescribed regime of 400,000 units in three divided dosages for two consecutive days only. Repeat every six weeks, several times, then once annually. Klinghardt says that using this protocol immediately following a vaccine reaction can prevent future problems. For other treatments, the reader is referred to the Defeat Autism Now! treatment manual.[22]
* *Borna virus* – This insidious bug attacks the limbic system and is thus responsible for psychiatric symptoms, especially manic depression. High levels of Borna viruses are apparent in the manic phase.[23] Klinghardt uses herbal anti-virals like olive leaf and mushroom extracts, as well as the drug Amantidine for at least four months.
* *Giardia, amoebas and protozoa* – Klinghardt treats these and other bugs with rizoles, a new class of bio-active compounds created by ozonating plant oils, including clove, wormwood, marjoram, cumin and others, for several weeks. Ozone, a form of oxygen therapy, kills anaerobes, bugs that live without oxygen.
* *Parasites* – like roundworms, threadworms, tapeworms and liver flukes are all very hearty bugs that should never be underestimated. Rizoles are good for treating all worms, cysts and larvae. He also uses Alinia, which crosses the blood brain barrier, Albendazole[24] and Biltrocide in high doses to attack these critters.

- *Herpes viruses* – Treatment depends upon type. Some respond well to Heel homeopathics, chlorella, freeze-dried garlic and ozonated oils.
- *Strep infections and consequences (chorea minor)* – Use homeopathic Sanum remedies.
- *Molds and fungi* – Many of today's homes have elevated levels of aspergillus, cladosporium, stachybotrys and other potentially deadly molds caused by poor building plan and materials. To test a home for mold, order mold test plates from <www.moldlabintl.com>.

Propolis, a waxy balsamic resinous substance that forms inside beehives in Somalia, Eritrea, Saudia Arabia and India is a potent anti-microbial. The word propolis is made up of two Greek words: "pro" meaning "in front or in defense of," and "polis," which means "town." Propolis is thus the town of the bees, or a beehive. Rich in flavonoids, hydroxyacids, terpenes, aromatic alcohols and essential oils, propolis kills molds, and has a fantastic long-term anti-inflammatory effect. Its anti-microbial properties were discovered several centuries BC.[25]

Propolis can be taken orally or applied externally. It can also be put in a vaporizer in the home and car to eliminate most bacteria, viruses, fungi and mold from the air in an all-natural way. Putting propolis in a vaporizer heats it and releases it into the environment to do its job.

Every home of a child with autism should have an indoor air quality inspection by a qualified inspector. (Go to <www.buildingbiology.net> to find one.) If you suspect mold, Klinghardt recommends that, at the minimum, change bedding and vacuum often. Mold infestations can be so bad that a family may have to move.

Klinghardt's patients benefit from another of his inventions, "Matrix microbes." Put them in a spray bottle, and use nasally or orally; the brain absorbs these "good bugs" very quickly. Spritzing the entire house twice a week competes with the "bad bugs" to create a healthy environment home. The fulvic acid in Matrix microbes is death to many viruses.

Klinghardt has pioneered the use of micro-current technology to inhibit microbial growth. His "KMT 24" makes the body a hostile environment for the bugs that cause infections. This sophisticated instrument is a mini-computer with six different programs of carefully selected frequencies, sequences, wave characteristics and amperage to target specific infections and mobilize heavy metals. Some programs utilize microbial inhibition frequencies developed during the genome project; others are proprietary to Klinghardt.

Patients use the KMT 24 for six days while sleeping, then take a one day break. Klinghardt uses two cell signal enhancers, one on each side of the brain, to magnify microbial currents from the machine to create a huge field, which pulses at a stable rhythm. Bugs must have a chaotic rhythm to survive. The stable rhythm from the KMT 24, a type of biofeedback, destroys the bugs, molds, Lyme, viruses, microplasma, etc. and entrains the body's brain waves. Use of it shortens treatment time, although sometimes, seizures may be a reaction.

Klinghardt has also recorded CDs with the strange vibrations of various bugs in action recorded underground. The patient plays the CD while sleeping, and the bugs respond as if they are being attacked, dying in the process. This is an extremely effective treatment for viruses.

Rizoles, Propolis vaporizers for home and car, Matrix microbes, KMT 24 and CDs are all available from <www.biopureus.com>.

5. Restoration of Damaged Organ Systems
The final phase is brain and system repair. Some effective strategies for restoring the body's regulation follow.

- *Psychokinesiology* Klinghardt has developed an elegant, extremely effective, short-term psychotherapy he calls psychokinesiology (PK).[26] The core of this approach is the patient's continuous dialogue with the subconscious mind.

Using ART, the muscle test engages the subconscious mind in a conversation, and reveals unresolved deep seated conflicts and post-traumatic stress states. Underlying causes of many long standing illnesses, psychological problems, chronic pain, and other issues reveal themselves. The therapist uses quick techniques such as tapping on acupuncture points to relieve stress on the organs, engaging the patient in repetitive eye movements while wearing colored glasses, and other methods, to allow processing of the material in a way that is healing to both the patient and the family.

Klinghardt believes that PK is crucial in treating patients with autism and related disorders, as well as their family members. He finds that in many cases treating patients with PK early on unloads emotional material which allows them to respond dramatically to other therapies. In fact, many aspects of their biochemistry, including blood pH, hormone and mineral levels, move in a direction toward normal after successful PK treatments. Results are often permanent.

In the past decade, PK has become the fastest growing technique in humanistic psychology in Europe. Klinghardt teaches PK techniques in workshops several times a year. Go to <www.klinghardt.org> to see his schedule.

- *Family Constellations* Family constellations are another of the most popular therapeutic approaches in Europe today, and are just beginning to make their way to the United States. Family Constellations work at the Fourth or Intuitive level of healing, an area previously ignored by more familiar interventions. Growing out of the family systems movement of the 1950s, this approach begins with the idea that instead of originating in an individual's life history from birth to the present, dysfunction and suffering often relate to painful events in the family's past.

Nothing is more important to a child than belonging. Sometimes a child's way of being connected, though, is to suffer like those who came before him. A child may become "entangled" in the difficult fate of a past family member, and unconsciously draw unhappiness, failure, addiction or illness into his own life.

While parents' deepest wishes are that their children thrive and their relationships work, Dr. Bert Hellinger, a renowned German psychoanalyst, believes that sometimes an individual's future may be out of his/her control. An entanglement with a deceased relative from a past generation may be at play, sealing an unhappy fate, with a child as the victim. Family constellations can serve to reverse illness, failure and conflict by revealing hidden dynamics and pointing the way toward resolution. For a family whose child or children have autism, a constellation can break an energetic bond of pain and suffering, allowing a child to heal.

Families of children at the severe end of the autism spectrum know all too well how the daily issues they confront constitute a particularly difficult fate for their families. Klinghardt believes that their large energetic field gives children on the autism spectrum an extraordinary energetic sensitivity that makes them particularly vulnerable to disturbances in the energy field of the extended family, including unhealed trans-generational issues.

Toxins prevent the physical body from receiving and processing perceptions and communications. Heightened energetic sensitivities further perpetuate illness. Furthermore, it is as though the soul is outside the body looking for a place to dock, and can't find one, because receptors are corrupted. Klinghardt recommends two or three sessions of Family

Constellation work to free up the system to release more toxins. Then other interventions suddenly become more effective.

Family Constellations usually take place in groups. An individual chooses representatives for members of his/her family from the circle of participants and positions them in a way that seems right. In a short time the representatives begin to experience physical sensations, emotions or urges, belonging not to themselves but to the family members they represent. It is as though they have become antennae, receiving information from a "family soul" mysteriously present in the room. Facilitators refer to this as the "knowing field."

Through observations, questions, trial statements and movements, the facilitator and client come to see the issue in a new way and create a resolution that enables the client to break his/her connection with difficulties in the family's past. As the hidden dynamic becomes clear, and movements of peace and reconciliation arise, the genuine love and strength in a family begin to flow in a healthy way.

An Example

The family history of one boy with autism was full of turmoil and pain on both sides. The father was excessively involved with his own mother; the boy's mother, an immigrant, had been unable to establish roots in her husband's country; and a decision to abort a child from a former relationship had been made with too little respect and seriousness to bring the event to a healthy closure.

As the constellation unfolded, the body language of the boy's representative showed how he was tied to those issues. To lighten the burden on their son, the father needed to free himself from his attachment to his own mother and become more available to his current family. The mother needed to develop a sense of rootedness in and respect for her new country. Together they needed to honor the soul of the aborted child by creating a place for it in their hearts.

Klinghardt suggests that families of children with autism put prodigous effort into healing their own families. The "family" includes children who have died early, aborted children, husbands excluded after a divorce, mothers who died at childbirth, and men who died in wars. Healing involves relating and communicating to everybody who is alive, as well as holding a loving memory of those who are gone. Don't rest until love and respect flows among everybody in the present and at least two generations prior.

Six Hellinger Institutes and independent groups offer family constellations across the United States. Klinghardt does "Healing Evenings" about once a month when he facilitates constellations. Hellinger's work is available in many books published by Zeig Tucker & Theisen, and continues to evolve from a lifetime of rich experience, including years as a priest and living with the Zulu tribe in Africa. To learn more about Family constellations, read Ulsmer's *Healing the Power of the Past*[27] and visit <www.hellinger.com>.

- *Homeopathy* In Chapter 12 the authors describe various methods of using homeopathy to treat those with autism spectrum disorders. In the Klinghardt model, practitioners use Reckeweg's Heel remedies from Germany at all six stages of his protocol to assist in regulating and balancing patients' systems. These medicines have many advantages and require little training to use correctly. They are inexpensive, have many years of support behind them, proving their effectiveness and safety. However, classical homeopaths, who use single remedies, are generally not in favor of these products. Heel remedies support each stage of healing.

At *Stage 1* they prepare and strengthen lymphatic and organ drainage in preparation for a dumping of mercury and other toxins from their hiding places. This stage lasts about two months.

At *Stage 2* Heel remedies assist in the metal detoxification program by mobilizing mercury and other toxins.

At *Stage 3* they help the cells wake up and regain their ability to communicate. This phase should start after at least three months into the program.

At *Stage 4* certain Heel remedies help clear infections.

Stage 5 takes place at least four months after the start to assist in brain and system repair.

Heel remedies come in a saline solution, which holds the energy very strongly for hundreds of years if stored in glass, not plastic. The remedies can be ingested, squirted up the nose or into the mouth using a syringe. Klinghardt has developed combinations of Heel products for each step of the way, always individualizing for unique issues with each patient. Heel remedies are available from <www.biopureus.com>.

- *Futures Unlimited* The late Ed Snapp, PT developed a non-invasive, non-traumatic program that creates an intrauterine environment in which a child's central nervous system can regress to a stage where new growth is possible. Called "Chronologically Controlled Developmental Therapy" (CCDT), it is based on the following premise: when a human being experiences a toxic injury to the brain, the nervous system is traumatized throughout. While the damaged tissue may recover, the trauma from the injury remains.

The treatment approach is directed toward the stimulation of the nervous system to allow the body to define its own dysfunction, lack of coordination, developmental failure and to make its own corrections. The body then regains lost sensory and motor information that is stored in the DNA, and reintegrates that memory into the traumatized system. The prime modalities include a flotations tank, sensory stimulation, therapeutic massage and exercise. Each modality is performed in a strictly controlled sequence.

Klinghardt has seen dramatic results in his patients who include this intervention in the first nine months of their program. To learn more, go to <www.futuresunlimited.com>.

Many of the adjunct therapies included in other chapters of this book are also a part of the Klinghardt protocol. In addition to improved auditory processing with Tomatis therapy, he has observed that Herpes viruses often disappear, hormones balance and posture changes. Other therapies Klinghardt endorses are HANDLE (Chapter 7) and vision therapy, including color therapy and syntonics.

Summary

Dr. Dietrich Klinghardt brings to autism a diagnostic and treatment protocol that is fully compatible with this book's other interventions and effective treatment modalities. Klinghardt adds some unique observations and interventions that complete a truly integrative and holistic model. He encourages families to focus not on defective genes, but rather to address toxic insults at the emotional, intuitive, and energetic, as well as the physical level. His optimistic approach toward a postive outcome leads to recovery, not despair, down the road.

Autism starts in a womb that lives in a physical home. Klinghardt notes a huge difference between how homes are built in the United States and in his native Germany. Here, many people live in cardboard boxes with plastic wrapped around them. Our houses cannot breathe; thus they build up moisture, mold and toxic chemicals. Frequently builders do not follow codes for proper ventilation and electrical wiring. Building materials off-gas and electro-smog from alarm systems, stereos, high speed internet and phone systems pervade the living space.

Every home should, at a minimum,
- have air and water filters, and be checked for geopathic stress. Remove or mitigate the results of cordless phones, cell phones, computers and other electronic devices.
- be free of chemicals from cleaning, personal care products, furniture, carpeting and bedding. Vacuum frequently with a high quality product. Run pillows through wash and dry cycle.

Klinghardt strongly recommends that every woman undergo a metal detoxification program, including having any mercury-containing amalgams removed by a biological dentist, well before becoming pregnant. A sound pre-natal, natal and nursing diet should consist of fresh, organic foods with an abundance of washed, organic fruits, vegetables and essential fats. All babies should receive cranio work immediately following delivery to assure the integrity of the body's structure. All new mothers should screen their breast milk and take 10 tablets of chlorella four times a day while nursing. New parents should fully educate themselves about vaccines and their side effects.

Once a child is diagnosed with autism or one of the other conditions on the autism spectrum, the healing practitioner must address all seven stressors at all levels of healing for complete healing to take place. The easiest way to diagnose which stressors are primary, what interventions are necessary and to monitor recovery, is through autonomic response testing, an eloquent and sophisticated version of kinesiology. Through it, the body will reveal what is wrong, and what procedures it is ready for and when.

As a child heals, Klinghardt's protocol is useful in sequencing "next steps." It is a unique and brilliant model applicable to any medical condition, not just autism.

References

1. Mercola J. www.mercola.com (Accessed March 28, 2007)

2. Mutter J. Mercury and Autism: accelerating evidence. Neuroendocrinal Letters 2005. Freiberg, Germany: 26(5):439-46.

3. Pendergrass JC, Haley BE, Vimy MJ, Winfield SA, et al. Neurotoxicology.1997;18:315-24.

4. KEMI (Swedish Chemicals Agency). Phase out of PBDEs and PBBs: Report on a governmental commission. Solna, Sweden, 1999.

5. Palmer RF., Blanchard S, Stein Z, Mandell D and Miller C. Environmental mercury release, special education rates, and autism disorder: an ecological study of Texas. Health & Place , June 2006 12:203-09.

6. Loesche WJ, Schork A, Terpenning MS, Chen Y-M, Kerr C, et al. The relationship between dental disease and cerebral vascular accident in elderly United States veterans. Ann Periodontal 1998; 3:161-74.

7. Koehler G. The Handbook of Homeopathy: Its Principles and Practice. Rochester, VT: Healing Arts Press, 1986.

8. Jung CG, Campbell J. Translated by RFC Hull. The Portable Jung. New York, NY: Viking Penguin, 1971.

9. Bowen M. Family Therapy in Clinical Practice. New York, NY: Aronson, 1978.

10. Hellinger, B., Weber, G., Beaumont, H. Love's hidden symmetry: What makes love work in relationships. Phoenix, AZ: Zeig, Tucker & Co, 1998.

11. Ramachandran, VS, Oberman, LM. Broken Mirrors: A Theory of Autism. Sci Am November 2006:63-69.

12. Reiter RJ, Robinson J. Melatonin: Your body's natural wonder drug. New York: Bantam Books, 1995.

13. Popp FA. Electromagnetic Bio-Information. Munich: Urban and Schwarzenberg, 1979.

14. www.dromura.net. (Accessed September 24, 2007)

15. http://www.wholywater.com/fluoride.html. (Accessed June 18, 2007)

16. Yaimouyiannis J. Fluoride: The Aging Factor, Delaware, Ohio, Health Action Press, 1993:14.

17. Clark DC. *Appropriate uses of fluorides for children: guidelines from the Canadian Workshop on the Evaluation of Current Recommendations Concerning Fluorides. CMAJ Dec.15, 1993;149:1787-93.*

18. Waldbott G. *Fluoride: The Great Dilemma, Lawrence, KS: Coronado Press, 1978.*

19. Sener G, Sehirli O, Tozan A, Ayanoglu-Dülger G. *Melatonin protects against mercury induced oxidative tissue damage. Basic Clin Pharmacol Toxicol 2003;93:290-96.*

20. Cowan E. *Plant Spirit Medicine: The Healing Power of Plants. Columbus, NC: Swan Raven & Co, 2000.*

21. www.neuraltherapy.com *Lyme disease: A look beyond antibiotics. 1/7/05. (Accessed October 28, 2005)*

22. Pangborn J, Baker SM. *Autism: Effective Biomedical Treatments. San Diego, CA: Autism Research Institute, 2005.*

23. Bode L, Ludwig H. *Borna disease virus infection, a human mental health risk. Clin MicrobiolRev 2003; 16:534-45.*

24. Correspondance. *Neurocysticerosis uncovered by single dose albendazole. N E J Med 2007;356:12, 1277-78.*

25. Ota C, Unterkircher C, Fantinato V, Shimizu, MT. *Antifungal activity of propolis on different species of Candida. Mycoses 2001;44:375-78.*

26. Klinghardt D. *Psychokinesiology: a new approach in psychosomatic medicine. www.neuraltherapy.com (Accessed September 24, 2007)*

27. Ulsamer B. *The healing the power of the past: the systemic therapy of Bert Hellinger. Nevada City, CA: Underwood Books, 2005.*

Chapter 17
Prioritizing Therapies for Children with Autism Spectrum Disorders

Patricia S. Lemer, M.Ed., NCC

The previous chapters provide many pieces of a complex puzzle. How does a parent with a newly diagnosed child or one who has "tried everything" with a teenager, put this 1000 piece puzzle together? How does someone who has been told that autism is an immutable psychiatric brain disorder for which no "cure" exists change thinking to viewing it as biological and energetic imbalances that interfere with all aspects of cognitive, motor, sensory, language, social-emotional and purposeful functioning?

This chapter is a road map to the bright future that is every child's birthright. Thanks to Jenny McCathy and the publication of her book, *Louder than Words,*[1] more and more people are seriously considering therapies that go beyond simply helping our children compensate. Put your big toe into the water and begin now!

Where to Start?

In his brilliant book, *The Four Pillars of Healing,*[2] Leo Galland, MD, likens bringing a body back to health to restoring a fine painting: in both cases, you must know the history. In the book's introduction, Galland takes the reader to an art restoration center in Florence, where experts are learning about the environmental history of a fifteenth century masterpiece. How many damp basements and fires did it survive? What pigments did the artist use to paint it? What solvents did historians apply during its last restoration?

A child diagnosed with autism demands and deserves at least as careful a look as a painting. In order to reveal a child's true abilities and allow them to emerge, one must know his/her history. Galland views disease as the appearance of symptoms related to an accumulation of load factors in the body. Peel back and treat each layer, one by one, until a person is well.

A large subgroup of kids is physically sick well before they "have" autism. These kids have usually gotten sick from the outside in: first skin, then digestive, respiratory and nervous systems, and finally cognitive factors show imbalances. Most children diagnosed with autism, and those with attention deficits and learning disabilities, to a lesser degree, follow this pattern, which is described in Chapter 12. Many doctors now recognize their ear infections, allergies, sleep disturbances, constipation, diarrhea, skin problems, or other symptoms as risk factors for autism spectrum disorders.

Wellness progresses from the inside out. During treatment, parents often report that their children become more cognitively aware, and begin speaking well before their respiratory and gut symptoms resolve. The final phase of healing usually includes some skin eruptions, such as pimples and even boils, along with growth in complex cognitive skills such as abstract thinking and relating socially.

Autism did not just happen overnight, although it may seem, in some cases, as if the child did in fact go from "fine" to "autistic." What was occurring inside the gut, the immune system, and brain were slow processes that may not have been apparent. As problems accumulated and were possibly exacerbated by medical treatments and practices, such as antibiotics, back sleeping, restricted movement and limited diets, outward manifestations appeared. This process could have taken months, even years. Getting well will take at least as long as getting sick. Reversing autism follows a different path for each child because of biological uniqueness.

What a Diagnosis Says

Once a child receives a diagnosis, parents often think that the next step is easy: just treat the problem. However, a diagnosis of one of the pervasive developmental disorders, whether it is autism, ADD, LD, Asperger syndrome, PDD-NOS or any other, merely says that a child's symptoms match a specific cluster of signs. A diagnosis does not prescribe treatment. Individuals with the same diagnosis display similar symptoms; however, they do not necessarily require the same treatments.

Consider the following example:

Symptom: A pounding pain in the right front temporal lobe

Diagnosis: Headache

Possible Causes	Treatment for that cause
Tension and Stress	Aspirin, bed rest
Brain tumor	Surgery
MSG poisoning	Alka-Selzer Gold
Nagging spouse	Divorce

If a person with a headache has not ingested Chinese food, gefilte fish, or another food containing MSG, or is unmarried, causes can be narrowed down to stress and a brain tumor. While this example might seem frivolous, it can easily be applied to those with autism spectrum disorders.

Every Child is Unique

Children with autism diagnoses vary markedly despite similar behavioral symptoms [3]. Sidney Baker, MD, co-founder of Defeat Autism Now! urges doctors and therapists to treat each child on the autism spectrum as a unique individual with a unique health and developmental history, because the causes of the symptoms in all those diagnosed with "autism" are not the same. Determining appropriate treatments and their sequence requires knowing the multiple causes of symptoms in each patient. Baker's guidelines for professionals are in Part 3 of Chapter 6. All parents should share these with anyone working with their children.

Look at ALL Total Load Factors

Recall the concept of "Total Load" presented in Chapter 3. Remember that the body is like a bridge, and can handle only a limited number of stressors, and that it is the cumulative effect of stress factors that overloads it.

The *only* way to determine possible cause(s) of an individual's autism is to take a complete history of *all* possible Total Load factors, including genetic, pre-natal, natal, environmental, developmental and medical concerns. This process could take many hours, a sharp memory and biochemical understanding. One family traced their son's autism back to mold exposure in their air-tight home. Another found the same chemicals in their child's blood as the exterminator used for clearing their house of termites. Yet another discovered a new cell phone tower not far from their home. While no chemical or electro-magnetic field alone is the "cause" of autism, in an immune compromised body, any one could be a trigger that is the "straw that breaks the back" of a child's body's ability to cope.

Genetics Loads the Gun, Environment Pulls the Trigger

Not all individuals exposed to the environmental chemical soup end up with autism. Experts are now able to determine which factors are key in this regard. We know that genetic load factors include a family history of immune system dysfunction such as chronic fatigue, fibro-myalgia, familial allergies, and endocrine deficiencies, including thyroid dysfunction.

Environmental insults are now thought to play a huge role. These are enumerated in Chapter 3. As a review, they include, but are not limited to birth trauma, mercury, aluminum, lead and other heavy metal exposure from the mother's dental amalgams, Rhogam, fish, vaccines, and the air, allergy-prone foods, including wheat and dairy, aggressive use of medications, pesticides, flame retardants, plasticizers, toys, mattresses, water, etc.

Recall the Autism Spectrum Disorder Continuum presented in Chapter 1 with ADD on the least severe end and full-blown autism at the most severe extreme. This continuum can easily look like "alphabet soup" to a confused parent. Usually, the broader the exposure to Total Load factors, the more severe the diagnosis. The sophisticated laboratory tests recommended in Chapters 3 and 6 can assist in looking at both genetic and environmental factors.

Whom to Turn to: Whom to Trust

Autism has become a business in a thriving marketplace of interventions delivered by talented and experienced practitioners, most of whom have something to offer a child with an autism spectrum diagnosis. New approaches are emerging every day, claiming to be the missing link for eliminating toxic metals, healing a leaky gut, enhancing social skills, improving eye contact, increasing expressive language or a plethora of other miracles.

- *Pediatricians?* Most families suspect that "something" is wrong with their children well before getting a formal diagnosis. Many have tried unsuccessfully to convince their pediatricians to refer their offspring for screenings or for early intervention. In the past, their pleas often fell on deaf ears.

In Fall 2007, however, the American Academy of Pediatrics (AAP) strongly urged their member physicians to routinely screen babies for autism at 18 and 24 months, and not wait for a diagnosis before referring them for services[4]. Unfortunately, those screenings have two drawbacks: they come just at the time that the vaccine schedule accelerates, and the recommended referral is for palliative therapies that treat symptoms, not causes.

The good news is that doctors were urged to work together with their patients as partners and to take parents concerns seriously. The AAP suggested that they consider requests for alternative treatments and individualized vaccine schedules, rather than "fire" families from their practices if they did not conform. While these mandates should help toward the goal of "early" diagnosis, some fear they may also lead to "over" diagnosis.

- *Friends and Family?* Well-meaning relatives and parents encourage each other to "try" therapies that they have heard about or personally found helpful. This "buffet" dining approach, which includes many side dishes, and has no main course can waste both time and money. Simply taking therapies "off the rack" like a dress in a department store is like going into the wilderness without a compass.

- *The Internet?* The Internet has opened up a global society, and everyone has a website. The discovery of new exciting therapies with the potential to change children's lives spreads faster than California wildfires. How do you know who is legitimate and who is not?

- *A Case Manager?* For almost 30 years I served as a case manager to families of children with special needs. I attended IEP meetings, advocated for services at due process hearings, and referred families to private practitioners. Living in metropolitan Washington, DC, I was fortunate to be surrounded by extraordinarily talented individuals in many specialities. I had no vested interest in any particular services, although I admittedly did have my biases! Often families would comment up front that they heard I recommended vision therapy for everyone who consulted with me. Of course I did! Every child with special needs should have a developmental vision exam.

Some mental health professionals and developmental pediatricians can serve as professional case managers; ask around. Go to <www.hpakids.org>, the home of the Holistic Pediatric Association (HPA): the Alliance for Holistic Family Health and Wellness, and search their database. HPA is a 501-c3 non-profit, educational organization whose mission is to unite parents and health professionals in the common goal of improving and transforming family health care into a safe, nurturing, and sensible holistic system. They empower parents to trust their natural wisdom and make informed choices on behalf of their children.

Trying to figure out "next steps" or going to an IEP meeting alone can be daunting. When the school system fills a conference table with in an army of "big guns," having your own expert is reassuring. It is truly amazing how an educational team sits up and takes notice when a physician speaks. If you cannot find a paid professional, take a friend who has been through the process. A grandparent or other relative, a private therapist, a neighbor or babysitter can also fill the bill.

To help guide you, Developmental Delay Resources (DDR), the organization Lemer and Dorfman co-founded, offers local referrals to therapists, clinics and other specialists from their database of over 20,000 resources. Their published annual Networking Directory is available by calling 800-497-0944 or emailing to devdelay@mindspring.com.

Follow a Prioritized Model of Therapies

What *every* child with an autism spectrum diagnosis requires is a set of basic, general principles that are good for anyone and everyone interested in disease-free living, PLUS a therapy plan customized for that individual child's needs. The general principles form a strong, unbendable foundation for health. They are appropriate no matter whether the diagnosis is at the mild, moderate or severe end of the autism spectrum, or is even a degenerative disease of modern society. The therapy plan is unique for a specific child. It must be monitored by a health care professional, and will change daily, weekly, monthly, and yearly as the child responds, regresses, progresses, and heals.

The premise that the body's top priority is staying well, is the foundation for developing a hierarchy of therapies. The relationship between symptoms and treatments is not linear, but rather a complex matrix with multiple variables. As treatments reduce specific individual load factors, the body then uses newly freed up energy to address others.

Optometrists, CranioSacral practitioners, and others have told me that their patient's allergies often get better following vision and craniosacral therapy. Likewise, visual skills and performance in many other areas improves with detoxification, especially of mercury. Language often emerges following dietary modification and motor skills improve following VT. Making a step-by-step, "one size fits all" treatment plan is thus impossible. One must take a "wait and see" attitude following each intervention. The ultimate goal is to remove the largest load factors first, freeing up the most energy possible.

At first, sensory, language, social-emotional and academic development must take a back seat to biological issues. Once the body is putting less energy into digestion, circulation, respiration and detoxification, a team of experts can develop the specifics of a hierarchy of adjunct therapies. While it may sound crazy to wait, even for a short time, this plan will waste less time and money in the long term. Allowing the body to use its own wisdom to heal may result in bypassing some therapies altogether.

Step One- Immediately Eliminate ALL Possible Toxic Exposures

As soon as autism or any other spectrum diagnosis is suspected, eliminating all exposures to toxins is essential! Toxins can come from anything a child eats, drinks, breathes, puts on his/her skin, in the mouth, in the home, school, or other locations that the child frequents. Foods, personal care products, household cleaners, electro-magnetic fields, and even psychologically abusive people can all be toxic. Figure 17-1 shows steps to take to reduce toxic experience. An excellent general overview on eliminating toxins is *Chemical-Free Kids: How to Safeguard Your Child's Diet and Environment*[5] by Allan Magaziner, DO. These steps are a must:

Figure 17-1
Steps to Reduce Toxic Exposures
Clean up the existing diet
Eliminate any tobacco exposure
Use chemical-free alternatives for
  o   art supplies
  o   bedding
  o   cleaning and laundering products
  o   construction and remodeling
  o   personal care products
  o   pest control
Mitigate electromagnetic fields
Boost, not weaken the immune system

- *Clean up the existing diet*
  o Eat fresh, unrefined, mostly organic foods in season. Minimize the use of canned, frozen, pre-prepared and processed foods. Rediscover your kitchen. Take cooking classes; buy cookbooks. Cook food with gas or electric stoves, avoiding microwave ovens. Never microwave food in plastic containers.
  o Vary a healthy balance of high quality protein, carbohydrates and fats. Eat protein for breakfast. Focus on complex carbohydrates, especially fruits and vegetables, rather than processed products. Eliminate trans-fats and remember to include fat sources that supply essential Omega 3 fats. Drink only filtered, natural spring, and non-fluoridated water. Rotate grains, meats, fruits, and vegetable families. For specific guidelines, refer back to Chapter 5.

Expensive you say? Not if you eat REAL food: protein, vegetables and rice.

Hard to do? Maybe a little, at first, but SO much support is available online, from local Food Co-ops, stores like Trader Joe's, Whole Foods and Wild Oats.

- *Eliminate tobacco exposure.* If any family members are still smokers, insist that they smoke well away from the house. Stay clear of restaurants and bars that permit smoking. Adults carry second-hand smoke into the house on their clothing.

- *If remodeling, buy recycled, chemical-free products that do not off-gas* for both the home and school. Building materials are major sources of neurotoxins and other dangers. Use no-VOC paints and wood that is not treated with formaldehyde, especially when preparing a baby's room. Siding, cabinets, carpeting, glue, insulation and other materials can "out-gas" for years. Be sure that renovation doesn't occur when people are in residence. Go to <www.ecobuilding.org> for fact sheets on remodeling from foundation to roof from the Northwest Eco-Building Guild. Spending money on air filters and purifiers is a waste unless the toxins are eliminated in the first place.[6]

- *Watch those art supplies*
  o Use only lead- and asbestos-free crayons and magic markers denoted "non-toxic."
  o Avoid oil-based paints, chalk and spray adhesives around children, as they contain toxic metals to heighten color and add stickiness, and chalk dust contains talc.
  o Buy only water-based glues and paste.

- *Use alternative methods to banish pests*
  o Keep pests outside the home and school. Remember that pesticides used outdoors are tracked indoors. Copy the Japanese and leave your shoes at the door.

- o Utilize integrated pest management systems instead of pesticides to eliminate them. Protect pets with natural bug repellants, such as diatomaceous earth, a fine white powder, made from ground up fossilized remains of diatoms, a kind of sea algae.

- *Buy "green" cleaning products*
  - o Use toxin- and perfume-free cleaning and laundering products such as vinegar, baking soda, natural laundry and dishwasher soaps, bathroom cleaners and detergents. No dryer sheets or fabric softeners. Minimize dry-cleaning. If clothes are not washable, at least air them out before bringing them indoors, to let the chemicals dissipate.
  - o Try Deirdre Imus' Greening the Cleaning® products, Mrs. Meyer's Clean Day, and Seventh Generation items, now widely available. Seventh Generation also manufactures many paper products, bath and facial tissue, diapers, baby wipes, and other essentials that are both good for you and your family, as well as for the environment.

- *Use natural fibers for any product that touches the skin.* All clothing and bedding should be 100% natural, and organic when possible. Most cosmetics are full of poisons, such as lead and mercury. Join the Safe Cosmetics Campaign at <www.safecosmetics.org> to work with manufacturers who encourage reformulations and safer ingredients. Some companies that are committed to safe products are Aubrey Organics, Desert Essence, Dr. Bronner's, Pangea Organics, and Terressentials.

  - o Avoid flame retardants in mattresses and sleepwear. Buy only organic for the whole family, especially the new baby. Replace electric and synthetic blankets with natural bedding. Some sources are <www.lifekind.com>, <www.greensleep.com> and <www.nontoxic.com> .
  - o Watch out for phthalates, plasticizers that add texture and luster to hair spray, deodorant, nail polish, lipstick, perfume, and other personal care products. Lotions and creams are especially problematic. Phthalates can be absorbed through the skin, inhaled through off-gassing, and ingested by children mouthing products. Hundreds of studies have shown that they can damage the liver, kidneys, lungs and the reproductive system. In pregnant women, phthalates pass through the placenta to be absorbed by the fetus. Later they show up in breast milk of nursing mothers, whose babies ingest them. In male fetuses and infants, phthalates can cause testicular atrophy, leading to a reduced sperm count.[7]

- *Reduce exposure to electromagnetic fields (EMFs)*
  - o Remove all electrical appliances from everyone's bedrooms, including TVs, computers, cordless phones, routers, cell phones and their chargers. Use a battery or wind-up alarm clock. Turn off Wi-Fi at night, or, better yet, switch to DSL. Make sure you know what is on the other side of the wall from the heads of all beds. If a TV is on that wall, then move it or the bed.
  - o Never use laptops on the lap.
  - o Do not use fluorescent lighting of any kind. Compact fluorescent energy efficient bulbs emit radio frequencies and are difficult to dispose of because of their mercury content. Use ordinary full spectrum light bulbs throughout the house EXCEPT in the bedroom, where you can use normal incandescent bulbs.
  - o Keep the family's cell phone use to an absolute minimum. Try not to use the phone in the car, and at home use only corded phones.
  - o Have your home inspected by a trained Building Biology Inspector. Find one near you at <www.buildingbiology.net>.

To learn more, read *Electromagnetic Fields: A Consumer Guide to the Issues* and *How to Protect Ourselves*[8] and *Cell Tower: Wireless Convenience* or *Environmental Hazard?* by B. Blake Levitt.[9]

- *Boost, not weaken the immune system*

The history of a child whose body's immune system has become exhausted from too many load factors usually has several of the following signs:

- o Immediate relative with auto-immune disorder; allergies (especially to cow's milk), diabetes
- o Colic, reflux, eczema, thrush, asthma, leaky gut
- o Over three ear/sinus/strep/yeast infections
- o Long bout with one illness
- o Heavy use of antibiotics, sugar cravings
- o Dark circles, red ears and cheeks
- o Regression in skills between 15 and 30 months
- o Hyperactivity, sleep disturbances, mood swings

Why is this recommendation under the section about reducing exposures? Because once a child has an autism spectrum diagnosis, parents and their physicians have to make the very difficult decision about whether to give additional vaccinations. Revaccinating a child who has had a "warning" vaccine reaction, or has regressed following vaccination is extremely risky. Also, vaccines without mercury still include potentially dangerous substances that add to the load of what the body must detoxify.

Doctors need to listen to and respond to parental concerns, making fathers and mothers, who wish it, an integral part of the treatment team. Physicians are no longer considered authority figures by this generation of parents who feel that they know their kids best. They recognize when their kids are not right, and have good hunches about what they need.

If necessary, a well-trained nurse practitioner or physician's assistant can help, by taking a child's complete history of prenatal, natal and environmental factors, and asking about what a child is eating, drinking and breathing, how much sleep, screen time and exercise a child is getting. After meeting with the doctor, the assistant can pick up where the doctor left off, and encourage a healthy diet, sufficient sleep, good hydration and daily exercise.

See the section entitled "Making a Vaccination Decision: Before You Vaccinate, Ask Eight" in Chapter 4 for guidelines. If parents ask physicians to work with them on a modified vaccination schedule, they should learn about supplements that are immune system boosters to use alone, or before and after vaccination, and cooperate, rather than chastise.

Remember that exposures from air, food, water, dust and all other sources are cumulative, and add incrementally to an individual's Total Load. Read labels on each and every product you bring into your home. No amount of cleanliness and convenience is worth risking your family's health. Unless you are conscious about ALL of the above steps, you could be spending thousands and thousands of dollars on fabulous therapies, and then returning your child's recovering body into a sick home or school.

Step Two – Address Structural Problems

The birth and peri-natal histories of children with underlying structural issues usually includes one or more of the following that cause(s) organs, fluids, bones and connective tissues to be out of balance:

- Long labor, breech presentation, forceps or vacuum aspiration, premature and/or traumatic birth, C-section
- Delay in sucking, reflux, vomiting or spitting
- Strabismus, nystagmus, reduced acuity
- Missing stages in motor development in the first year of life

Therapies in Figure 17-2 are described in Chapters 3 and 16. They can restore the body's structural integrity by

Figure 17-2
Therapies Addressing Structural Issues
Chiropractic
Chiropractic Neurology
Osteopathy
Cranio – Sacral Therapy

- Releasing blockages in flow of internal fluids and energy
- Balancing the relationships among organs
- Preparing the body to absorb essential nutrients

Changing the body's structure changes its function, allowing normal development to proceed along a pre-programmed, prescribed sequential path. Unless health care professionals address structural issues early in treatment, these impediments can interfere with later steps, especially the absorption of vitamins and minerals, and the detoxification of metals, pesticides and other poisons.

At this point an optometrist should also become a member of the diagnostic and treatment team. Extreme or overt visual symptoms, such as an obvious strabismus, nystagmus, or reduced acuity could require direct intervention immediately. Subtle problems, easier for parents and professionals to overlook, such as fluctuating focus, dynamic asymmetries between the two eyes, trouble crossing the midline while tracking, or integrating central with peripheral vision, have a more profound impact on overall visual processing, and thus effect behavior and learning. These less obvious functions warrant adding an optometrist to the "Early Intervention Team" now.

However, visual symptoms, both extreme and subtle, could possibly be secondary to structural, reflex or toxicity issues. Thus, many behavioral optometrists collaborate with chiropractors, osteopaths, nutritionists, and practitioners using CranioSacral techniques[10]. Some optometrists have even received advanced training in some of these areas.

Three other therapeutic modalities that may also be extremely beneficial early on in treatment are:

- *Reflex integration* – In Chapter 8, the authors suggest combining structural therapies with a reflex integration program, especially in children whose health issues are stabilized.
- *Homeopathy* – In Chapter 12, Drs. Judyth Reichenberg-Ullman and Dr. Robert Ullman discuss how to use homeopathic medicines to address all aspects of a child's profile.
- *Family Constellations* – In Chapter 16, Dr. Dietrich Klinghardt supports doing a family constellation before beginning other therapies in families with traumatic histories. This intervention releases past generational stressors, thus allowing other therapies to work more efficiently.

The last two above are interventions that work at an energetic level. They can thus be introduced at any time during a child's therapeutic program.

Experience shows that, in a majority of cases, most interventions must wait until health improves and stabilizes. However, sometimes families can work on several therapies simultaneously, even though the scientific method stresses only one intervention at a time.

Step Three – Biomedical Intervention
A biomedical treatment approach includes further dietary modification and nutritional supplementation. Chapter 5 covers these subjects in depth. An excellent book on the subject is Kenneth Bock's *Healing the New Childhood Epidemics: Autism, ADHD, Asthma and Allergies.*[11] Subsets of his Healing Program are special diets and the use of substances that address gastrointestinal disturbances, aid in detoxification, and build the immune system.

Supplements can be delivered by mouth, suppository, IV, trans-dermally, homeopathically, or nasally. For every viable biological intervention, health care practitioners and parents must agree on both the right substances and delivery methods. Infinite permutations and combinations are possible, and each nutritionist and physician has his/her favorite company, products and delivery systems. All must be individualized for a particular child. Trial and error is the only method that really works, because kids differ so in their tastes, sensory preferences, willingness and motivation to comply. If a child rejects a doctor's favorite product, if a product is too costly, if the parent cannot get the product in, or for other reasons that interfere with compliance, ask if a substitute exists.

- *Removing possible offenders* is the next step in dietary modification after improving the quality of the present diet. Some families use simple elimination diets, followed by a challenge; others rely on laboratory testing. Dr. Doris Rapp's book has easy-to-use elimination diets for those preferring this method.[12] See the end of Chapter 3 for a detailed list of recommended laboratory tests.

- *Special diets* are the foundation of biomedical intervention for children on the autism spectrum. Eating out and eating pre-prepared foods make adhering to special diets extremely challenging. Parents of children on special diets must work hard to cook at home daily. All members of the immediate family, including grandparents, aunts, uncles and cousins, and anyone else who spends any time with a child must be "on board" for special diets to work. If just one person feels sorry for a child who cannot eat ice cream and cake at a birthday party, that individual can undermine the program.

Therapists, teachers and their assistants, shadows, and all members of the school family must also comply, including using "acceptable" substitutes for reinforcers. Fortunately, once they see the results, compliance should not be that difficult.

Review Chapter 5 for full descriptions of the most popular diets. See Figure 17-3 for a list of diets that can help those with autism spectrum disorders. This section provides a review and specific information on each.

> Figure 17-3
> **Special Diets for ASD**
> Body Ecology Diet (BED)
> Feingold Diet
> Gluten-free, Casein-free Diet (GF/CF)
> Specific Carbohydrate Diet (SCD)
> Yeast-free Diet

Feingold Diet – Eliminates artificial colors, flavors, excitotoxins, preservatives and naturally occurring salicylates. Go to <www.feingold.org> to join and take advantage of the extraordinary materials this organization has to offer. For $89/year, a family receives:

- o A *Member Handbook* with an extensive Foodlist of acceptable and non-acceptable food, a two-week menu plan, recipes, a diet diary form and more
- o A *Supplement Guide* of acceptable brands
- o A *Mail order guide* for hard-to-find products
- o A *Fast Food Guide*, based on information provided by popular fast food chains
- o *"Pure Facts Newsletter"* printed 10 times a year with updates to the Foodlist, new research, member issues, etc.
- o *Members Section on Website* that is password protected
- o *Help-Line* by both e-mail and phone at no charge
- o **Product Alerts** via e-mail

EVERY family that cares about health should belong to this organization and read *Why Can't My Child Behave?* by Jane Hersey,[13] a veteran Feingold volunteer.

GF/CF Diet – A GF/CF diet is the most important intervention for many children, with 80% show some improvement. Many doctors working with Defeat Autism Now! believe that every child with an autism diagnosis should be on a GF/CF diet for at least three months.

Help is available from many sources.

- o **Autism Network for Dietary Intervention (ANDI)** at <www.AutismNDI.com>. Its founders, both mothers of boys with autism, have written best-selling books that many find invaluable. Karyn Seroussi's *Unraveling the Mystery of Autism and Pervasive Developmental Disorders*[14] is her heart-warming story that gives many newly diagnosed families hope. In a straight forward fashion Seroussi tells parents the importance of going GF/CF.
- o **Cookbooks:** *Special Diets for Special Kids*, Volumes I and II[15] by ANDI co-founder, Lisa Lewis. Volume I outlines the theory behind the diet, and has recipes for kid standards such as GF/CF macaroni and cheese, pizza dough, and chicken nugget coating. Volume II is a continuation with hundreds of GF/CF recipes for those ready to branch out to everything from to healthy casseroles to imaginative breakfasts. *The Kid-Friendly ADHD and Autism Cookbook: The Ultimate Guide to the Gluten-Free, Casein-Free Diet* by developmental pediatrician Pamela Compart, MD and nutritionist Dana Laake [16] has an easy-to-understand explanation of the science behind the diet, as well as many kid-tested recipes.
- o **Pre-made mixes and products** that make GF/CF cooking a breeze. Some favorites are Miss Robens (www.allergygrocer.com), Kinnikinnick Foods and The Gluten Free Pantry (www.glutenfree.com) and Enjoy Life Foods (www.enjoylife.com). Websites on gluten- and dairy-free cooking, along with thousands of recipes are also available online.
- o **Sully's Living Without Magazine** is a quarterly publication offering tips and recipes in a beautiful format. To subscribe, go to <www.livingwithout.com>.

Yeast-free Diet is often done in conjunction with the GF/CF and Feingold diets because a common problem is that many additive- wheat- and dairy-free products, especially baked goods, contain considerable amounts of sugar, which feeds yeast. Thus, health care practitioners discourage these processed foods, as well as foods that contain yeast and mold, including breads, crackers, pastries, pretzels, cakes, cookies, rolls, mushrooms, cantaloupes, peanuts, all cheeses, buttermilk, vinegar, catsup, mayonnaise, olives, pickles, alcohol, malted products, as well as anything aged or fermented. Follow a guidebook, such as *Feast Without Yeast; 4 Stages to Better Health*,[17] *The Yeast Connection Handbook*,[18] or *The Yeast Connection Cookbook*.[19]

Specific Carbohydrate Diet (SCD) – This diet takes GF/CF and Yeast-free a step further for those kids who still have gut problems by eliminating many foods that feed micro-organisms.

- o **Allows** most fresh fruits & vegetables, beans, unprocessed meats, fish and poultry, natural cheeses, olive & coconut oils, and honey.
- o **Disallows** all grains, processed meats, soy products, cow's milk, sugars, canned fruit & vegetables.
- o **Includes** a specially fermented home-made goat milk yoghurt, in which the culturing changes the structure of the casein and renders it harmless. Most children tolerate the goat yogurt if they start out with a tiny amount and gradually increase it.

Read: *Breaking the Vicious Cycle*[20] and *We Band of Mothers: Autism, My Son and The Specific Carbohydrate Diet*,[21] and go to <www.pecanbread.com> to thoroughly understand this diet.

Body Ecology Diet (BED), developed by nutritional consultant Donna Gates is, in my opinion, the best diet of all. Donna views autism as a combination of disorders – all correctable. She believes that the intestinal-brain infection distances the child from his/her surroundings. The goal of the BED is to "bring the children back into our world and back to their true selves" with dietary intervention. The BED removes all of the most problematic foods: sugars, gluten, casein, processed foods, soy and canola oil, as well as includes the best quality, most nutritionally dense foods from all the food groups:

- o ***Plentiful, nutritionally dense, dark, leafy green and root vegetables,*** such as collard and mustard greens, kale, broccoli, onions, parsnips, winter squash and potatoes.
- o *Animal proteins* that are hormone and antibiotic-free, and easier-to-digest, such as fish, chicken, and softly scrambled eggs. Sometimes amino acid supplements may be needed to aid protein digestion.
- o *Four gluten-free grains:* quinoa, millet, amaranth and buckwheat, all of which are high in vegetable proteins.
- o *Organic, unrefined, virgin oils and fats:* coconut, cod liver, flaxseed, macadamia nut, olive and pumpkinseed oils, ghee, raw butter and cream. These provide monoun-saturated fats, antioxidants, zinc and omega 3 fats.
- o *Selected fruits:* berries, grapefruit, kiwi, green apples and pineapples, eaten with at least four ounces of coconut kefir (see below), to counteract the negative effect of fruits' natural sugars, which can feed a systemic fungal/yeast infection and cause the blood to remain too acidic.

Gates has established an online community of families interested in healing their children using the BED. She calls her group **BEDROK** for **B**ody **E**cology **D**iet **R**ecovering **O**ur **K**ids. The goals of the **BEDROK** program are to:

1. nourish the cells and tissues of the body with high quality, easily-digested foods that contain superior nutrition.

2. bring ALL infections and virus' under control.

3. open detoxification pathways, thus allowing the body to continually cleanse out toxins that have accumulated since conception.

4. create a strong, vital inner ecosystem in the intestines that ensures the digestion and absorption of foods, and corrects the nutrient deficiencies that accompany autism. This vibrant inner ecosystem also builds a healthy intestinal lining, and a strong immune system that protects a child from further infections.

The **BED**'s following seven principles encompass all the other diets.

- *Principle of Uniqueness* This principle is a foundation of the Defeat Autism Now! protocol. Individual dietary and nutritional needs change daily, with the seasons, as well as with load factors. Donna adds the principles of the original blood type diet[22] to help guide food choices that might be better for individuals from one blood group than another.

- *Principle of Expansion and Contraction* Based on the macrobiotic principles of yin and yang, which look at the energetic properties of food, this principle helps a person maintain dietary balance by avoiding foods and substances that are too contracting such as meat, eggs and salt or too expansive, such as sugar. The BED encourages primary food selection from the middle of this continuum, which includes many types of vegetables.

- *Principle of Acid and Alkaline* Keeping blood in a slightly alkaline condition is vital to restoring health. Too much acid encourages yeast overgrowth, viruses, parasites, and other unhealthy bugs to thrive. Every meal should contain 20% acid-forming foods and

80% alkaline-forming foods. To download a food chart showing the pH of many foods, go to <www.acidalkalinebalance.com>. Another good reference is the book *Alkalize or Die*.[23] To assure an alkaline gut, the BED uses Vitality SuperGreen® or other powdered nutrient-rich green drinks to alkalize the intestines and restore and maintain a healthy inner ecosystem.

- *Principle of Cleansing* This principle states that humans must continuously cleanse to remove the toxins of modern-day living. The BED is unique in recommending regular colon cleansing as an element to this most important principle.

- *Principle of Food Combining* The basic premise of this principle is that different nutrients require different conditions in the stomach to be properly digested. For example, protein requires a high-acid environment; starch requires an alkaline environment. Mixing starch and protein in a single meal does not allow the stomach to digest either properly. Three rules: Always eat

  o protein with non-starchy and/or ocean vegetables.
  o allowable grains (amaranth, quinoa, buckwheat and millet) and starchy vegetables (acorn and butternut squash, lima beans, peas, corn, water chestnuts, artichokes and red skin potatoes) with non-starchy and/or sea vegetables.
  o fruits alone, and on an empty stomach.

Separating starch and protein into separate meals and eating fruit separately increases the efficiency of digestion. Following this principle can often lead to great success with digestive issues.

- *Principle of 80/20* Two more rules:
  1. Eat until your stomach is 80% full, leaving 20% available for digestion. Overeating, until your stomach is 100% full slows digestion and furthers yeast overgrowth. Leaving a little room for the digestive juices to do their job is essential for efficient digestion. Limit a meal to one portion of grain or starchy vegetables, and if still hungry, eat more alkaline vegetables.

  2. 80% of your food should be land and/or ocean vegetables. The remaining 20% are animal protein (fish or poultry), an acceptable grain, and starchy vegetables.

- *Principle of Step-by-step* True healing takes place in small steps, which happen in their own time and order. The body goes through cycles of progress followed by periods of rest. Each step gets deeper and deeper into the body to pull out toxins and heal. Quick fixes, such as drugs halt the body's innate wisdom to cleanse, driving sickness deeper into the body, and opening the potential for more serious illness later. The toxins that have accumulated over years cannot be eliminated in days. To assist the body in healing, Gates makes the following suggestions:
  1. Eliminate all stressors
  2. Don't cheat on the diet
  3. Eat foods that aid in cleansing (see below).
  4. Eliminate medications that suppress healing
  5. Rest and sleep
  6. Use probiotics (See section on supplements)

The **BED** also includes unique "signature" foods that aid in detoxification and healing: kefir and fermented coconut pudding from young coconuts, cultured and sea vegetables, (together 75 - 80% of each meal), raw butter, Celtic sea salt and whey protein. These fermented and other important foods are the real "stars" of the **BEDROK** protocol that can put a big jump start on healing.

- *Young coconut kefir (yck)* and coconut pudding are made from the green or white, unripe baby versions of the mature fuzzy brown coconuts most people recognize. These gems are available in most health food or natural food stores. Their sterile pale "milk" and gelatinous "meat" are full of minerals and enzymes. Donna "kefirs" these parts of the coconut, using a special "starter" that she sells, to make a drink and pudding that most children love. She recommends drinking at least 1/4 -1/2 cup of the kefir in the morning upon rising, with meals, and at bedtime. The fermented meat, great for breakfast or a snack, provides a raw, easily-digested, vegetarian protein that contains valuable lauric (antimicrobial) and caprylic (antifungal) fatty acids.

- *Cultured vegetables (CVs)* aid in digestion, especially when eaten with meals containing animal protein. Ideally everyone should have some CVs or yck with every meal. Puree cultured vegetables for children who do not chew well. They taste tart and sour, and can be made more palatable by combining them with olive or pumpkinseed oil, raw cream, homemade mayonnaise, celtic seasalt, and/or stevia.

- *Raw Butter* is almost 100% milk fat, while over 50% of breast milk is raw fat. The goal is to duplicate the raw fat in a healthy mother's breast milk. Raw butter contains vitamins A, D, E and butyric acid. It is very healing to the mucosal lining of the gut, and helps the micro-flora adhere there and colonize. Butter is 99% casein-free; that's less casein than in human breast milk. If kids start on raw butter four to seven days after coconut kefir, the small amount of residual casein does not cause a problem for those following a GF/CF regimen. In fact, the butter seems to really jump-start the healing process. Find a reliable, local source for raw, organic, grass-fed butter.

- *Whey protein*, while a milk product, does not contain casein. Milk is made up of 20% whey protein and 80% casein. Whey protein increases glutathione levels in the liver, thus helping with detoxification. It is also great for muscle development. After being on yck for about two weeks, add one scoop of the undenatured whey protein to the Vitality SuperGreen drink.

The BED can be a very different way of eating for many people, especially those who subsist on a standard American diet replete with wheat and sugar. I have included so many details about this diet because just cleaning up the quality of the diet can result in some remarkable changes. While some families can make a transition to this healthy way of eating quickly, others may find it very challenging, especially for children who are picky eaters. However, the BED can do no harm, and the whole family is guaranteed to benefit from it.

Donna Gates has made her autism support program available to anyone serious about learning about the BED. She sells a 12-CD set entitled *The Natural Autism Solution: Dietary Secrets to Help Prevent and Overcome Autism, ADHD, Asperger's and other Epidemic Childhood Disorders* and teaches seminars on the subject. This product and a list of her trained BED coaches in almost every state are listed on the Body Ecology website at <www.bodyecologydiet.com>.

What's for Breakfast?

One of the most frequently asked questions from families new to special diets is, "What can we eat for breakfast?" For anyone used to juice, cereal and toast, breakfast can be a real challenge. Some guidelines:

- ***Think protein*** – Research now shows the importance of a good breakfast to prepare children for learning. [24] Nutritionist Kelly Dorfman says we have it backwards: eat your dinner for breakfast! Protein in the morning is the best gift to give your child; any animal or vegetable protein will do. Last night's leftovers, a turkey burger, lamb chop, salmon patty, scrambled eggs, lentil soup, bean burrito, or any other meal that gives you at least 10 grams of protein.

- *Think dense nutrition* – Donna Gates suggests a delicious breakfast soup made with fennel, broccoli, garlic and parsley, cooked in organic vegetable or chicken broth.

- *Think quick and easy* – Look in the freezer section for good quality gluten- and dairy-free waffles and pancakes. Up their protein with a nut butter spread. Try GF/CF cereals made with amaranth or quinoa, and added flaxseeds. Make high protein muffins with pre-made mixes from excellent suppliers. Use these substitutes at most twice a week.

- *Think portable* - Try some high protein GF/CF breakfast bars for a fast breakfast on days when time is a problem. A huge variety is available from good health food stores, Whole Foods, Trader Joe's, ANDI and Kirkman. Sample several until you find some whose taste you like.

- *Think drink* – Use nut and grain milks with protein powders to make a quick nutritious drinkable breakfast. Each of the above diets offers online recipes for a multitude of tastes from chocolate to fruity to nutty. Experiment with ingredients. No two batches will be the same.

- *Think EFAs* – Add flax, hemp, flavored cod liver, pumpkinseed or other high quality oils to whatever you make. They enhance texture and are close to tasteless.

Rotate four or five of the above breakfasts, never having the same breakfast two days in a row. Once your kids discover several acceptable alternatives, breakfast should be the best meal of the day!

In review, modifying and being flexible with diet is the essence of maximizing a child's ability. At the risk of using a cliché, "A car runs only as well as the gasoline in its tank." The human body, like a car, MUST have excellent fuel to run. As the now classic book on a biomedical approach to autism suggests[25], many of our children have "starving brains." We must change the way they eat for any and all of the excellent therapies they receive to work well.

Take the first big step to reversing and healing autism and other disorders by making a commitment to one or more of the above diets, and stick to it. Move to a different one if changes do not show up quickly. Get support from family members and the many resources available if you are having trouble. Good luck!

- *Nutritional supplementation* is the essential companion therapy to special diets because it closes the gap between what children eat and what their bodies and starving brains need to grow, develop and heal. Review Chapter 5 to understand why food alone cannot satisfy the omega 3 fatty acid and mineral deficiencies, immune system dysregulation, chronic diarrhea or constipation and heavy metal toxicity that a majority of kids have.

Putting together the right combination of supplements for a particular child is an art, not a science. Find a nutritionist or other health care provider familiar with autism spectrum disorders to guide you. Also, re-read the section on Klinghardt's use of Autonomic Response Testing (ART) in Chapter 16. ART is invaluable in determining appropriate detoxification techniques, as well as the body's readiness for any particular treatment at a given time. Parents are urged to learn how to use this sophisticated, non-invasive form of muscle testing to prioritize therapies, for "tweaking" diets, supplement dosages and frequencies, and other interventions. It is also extremely helpful in identifying toxic metals, pesticides, plastics and other problematic chemicals, as well as the best substance(s) to remove them.

Just as important as increasing the quality of food children eat is taking vitamins of good quality without artificial and non-essential fillers. Here are some guidelines.

Buy "pharmaceutical grade" vitamins from pharmacies, health care providers and others, by manufacturers who take pride in their products and know this population of kids. Many instances of "the supplement did not work" are due to poor quality products off the shelves of grocery and health food stores. Supplements are one instance where you really get what you pay for.

Remember EFAs must be ingested. Child who are not eating good fats must take them as supplements. See Chapter 5 for symptoms of EFA deficiencies, food sources, how to balance out omega 3 and 6 fats, and avoiding "bad" fats.

Use the proper form of a vitamin or mineral. Ask a knowledgeable health care practitioner to recommend the form and delivery system of a vitamin or mineral, to assure it is absorbable, and appropriate for a particular child. For instance, the most highly recommended form of B12 is injectable methylcobalamin, not oral cyanocobalamin, which is more available.

Start slowly and gradually increase dosages. Work with a health care practitioner to make sure that the initial dosage is not too powerful. Err on the side of caution by starting with a small amount and moving to a target dosage gradually.

Drop back the dosage or stop the supplement with negative symptoms such as irritability, diarrhea or constipation. All of these symptoms signal something is amiss. Decrease dosages until symptoms disappear.

Figure 17-4 shows minimum allowances of the top anti-oxidants, B vitamins, minerals and essential fatty acids for all children who have any types of developmental delays, whether diagnosed or not. [26] Make sure these allowances are in place before adding other supplements to bring dosages up to therapeutic levels.

Figure 17-4
Optimal Intake of Vitamins and Other Nutrients from Food & Supplements

NUTRIENTS	FUNCTION	<AGE 3	>AGE 3
Anti-Oxidants:			
Vit C	Protects against environmental toxins Supports immune system	100-250 mg	250-1000 mg
Vit E	Detoxifies; protects fat soluble tissues	30-100 I.U.	60-200 I.U.
B Vitamins:	Aid in growth, repair of neurological function	2-10x RDA	
Vit B6	Co-factor in over 300 reactions. Take w/Mg	25-50 mg	Up to 8 mg/lb
Vit B12	Facilitates methylation in detoxification	Up to 55 mcg/kg	
Minerals:			
Calcium (Ca)	Builds healthy bones and teeth		Total of 900 mg
Chromium (Ch)	Stabilizes blood sugar	50 mcg	50-150 mcg
Magnesium (Mg)	Maintains electrical balance Stabilizes cell membranes	100 mg	100-400 mg
Selenium (Se)	Displaces mercury	50 mcg	50-150 mcg
Zinc (Zn)	Strengthens immune function Improves smell, taste Calms nervous system	5-12 mg	12-20 mg
Essential Fatty Acids	Enhance cognitive/neurological function Calms nervous system	1 tsp flaxseed, or ½ teas. cod liver oil	1-2 teas. cod liver oil

- *Add other supplements* once a child is no longer nutritionally bereft. Again refer back to Chapters 5 and 6 to review specific recommendations from Defeat Autism Now! and nutritionist Kelly Dorfman for other supplements and occasional pharmaceuticals that
  - reduce inflammation
  - restore intestinal integrity
  - boost the immune system
  - repair the leaky gut
  - help with poor absorption
  - detoxify environmental chemicals

DMG, one of Dr. Rimland's favorite supplements, will probably be at the top of the list to add along with B_6 and magnesium. Other close contenders are folic acid, probiotics, digestive enzymes and anti-fungals.

The importance of working with a knowledgeable health care practitioner cannot be overemphasized. Although working independently, using a guidebook or recommendations taken from someone's website can be very tempting, experience in this field, even with just infrequent consultations is invaluable.

Step Four – Detoxification

Once diet and nutrition have stabilized the gut, a child is eating a wider variety of foods, including sufficient protein, taking a regime of vitamin and mineral supplements, and is generally healthier, the next step is ridding the body of the toxins that wreaked havoc there in the first place. Testing for toxicity can be tricky because most urine, hair, blood and stool tests pinpoint only recent exposures. Refer to the section entitled "Identifying Children who are Toxic" in Chapter 5 for recommendations on laboratory testing utilizing and the new porphyrin tests that show the presence of mercury.

Doctors and other health care practitioners are using many creative methods for ridding the body of unwanted substances, and assisting it in healing from the inside out. Figure 17-5 shows different methods for detoxification of various substances that interfere with function. *All detoxification requires strict supervision.*

| Figure 17-5 |
| **Methods of Detoxification** |
| Foods and Supplements |
| Chelation |
| Homotoxicology |
| Sweating in Sauna |

o *Diet and Supplements* – Some foods are natural detoxifiers. Garlic, chlorella and cilantro, among others, can often do the job slowly in less severe cases, and for those children whose bodies are not ready for more potent treatments.

o *Chelation programs,* like nutritional supplementation, vary markedly, depending upon which doctor or health care practitioner a family works with, and what type of testing was used to identify the culprits. ART is so valuable in this regard, as it asks a unique, individual body to expose what it is ready for at the present time, rather than depend upon standardized protocols and trial and error methods which can be expensive and potentially dangerous.

Some children, however, require more powerful treatments, such as intravenous glutathione, DMPS, TTFD, EDTA or other chelators, available only by prescription. All must be supported by strong nutritional programs to replenish minerals that chelators take with them along with the metals.

- *Homotoxicology* is fast becoming one of the most popular ways of removing toxins from the body because it is one of the least invasive, least costly, safest and most efficient methods we have today. See the section on this exciting rising therapy in Chapter 12.

Using special equipment, a homeopathic practitioner determines what order to detoxify the body using combination and low potency remedies that support and stimulate the body's own detoxification pathways. This energetic treatment first "opens the channels" to assure that the toxins are not reabsorbed, and then sequentially uses substances to rid the body of viruses, bacteria, parasites, metals, plastics, radiation, and other toxins. The body releases the substances naturally via sweat, urine, hair and stool. If done properly, the patient experiences no discomfort. Sometimes slight diarrhea or skin eruptions occur as substances pass out of the body.

Newly trained practitioners are entering this field weekly. To learn more about homotoxicology and its use with autism spectrum disorders, go to <www.HomeopathyHouston.com> and join Homeopathy-ADDthruAutism at Yahoo Groups. This listserv is hosted by mothers of children who have been using the Houston Homeopathic Method™.

- *Sweating* is one of the oldest, safest, most natural and least expensive ways to remove toxins. Saunas are finding their way into the homes of many health conscious people. Find one that is totally natural, with no off-gassing or toxic glues.

Detoxification should be part of everyone's daily routine because we are constantly being exposed to more chemicals and other toxins, and our bodies must rid themselves of them or we get sick. To learn more about this important subject and how to recover the health of loved ones and to protect your family, read *Detoxify or Die* by Sherry Rogers[27] and *7-Day Detox Miracle.*[28]

Step Five – Lay Neurological, Sensory and Motor Foundations for Learning
In Step Five, a similar approach to that taken in Step One is necessary to lay the highest quality foundations for learning and behavior in motor, sensory and neurological areas. Just as the recommendations early on were to assure that the existing environment was the best quality, at this point, we must assure that there are adequate movement opportunities. According to Carla Hannaford, author of *Smart Moves: Why Learning is Not All in Your Head,*[29] "Movement is not only essential for nerve net development and learning, but also for adequate heart and lung development to support brain function."

How much movement is enough? According to The National Association for Sport and Physical Education (NASPE), elementary age students need at least 60 minutes of moderate to vigorous activity each and every day, while middle and high school students need at least 30 minutes a day.[30] How is that possible when recess is disappearing,[31] and schools are limiting physical education (PE)?

Only one state, Illinois, requires PE for all 12 years of school. Twenty-seven states (58%) allow high school students to substitute other classes for physical education because they participate in the band or other school activities. Schools must start offering activities such as dance, martial arts and in-line skating, and not just competitive team sports such as football and basketball.[32]

Families have to pick up the slack; they cannot afford to wait until schools make necessary changes. Hike, go dancing, join the gym as a family, and walk or bike instead of getting into the car to go to places less than a mile away. Combined with healthier eating, this foundation can take off pounds in all generations. Everyone must find ways to make exercise a priority.

Time for More Therapies
During the many months when a child's developing body is attempting to recover its health and stay well, sensory, language, social-emotional, academic and other skills have all had to take a back seat to digestion, breathing and survival. Occasionally, resolving

biological problems alone frees up sufficient energy for development to accelerate and catch up without intervention.

Usually, though, integrating a multitude of sensory and behavioral interventions with biomedical modalities is necessary for most children to catch up. Therapies that resolve delays and assist in regaining skills in oral motor, gross motor, sensori-motor, visual, auditory, vestibular areas, and focus on reflex integration, are the next steps in laying a strong foundation for language and cognitive development. Some of the risk factors for children needing sensory interventions are listed in Figure 3-1 in Chapter 3.

In Chapters 7-11, the authors explain the importance of neurological, sensory and motor pathways for laying the foundations for language and socialization. Sleep problems, picky eating, and oral motor delays also respond particularly well to therapies that focus on this level. Those working with children who have the above issues should re-read the sections on these subjects in Chapter 7.

Another "good read" about the importance of strong neurological and sensory foundations for learning is *The Mislabeled Child: How Understanding Your Child's Unique Learning Style Can Open the Door to Success*.[33] The co-authors, physicians Brock and Fernette Eide, have provided an extremely user-friendly resource for those working with children on the high functioning end of the autism spectrum. They thoroughly understand their subject, and have aligned themselves with both occupational therapy and optometry. To learn more go to their websites <www.mislabeledchild.com> and <www.neurolearning.com>.

Take a Developmental Approach

The basic paradigm of this book views autism and related disorders as developmental problems, not as unchangeable neurological conditions. Therefore, the authors consider neural pathways immature, damaged, or inefficient, and believe that, as in any rehabilitation program, they can re-grow, heal and change.

Figure 17-6
Therapeutic Priorities Age 5 or Younger
Special diets, nutritional supplementation and detoxification
Structural therapies
Reflex Integration
Sensory-motor occupational therapy
Vision therapy
Sound therapy
Play therapy

All development, including motor, language, academic and social-emotional skills, follows a predictable hierarchy. Consider treating individuals with autism spectrum disorders as if they have the potential to be typical, yet are on developmentally different schedules than their age-level peers. This approach avoids unnecessary labelling, expensive "special" programs, and allows for customizing interventions according to a child's unique history. Figure 17-6 shows therapy priorities for children developmentally less than age five.

Choosing which of the next tier of therapies to combine with biomedical intervention for a particular child can be challenging. Look closely again at a child's individual history to design a program integrating multiple approaches from a variety of disciplines. Thinking is a "team sport" and thus requires many types of players.

- Occupational therapists (OTs) treat delays in sensory integration, motor planning, reflex integration, and motor coordination.
- Optometrists (ODs) treat delays in vision development, including problems related to eyesight, accommodation, convergence, binocularity, visual processing and eye health.
- Audiologists and sound therapists treat issues with auditory integration.

- Psychologists, mental health professionals and play therapists focus on social-emotional development and socialization.
- ABA specialists treat inappropriate behaviors, and train appropriate ones.
- Speech-language therapists (SLPs) work on articulation, communication and pragmatics.
- Developmental pediatricians treat children with growth, maturation and health issues.
- Educators work on reading, writing and arithmetic.

Where is a parent to turn? Each and every one of these experts can justify the need for the intervention he/she is most knowledgeable about. Here are some guidelines:

Find therapists who:
- *Work "bottom-up" and "inside-out"* In each discipline therapists who take a developmental approach get the best results. Ask around, the same names will come up again and again.
- *Co-treat* Teams of OTs and SLPs or OTs and ODs are fantastic because their talents are so synergistic. Speech-language therapy done in a swing, instead of sitting on a chair, stimulates the vestibular system and pushes the "on" button for talking. Walking rails and balls are common sights in many vision therapy rooms. Some feeding clinics offer teams composed of a nutritionist, OT and mental health professional to deal with the complex oral-motor and sensory issues inherent in picky eating. Other multi-disciplinary teams can offer one-stop shopping for both testing and treatment.

- *Collaborate* School-based therapists should communicate regularly with private providers, especially optometrists, and vice versa. Private therapists should touch base with a child's teacher, explain the goals of therapy, and maybe even spend a few minutes in the classroom. Understanding the learning environment and the demands being placed on a child can assist therapists in designing the best intervention programs.

- *Educate* Teach each therapist about the role of others. Help everyone see the benefits of special diets, a sensory diet, and therapeutic lenses that may have a "low" prescription. Buy teachers and therapists books and other educational materials, send them newsletters online, and help them understand why you are committed to and pursuing the outside therapies you are.
- *Cooperate* Do schoolwork with children nightly, and prescribed therapeutic home programs consistently to accelerate progress. Make children wear the lenses an optometrist prescribes. Reward kids for cooperating. I do not view this as bribery. Learning is children's work, and they should get paid to do it.

In Chapter 7, I describe the impact of dysfunctions in sensory integration, gross and fine motor coordination and praxis in children with autism. Review therapy strategies, and some of the exciting combination intervention programs listed there. The Alert program, HANDLE, Sensory Learning Institute, Tool Chest applications and others can all be of benefit. So can Brain Gym (see Chapter 13).

In Chapter 8, the authors from diverse backgrounds explain how over 100 reflexes emerge, become active, then integrate to lay the foundations for muscle tone, motor development, vestibular function, lateralization, binocularity, eye motor coordination, and visual perception. If conditions during the first year of life were not right for this process to take place, or if it was interrupted at any stage, intervention in this area is also is necessary.

Chapter 9, while primarily for optometrists treating those on the spectrum, can help parents, educators and therapists in other disciplines understand the extraordinary power of vision therapy (VT). Developmental optometrists have many methods of therapy. They may use special lenses and prisms, recommend therapeutic activities for home and school, or suggest that a child come to an office one or more times a week for intervention.

Choosing an Eye Doctor

EVERY child with an autism diagnosis should have an evaluation by a developmental optometrist, who has attended four years of optometry school, and taken advanced courses in vision therapy. The Optometric Extension Program Foundation (OEPF), the publisher of this book, offers post-graduate education to optometrists.They dispense free information about vision, and can make referrals to Clinical Associates in your area. Reach them at <www.oep.org>. The College of Optometrists in Vision Development (COVD) certifies developmental optometrists who have studied vision therapy, and who satisfy strict criteria. They also have excellent information about vision and can make referrals. Contact them at <www.covd.org >.

In Chapter 10, Dorinne Davis discusses the necessity for sound-based therapies and how to determine which one(s) is appropriate for an individual child. Refer back to that chapter for contact information on the various types of sound therapy.

In Chapter 11, I described in depth the complex programs conceived by Greenspan, Lewis, Guttstein, the Kaufman family, Miller, Prizant and Porges. These and the ABA programs in Chapter 14 are all developmental in nature. Some comprehend the essential role of each of the above areas better than others. However, they all build body awareness by moving from self to object to picture to symbol, and from concrete to abstract. That is why they are so effective. These remarkable therapies include hundreds of activities that gradually, systematically build the foundations for language and socialization.

Practitioners from a variety of disciplines, completing the DIR, ABLC, RDI, Son-Rise, Miller Method, SCERTS, Porges and CARD training programs are uniquely qualified to enter a child's life at this point. They bring with them the matchless combination of expertise from optometry, occupational and speech-language therapy, or educational kinesiology and play therapy training. Their individualized therapy programs are designed to give the brains of children with autism a second chance to develop critical neural connections.

How to Determine If a Treatment Really Helps

Stephen M. Edelson, Ph. D., Director of the Autism Research Institute (ARI) offers the following tips to help parents determine if a child is improving from a specific treatment:

1. ***Learn as much as possible about any new treatment before you try it*** Seek out criticisms as well as positive reports. When evaluating conflicting claims, compare studies and their methodologies. Examiner bias is rampant in research, especially if the funding source has a vested interest in the outcome. Be leery of any treatment that has been around for ten or more years with no research studies to support its effectiveness. The best sources for information are parents of kids like yours, not research studies that average outcomes of a varied group of subjects.

2. ***Control timing*** Give a new treatment six weeks to two months to determine whether or not it is helpful before beginning a new one. However, if it is obvious that the child is improving even after a week or two, then it is okay to start another one.

3. ***Keep new interventions confidential at first*** If possible, tell no one when a child starts a new treatment. This includes teachers, friends, neighbors, and relatives. Obviously this is difficult with diets. If a noteworthy change occurs, people in contact with the child are likely to say something about it. Do not ask, "Have you noticed any changes in my child?" Spontaneous statements regarding the child's improvement are more credible than responses to hopeful questions.

4. *Use objective measures*   Structured observation brings the nature of behavioral changes into clear focus. Consider completing the Autism Treatment Evaluation Checklist (ATEC), designed specially to evaluate treatment effectiveness, monthly prior to initiating a new intervention and again six weeks after. This free checklist can be down-loaded in English, Spanish, French, Italian and Russian from <www.autism.com/ari/atec/atec-online.htm>. Remember that growth due to maturation takes place gradually; effective interventions, especially diets, can produce sudden improvements. Some kids go from a few words to speaking in sentences when off gluten and casein.

5. *Keep good records*   Ask people who know that the child is receiving a specific treatment to compile a list of changes they notice. Compare their observations after a month or two. If different people report similar changes, you can consider the changes real. Be sure to keep records of these observations. You may not remember what the child's behavior was like before the treatment, especially if the old behavior was undesirable.

6. *Expect the unexpected*   Once in awhile a child will do something out-of-the-ordinary. If a child improves soon after an intervention is begun, his/her behavior will likely lead to more 'surprises' than usual - hopefully good ones!

Remember too that no treatment helps everyone. Careful observation along with a critical perspective allows parents and others to know when a treatment is truly beneficial.[34]

For older children who are developing slowly, and not yet reading or writing, strongly consider the possibility of avoiding special education for a period of time, while taking the above steps. Not pushing academics until a child is age seven or even eight, while providing appropriate therapies to lay foundation skills can have miraculous results. A forgiving, developmental or ungraded educational setting or homeschooling may be preferable to a special education placement that teaches developmentally inappropriate skills. These choices may be better equipped to offering a child in transition, the "gift of time."

Waldorf and Montessori curricula are developmental and attract families looking for forgiving options, although neither approach likes to be associated with kids who have special needs. Homeschooling is not the socially isolated, limited choice that it used to be. Once the home of the religious right, it now is attracting families with and without children on the autism spectrum who refuse to vaccinate their children according to the prescribed vaccine schedule, large families, and "stay-at-home moms" with education degrees.

School systems still have the obligation to provide related services at no cost to children who qualify for special education, even if the children attend private, parochial and home schools. The children must be registered, but do not have to attend, the local school. Depending upon the age of the child and the jurisdiction, services may take place at the school, in the child's home, or at another location.

Step Six - Focus on Academic Programs and Social Skills
When are children really ready to read, write and do mathematics? When all sensory systems are strong, and they show interest in and begin to participate in those activities spontaneously.

The Optometric Extension Program (OEP), the publisher of this book, distributes over 20 pamphlets, several of which focus on academics. "Does Your Child Have a Learning-Related Visual Problem?" "Educators Guide and Checklist to Classroom Vision Problems," "Is Your Child Ready to Learn?" "Vision in the Classroom," and "When a Bright Child has Trouble Reading," are available online at <www.oep.org>.

The College of Optometrists in Vision Development (COVD) has "White Papers" written for patients, parents, educators, and other health care professionals on a variety of topics related to learning. Some of COVD's offerings are "Vision and Learning," Vision and Dyslexia," and "Vision Based Learning Problems: The Role of the Optometrist on the Multidisciplinary Team." Go to <www.covd.org> and then search "White Papers."

Positioning and Lighting

Schools and families need to take into account both positioning and lighting for all academics. Assure that desks and chairs are the right size for each student; one size does not fit all. Each should be adjustable, so that a child's feet are fully on the floor at right angles to the waist, and the desk meets the student's body slightly above the waist. Desks and chairs that do not match in size, and that are too high or low, can make learning more difficult.

Use of ergonomically validated lighting systems can increase the speed with which students perform reading and writing tasks.[35] Lights must not have glare or buzz. One student with special needs I know had her first seizure in fourth grade. When the father, an optometrist, came to the school to pick her up, he noticed that the fluorescent light had a strobe effect. Removing her from that classroom cured her "seizure disorder."

Look for lights without too much blue. Full spectrum lights, according to lighting expert Robin Mumford, are "like the whole orchestra playing off key." What good lighting offers is the few notes that make a chord. He has designed some great products for ceiling, floor and desk lighting called RobinSpring. No website yet; however, you can learn more by emailing him at mumford.robin@gmail.com.

ACADEMICS
Reading

Think of reading as language on paper. Reading aloud to children is one of the great pleasures of parenthood that can begin almost at the day of birth. Children enrich their vocabularies by pairing words with pictures, objects and concepts.

- ***Reading readiness*** Some children with autism read very early. Extremely early reading, called hyperlexia, is a sign of uneven development, especially in the area of vision. Early reading should be discouraged; it is not a sign of a budding genius. As explained above, pre-school children need to develop large motor skills first, then smaller ones.

Children who are visually ready for reading have strong motor foundations, can move eyes across the page without upper body or head movements, and cannot only recognize words, but read with understanding. They use their eyes together as a team, can change focus easily from the book to the teacher, and can perceive just-noticeable differences among visually similar objects and words.

Achievers Unlimited of Wisconsin, Inc. is a team of vision therapists, occupational therapists and educators, headed by Donna Wendelburg, MS, who collaborate with optometrists to educate the public about the role of vision and motor skills in acquiring academics. They have a number of publications, including a "how-to" book for those working with children on the autism spectrum. Called "Begin Where they Are," it is a wonderful resource for those who need ideas for activities to play with children who are at the more severe end of the spectrum. Go to <www.achieverswisconsin.org> to learn more about Achievers' workbooks and workshops.

Scott Theirl, DC, a chiropractic neurologist in New York City, has developed the SuperFit Reading Kit, which uses eye movement exercises to pave the way for and enhance learning. Dr. Theirl works closely with developmental optometrists and recommends that all of his patients receive developmental vision evaluations. Starting with colors, pictures and letters, and moving on to words, the SuperFit Reading Kit can be an adjunct to vision therapy. For more information, go to <www.superfitbrain.com>.

OEP also distributes many books and workbooks, written by optometrists, for teachers and parents to use for establishing the visual and motor foundations for reading. These books are not substitutes for working with an optometrist. However, they provide a comprehensive readiness program covering a multitude of activities that are generally recommended for pre-readers.

Two that are especially helpful with students on the autism spectrum:

Developing Your Child for Success[36] is divided into eight sections of activities, each focusing on a developmental area: Over 600 activities are divided into eight categories: motor, visual motor, ocular motor, vision, laterality, directionality, sequential processing and simultaneous processing. In each section, the activities go from easy to more difficult, so that the book is applicable for developmentally age five up. Separate workbooks are also available for the remediation of common visual and motor issues, such as reversals, that interfere with learning.

Classroom Visual Activities[37] includes many activities to be done standing and at a chalkboard that integrate the eyes and hands, as well as the two sides of the body.

Go to <www.oep.org> to order the above books.

Many of the Brain Gym® activities described in Chapter 13 can also lay the foundations for reading and writing. Another fantastic program for developing reading readiness is S'Cool Moves for Learning, created by reading specialist Debra Em Wilson. S'cool Moves activities bridge occupational and vision therapy with the classroom and home. Activities incorporate movement, vision, sensory experiences in an extremely well-conceived group of products, including a book, booklets, and DVDs. Go to <www.schoolmoves.com>.

- **Choosing a reading program** The best reading programs contain subject matter that is developmentally appropriate. For older children who are slow to read, look for "high interest, low level" readers. Many are available from specialized publishers.

One of my favorite reading programs for students on the autism spectrum is from *Lindamood-Bell® Learning Processes*. This company has over 20 years experience in developing reading programs that improve sensory-cognitive processing of language for students with all types of learning issues, including those on the autism spectrum. Many schools have chosen Lindamood-Bell® programs for children in special education, and for those that have not, over 30 Lindamood-Bell® centers are located throughout this country and in England. To learn more, go to <www.lindamoodbell.com>.

- **Tutoring** In the same way that parents are very concerned when their young children are not talking, they become anxious about late readers. The panacea is often hiring a reading tutor. In my developmental model of autism and related disorders, tutoring is inappropriate until at least age eight, or when foundational skills are at a five to six year level. Spend the time and money instead on those therapies included in Step Five above. For older children, find a tutor who uses a combination of reading methods, rather than one who recommends only phonics.

Mathematics

The foundation for understanding numbers is also based in sensory experiences. According to Harry Wachs, OD, a child learns concepts such as same/different, greater/smaller and first/last through touch, movement, pressure, vision, and even taste and smell, by creating images in his mind's eye. Rote learning of number facts or rote counting is not the same. Wachs cites three foundational skills based on Piagetian conservation principles, all essential for successful understanding of mathematics:

1. *Visual thinking* concepts, such as part-whole, figure-ground, perspective, and time perception. Activities using parquetry blocks and pegboards can enhance visual thinking.

2. *Numerical literacy* includes the ability to read numerals, position commas, and understand place value. "Base Ten" blocks, available commercially can assist in building skills in this area.

3. *Visual logic* adds the component of logical reasoning to visual thinking. A child needs to understand one-to-one correspondence, order, conservation of mass, weight, volume, number and linear length, as well as classification, seriation, and probability to learn traditional academic arithmetic or geometry. Children with poorly developed visual logic might master basic computations but will be unable to solve word problems.

To learn more about the relationship between vision and mathematical thinking, along with hundreds of games designed to develop these skills, read *Thinking Goes To School*, co-written by Wachs and Hans G. Furth.[38]

Programs focusing on teaching mathematics must adhere to these concepts for children with and without issues to fully comprehend mathematics. Any programs that require the use of manipulative materials, number lines and concrete materials are the best choices. Activities that include estimation of time, money and measurement are preferable to drill with paper and pencil.

Organzational and Study Skills

If good organizational and study skills are goals for a secondary school aged child with attention deficits or autism, then working with mathematics concepts is the way to go. Comprehending mathematics is closely aligned with the understanding of time and space, both visual concepts.

Students who are well organized, are usually good in math, and are able to develop their own study methods. While courses in study skills can offer some kids a few tools to help them get organized, most disorganized students have underlying visual spatial issues, and thus cannot conform to someone else's timelines and structuring of space.

Better to provide students with the tools to organize themselves, such as a watch with a built-in stop watch, alarm clock, calendar (weekly and monthly), organizer, measuring tape, allowance (in a denomination that is easily broken down, such as one dollar) and pedometer.

Handwriting

Writing is a complex process that requires the integration of touch, proprioception, kinesthesia, vision, motor coordination and language. All the senses must be well-developed and integrate with each other to produce the memory, motor coordination, perception and attention necessary to put thoughts on paper. Until young bodies are motorically and visually ready, teachers and parents should not demand paper and pencil results.

Writing is dependent on vision and motor skills working in concert. Reread the section on Piaget's developmental hierarchy in Chapter 7 to understand the role of each. Children having difficulty with handwriting should have developmental evaluations by both an occupational therapist and an optometrist.

For children who are struggling, occupational therapists can provide special handwriting aids such as special papers, grippers, slant boards, cushions and writing implements. One vendor carrying many products is Therapro, at <www.theraproducts.com>. The need for these, however, usually means that the demands exceed a child's maturity levels. Better to fall back and work at a level at which a child is comfortable, while remediating visual and motor weaknesses.

Social/Emotional Skills

The body, in its wisdom, prioritizes social skills after building up the immune system, strengthening motor skills, and developing language, reading, writing and mathematics skills. The ability to interact appropriately with others is usually the final step in development, although it, like language and academics, is frequently highly prized by parents and teachers, and often pushed prematurely.

Adults' impatience is understandable, since Daniel Goleman, author of *Emotional Intelligence*[39] and *Social Intelligence*[40] believes that emotional and social intelligence are better predictors of success in life than SAT scores. They realize that almost 90% of people with disabilities lose jobs because of poor social-emotional skills.[41]

In Chapter 11 I described the role of efficient sensory processing in interacting appropriately with others. Social skills groups and play therapies that respect a child's over- and under-responsivity are most likely to be successful because they integrate sensory and movement experiences into their programs.

What about self-esteem? How does someone come to feel good about himself? By parents and teachers telling him he has done a good job? Unlikely. The intrinsic rewards of enjoying learned skills, such as reading and playing soccer, far surpass the value of extrinsic rewards such as stickers or trophies. Self esteem comes from the inside out. Instead of praising or rewarding a child for a "good job," consider asking him to evaluate the work himself. You might be in for a surprise!

> Figure 17-7
> **Therapeutic Priorities for Older Children**
> Revisit nutritional needs with hormonal changes
> Vision Therapy
> Pragmatic language
> Social-emotional skills

Figure 17-7 lists therapeutic priorities for older children. Remember that as kids get older, taller and heavier, their nutritional needs change. Be sure and revisit dosages and frequencies as hormones rage. Once a child is ready for academics, vision therapy might need to continue with the emphasis moving from tracking and eye teaming to visual thinking.

Once kids are speaking well with lengthy sentences and a rich vocabulary, language needs change too. Important aspects of strong social-emotional ability are special language skills called "pragmatics." A few areas that could benefit from help in the late elementary and secondary years are knowing when it is your turn to talk, making conversation, asking for what you need, and knowing how to phrase what you want to say. Social Stories, described in Chapter 11 can help in this regard.

Adjunct Therapies

Special programs abound that schools and families can integrate into the day-to-day routines to help those with autism maximize their potential. Each of the following are like condiments that complement a meal making it that much better.

- **Brain Gym®** Refer back to Chapter 13 to learn how this program can be a superb adjunct to other therapies for those on the autism spectrum. Brain Gym® activities are quick, easy to learn, powerful, and noninvasive. They require no fancy equipment and can easily be completed in a few minutes several times a day at home and school.

- *Hypotherapy* Horses are a terrific way for those on the autism spectrum to gain self confidence and motor control. Refer to Chapter 15, Healing with Animals, to determine if this is appropriate for an individual child.
- *Martial arts* such as karate, Aikido, Tae Kwon Do, T'ai chi and judo can all benefit those with language, learning and behavioral issues because they help with body control. Find local resources that have experience with students with special needs.
- *Neurofeedback* In Chapter 14, the authors address how several types of neurofeedback can calm individuals on the spectrum. This adjunct therapy is a tool in the tool chests of several different disciplines, mostly mental health professionals. Again, local resources may be available.

Planning for Adulthood

Careers: In her book, *Developing Talents: Career Planning, Including Higher Education, for Students with Autism and Asperger Syndrome,*[42] Temple Grandin, PhD., one of the most accomplished and well-known adults with autism in the world, describes how parents and teachers can nurture and turn talents, interests and even obsessions, into paid work. Read the delightful autobiography *Look Me in the Eye* by John Elder Robison,[43] a multi-talented man who did not receive an Asperger diagnosis until well into adulthood, to learn how he did just that. Robison worked in the music field for years, and now runs a very successful, high-end automobile repair business.

Figure 17-8
Careers well-suited to those with Autism
Animal handler
Artist
Auto mechanic
Computer programmer or technician
Crafts
Drafting
Engineering
Graphic design
Landscaping
Theatre lighting and sound
Music
Web design

While the importance of finding hobbies and leisure time activities other than watching television and playing video games cannot be over-emphasized, adults with autism can often turn their strong interests in computer technology, music videos, car parts, collecting, classifying and categorizing into meaningful careers. Obviously, individuals with autism differ in career choices as in every other aspect of their being. However, Grandin believes that some jobs are particularly well-suited to individuals on the spectrum. They are listed in Figure 17-8.

Estate Planning Even though some might find the subject uncomfortable, planning for the day when parents are no longer alive, is an essential step for families of children with special needs. Despite prodigious efforts, some children with autism will not be able to live independently as adults. Who will care for them? Where will funding come from? What will be the role of siblings and other family members?

Planning for the future of an individual with special needs requires knowledge of federal laws pertaining to government benefit eligibility and legal documents such as special needs trusts and guardianships. Fortunately, many resources are available in this area. Many attorneys know how to set up special needs trusts. Some insurance companies like MetLife's **D**ivision of **E**state Planning for **S**pecial **K**ids (Met**DESK®)** guides families through the steps necessary to provide lifetime quality care. Special MetDESK agents are available nationwide. To find one, go to <www.metlife.com/desk>.

Summary and Conclusions

Prioritizing therapies for children, adolescents and adults on the autism spectrum is a challenging task, not unlike putting together a jigsaw puzzle. Everyone a parent speaks with has an opinion on what to do, and professionals in a myriad of disciplines make recommendations to work in areas they know best. Because each child is a unique individual with a unique history, no one-size-fits-all program works. Furthermore, therapy is never linear. If only it were possible to do A, then B, then C, etc.

A good portion of this chapter includes steps families can take to improve the quality of what they eat (varied, unprocessed, organic, in season) products they already use (cleaners, personal care items, construction materials) and activities they participate in on a daily basis (cooking, using technology, learning). Just making the changes suggested in the early sections of the chapter could result in extraordinary benefits in everyone's health, without an IEP, the right health insurance, or expensive out-of-pocket therapies.

When one takes a developmental approach and treats autism, attention deficit disorder, Asperger syndrome and other pervasive developmental disorders as lags in development instead of different frank conditions, the job of remediation is not so onerous. Causes and treatments fall into categories fairly neatly, and these line up into first, next, and onward.

In all circumstances, health care professionals must resolve children's biological and nutritional issues first. Second are therapies that lay pathways for sensory, motor, visual and neurological foundations for language, learning and behavior. Last come academic and social skills interventions that depend on true sensory and cognitive integration. Because some programs integrate many theories and concepts, they could be used early on in treatment. Others that focus on single dimensional issues, must wait.

Vision issues are frequently missed and misunderstood in autism. Because many on the autism spectrum see well and appear to depend upon their visual skills, adults erroneously assume that "vision" is fine or even a strength. Every child with an autism spectrum diagnosis must have a comprehensive, developmental vision evaluation to determine the status of the many skills that allow them to consistently and efficiently focus on and give meaning to what they see.

Since visual skills are an inherent component of every single aspect of learning, socialization, behavior and cognition, vision therapy should be a primary part of every intervention program. Treatment may not be direct or one-on-one. However, some aspect of vision intervention will benefit every other therapy, and vice versa.

At the risk of offending therapists who are providing excellent programs in many areas to those with autism, Figure 17-9 offers an extremely general chart that simplifies where to look for interventions at what developmental age. To thoroughly understand treatment in each area, PLEASE read the chapters describing each therapy. Only then can a well conceived program be put into gear.

Figure 17-9
Appropriate therapies for each developmental age level

Age	Primary	Secondary	Extra Fun Activities
0-3	Diet & Nutrition SI-based OT/PT w/reflexes Structural therapy Vision therapy	Speech/Language Play therapy	Movement games
4-7	All of the above plus Speech/Language	Play therapy S'Cool Moves	Music therapy
8-12	All of the above plus Academics and Social/Emot.	Speech/Language Brain Gym	Martial Arts Hippotherapy
13-18	Psychological Academic	Vision therapy Nutrition	Neurofeedback
19-Adult	Social skills Vocational	Academic Diet & Nutrition	Hobbies

Families and schools should work together collaboratively on designing an appropriate program for a child. Schools must continuously remind parents that their obligation is "appropriate," not best. Parents must remind school systems that they have rights to a variety of related services and programs, and that requests for testing be carried out in a timely fashion. Most parents today are prepared to execute their rights, if necessary.

Make prioritizing therapies a priority. Revisit a child's needs at least four times a year. That way, a good balance is assured.

References

1. McCarthy J. *Louder Than Words: A Mother's Journey in Healing Autism.* New York, NY: Penguin Group, 2007.

2. Galland L. *The Four Pillars of Healing.* New York: Random House, 1997:xiii-xvi.

3. Baker SM, Pangborn J. *Biomedical assessment options for children with autism and related problems DAN! Consensus Report,* ARI (Oct 2002).

4. Johnson C, Myers S. *Identification and evaluation of children with autism spectrum disorders.* Elk Grove Village, IL: American Academy of Pediatrics, October 29, 2007.

5. Magaziner A. Bonvie L, Zolezzi A. *Chemical-free Kids: How To Safeguard Your Child's Diet And Environment.* New York, NY: Kensington Publishing Group, 2003.

6. May JC. *My House Is Killing Me.* Baltimore, MD: Johns Hopkins University Press, 2001:264.

7. Schettler T. *Human exposure to phthalates via consumer products.* Intl JAndrolo 2006;29:134-39.

8. Levitt BB. *Electromagnetic Fields: A Consumer Guide to the Issues and How to Protect Ourselves.Safe.* New York, NY: Harcourt Brace, 1995.

9. Levitt BB. *Cell Tower: Wireless Convenience or Environmental Hazard?* Sheffield, MA: Safe Goods Publishing, 2001.

10. Frey KI. *Craniosacral therapy and the visual system.* J Behav Optom 1999;10:31-35.

11. Bock, K. *Healing the New Childhood Epidemics: Autism, ADHD, Asthma, Allergies.* New York, Ballantine Books, 2007.

12. Rapp, DJ. *Is this your child?* New York, NY: Morrow, 1991.

13. Hersey J. *Why Can't My Child Behave? Why Can't She Cope? Why Can't He Learn?* Alexandria, VA: Pear Tree Press, 2002.

14. Seroussi K. *Unraveling the Mystery of Autism and Pervasive Developmental Disorders: A Mother's Story of Research and Recovery.* New York, NY: Broadway Books, 2002.

15. Lewis L. *Special Diets for Special Kids, volumes 1 and 2.* Dallas, TX: Future Horizons, 1999, 2001.

16. Compart P,. Laake D. *The Kid-Friendly ADHD and Autism Cookbook: The Ultimate Guide to the Gluten-Free, Casein-Free Diet,* Gloucester, MA: Quayside Publishing, 2006.

17. Semon B, Kronblum L. *Feast without Yeast: 4 Stages to Better Health.* Glendale, WI, Wisconsin Institute of Nutrition, 1999.

18. Crook WG. *The Yeast Connection Handbook.* Jackson, TN: Professional Books. 1996.

19. Crook WG, Jones MH. *The Yeast Connection Cookbook.* Jackson, TN, Professional Books, 2001.

20. Gottschall E. *Breaking the Vicious Cycle:intestinal Health Through Diet.* Baltimore, Ontario, Canada: The Kirkton Press, 2004.

21. Chinitz J. *We Band of Mothers: Autism, My Son and the Specific Carbohydrate Diet.* San Diego, CA: Autism Research Institute, 2007.

22. D'Adamo J. *The D'Adamo Diet.* Toronto, Ontario, Canada: McGraw-Hill Ryerson, 1989.

23. Baroody TA. *Alkalize or Die.* Waynesville, NC: Holographic Health Press, 2002.

24. Ingwersen J, Defeyter NA, Kennedy, DO, Wesnes, KA, et al. *A low glycaemic index breakfast cereal preferentially prevents children's cognitive performance from declining throughout the morning.* Appetite, 2007;49:240-44.

25. McCandless J. *Children with Starving Brains, 2nd edition.* Putney, VT: Bramble Books, 2005.

26. Dorfman K. *Is your child malnourished?* "New Developments" Newsletter 2001 Spring;6:4,7.

27. Rogers SA. *Detoxify or Die.* Vineland, NJ: Prestige Pub, 2002.

28. Bennett P, Barrie S, Faye S. *7-day Detox Miracle.* Roseville, CA: Prima Publishing, 2001.

29. Hannaford C. *Smart Moves: Why Learning is Not All in Your Head.* Salt Lake City, Utah: Great River Books, 2005:158.

30. National Assoc. for Sport and Physical Education. *Shape of the Nation Report.* Reston, Virginia: Executive Summary, 2001:6.

31. Bonde D. *Recess: Disappearing from the schedules of american children.* Torrington, Wyoming: The Blazing Sun, January 26, 2007.

32. Mercola J. http://www.mercola.com/2001/oct/20/physical_education.htm Accessed January 2, 2008.

33. Eide B, Eide F. *The Mislabeled Child: How Understanding Your Child's Unique Learning Style Can Open the Door to Success.* New York: Hyperion, 2006.

34. Edelson SM. *How to determine if a treatment really helped.* http://www.autism.org/determine.html, (Accessed December 29, 2007)

35. Mumford RB. *Improving visual efficiency with selected lighting.* JOVD 2002;3:1-7.

36. Lane KA. *Developing Your Child for Success.* Lewisville, TX: Learning Potentials Pub, 1991.

37. Richards RG, Remick KM. *CVA - Classroom Visual Activities: A Manual to Enhance the Development of Visual Skills.* Novato, California: Academic Therapy Publications, 1988.

38. Furth HG, Wachs H. *Thinking Goes to School: Piaget's Theory in Practice.* New York: Oxford University Press, 1975.

39. Goleman D. *Emotional Intelligence: Why It Can Matter More Than IQ.* New York, NY: Bantam Books, 1995.

40. Goleman D. *Social Intelligence: The Revolutionary Science Of Human Relationships.* New York, NY: Bantam Books, 2007.

41. Elksnin N, Elksnin LK. *Adolescents with disabilities: The need for occupational social skills training.* Exceptionality 2001;9: 91-105.

42. Grandin T, Dufy K. *Developing Talents: Career Planning, Including Higher Education, for Students with Autism and Asperger Syndrome.* Shawnee Mission, KS, Autism Asperger Publishing Company, 2004

43. Robison JE. *Look Me in the Eye.* New York, NY: Random House, 2007.

Testimonials

"At last! A very comprehensive reference about working with patients diagnosed with ADD, learning disabilities and autism. This handbook is not only for optometrists who want to know how to examine and treat individuals with these diagnoses, but also for parents, teachers and other professionals. Thank you OEP for publishing Patty's treatment model. I have watched it evolve for over 20 years, and believe that this book may be just what optometry needs to further educate the public about the important role of visual dysfunction in learning and behavior problems."

Lynn F. Hellerstein, O.D., FCOVD, FAAO
Englewood, CO
Past President, College of Optometrists in Vision Development (COVD)

"For anyone who has been a member of Patricia Lemer's Developmental Delay Resources (DDR), the wealth of information that Patty and her colleagues have to share regarding autism will come as no surprise. As good as DDR's newsletters, workshops and website (www.devdelay) are at integrating conventional and holistic approaches, no book to date has provided a cohesive trans-disciplinary framework in caring for the child with autism – particularly one that features optometry. This phenomenal book fills that gap in providing the reader with a centralized source of timely and well-considered information. Ms. Lemer and her collaborators probe deeply into the substance behind tightly held conventional wisdom. Reading Envisioning a Bright Future will energize you; keep it on your desk to guide you in weighing interventions that make a difference."

Leonard J. Press, O.D., FCOVD, FAAO
Past President, College of Optometrists in Vision Development (COVD)
Optometric Director, The Vision & Learning Center
Fair Lawn, New Jersey

"Optometry has only recently become involved with autism, and Patricia S. Lemer has been an important catalyst to foster this involvement. Her multifaceted career gave her appreciation for the role of vision and visual dysfunction in human behavior, particularly learning. The Optometric Extension Program has given her the opportunity to educate optometrists about the autism spectrum from the lecture platform over a number of years. In publishing this book it has extended Ms. Lemer's role considerably. The chapters provide a panoramic view of the autism spectrum for a diverse readership. It offers a superbly conceived and organized resource for educators, parents, and a wide range of health care professionals. Its presentations of management options and particularly the role that optometry plays in the care of patients with autism are invaluable."

Irwin B. Suchoff, OD, DOS, FAAO, FCOVD-A
Emeritus Distinguished Service Professor
State University of New York, State College of Optometry
Emeritus Editor, Journal of Behavioral Optometry (JBO)

Index

amoebas, 348
Amoxicillin, 271
Anafranil, 14, 15t, 16
analglyphs, 207
Angelman's syndrome, 286
Angels in the Snow reflex integration program (Berne), 189
angels in the snow (visual activity), 201, 211
animal-assisted therapy, 323–31
animal proteins, 365
anterior deltoid muscle, 282
anthrax vaccine, 97
anti-anxiety agents, 15t, 16
antibiotics
    alternatives to, 49
    disease prevalence in those not exposed to, 81
    emergence of, 80
    and endotoxin, 91
    resistance to, 106
    vaccines, interaction with, 71, 72, 89, 94
antibiotics, over-use of
    as autism spectrum disorder risk factor, 45f
    developmental delays linked to, 3, 46
    digestive system, effect on, 51, 126–27
    effects and recovery from, viii–ix
    immune system, effect on, viii, 50, 81, 361
    prevalence of, 2
    vestibular problems linked to, 23
    vision problems, link to, 29
anti-convulsants, 15t
anti-depressants, 15t, 16
anti-fungals, 126, 147–48, 152, 308, 370
anti-hypertensives, 15t
anti-oxidants, 58, 127, 130, 131, 149, 369, 369f
anti-psychotics, 15, 15t, 16
anti-viral measures, 144, 148
anxiety
    eliminating, focus on, 14
    preparing for situations producing, 167
    reducing, 262, 297
    sound-based therapy impact on, 221, 234
    vision therapy role in reducing, 203, 204
AOA (American Optometric Association), 21
AOTA (American Occupational Therapy Association), 155
Apell, Richard, 202
Apgar scores, 29
aphasia, developmental, 7
Applied Behavior Analysis (ABA)
    and autism, 311–13, 320
    case studies, 307, 314
    components of, 311, 373
    effectiveness of, 308
    historic developments in, 306–9
    innovations in, 316–20
    other therapies combined with, 309, 311, 313–16
    overview of, 297, 306, 374
    terminology of, 310–11
    types of, 316–20
Applied Psychoneurobiology (APN), 334, 337
apprentice level of relationship curriculum, 253, 254
apraxia, 224
arabinose, 52
Arching Cat (Physical Moro) reflex integration program, 187, 191

arching of back, 182
arithmetic difficulties, 28
Armstrong, Thomas, 11, 13
arthritis, 60, 67t, 83–84, 87, 88, 96, 97
Arthrostim™, 344
ASA (Autism Society of America), 76, 138, 308
ASL (American Sign Language), 260
aspartame, 54, 225
Asperger, Hans, 6, 85–86
Asperger syndrome (AS)
    adaptive behaviors in, 6
    animal-assisted therapy for persons with, 323
    Applied Behavior Analysis (ABA) for persons with, 317
    as autism spectrum disorder, 1
    brainwave patterns in, 299f
    case studies, 269–70, 304
    characteristics and symptoms of, 6–7
    classification of, 5, 6
    conversation, difficulty making, 24
    as developmental issue, 381
    EEG neurofeedback for persons with, 301
    employment for persons with, 380
    homeopathy treatment for, 267, 269–70
    hypersensitivity in, 283
    and sensory issues, 168
    vision problems in patients with, 39
asprin, 116
Association for Science in Autism Treatment (ASAT), 309
asthma
    as autism spectrum disorder risk factor, 45f
    digestion problems related to, 53
    immune problems linked to, 361
    language delays following symptom of, 265
    of mother, 29
    protection against, 81
    regression following development of, 79
    toxins linked to, 60
    vaccines linked to, 83, 88, 98
    visual development disrupted by, 27
astigmatism, 31
asymmetrical tonic neck reflex (ATNR), 24, 177, 178, 178t, 182–83, 185, 191–92
ataxia, 85
athletic skills, 183, 215t
Ativan, 15t
Atlanta, Georgia, autism prevalence in, 10

ATNR Eyes and Knees reflex integration program (O'Hara), 192
ATNR Eyes reflex integration program (O'Hara), 191
ATNR reflex integration program (Berne), 191
atropine, 126
attention
    to detail, 179, 319
    EEG neurofeedback effect on, 303, 304
    enhancing, 313
    glasses impact on, 38
    hyperbaric oxygen impact on, 134
    lens impact on, 36
    maintaining and shifting, difficulties with, 219
    nutritional supplement impact on, 126
    paying, 166, 204–5, 221
    reflex impact on, 181

vaccines linked to, 83–84, 88, 89, 94, 95–96
autonomic nervous system dysfunction, 338
Autonomic Response Testing (ART), 334, 340–42, 353, 368
Awakening Ashley: Mozards Knocks Autism on its Ear (Ruben), 222
Ayres, A. Jean, 158, 159, 161, 290, 292

B
bacteria
  beneficial, 127
  and brain inflammation, 88–91
  in digestive tracts, viii–ix
  exposure to, 97, 99
  mutations of, 106
  treating infections of, 348
  in utero, 72
bacterial dysbiosis, treating, 144, 147, 149
Baker, Sidney, 3, 54, 59, 140, 141, 144, 148, 356
balance
  assessment of, 33
  brain function and, 283
  developing, 161, 193
  dysfunction of, 300
  emotional security and, 240
  evaluating, 164, 165
  glasses impact on, 38
  hippotherapy impact on, 326
  as learning prerequisite, 185
  lense impact on, 36
  problems with, 155, 159, 180, 182, 183, 184
  relationship-based therapies and, 245
  sound-based therapy impact on, 221
  sound stimulation effect on, 217, 218
  toxicity impact on, 60
  vestibular intervention impact on, 157
balance/vision/movement coordination, 193
balloons, activities with, 201
ball playing. *See also* Marsden ball
  difficulties of, 200
  reflex impact on, 182, 184
  in relationship-based therapies, 248
  skills in, 182, 183, 184
  as visual activity, 201, 207
  visual aid use effect on, 205
Balsley, John, 248
Barrie, S., 59
Baryta carbonica (barium carbonate), 268, 269
Baryta sulphuricum (barium sulfate), 269
Bates, William, 294
Bauman, Margaret, 93, 276
beanbag games as visual activity, 201, 205
Bear-Walk Soccer Drill (integration program) (Cheatum and Hammond), 193
Beck, Victoria, 126
BEDROK (Body Ecology Diet Recovering Our Kids) program, 365
bedtime routines, 169
bed-wetting, 181, 190
behavior
  adaptive, 6
  as communication, 158
  compensatory, 26, 204
  coping, role in, 243, 262
  and diet, 152

difficult, managing, 198, 199
  fearless, 28
  generalizing, 311
  hearing effect on, 219–20
  homeopathic therapy impact on, 271, 275
  inflexible, 25
  management, applied, 14, 16
  meaning underlying, 259
  medications modifying, 16, 17t
  in mercury poisoning *versus* autism, 66t
  movement role in, 371
  music impact on, 231
  neurofeedback effect on, 299, 300
  observed as autism diagnostic criteria, 10
  regression in, 7
  relational deficits as cause of, 255
  relationship-based therapies and, 241
  repetitive and stereotyped, 5, 6, 239
  sensory-avoiding, 159, 160–61
  sensory intervention programs and, 168
  sensory roots of, 167, 172
  sensory-seeking, 159, 160–61
  skill deficit, selecting, 311
  sound-based therapy impact on, 233
  spontaneous interactive, developing, 243
  stereotypical, 306, 307
  strabismus effect on, 208–9
  target, 310, 311
  therapies and interventions, 29, 313, 318, 372 (*see also* Applied Behavior Analysis (ABA))
  transfering and generalizing, 306
  undesirable, reducing, 16, 311
  unusual, homeopath interest in, 267
  vision role in, 37, 211, 381
  visual dysfunction relationship to, 26, 27, 39, 200
Behavioral Language Assessment, 320
behavioral optometry, 281, 300, 362
behavior problems
  animal-assisted therapy for, 324, 330
  deficits, symptom relief *versus* causes, 14, 16
  immune system dysfunction as factor in, 60
Bell retinoscopy, 31
Bender, Miriam, 176–77, 183
Bennett, S., 59
Berard, Guy, 219–20, 222, 225, 226, 232
Berard Auditory Integration Training (AIT). *See* Auditory Integration Training (AIT)
Berard sound-based therapy spinoffs, 229, 231–32
Bernard, Sallie, 56, 63–68, 92
Berne, Samuel, 178, 185, 186, 187, 188, 189, 190, 191, 192, 290
Bethanechol, 126
Bettelheim, Bruno, 1, 3
Beyond the Wall (Shore), 235–36
BG (case study), 212
BGC machine, 231
bike riding, 291
bilateral movements, reflex impact on, 182, 184
Billie (case study), 307
binocularity
  communication, role in, 284
  coordination, 175
  developing, 193, 200
  dysfunction, 241, 277, 284, 372
  enhancing, 189, 207

capryllic acid, 147–48
carbohydrates, complex, prohibiting, 117
Carbone, Vincent, 319, 320
Carcinosin, 272
CARD (Center for Autism and Related Disorders)
    programs, 306, 309, 313, 317–18, 374
caregivers, relationships with, 243
Carson, Rachel, 12
casein
    avoidance trial, 144, 145–46, 147, 150
    intolerance for, 83
    problems breaking down, 53
    response, testing, 61
    sensitivity to, 58, 117
    sources of, 116
casein-free gluten-free diet. *See* gluten-free casein-free
    (GF/CF) diet
case managers, 357–58
case studies of vaccine reactions, 71–72, 74–75
Cassily, James, 229, 233
CAT scans, 300
cause and effect, understanding, 317
Celexa, 15t
celiac disease, 85–86, 145
cell signaling, 274–75, 276
cell signaling growth factors, 278
cellular *versus* humoral immunity, 82, 83
Celtic sea salt, 366
Center for Autism and Related Disorders, 306, 309, 313,
    317–18, 374
centering dimension of brain function, 283–84, 292
central and peripheral vision, integration of, 26, 28, 35,
    39, 362
central nervous system
    growth of, treatment promoting, 352
    messages delivered to, 156
    structural pathology of, 67t
central/peripheral awareness, 200
cerebral palsy
    versus autism, prevalence of, 9
    therapies and interventions for, 194
cerebrospinal fluid, 47–48
cervical and lumbar spines, integration of, 188
chaining, 310
challenger level of relationship curriculum, 253, 254
change, resistance to, 25
Cheatum, Billye Ann, 23, 184, 185, 189, 192, 193
cheiroscope, 32
chelation, 129–34, 370
Chelsey (case study), 142
chemicals
    eliminating and detoxifying, 359, 370
    as endocrine disruptors, 55
    exposure to, 54, 97, 338
    sensitivities to, 45f, 46
    toxins and autism, 72, 353, 356, 357
chemokines, 47–48
Chess, S., 87
chickenpox, 87
chickenpox vaccine, 55, 87
child-animal bonds, 323, 325
childhood cancer *versus* autism, prevalence of, 9
Childhood Disintegrative Disorder (CDD), classification
    of, 5, 7
Children's Center for Neurodevelopmental Studies, 165

children with disabilities
    audiograms of, 220
    Brain Gym for, 285–86
Children with Starving Brains (McCandless), 62, 116,
    129, 142
child's desire, helping with, 244
child's lead, following, 242, 243–44, 249, 255, 266
Child With Special Needs, The (Greenspan and Wieder),
    241
Chinese medicine, traditional, 337
chiropractic neurology, 47
chiropractic therapy
    healing, approach to, 334
    history of, 29, 46
    referrals for, 25, 39
chlorella, 130, 132
choice, allowing, 313
choline compounds, 126, 127–28
Chretien, Kristina, 260
Chris (case study), 71–72
chromium, 123, 369f
chromosome damage, 96–97
chronic disease
    epidemic of, 73
    prevalence of, 77, 106
    vaccine link to, 81, 82, 83, 105
Chronologically Controlled Developmental Therapy
    (CCDT), 352
Clark, Bill, 231
Clark Method of therapy, 231
Classen, Barthelow, 83
classical conditioning, 297
Classroom Visual Activities, 377
class size, increase in, x
cleaning products, environment-friendly, 360
cleansing, dietary principle of, 366
Clear-Brain Buttons, 284–85
clinical ecology, 13
clinical research studies, 265
clinoptilolite, 132
Clonodine, 14, 15t
closing one eye, 28
Clostridia, 52
clothing, hypersensitivity to, 157t
clothing and bedding, natural, 360
Clozaril, 15t
clumsiness, 184, 185
Coalition of SafeMinds (Sensible Action For Ending
    Mercury-Induced Neurological Deficits), 57, 92, 93
cod liver oil, 124, 126, 148
cognition, regression in, 7
cognitive deficits
    as brain inflammation effect, 85
    immune system dysfunction as factor in, 60
    in mercury poisoning *versus* autism, 66t
    physical problems followed by, 265
    range of, 1
cognitive development, 22, 25, 29
cognitive-developmental theory, 258
cognitive function, 155, 236, 299–300, 381
cognitive integration, 381
cognitive skills, 33, 175, 243
Colburn, Theo, 12, 55, 57
colitis, 86
collaboration, 373, 382

Delacato, Carl, 155, 185
delta waves, 299
demyelination, 85, 86, 88, 90
Dennison, Gail, 282, 283, 284, 285, 287, 290, 292, 294–95
Dennison, Paul, 281, 282, 283, 284, 285, 287, 289, 290, 292, 294–95
Dennison Laterality Repatterning, 289–90
Depakote, 15t
depression, eliminating, 14
depth awareness, assessing, 34
depth perception
    developing, 175, 195
    patterns blocking, 282
    problems with, 28, 181, 183
    requirements for, 241
    and strabismus, 207
descripitive sentences in social stories, 256, 257
design copying, 165
detoxification
    benefits of, 358
    foods aiding, 366–67
    homotoxicology, 276–78
    methods of, 370–71, 370f
    monitoring, 62–63
    nutritional supplement role in, 125, 370
    pathways, faulty, viii, 61, 117, 118, 120, 153
    pathways, opening, 365
    process of, 59–60, 150
    sensory processing energy released through, 240
    sound-based therapy and, 226, 227
    treatments aiding, 115, 125, 128–34, 144t, 150, 278, 320, 345, 362, 368 (*see also* metals, toxic: removing)
Detoxification and Healing: The Key to Optimal Health (Baker), 54, 59
DETP (Diagnostic Evaluation for Therapy Protocol), 221, 223, 226
Developing Talents: Career Planning, Including Higher Education, for Students with Autism and Asperger Syndrome (Grandin), 380
Developing Your Child for Success, 377
development
    adjunct therapies for, 151
    Applied Behavior Analysis (ABA) impact on, 316
    assessment of, 39
    information and history of, 29, 47
    missed stages, replicating, 185
    Piaget's hierarchy, 162–63, 378
    prerequisites of, 258
    reflex role in, 183, 195
    stages of, 241, 245
    stimulating, 39
    therapies and interventions for, 371–73, 372f
    vision and motion as components in, 155
    vision therapy based on, 206, 207
Developmental Coordination Disorder, 159
Developmental Delay Resources (DDR) (*formerly* Developmental Delay Registry), 2, 76, 170, 358
developmental delays
    antibiotic overuse linked to, 3, 46
    autism spectrum disorders approached as, 381
    brain inflammation as factor in, 84
    causes of, 371–72
    listening therapy for, 224
    in older children, 375

sensory and behavioral interventions for, 372
sound-based therapies for, 229, 237
vaccines linked to, 72, 75–76
developmental disabilities and disorders
    Applied Behavior Analysis (ABA) impact on, 307
    immune-mediated, 73
    prevalence by type, 9
    risk factors for, 45, 46
    sound-based therapies for, 233, 261–62
Developmental-Individual Difference-Relationship Based model, 234, 241–48, 253, 262, 319, 374
developmental milestones, 29, 46, 79
developmental optometry, 155, 172
Dexedrine, 15t
DHA (docosahexaenoic acid), 120
diabetes
    versus autism, prevalence of, 9
    digestion problems related to, 53
    etiology of, 83
    family history of, 361
    gestational, 29
    vaccines linked to, 83, 98
Diagnosis Autism: Now What? 10 Steps to Improve Treatment Outcomes, a Parent-Physician Team Approach (Kaplan), 100
diagnosis of autism, 39
diagnosis of autism spectrum disorders
    academics, premature pushing, role in, 162
    Applied Behavior Analysis (ABA) following, 312
    behavior observation as basis for, 10
    costs of, 13
    overdiagnosis, possibility of, 9
    overview, 4–7
    physical symptoms prior to, 355
    prerequisite tests for, 144, 145
    treatment independent of, 356
Diagnostic Evaluation for Therapy Protocol (DETP), 221, 223, 226
diarrhea
    in autism patients, 51–52
    in detoxofication process, 371
    food allergies and, 53
    food limitations in correcting, 368
    supplements and, 369
Dickson, Debra, 169
diet
    autism treatment through, 75, 116–19, 134, 140, 141, 144, 145, 148, 153, 320, 342, 359, 362, 363–68, 381
    and behavior, 152
    chelation preparation, role in, 130
    detoxification following establishment of, 370
    ear infection prevention through, 49
    guidelines, general, 119
    homeopathy combined with, 265, 266, 277
    hyperactivity linked to, 53
    immune system enhancement through, 47
    and language development, 358
    as multidisciplary package component, 39
    parent ratings of, 17t
    of parents, 29
    for picky eaters, 170–71
    and relationship-based therapies, 256
    self-restricted of children with behavioral and developmental problems, 120
    types of, 115, 116–19

essential fatty acids (EFAs), 120–21, 130, 334, 368, 369, 369f

Essential Glutathione™, 131

estate planning, 380

ethylenediamine tetra-acetic acid (EDTA), 133, 370

etiology of autism spectrum disorders, 10–13, 14, 63, 72, 96, 106, 137, 152, 333–34. *See also* load factors; risk factors for autism spectrum disorders; total load theory; vaccines: autism linked to

Eurhythmics (Dalcroze Method), 235

European Union, 13

Every Day a Miracle: Success Stories with Sound Therapy (Davis), 221

evidence-based literature, 319

Evidence of Harm: Mercury in Vaccines and the Autism Epidemic, a Medical Controversy (Kirby), 57, 73, 93

excitotoxins, 54–55

exercise, importance of, 371

exophoria, 36

exotropia, 22, 34, 35, 36, 205

expansion activities, 310

expansion and contraction, dietary principle of, 365

experiences and emotions, relationship between, 243

experience sharing, 250, 252, 253

explorer level of relationship curriculum, 253, 254

extended family, reduced contact with, xi

eye alignment
    assessing, 31–32
    glasses impact on, 38

eye contact
    dietary modification impact on, 116
    EEG neurofeedback impact on, 304
    glasses impact on, 38
    homeopathic therapy impact on, 270, 273
    improving, 14, 27, 255
    increasing, 313
    lens impact on, 36
    poor, 5, 21, 25, 28, 28t, 39, 180, 239, 241, 314, 315
    relationship-based therapy impact on, 249
    sound-based therapy impact on, 221
    vestibular stimulation impact on, 157
    vision therapy impact on, 199, 200

eye control, 180

eye coordination, 175

eye health, mineral role in, 121

eye motor coordination, reflex role in, 373

eye movements, abnormal
    auditory dependence, increased in compensation for, 34
    in autism patients, 22, 27
    and cognition, 25
    as medication side effect, 15t, 16
    reading, interference with, 162
    reflexes, primitive or retained role in, 176
    reflex role in, 186
    vestibular problems as factor in, 23

eye movements, testing, 30–31, 32

eyes
    closing, 304
    muscles of, vestibular system connected to, 156

eye surgery, 207, 208, 209

F

facial development, structural abnormalities in, 338–39

Faddick, Chris, 229, 230

fading a prompt, 310, 319

families, changes in, xi–xii, 11

Families for Early Autism Treatment (FEAT), 9, 76

family constellations, 337, 342, 347, 350–51, 362

family healing, 351

family issues, transgenerational, unhealed, 338, 340, 347, 350, 351

Family Systems Theory, 337

far infrared sauna, 133–34, 347

fast food, increase in, xi

Fast ForWord sound-based therapy, 222, 229, 232

fatty acids
    analysis of, 63, 149
    essential, 120–21, 130, 334, 368, 369, 369f
    problems with, 62
    short chain, 127

Fay, Temple, 185

feelings
    expressing, 268, 291
    range of, understanding, 241
    sensory impressions tied to, 242

Feingold, Benjamin, 116

Feingold diet, 115, 116–17, 363

Feldenkrais, Moshe, 210

Feldenkrais Method, 210

Fetal Fling reflex integration program (Marusich), 186

fevers, chronic unexplained, 45f

fibroblast growth factor-2 (FGF2), 275–76

fidgeting, reducing, 190

FightingAutism (organization), 10

fight or flight response, 179, 283, 288

figure-ground perception, 165

figure/ground problems, 181

filters, 22

filters, colored, 37

fine motor abilities, 22, 26, 33–35, 39, 127, 205, 218, 312, 328

fine motor activities, 205, 211

fine motor delays and deficits, 72, 159, 161, 225

fish
    consumption, excessive, 45f
    as environmental insult, 357
    mercury in, 334
    oil, 121

Fisher, Barbara Lee, 71–72, 73, 74, 89, 99, 100

Fishman, Beth, 155

Fitzpatrick, Stephanie, 325

five-year-old boy (case study), 211

fixation
    activities requiring, 200
    assessing, 31, 34
    developing and improving, 184, 206–7
    poor, 28, 30, 179, 180

Flach, Frederic, 202

flame retardants, 12, 18, 54, 55

flashlight tag (visual activity), 201, 207

flexibility
    EEG neurofeedback effect on, 303
    hippotherapy impact on, 326

flippers, 36, 37, 199, 200, 207

FloorTime. *See* DIR (Developmental-Individual Difference-Relationship Based)/Floortime model

Flowers, Janet, 328

fluid transitions, 250

fluoride, 119, 343

human-animal interactions, 323, 324, 326, 327–28, 330–31. *See also* animal-assisted therapy
hydrogenated fats, 120
hydrolyzed vegetable protein, 54
hydroxy- B12, 343
hygiene hypothesis, 81, 83
hyperactivity. *See also* Attention Deficit Disorder with hyperactivity (ADHD)
  as autism spectrum disorder risk factor, 45f, 361
  as compensatory behavior, 299
  diet linked to, 53, 118
  eliminating, focus on, 14
  as energy issue, 338
  hyperbaric oxygen impact on, 134
  immune responses and, 48
  nutritional supplements linked to, 126
  physical symptoms preceding, 265
  sound-based therapy impact on, 221
  and survival state, 60, 211
  treating, 126
  vaccines linked to, 76
  visual therapy and, 205
hyperbaric oxygen therapy (HBOT), 134
hyperlexia, 376
hyperopia, 22, 31
hypersensitivity to sounds, tastes, smells, and sights, 6, 23, 39, 159, 160, 160t. *See also* light: hypersensitivity to; odors, hypersensitivity to; sound hypersensitivity; tactile sensitivity
hypertropia, 36
hyperventilation, 210
hyper-vigilance, 218, 283
hypnosis
hyposensitivity to sounds, tastes, smells, and sights, 23, 39, 159, 160, 160t
Hyson, Michael, 327

I

I Am the Child (Koester), 286
ideas, difficulty combining and organizing, 319
IgE scratch tests, 61
illness, frequent, 29
immune dificiency panel, 62
immune system
  abnormalities and dysfunctions of, 18, 46, 47–53, 67t, 72, 74, 76, 77, 82, 92, 95, 98, 102, 105
  antibiotic effects on, 50
  assessment of, 61, 62
  boosting, 361, 370
  brain, developing interaction with, 82
  building, 362
  compromised, viii, 60, 130–31, 355, 357, 368
  digestion impact on, 127
  enhancing, 47, 115
  function of, 48, 82
  load factors, 60
  maternal transfered to infant, 128
  opioid excess effect on, 53
  responses, measuring, 49
  restoring, 342
  social and communication skills, prerequisite for, 262
  stress, signs of, xii
  support, providing, 144, 148
  testing, 147
  toxic metal interaction with, 334

  vaccine effect on, 81, 82–83, 97, 98, 105
immunizations. *See* vaccines
Impossible Cure, The (Lansky), 265, 271
inactivated polio vaccine (IPV), 87
Incao, Philip, 82
incidental teaching (term), 312
inclusion, increase in, x, 7–8
independence, developing, 317, 325
independent living, 251, 329
In-Depth Balance, 293, 295
In-Depth Menu, 293–94
Individualized Education Plan (IEP), 325
Individualized Education Program (IEP), 8
Individuals with Disabilities Education Act (IDEA), 1990, 7–8
Infantile Autism: The Syndrome and its Implications for a Neural Theory of Behavior (Rimland), 137–38
infants
  focusing of, 175, 184, 195
  learning in, 176
  reflex development in, 195
infections
  and autism, 148, 361
  diet role in controlling, 365
  immune system problems, xii, 18
  protection against, 127
  and reflexes, 179
  response to, 131
  secondary, treatments for, 342
  as strabismus factor, 208
  testing for, 341
  toxin role in, 340
  treating, 342
infectious diseases
  immune system dysfunction caused by, 95
  prevention of, 81, 106
  symptoms of, 103
inflammation, 48, 51, 52, 83–85, 95, 105, 131, 370. *See also* brain: inflammation of
inflammatory bowel disease (IBD), 51, 85
inflammatory bowel disorders, 83
inflammatory immune response, 82–83, 91
influenza, 87
influenza vaccine, 18, 87–88, 91, 92
information processing
  relationship-based therapy impact on, 277
  sequence of, 22
  social referencing as form of, 252
  visual dysfunction, role in, 26
informed consent, 73, 74, 105, 106
infrared sauna, 133–34
In Harm's Way: Toxic Threats to Child Development (Greater Boston Physicians for Social Responsibility (GBPSR)), 54
insomnia, eliminating, 14
Institute for Neuro-Physiological Psychology (INPP), 177
intake forms, 29, 41–44
Integrating Mind, Brain and Body (Rowley), 201
intelligence, impaired, causes of, 12–13
interaction. *See also* social interaction; two-way interaction
  assessment of, 33
  reduced, xi
  tailoring, 244

optometry and autism, cross-education concerning, 18
optometry/neuofeedback practitioners, 304
sound-based therapies, 216, 226
therapies, selecting, 39
visual symptoms, secondary, 362
multiple myeloma cancer, 97
multiple sclerosis (MS), 81, 84, 88
multi-sensory processing, 163, 236
Mumper, Elizabeth, 134
mumps and mumps vaccine, 86, 103, 106
muscle checking, 282, 288, 291
muscle tension, 128, 180
muscle testing, 50, 337, 340, 341, 342, 368
muscular dystrophy, 8
music
    decreased time for, x
    healing, role in, 337
    therapy, use in, 29, 224, 226, 231, 232, 234–36
musical giftedness, 235–36
MX Pro sound-based therapy, 229, 230–31
myopia, 31
My Social Stories Book (Gray), 257–58

N
N acetylcysteine (NAC), 150
Naltrexone (LDN), 343
Nathanson, David F., 327–28
National Alliance for Autism Research (NAAR), 11, 18
National Association for Child Development (NACD), 230
National Center on Birth Defects and Developmental Disabilities (NCBDDD), 10
National Childhood Vaccine Injury Act, 1986, 74, 79
National Service Dogs (organization), 330
National Vaccine Information Center, 74, 75, 76, 81, 102, 103
Natural Medicine Guide to Autism, The, 265
nature *versus* nurture role in autism, 10–12
near point of convergence (NPC), testing for, 32
negative reinforcement, 310
negative space activity, 248
Nelson, Karin, 93
nervous system
    brain wave regulation of, 218
    development, immature, 119
    functioning, brain inflammation effect on, 85
    restoring, 342
    strengthening, 345
Neubrander, James, 125, 149
neural function, improving, 299
neural therapy, 334, 336, 337
neurochemistry, abnormal in mercury poisoning *versus* autism, 66t
"Neuro-Developmental Delay (NDD)" (term), 177
neurofeedback, 297–98, 299–301, 302–5, 306, 380
neuroimmune disorders, 82, 94, 99
neuroleptics, 15, 15t, 16
"neurological abnormalities" hypothesis, 10, 13
neurological damage, vaccines linked to, 90
neurological development, 371
neurological disorders, 102, 194
neurological flexibility, 176
neuromuscular deformity, vaccine-related, 86
neuro-physiology, abnormal in mercury poisoning *versus* autism, 66t

Nizoral, 118
Noah (case study), 330
"No Child Left Behind" initiative, x
nonverbal cues, difficulty reading, 6
non-verbal learning disabilities (NLD)
    as autism spectrum disorder, 1
    vision problems in patients with, 39
nonverbal skills and cognition, 25
Nordoff, Paul, 236
Nordoff-Robbins Method of music therapy, 236
norepinephrine re uptake inhibitor, 15t
North American Riding for the Handicapped Association, 326
nosodes, 272–73, 276, 277, 278
nourishment level, evaluating, 119–20
novice level of relationship curriculum, 253
Nsouli, Talal, 49
numerical literacy, 378
nutrition, optimal, 119, 120–23, 129, 130, 134
nutritional counseling, 115
nutritional deficiencies
    and autism, 72
    correcting, 120, 365, 381
    sensory and oral motor aspects of, 169
    sound-based therapy and, 227, 228
    as stress area, 338, 343
    and vaccine reactions, 102
nutritional referrals, 25, 38
nutritional supplements
    autism treatment through, 75, 363
    bacteria-containing, 118
    as chelation preparation, 129–30, 133
    detoxification and, 370
    diet, special combined with, 368–70
    effectiveness of, 152
    homeopathy combined with, 265, 266, 276, 277
    immune system enhancement through, 47
    minerals, 120–23
    miscellaneous, 126–28
    as multidisciplary package component, 29
    non-drug, parent ratings of, 17t
    overview of, 115
    recommendations for, 144, 146, 148–49, 343
    secretin, 125–26
    substitution approach to healing, component of, 334
    visual function, effect on, 29
    vitamins, 121, 122, 123–25
nutritional therapy
    history of, 29
nystagmus, 165, 362
Nystatin, 118, 147–48

O
objects, bumping into, 28t
objects *versus* people in autism, 250, 254
obsessive compulsive disorder (OCD), 49, 283
occlusion, 21–22, 37, 206–7, 208, 209
occupational hazards, 45f
occupational therapy
    animal use in, 324, 325
    autism spectrum disorders, approach to, 172
    benefits of, 35, 39
    in case studies, 314
    effectiveness, factors affecting, 240
    evaluations, 163, 165, 378